CONCISE GUIDE TO MEDICINES & DRUGS

Chief Medical Editor
Dr Kevin M O'Shaughnessy MA BM BCh DPhil FRCP FBPhS

DK

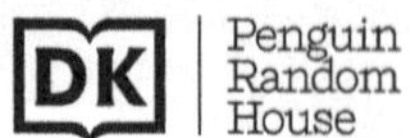

DK UK

Consulting Editor Martyn Page
Senior Editor Katie John
Managing Editor Angeles Gavira
Managing Art Editor Michael Duffy
Jacket Design Development Manager Sophia MTT
Jacket Designer Stephanie Cheng Hui Tan
Production Editor Kavita Varma
Senior Producer Controller Meskerem Berhane
Art Director Karen Self
Associate Publishing Director Liz Wheeler
Publishing Director Jonathan Metcalf

DK INDIA

Assistant Editor Aashirwad Jain
DTP Designer Anita Yadav
Senior DTP Jacket Designer Harish Aggarwal
Managing Jackets Editor Saloni Singh
Editorial Manager Rohan Sinha
Preproduction Manager Balwant Singh

This edition published in 2021
First published in Great Britain in 2001 by
Dorling Kindersley Limited

DK, One Embassy Gardens, 8 Viaduct Gardens, London, SW11 7BW

The authorised representative in the EEA is Dorling Kindersley
Verlag GmbH. Arnulfstr. 124, 80636 Munich, Germany

Concise Guide to Medicines and Drugs is based on
New Guide to Medicines and Drugs (11th edition)

2 4 6 8 10 9 7 5 3 1
001–323212–Dec/21

A CIP catalogue record for this book is available from the British Library
ISBN: 978-0-2414-9032-7

Printed in Great Britain

For the curious
www.dk.com

A NOTE ON GENDER IDENTITIES

DK recognizes all gender identities, and acknowledges that the sex someone was assigned at birth, based on their sexual organs, may not align with their gender identity. People may identify as any gender (including genders outside the male/female binary) or as no gender, and their gender identity may change during their lifetime. As gender language, and its use in our society, evolves, the scientific and medical communities continue to reassess their own phrasing. Please note, this book uses "women" to refer to people who were assigned as female at birth on the basis of their sexual organs, and "men" to refer to people who were assigned male at birth on the basis of their sexual organs.

This book was made with Forest Stewardship Council™ certified paper – one small step in DK's commitment to a sustainable future. For more information go to www.dk.com/our-green-pledge

CONTENTS

READER NOTICE

INTRODUCTION

Concise Guide to Medicines and Drugs provides clear information and practical advice on drugs and medicines that can be readily understood by a non-medical reader. The text reflects current medical knowledge and standard medical practice in the UK. It is intended to complement and reinforce the advice of your doctor.

The book is divided into three parts. The first part covers the major groups of drugs. The second part gives detailed information about 285 individual drugs, arranged alphabetically. The third part consists of the drug finder and index.

PART 1: MAJOR DRUG GROUPS

This part of the book is subdivided into sections on each body system or major disease grouping. It contains descriptions of the principal drug groups and information on the uses, actions, effects, and risks associated with each. Common drugs in each group are listed to allow cross-reference to Part 2.

PART 2: A–Z OF DRUGS

This part consists of profiles of 285 key drugs. Each profile gives detailed information and practical advice and is intended to provide reference and guidance for non-medical readers taking drug treatment. It is impossible, however, to take into account every variation in individual circumstances; readers should always follow a doctor's or pharmacist's instructions where they differ from the advice in this section.

The drugs have been selected to provide representative coverage of the principal classes of drugs in medical use today. For some disorders, a number of drugs are available and the most commonly used drugs have been chosen. Emphasis has also been placed on the drugs likely to be used in the home, although in a few cases drugs administered only in hospital have been included when the drug has been judged to be of sufficient general interest.

HOW TO UNDERSTAND THE PROFILES

For ease of reference, the information on each drug is arranged in a consistent format under standard headings.

Drug name Tells you the drug's generic name, brand names under which the drug is marketed, and combined preparations that contain the drug.

Quick reference Summarizes important facts regarding the drug.

General information Gives a brief summary of the drug's important characteristics.

Information for users Practical information on how and when to take the drug, the usual recommended dosage, how soon it takes effect, how long it is active, and advice on diet, storage, and missed doses.

Overdose action Indicates the symptoms that may occur if an overdose has been taken and tells you what immediate action is required.

Possible adverse effects Indicates adverse effects that may be experienced with the drug.

Interactions Tells you how the drug may interact with other drugs or substances taken at the same time.

Special precautions Describes circumstances in which the drug should be taken with special caution or in which it might not be suitable.

Prolonged use Tells you what effects the drug may have when taken long term and what monitoring may be advised.

PART 3: DRUG FINDER AND INDEX

The combined drug finder and index provides basic information on over 3,000 generic and brand-name drugs and drug groups and directs you to further information about them throughout the book.

PART 1

MAJOR DRUG GROUPS

Subdivided into sections dealing with each body system (such as heart and circulation) or major disease grouping (such as malignant and immune disease), this part of the book contains descriptions of the principal classes of drugs (such as corticosteroids), with information on the uses, actions, effects, and risks associated with each group of drugs. Individual drugs common to each group are listed to allow cross-reference to Part 2.

BRAIN AND NERVOUS SYSTEM

The human brain contains more than 100 billion nerve cells (neurons). These nerve cells receive electrochemical impulses from everywhere in the body. They interpret these impulses and send responsive signals back to various glands and muscles. The brain functions continuously as a switchboard for the human communications system. At the same time, it serves as the seat of emotions and mood, of memory, personality, and thought. Extending from the brain is an additional, large rod-shaped cluster of nerve cells that forms the spinal cord. Together, these two elements comprise the central nervous system.

Radiating from the central nervous system is the peripheral nervous system, which has three parts. One branches off the spinal cord and extends to skin and muscles throughout the body. Another, in the head, links the brain to the eyes, ears, nose, and taste buds. The third is a semi-independent network called the autonomic, or involuntary, nervous system. This is the part of the nervous system that controls unconscious body functions such as breathing, digestion, and glandular activity (see below).

Signals traverse the nervous system by electrical and chemical means. Electrical impulses carry signals from one end of a neuron to the other. To cross the gap between neurons, chemical neurotransmitters are released from one cell to bind on to the receptor sites of nearby cells. Excitatory transmitters stimulate action; inhibitory transmitters reduce it.

WHAT CAN GO WRONG

Disorders of the brain and nervous system may manifest as physical impairments, such as epilepsy or strokes, or mental and emotional impairments (for example, schizophrenia or depression).

Illnesses causing physical impairments can result from different types of disorder of the brain and nervous system. Death of nerve cells due to poor circulation can result in paralysis, while electrical disturbances of certain nerve cells cause the seizures of epilepsy. Temporary changes in blood circulation within and around the brain are associated with migraine. Parkinson's disease is caused by a lack of dopamine, a neurotransmitter that is produced by specialized brain cells.

The causes of disorders that trigger mental and emotional impairment are not known, but these illnesses are thought to result from the defective functioning of nerve cells and neurotransmitters.

WHY DRUGS ARE USED

By and large, the drugs described in this section do not eliminate nervous system disorders. Their function is to correct or modify the communication of the signals that traverse the nervous system. By doing so they can relieve symptoms or restore normal functioning and behaviour. In some cases, such as anxiety and insomnia, drugs are used to lower the level of activity in the brain. In other disorders (depression, for example) drugs are given to encourage the opposite effect, increasing the level of activity.

Drugs that act on the nervous system are also used for conditions that outwardly have nothing to do with nervous system disorders. Vomiting, for example, may be treated with drugs that directly affect the vomiting centre in the brain or block stimulatory nerve signals to the vomiting centre.

AUTONOMIC NERVOUS SYSTEM

The autonomic, or involuntary, nervous system governs the actions of the muscles of the organs and glands. Such vital functions as heart beat and digestion continue without conscious direction, whether we are awake or asleep.

The autonomic nervous system is divided into two parts, the effects of one generally balancing those of the other. The sympathetic nervous system has an excitatory effect. For example, it widens the airways to the lungs, increases the heart rate, and increases the flow of blood to the arms and legs. The parasympathetic system, by contrast, has an opposing effect. It slows the heart rate, narrows the large airways, and redirects blood from the limbs to the gut.

Although the functional pace of most organs results from the interplay between the two systems, the muscles in the blood vessel walls respond only to the signals of the sympathetic nervous system. Whether a vessel is dilated or constricted is determined by the relative stimulation of two sets of receptor sites: alpha sites and beta sites.

Blood vessels in the skin These are constricted by stimulation of alpha receptors by the sympathetic system; the parasympathetic has no effect on them.

The heart The rate and strength of the heart beat are increased by the sympathetic and reduced by the parasympathetic.

The pupils These are dilated by the sympathetic and constricted by the parasympathetic.

The airways The bronchial muscles are relaxed and widened by the sympathetic and contracted and narrowed by the parasympathetic.

Intestines The activity of the intestinal wall muscles is reduced by the sympathetic and increased by the parasympathetic.

NEUROTRANSMITTERS

The parasympathetic system depends on the neurotransmitter acetylcholine to transmit signals between cells. The sympathetic system relies on epinephrine (adrenaline) and norepinephrine (noradrenaline), substances that act as both hormones and neurotransmitters.

DRUGS THAT ACT ON THE SYMPATHETIC NERVOUS SYSTEM

The drugs that stimulate the sympathetic nervous system are called adrenergics (or sympathomimetics). They either promote the release of epinephrine and norepinephrine or mimic their effects. Drugs that interfere with the action of the sympathetic nervous system are called sympatholytics. Alpha blockers act on alpha receptors; beta blockers act on beta receptors (see also Beta blockers, p.28).

DRUGS THAT ACT ON THE PARASYMPATHETIC NERVOUS SYSTEM

Drugs that stimulate the parasympathetic system are called cholinergics (or parasympathomimetics); drugs that oppose its action are called anticholinergics. Many prescribed drugs have anticholinergic properties.

MAJOR DRUG GROUPS

- Analgesics
- Sleeping drugs
- Anti-anxiety drugs
- Antidepressant drugs
- Antipsychotic drugs
- Antimanic drugs
- Anticonvulsant drugs
- Drugs for parkinsonism
- Drugs for dementia
- Nervous system stimulants
- Drugs for migraine
- Anti-emetics

Analgesics

Analgesics (painkillers) are drugs that relieve pain. As pain is not a disease but a symptom, long-term relief depends on treatment of the underlying cause. For example, toothache can be relieved by drugs but can be cured only by appropriate dental treatment. If the underlying disorder is irreversible, such as some rheumatic conditions, long-term analgesic treatment may be necessary.

Damage to body tissues as a result of disease or injury is detected by nerve endings that transmit signals to the brain. Interpretation of these sensations can be affected by a person's psychological state, so that pain is worsened by anxiety and fear, for example. Often an explanation of the cause of discomfort can make pain easier to bear or even relieve it altogether. Anti-anxiety drugs (see p.11) are helpful when pain is accompanied by anxiety; some of these drugs are also used to reduce painful muscle spasms. Some antidepressants (see p.12) block the transmission of impulses signalling pain and are particularly useful for nerve pains (neuralgia), which do not always respond to analgesics.

TYPES OF ANALGESIC

Analgesics are divided into the opioids (with similar properties to drugs derived from opium, such as morphine) and non-opioids, which include all the other analgesics, such as paracetamol, nefopam, and non-steroidal anti-inflammatory drugs (NSAIDs), the most well known of which is aspirin. The non-opioids are all less powerful as painkillers than the opioids. Local anaesthetics (see opposite) are also used to relieve pain.

Opioid drugs and paracetamol act directly on the brain and spinal cord to alter the perception of pain. Opioids act like endorphins, hormones naturally produced in the brain that stop the cell-to-cell transmission of pain sensation. NSAIDs block the formation of pain-modulating substances (e.g. prostaglandins) at nerve endings at the site of pain.

When pain is treated under medical supervision, it is common to start with paracetamol or an NSAID; if neither gives adequate relief, they may be combined. A mild opioid such as codeine may also be used. If the less powerful drugs are ineffective, a strong opioid such as morphine may be given. As there is now a wide variety of oral analgesic formulations, injections are seldom necessary to control even the most severe pain.

When using an over-the-counter preparation (for example, taking paracetamol for a headache) you should seek medical advice if pain persists for longer than 48 hours, recurs, or is worse or different from previous pain.

NON-OPIOID ANALGESICS

Paracetamol This analgesic is believed to act by reducing the production of chemicals called prostaglandins in the brain. However, paracetamol does not affect prostaglandin production in the rest of the body, so it does not reduce inflammation, although it can reduce fever. Paracetamol can be used for everyday aches and pains, such as headaches, toothache, and joint pains.

As well as being the most widely used analgesic, it is one of the safest when taken correctly. It does not usually irritate the stomach, and allergic reactions are rare. However, an overdose can cause severe and possibly fatal liver or kidney damage. Its toxic potential may be increased in heavy drinkers.

Non-steroidal anti-inflammatory drugs (NSAIDs): aspirin Used for many years to relieve pain and reduce fever, aspirin also reduces inflammation by blocking the production of prostaglandins, which contribute to the swelling and pain in inflamed tissue. Aspirin is useful for headaches, toothache, mild rheumatic pain, sore throat, and discomfort caused by feverish illnesses. When given regularly, it can also relieve the pain and inflammation of chronic rheumatoid arthritis (see Antirheumatic drugs, p.49).

Aspirin is found in combination with other substances in a variety of medicines (see Cold cures, p.26). It is also used in the treatment of some blood disorders, since aspirin helps to prevent abnormal clotting of blood by preventing platelets from sticking together (see Drugs that affect blood clotting, p.36).

Aspirin in the form of soluble tablets, dissolved in water before being taken, is absorbed into the bloodstream more quickly, thereby relieving pain faster than tablets. Soluble aspirin is not less irritating to the stomach lining, however.

Aspirin is available in many forms, all of which have a similar effect, but because the amount of aspirin in a tablet of each type varies, it is important to read the packet for the correct dose. Aspirin is not recommended for children under 16 years because its use has been linked to Reye's syndrome, a rare but potentially fatal liver and brain disorder.

Other non-steroidal anti-inflammatory drugs (NSAIDs) These drugs can relieve both pain and inflammation. NSAIDs are related to aspirin and also work by blocking the production of prostaglandins. They are most commonly used to treat muscle and joint pain and may also be prescribed for other types of pain including period pain. For further information on these drugs, see p.48.

COMBINED ANALGESICS

Mild opioids, such as codeine, are often found in combination preparations with non-opioids, such as paracetamol. The prefix "co-" is used to denote a drug combination. Although both opioids and paracetamol act centrally, these mixtures have the advantage of combining different mechanisms of action. Another advantage of combining analgesics is that the reductions in dose of the components may reduce the side effects of the preparation. Combinations can be helpful in reducing the number of tablets taken during long-term treatment.

OPIOID ANALGESICS

These drugs are related to opium, an extract of poppy seeds. They act directly on several sites in the central nervous system to block the transmission of pain signals. Because they act directly on the parts of the brain where pain is perceived, opioids are the strongest analgesics and are therefore used to treat the pain arising from surgery, serious injury, and cancer. These drugs are particularly valuable for relieving severe pain during terminal illnesses. In addition, their ability to produce a state of relaxation and euphoria is often of help in relieving the stress that accompanies severe pain.

Morphine is the best-known opioid analgesic. Others include diamorphine (heroin) and pethidine. The use of these powerful opioids is strictly controlled because the euphoria produced can lead to misuse and addiction. When they are given under medical supervision to treat severe pain, though, the risk of addiction is negligible.

Opioid analgesics may prevent clear thought and cloud consciousness. Other possible adverse effects include nausea and vomiting, constipation, drowsiness, and depressed breathing. When they are taken in overdose, these drugs may induce a deep coma and lead to fatal breathing difficulties.

In addition to the powerful opioids, there are some less powerful drugs in this group that are used to relieve mild to moderate pain. They include codeine and tramadol. The opioids' normally unwanted side effects of depressing respiration and causing constipation make them useful as cough suppressants (p.26) and antidiarrhoeal drugs (p.42).

LOCAL ANAESTHETICS

These drugs are used to prevent pain, usually in minor surgical procedures (for example, dental treatment and stitching cuts). They can also be injected into the space around the spinal cord to numb the lower half of the body. This is called spinal or epidural anaesthesia and can be used for some major operations in people who are not fit for a general anaesthetic. Epidural anaesthesia is also used during childbirth.

Local anaesthetics block the passage of nerve impulses at the site of administration, deadening all feeling conveyed by the nerves with which they come into contact. They do not interfere with consciousness, however. Local anaesthetics are usually given by injection but can also be applied to the skin, mouth, and other areas lined with mucous membrane (such as the vagina), or the eye to relieve pain. Some local anaesthetics are formulated for injection together with epinephrine (adrenaline). Epinephrine constricts the blood vessels and prevents the local anaesthetic from being absorbed into the bloodstream. This action keeps the anaesthetic at the site, thus prolonging its effect.

Local anaesthetic creams are often used to numb the skin before injections in children and people with a fear of needles.

COMMON DRUGS

Opioids Buprenorphine, Co-codamol, Codeine*, Co-dydramol, Diamorphine (heroin), Dihydrocodeine*, Dipipanone, Fentanyl, Meptazinol, Methadone*, Morphine*, Oxycodone, Pethidine, Tramadol*

NSAIDs (see p.48) Aspirin*, Diclofenac*, Etodolac, Fenbufen, Fenoprofen, Ibuprofen*, Indometacin, Ketoprofen*, Mefenamic acid*, Naproxen*, Piroxicam*

Other non-opioids Nefopam, Paracetamol*

Local anaesthetics Bupivacaine, Lidocaine

* **See Part 2**

Sleeping drugs

Difficulty in getting to sleep or staying asleep (insomnia) has many causes. Most people have sleepless nights from time to time, usually due to a temporary worry or discomfort from a minor illness. Persistent sleeplessness can be caused by psychological problems including anxiety or depression, or the pain and discomfort of a physical disorder.

WHY THEY ARE USED

For occasional sleeplessness, simple, common remedies to promote relaxation, such as taking a warm bath or a hot milk drink before bedtime, are usually the best treatment. Sleeping drugs (also known as hypnotics) are normally prescribed only when these self-help remedies have failed, and when lack of sleep is beginning to affect general health. They are used to re-establish the habit of sleeping, and should be used in the smallest dose and for the shortest possible time (not more than 3 weeks). It is best not to take sleeping tablets every night (see Risks and special precautions, right). Do not use alcohol to help you get to sleep as it can cause disturbed sleep and insomnia. Long-term treatment of sleeplessness depends on resolving the underlying cause.

TYPES OF SLEEPING DRUG

Benzodiazepines are the most commonly used class of sleeping drug because they have comparatively few adverse effects and are relatively safe in overdose. They are also used to treat anxiety (see opposite).

Barbiturates are now almost never used because of the risks of misuse, dependence, and toxicity in overdose. There is also a risk of prolonged sedation ("hangover").

Chloral derivatives effectively promote sleep but are little used now. If prescribed, triclofos causes fewer gastrointestinal side effects than chloral hydrate.

Other non-benzodiazepine sleeping drugs Zopiclone, zaleplon, and zolpidem are non-benzodiazepine sleeping drugs that work in a similar way to benzodiazepines. They are not intended for long-term use, and withdrawal symptoms have been reported.

Antihistamines are widely used to treat allergic symptoms (see p.56). Because these drugs also cause drowsiness, they are sometimes used to promote sleep.

Antidepressant drugs may be used to promote sleep in depressed people (see p.12) as well as being effective in treating underlying depressive illness.

HOW THEY WORK

Most sleeping drugs promote sleep by depressing brain function. The drugs interfere with chemical activity in the brain and nervous system by reducing communication between nerve cells. This leads to reduced brain activity, allowing you to fall asleep more easily, but the nature of the sleep is affected by the drug. The main class of sleeping drugs, the benzodiazepines, is described in Anti-anxiety drugs, opposite.

HOW THEY AFFECT YOU

A sleeping drug rapidly produces drowsiness and slowed reactions. Some people find that the drug makes them appear to be drunk, their speech slurred, especially if they delay going to bed after taking their dose. Most people find that they usually fall asleep within about an hour of taking the drug.

Because the sleep induced by drugs is not the same as normal sleep, many people find that they do not feel as well rested by it as by a night of natural sleep. This is the result of suppressed brain activity. Sleeping drugs also suppress the sleep during which dreams occur; both dream sleep and non-dream sleep are essential for a good night's sleep.

Some people experience a variety of hangover effects the following day. Some benzodiazepines may produce minor side effects, such as daytime drowsiness, dizziness, and unsteadiness, that can impair the ability to drive or operate machinery. Older people are likely to become confused, and the selection of an appropriate drug is important for them.

RISKS AND SPECIAL PRECAUTIONS

Sleeping drugs become less effective after the first few nights and there may be a temptation to increase the dose. Apart from the antihistamines, most sleeping drugs can produce psychological and physical dependence when taken regularly for more than a few weeks, especially if they are taken in larger-than-normal doses.

When sleeping drugs are suddenly withdrawn, anxiety, seizures, and hallucinations sometimes occur. Nightmares and vivid dreams may be a problem because the time spent in dream sleep increases. Sleeplessness will recur and may lead to a temptation to use sleeping drugs again. Anyone who wishes to stop taking sleeping drugs, particularly after prolonged use, should seek their doctor's advice to prevent these withdrawal symptoms from occurring.

COMMON DRUGS

Benzodiazepines Flurazepam, Loprazolam, Lormetazepam, Nitrazepam*, Temazepam*

Other non-benzodiazepine sleeping drugs Clomethiazole, Promethazine*, Zaleplon, Zolpidem, Zopiclone*

* **See Part 2**

Anti-anxiety drugs

A certain amount of stress can be beneficial, providing a stimulus to action. But too much will often result in anxiety, which might be described as fear or apprehension that is not caused by real danger.

Clinically, anxiety arises when the balance of certain chemicals in the brain is disturbed. The fearful feelings increase brain activity, stimulating the sympathetic nervous system (see Autonomic nervous system, p.6) and often triggering physical symptoms such as breathlessness, shaking, palpitations, digestive distress, and headaches.

WHY THEY ARE USED

Anti-anxiety drugs (also known as anxiolytics or minor tranquillizers) are prescribed for short-term relief of severe anxiety and nervousness caused by psychological problems. However, these drugs cannot resolve the causes. Tackling the underlying problem through counselling and perhaps psychotherapy offers the best hope of a long-term solution. Anti-anxiety drugs are also used in hospitals to calm and relax people undergoing uncomfortable medical procedures.

There are two main classes of drug for relieving anxiety: benzodiazepines and beta blockers. Benzodiazepines, which are the most widely used, are given as regular treatment for short periods to promote relaxation. Most have a strong sedative effect, helping to relieve the insomnia that accompanies anxiety (see also Sleeping drugs, p.9).

Beta blockers are mainly used to reduce physical symptoms of anxiety, such as shaking and palpitations. These drugs are commonly prescribed for people who feel excessively anxious in certain situations, such as interviews or public appearances.

Many antidepressants (see p.12), including SSRIs, clomipramine, and venlafaxine, are also useful in some anxiety disorders.

HOW THEY WORK

Benzodiazepines and related drugs depress activity in the part of the brain that controls emotion by promoting the action of the neurotransmitter gamma-aminobutyric acid (GABA), which binds to neurons, blocking transmission of electrical impulses and thus reducing communication between brain cells. Benzodiazepines increase the inhibitory effect of GABA on brain cells, preventing the excessive brain activity that causes anxiety.

Buspirone is different from other anti-anxiety drugs; it binds mainly to serotonin (another neurotransmitter) receptors and does not cause drowsiness. Its effect is not felt for at least 2 weeks after starting treatment.

Beta blockers block the action of the neurotransmitter norepinephrine (see p.7) in the body, reducing the physical symptoms of anxiety. These symptoms are produced by an increase in the activity of the sympathetic nervous system; sympathetic nerve endings release norepinephrine, which stimulates the heart, digestive system, and other organs. For more information on beta blockers, see p.28.

HOW THEY AFFECT YOU

Benzodiazepines and related drugs reduce feelings of restlessness and agitation, slow mental activity, and often produce drowsiness. They are said to reduce motivation and, if they are taken in large doses, may lead to apathy. They also have a relaxing effect on the muscles, and some benzodiazepines are used specifically for that purpose (see Muscle relaxants, p.53).

Minor adverse effects of these drugs include dizziness and forgetfulness. The latter can be useful when benzodiazepines are used as sedatives for invasive procedures such as endoscopy. However, people who drive or operate machinery should be aware that their reactions may be slowed by the drug. Because the brain soon becomes tolerant to and dependent on their effects, benzodiazepines are usually effective for only a few weeks at a time.

Beta blockers reduce the physical symptoms associated with anxiety, which may promote greater mental calmness. Because they do not cause drowsiness, they are safer for people who need to drive.

RISKS AND SPECIAL PRECAUTIONS

Benzodiazepines are safe for most people and less dangerous in overdose than other sedative drugs. The main risk is psychological and physical dependence, especially for regular users or with larger-than-average doses. For this reason, they are usually given for courses of 2 weeks or less. If they have been used for longer, they should be withdrawn gradually under medical supervision. If they are stopped suddenly, withdrawal symptoms, such as excessive anxiety, nightmares, and restlessness, may occur.

Benzodiazepines have been misused for their sedative effect, and are therefore prescribed with caution for people with a history of drug or alcohol abuse.

COMMON DRUGS

Benzodiazepines Alprazolam, Chlordiazepoxide, Diazepam/Lorazepam*, Oxazepam

Beta blockers Atenolol*, Bisoprolol*, Oxprenolol, Propranolol*

Other non-benzodiazepines Buspirone

* **See Part 2**

Antidepressant drugs

Occasional moods of discouragement or sadness are normal and usually pass quickly. However, more severe depression that is accompanied by despair, lethargy, loss of sex drive, and often poor appetite may call for medical attention. This kind of depression can arise from life stresses such as the death of someone close, an illness, or sometimes from no apparent cause.

There are three main types of drug for depression: tricyclic antidepressants (TCAs), selective serotonin re-uptake inhibitors (SSRIs), and monoamine oxidase inhibitors (MAOIs). In addition to these drug groups, lithium may be prescribed to treat severe depression. Several other antidepressants may also be prescribed (see right).

WHY THEY ARE USED

Minor depression does not usually require drug treatment; support and help in coming to terms with the cause is often all that is needed. Moderate or severe depression usually requires drug treatment, which is effective in most cases.

Antidepressants may have to be taken for many months. Treatment should not be stopped too soon because symptoms are likely to reappear. When the treatment is stopped, the dose should be reduced gradually over several weeks because withdrawal symptoms may occur if the drugs are stopped suddenly.

TYPES OF ANTIDEPRESSANT

Treatment usually begins with either a TCA or an SSRI.

TCAs Some TCAs (such as amitriptyline) cause drowsiness, which is useful for sleep problems in depression. TCAs also cause anticholinergic effects (see Drugs that act on the parasympathetic nervous system, p.7), including blurred vision, dry mouth, and urinary difficulties.

SSRIs These drugs generally have fewer side effects than TCAs. The main unwanted effects are nausea and vomiting. Anxiety, headache, and restlessness may also occur at the beginning of treatment.

MAOIs These are especially effective in people who are anxious as well as depressed, or those who have phobias.

Lithium Salts of this metallic element are used to treat bipolar disorder (see Antimanic drugs, p.14). In some cases, lithium is given together with an antidepressant drug for treating resistant depression.

Other antidepressants These include venlafaxine, duloxetine, flupentixol, mirtazapine, mianserin, and trazodone.

HOW THEY WORK

Normally, the brain cells release sufficient quantities of certain chemicals (known as neurotransmitters) in the brain to stimulate neighbouring cells. The neurotransmitters are constantly reabsorbed into the brain cells, where they are broken down by an enzyme called monoamine oxidase. Depression is thought to be caused by a reduction in the level of neurotransmitters in the brain. Antidepressants raise the level of these neurotransmitters.

TCAs and venlafaxine work by blocking the re-uptake of the neurotransmitters serotonin and norepinephrine (noradrenaline), thereby increasing the level of these neurotransmitters in the brain.

SSRIs act by blocking the re-uptake of only one neurotransmitter, serotonin.

MAOIs act by blocking the breakdown of neurotransmitters, mainly serotonin and norepinephrine.

HOW THEY AFFECT YOU

The antidepressant effect of these drugs starts after 10 to 14 days of treatment, and it may be 6 to 8 weeks before the full effect is seen. However, side effects may happen at once. Tolerance to these side effects usually occurs and treatment should be continued.

RISKS AND SPECIAL PRECAUTIONS

Overdose can be dangerous: tricyclic antidepressants can produce coma, seizures, and disturbed heart rhythm, which may be fatal; MAOIs can also cause muscle spasms and even death. Both are prescribed with caution for people with heart problems or epilepsy.

When MAOIs are taken with certain drugs or foods rich in tyramine (for example, cheese, meat, yeast extracts, and red wine), they can produce a dramatic rise in blood pressure, with headache or vomiting. People taking MAOIs are given a card that lists prohibited drugs and foods. Because of this adverse interaction, MAOIs are used much less frequently today, and SSRIs or tricyclics are prescribed in preference to them, although SSRIs are not generally prescribed to anyone under the age of 18.

COMMON DRUGS

Tricyclics Amitriptyline*, Clomipramine*, Dosulepin*, Doxepin, Imipramine*, Lofepramine*, Nortriptyline, Trimipramine

SSRIs Citalopram/Escitalopram*, Fluoxetine*, Fluvoxamine, Paroxetine*, Sertraline*

MAOIs Isocarboxazid, Moclobemide, Phenelzine*, Tranylcypromine

Other drugs Duloxetine, Flupentixol*, Mianserin, Mirtazapine* Reboxetine, Trazodone, Tryptophan, Venlafaxine*

* **See Part 2**

Antipsychotic drugs

Psychosis is a term used to describe mental disorders that prevent an affected person from thinking clearly, recognizing reality, and acting rationally. These disorders include schizophrenia and bipolar disorder (manic-depressive illness). The precise causes of these disorders are unknown, although several factors, including stress, heredity, and brain injury, may be involved. Temporary psychosis can also arise as a result of alcohol withdrawal or the misuse of mind-altering drugs. Various drugs are used to treat psychotic disorders (see Common drugs, p.14), most of which have similar actions and effects. One exception is lithium, which is particularly useful for bipolar disorder (see Antimanic drugs, p.14).

WHY THEY ARE USED

A person with a psychotic illness may recover spontaneously, so drugs will not always be prescribed. Long-term treatment is started only when normal life is seriously disrupted. Antipsychotic drugs (also called major tranquillizers or neuroleptics) do not cure the disorder, but they help to control symptoms.

By controlling the symptoms of psychosis, antipsychotics make it possible for many people to live in the community and only be admitted to hospital for acute episodes.

The drug given to a particular individual depends on the nature of their illness and the expected adverse effects of that drug. Drugs differ in the amount of sedation produced; the need for sedation also influences the choice of drug.

Antipsychotic drugs may be given to calm or sedate a person who is highly agitated or aggressive, whatever the cause. Some antipsychotic drugs also have a powerful action against nausea and vomiting (see p.19), and are therefore sometimes used as premedication before surgery.

HOW THEY WORK

It is thought that some mental illnesses are caused by an increase in communication between brain cells due to overactivity of an excitatory chemical called dopamine. This may disturb thought processes and produce abnormal behaviour. Dopamine combines with receptors on the brain cells. Antipsychotic drugs reduce the transmission of nerve signals by binding to these receptors, thereby making the brain cells less sensitive to dopamine. Some newer antipsychotics, such as clozapine, risperidone, and sertindole, also bind to receptors for serotonin.

HOW THEY AFFECT YOU

Because antipsychotics depress the action of dopamine, they can disturb its balance with another chemical in the brain, acetylcholine. If an imbalance occurs, extrapyramidal side effects (EPSE) may appear, including restlessness, disorders of movement, and parkinsonism (see Drugs for parkinsonism, p.16).

In these circumstances, a change to a different type of antipsychotic may be necessary. If this is not possible, an anticholinergic drug (see p.16) may be prescribed.

Antipsychotics may block the action of the neurotransmitter norepinephrine (see p.7). This lowers blood pressure, especially when you stand up, causing dizziness. It may also prevent ejaculation.

RISKS AND SPECIAL PRECAUTIONS

It is important to continue taking these drugs even if all symptoms have gone, because the symptoms are controlled only by taking the prescribed dose.

Because antipsychotic drugs can have permanent as well as temporary side effects, the minimum necessary dosage is used. This minimum dose is found by starting with a low dose and increasing it until the symptoms are controlled. Sudden withdrawal after more than a few weeks can cause nausea, sweating, headache, and restlessness. Therefore, the dose is reduced gradually when treatment needs to be stopped.

The most serious long-term risk of antipsychotic treatment is a disorder known as tardive dyskinesia, which may develop after 1 to 5 years. This consists of repeated jerking movements of the mouth, tongue, and face, and sometimes of the hands and feet. The condition is less common with the newer antipsychotics (atypical antipsychotics) than the older drugs (typical antipsychotics).

HOW THEY ARE ADMINISTERED

Antipsychotics may be given by mouth as tablets, capsules, or syrup, or by injection. They can also be given as an intramuscular depot injection, which releases the drug slowly over several weeks.

COMMON DRUGS

Typical antipsychotics Benperidol, Chlorpromazine*, Flupentixol*, Fluphenazine, Haloperidol*, Levomepromazine, Pericyazine, Perphenazine, Pimozide, Pipotiazine, Prochlorperazine*, Promazine*, Trifluoperazine, Zuclopenthixol

Atypical antipsychotics Amisulpride*, Aripiprazole, Clozapine*, Olanzapine*, Quetiapine*, Risperidone*, Sertindole, Zotepine

* **See Part 2**

Antimanic drugs

Changes in mood are normal, but if mood swings become grossly exaggerated, with peaks of elation or mania alternating with troughs of depression, it becomes an illness known as bipolar disorder or manic depressive illness. This is usually treated with salts of lithium (p.299), a drug that reduces the intensity of the mania, lifts the depression, and lessens the frequency of mood swings. Because it may take weeks or even months before the lithium starts to work, an antipsychotic may be prescribed with lithium at first to give immediate relief of symptoms.

Lithium can be toxic if blood levels of the drug rise too high. Regular checks on the blood concentration of lithium should therefore be carried out during treatment. Symptoms of lithium poisoning include blurred vision, tremor, vomiting, and diarrhoea.

COMMON DRUGS

Carbamazepine*, Lithium*, Sodium valproate*

* **See Part 2**

Anticonvulsant drugs

Electrical signals from nerve cells in the brain are normally finely coordinated to produce smooth movements of the arms and legs, but these signals can become irregular and chaotic, and trigger the disorderly muscular activity and mental changes that are characteristic of a seizure (also called a fit or convulsion). The most common cause of seizures is epilepsy, which occurs as a result of brain disease or injury. In epilepsy, a seizure may be triggered by an outside stimulus such as a flashing light. Seizures can also result from the toxic effects of certain drugs and, in young children, a high temperature.

Anticonvulsant drugs are used both to reduce the risk of an epileptic seizure and to stop one that is in progress.

WHY THEY ARE USED

Isolated seizures seldom require drug treatment, but anticonvulsant drugs are the usual treatment for controlling seizures caused by epilepsy. In most cases, they permit a person with epilepsy to lead a normal life.

Most people with epilepsy need to take anticonvulsants on a regular basis to prevent seizures. Usually a single drug is used, and treatment continues until there have been no attacks for at least 2 years.

If one drug is not effective, a different one will be tried. Occasionally, it is necessary to take a combination of drugs. Even when receiving treatment, a person can still have seizures. Repeated seizures or status epilepticus can be halted by injection of diazepam or a similar drug.

The choice of anticonvulsant depends on the type of epilepsy, the patient's age, and their particular response to individual drugs.

Generalized epilepsy In these forms of epilepsy, there is widespread disturbance of electrical activity in the brain, and loss of consciousness occurs at the outset. In its simplest form, a momentary loss of consciousness occurs during which the person may stare into space. This is called an absence seizure, and mainly affects children. Seizures do not occur.

Another form of generalized epilepsy causes a brief jerk of a limb (myoclonus).

The most severe type is a tonic-clonic (grand mal) seizure, which is characterized by loss of consciousness and seizures that may last for a few minutes.

Affected people may have one or more of these types of generalized epilepsy. Sodium valproate, lamotrigine, topiramate, levetiracetam, or the benzodiazepines are normally used for these types of epilepsy.

Partial (focal) epilepsy These types are caused by an electrical disturbance in only one part of the brain. The result is a disturbance of function, such as an abnormal sensation or movement of a limb, without loss of consciousness. In a simple partial seizure, this may precede a more serious attack associated with loss of consciousness (complex partial seizure), which may in turn progress to a generalized convulsive seizure.

Carbamazepine, lamotrigine, or phenytoin may be prescribed for this type of epilepsy.

Status epilepticus Repeated attacks without full recovery between, or a single attack lasting more than 10 minutes, occur in this form of epilepsy. Emergency treatment is required.

HOW THEY WORK

Brain cells bring about body movement by electrical activity that passes through the nerves to the muscles. In an epileptic seizure, uncontrolled electrical activity starts in one part of the brain and spreads to other parts, causing uncontrolled stimulation of brain cells. Most anticonvulsants have an inhibitory effect on brain cells and damp down electrical activity, preventing the excessive build-up that causes epileptic seizures.

HOW THEY AFFECT YOU

Ideally, the only effect an anticonvulsant should have is to reduce or prevent epileptic seizures. Unfortunately, no drug prevents seizures without potentially affecting normal brain function, often leading to poor memory, inability to concentrate, lack of coordination, and lethargy. It is important, therefore, to find a drug and dosage sufficient to prevent seizures without causing unacceptable side effects. The dose has to be carefully tailored to the individual. It is usual to start with a low dose of a selected drug and to increase it gradually until a balance is achieved between control of seizures and the occurrence of side effects, many of which wear off after the first weeks of treatment.

Blood tests are used to monitor levels of some anticonvulsants in the body as an aid to dose adjustment.

RISKS AND SPECIAL PRECAUTIONS

Each anticonvulsant has its own specific adverse effects and risks. In addition, some affect the liver's ability to break down other drugs and may influence the action of other drugs that you take. Doctors try to prescribe the minimum number of anticonvulsants needed to control the seizures, to reduce the risk of such interactions occurring.

Some anticonvulsants pose risks to a developing baby; if you are hoping to become pregnant, you should discuss the risks, and whether your medication should be changed, with your doctor. People taking anticonvulsants need to take them regularly as prescribed. If levels of anticonvulsant in the body fall suddenly, seizures are very likely to occur. The dose should not be reduced or treatment stopped, except on a doctor's advice. Certain driving restrictions may apply if you have had a seizure; in the UK, you need to report this to the Driver and Vehicle Licensing Agency (DVLA).

If anticonvulsant drug treatment needs to be stopped, the dose should be reduced gradually. People on anticonvulsant therapy are advised to carry an identification tag giving full details of their condition and treatment.

COMMON DRUGS

Carbamazepine*, Clobazam, Clonazepam*, Diazepam*, Ethosuximide, Gabapentin*, Lamotrigine*, Levetiracetam*, Lorazepam, Midazolam, Oxcarbazepine, Phenobarbital*, Phenytoin*, Primidone, Sodium valproate*, Tiagabine, Topiramate, Vigabatrin

* **See Part 2**

Drugs for parkinsonism

Parkinsonism is a general term used to describe shaking of the head and limbs, muscular stiffness, an expressionless face, and inability to control or initiate movement. It is caused by an imbalance of chemicals in the brain; the effect of acetylcholine is increased by a reduction in the action of dopamine.

The most common cause of parkinsonism is Parkinson's disease, degeneration of the dopamine-producing cells in the brain. Other causes include the side effects of certain drugs, notably antipsychotics (see p.13), and narrowing of the blood vessels in the brain.

WHY THEY ARE USED

Drugs can relieve the symptoms of parkinsonism but, unfortunately, the degeneration of brain cells in Parkinson's disease cannot be halted, although drugs can minimize the symptoms for many years.

HOW THEY WORK

Drugs to treat parkinsonism restore the balance between the chemicals dopamine and acetylcholine. They fall into two main groups: those that reduce the effect of acetylcholine (anticholinergic drugs) and those that boost the effect of dopamine.

Anticholinergics combine with receptors on brain cells, preventing acetylcholine from binding to them. This action reduces acetylcholine's relative overactivity and restores the balance with dopamine.

Dopamine cannot pass from the blood to the brain, and therefore cannot be given to boost its levels in the brain. Instead, levodopa (L-dopa), the chemical from which it is naturally produced in the brain, is combined with carbidopa (as co-careldopa) or benserazide (as co-beneldopa) to prevent it from being converted to dopamine before it reaches the brain. Amantadine (also used as an antiviral, see p.67) boosts dopamine levels in the brain by stimulating its release. The action of dopamine can also be boosted by other drugs, including bromocriptine, pergolide, or apomorphine (injection only), which mimic the action of dopamine.

CHOICE OF DRUG

Anticholinergics are used to treat parkinsonism due to antipsychotic drugs, which have dopamine-blocking properties. These drugs are not generally used to treat parkinsonism of unknown cause because they are less effective and may increase cognitive impairment. L-dopa is usually given when the disease impairs walking; its effectiveness usually wanes after 2 to 5 years, in which case other dopamine-boosting drugs may also be prescribed.

COMMON DRUGS

Dopamine-boosting drugs Amantadine, Apomorphine, Bromocriptine*, Cabergoline, Entacapone, Levodopa* (as co-beneldopa/co-careldopa), Pergolide, Pramipexole, Rasagiline, Ropinirole*, Selegiline

Anticholinergic drugs Orphenadrine*, Procyclidine*, Trihexyphenidyl/benzhexol

* **See Part 2**

Drugs for dementia

Dementia is a decline in mental function severe enough to affect normal social or occupational activities. It can be sudden and irreversible, for example due to a stroke or head injury. It can also develop gradually and may be a feature of disorders such as poor circulation in the brain, multiple sclerosis, and Alzheimer's disease. Much research is in progress on the cause of Alzheimer's disease, the single most common cause of dementia.

WHY THEY ARE USED

Drugs called acetylcholinesterase inhibitors have been found to improve the symptoms of dementia in Alzheimer's disease, although they do not prevent its long-term progression.

HOW THEY WORK

In healthy people, acetylcholinesterase (an enzyme in the brain) breaks down the neurotransmitter acetylcholine, balancing its levels and limiting its effects. In Alzheimer's disease there is a deficiency of acetylcholine. Acetylcholinesterase inhibitors block the action of acetylcholinesterase, raising brain levels of acetylcholine, thus increasing alertness and slowing the rate of deterioration.

HOW THEY AFFECT YOU

Following assessment by a specialist of mental function, drug treatment is started at a low dose and increased gradually to minimize side effects. Any improvements should begin to appear in about 3 weeks. Assessment is repeated at 6-monthly intervals to determine if the treatment is beneficial.

RISKS AND SPECIAL PRECAUTIONS

It is important to continue taking these drugs if they prove effective, because there is a gradual loss of improvement after treatment is stopped. Side effects include urinary difficulties, nausea, vomiting, and diarrhoea. These drugs may increase the risk of seizures in some people.

COMMON DRUGS

Acetylcholinesterase inhibitors Donepezil*, Galantamine, Memantine, Rivastigmine*

* **See Part 2**

Nervous system stimulants

A person's state of mental alertness varies throughout the day and is under the control of chemicals in the brain, some of which are depressant, causing drowsiness, and others stimulant, heightening awareness.

It is thought that an increase in the activity of the depressant chemicals may be responsible for a condition called narcolepsy, which is a tendency to fall asleep during the day for no obvious reason. In this case, the nervous system stimulants are given to increase wakefulness. These include the amfetamines (usually dexamfetamine), the related drug methylphenidate, and modafinil. Amfetamines are used less often now due to the risk of dependence. A common home remedy for increasing alertness is caffeine, a mild stimulant that is present in coffee, tea, and cola. Respiratory stimulants related to caffeine are used to improve breathing.

WHY THEY ARE USED

In adults who have narcolepsy, some of these drugs prevent excessive drowsiness during the day. Stimulants do not cure narcolepsy and, since the disorder usually lasts throughout the affected person's lifetime, may have to be taken indefinitely. Methylphenidate or dexamfetamine are sometimes given to people who have attention deficit hyperactivity disorder (ADHD).

Stimulants were once used as part of the treatment for obesity because reduced appetite is a side effect of amfetamines, but they are no longer thought to be appropriate for weight reduction. Diet is now the main treatment, together with orlistat if necessary.

Caffeine is added to some analgesics to counteract the effects of caffeine withdrawal, which can cause headaches, but no clear medical justification exists for this.

Respiratory stimulants, such as theophylline, aminophylline, and doxapram, are used to improve breathing. They act on the respiratory centre, the part of the brain that controls breathing. Respiratory stimulants are sometimes used in hospitals to help people who have difficulty in breathing, mainly very young babies and adults who have severe chest infections.

Apart from their use in narcolepsy, nervous system stimulants are not useful in the long term because the brain soon develops tolerance to them.

HOW THEY WORK

The level of wakefulness is controlled by a part of the brain stem called the reticular activating system (RAS). Activity in this area depends on the balance between chemicals, some of which are excitatory (including norepinephrine (noradrenaline)) and some inhibitory, such as gamma aminobutyric acid (GABA). Stimulants promote release of norepinephrine, increasing activity in the RAS and other parts of the brain and so raising levels of alertness.

HOW THEY AFFECT YOU

In adults, the central nervous system stimulants taken in the prescribed dose for narcolepsy increase wakefulness, thereby allowing normal concentration and thought processes to occur. They may also reduce appetite and cause tremors. In hyperactive children, they reduce the general level of activity to a more normal level and increase the attention span.

RISKS AND SPECIAL PRECAUTIONS

Some people, especially older adults or those with previous psychiatric problems, are particularly sensitive to stimulants and may experience adverse effects, even with comparatively low doses. Stimulants need to be used with caution in children because they can retard growth if taken for prolonged periods. An excess of these drugs given to a child may depress the nervous system, producing drowsiness or even loss of consciousness. Palpitations may also occur.

These drugs reduce the level of natural stimulants in the brain, so after regular use for a few weeks a person may become physically dependent on them for normal function. If they are abruptly withdrawn, the excess of natural inhibitory chemicals in the brain depresses central nervous system activity, producing withdrawal symptoms. These may include lethargy, depression, increased appetite, and difficulty in staying awake.

Stimulants can produce overactivity in the brain if used inappropriately or in excess, resulting in extreme restlessness, sleeplessness, nervousness, or anxiety. They also stimulate the sympathetic branch of the nervous system (see p.6), causing shaking, sweating, and palpitations. More serious risks of exceeding the prescribed dose are seizures and a major disturbance in mental functioning that may result in delusions and hallucinations. Because these drugs have been misused, amfetamines and methylphenidate are classified as controlled drugs.

COMMON DRUGS

Respiratory stimulants Doxapram, Theophylline/aminophylline*

Other drugs Atomoxetine, Caffeine, Dexamfetamine, Methylphenidate*, Modafinil*

* **See Part 2**

Drugs for migraine

Migraine is a term applied to recurrent severe headaches that affect only one side of the head and are caused by changes in the blood vessels around the brain and scalp. They may be accompanied by nausea and vomiting and preceded by warning signs, usually an impression of flashing lights or numbness and tingling in the arms. Occasionally, speech may be impaired, or the attack may be disabling.

The underlying cause of migraine is uncertain, but an attack may be triggered by a blow to the head, physical exertion, certain foods and drugs, or emotional factors such as excitement, tension, or shock. A family history of migraine also increases the chance of an individual developing it.

WHY THEY ARE USED

Drugs are used either to relieve symptoms or to prevent attacks. Different drugs are used in each approach, but none cures the underlying disorder. However, a susceptibility to migraine headaches can clear up spontaneously, and if you are taking drugs regularly, your doctor may recommend that you stop them after a few months to see if this has happened.

In most people, migraine headaches can be relieved by a mild analgesic (painkiller), such as paracetamol or a non-steroidal anti-inflammatory drug (NSAID), or a stronger one like codeine (see Analgesics, p.7). If nausea and vomiting accompany the migraine, tablets may not be absorbed sufficiently from the gut. Absorption can be increased if they are taken as soluble tablets in water or with an anti-emetic (see below).

Some drugs used to relieve attacks can be given by injection, inhaler, nasal spray, or suppository. Preparations that contain caffeine should be avoided since headaches may occur with excessive use or on stopping treatment. 5HT1 agonists (such as sumatriptan) are used if analgesics are not effective. Ergotamine is used much less often now.

The factors that trigger an individual's attacks should be identified and avoided. Anti-anxiety drugs are not usually prescribed if stress is a precipitating factor because of the potential for dependence. If the attacks occur more often than once a month and significantly disrupt daily life, drugs to prevent migraine may be taken every day. The drugs used to prevent migraine are beta blockers (see p.28), such as metoprolol or propranolol, and pizotifen (an antihistamine and serotonin blocker). Other drugs that have been used include amitriptyline (an antidepressant, see p.12), verapamil, and cyproheptadine.

HOW THEY WORK

The symptoms of a migraine attack begin when blood vessels surrounding the brain constrict, producing the typical migraine warning signs. The constriction is thought to be due to certain chemicals found in food or produced by the body. The neurotransmitter serotonin causes large blood vessels in the brain to constrict. Pizotifen and propranolol block the effect of chemicals on blood vessels, thereby preventing attacks.

The next stage of a migraine attack occurs when blood vessels in the scalp and around the eyes dilate (widen). As a result, chemicals called prostaglandins are released, producing pain. Aspirin and paracetamol relieve this pain by blocking prostaglandins. Codeine acts directly on the brain, altering pain perception (see Analgesics, p.7). Ergotamine and 5HT1 agonists relieve pain by narrowing dilated blood vessels in the scalp.

HOW THEY AFFECT YOU

Each drug has its own adverse effects. 5HT1 agonists may cause chest tightness and drowsiness. Ergotamine may cause drowsiness, tingling sensations in the skin, cramps, and weakness in the legs, and vomiting may be made worse. Pizotifen may cause drowsiness and weight gain. For effects of propranolol, see p.28, and for analgesics, see p.7.

RISKS AND SPECIAL PRECAUTIONS

5HT1 agonists should not usually be used by people with high blood pressure, angina, or coronary heart disease. Ergotamine can damage blood vessels by prolonged overconstriction, so the drug should be used with caution by those with poor circulation. Excessive use can lead to dependence and many adverse effects, including headache. You should not take more than your doctor advises in any one week.

HOW THEY ARE ADMINISTERED

These drugs are usually taken by mouth as tablets or capsules. Sumatriptan can also be taken as an injection or a nasal spray. Ergotamine can be taken as suppositories, or as tablets that dissolve under the tongue.

COMMON DRUGS

Drugs to prevent migraine Amitriptyline*, Cyproheptadine, Fremanezumab, Pizotifen*, Propranolol*, Sodium valproate*, Verapamil*
5HT1 agonists Almotriptan, Eletriptan, Frovatriptan, Naratriptan, Rizatriptan, Sumatriptan*, Zolmitriptan
Other drugs to relieve migraine Codeine*, Ergotamine*, NSAIDs (see p.48), Paracetamol*, Tolfenamic acid
* **See Part 2**

Anti-emetics

Drugs used to treat or prevent vomiting or the feeling of sickness (nausea) are known as anti-emetics. Vomiting is a reflex action for getting rid of harmful substances, but it may also be a symptom of disease. Vomiting and nausea are often caused by a digestive tract infection, travel sickness, pregnancy, or vertigo (a balance disorder involving the inner ear). They can also occur as a side effect of some drugs, especially those used for cancer, radiotherapy, or general anaesthesia.

Commonly used anti-emetics include metoclopramide, domperidone, haloperidol, cyclizine, ondansetron, granisetron, prochlorperazine, promethazine, and cinnarizine. The phenothiazine and butyrophenone drug groups are also used as antihistamines (see p.56) and to treat some types of mental illness (see Antipsychotic drugs, p.13).

WHY THEY ARE USED

Doctors usually diagnose the cause of vomiting before prescribing an anti-emetic because the vomiting may be caused by an infection of the digestive tract or some other condition of the abdomen that might require treatment such as surgery. Treating only the vomiting and nausea might delay diagnosis, correct treatment, and recovery.

Anti-emetics may be taken to prevent travel sickness (using one of the antihistamines) or to relieve vomiting resulting from anticancer treatment (see p.94) and other drug treatments (metoclopramide, haloperidol, domperidone, ondansetron, and prochlorperazine, for example).

Vertigo is a spinning sensation in the head, often accompanied by nausea and vomiting. It is usually caused by a disease affecting the organ of balance in the inner ear. Anti-emetics are prescribed to relieve the symptoms.

Ménière's disease is a disorder in which excess fluid builds up in the inner ear, causing vertigo, noises in the ear, and gradual deafness. It is usually treated with cinnarizine, betahistine, prochlorperazine, or an anti-anxiety drug (see p.11). A diuretic (see p.30) may also be given to reduce the excess fluid in the inner ear.

Anti-emetics are also occasionally used to relieve severe vomiting during pregnancy. You should not take an anti-emetic during pregnancy except on medical advice.

You should not take any anti-emetic drug for longer than a couple of days without consulting your doctor.

HOW THEY WORK

Nausea and vomiting occur when the vomiting centre in the brain is stimulated by signals from three places in the body: the digestive tract, the part of the inner ear controlling balance, and the brain itself via thoughts and emotions and via its chemoreceptor trigger zone, which responds to harmful substances in the blood. Anti-emetic drugs may act at one or more of these places. Some help the stomach to empty its contents into the intestine. A combination of drugs may be used that works at different sites and has an additive effect.

HOW THEY AFFECT YOU

As well as treating vomiting and nausea, many anti-emetic drugs may make you feel drowsy. However, for preventing travel sickness on long journeys, a sedating antihistamine may be an advantage.

Some anti-emetic drugs (in particular, the phenothiazines and antihistamines) can block the parasympathetic nervous system (see Autonomic nervous system, p.6), causing a dry mouth, blurred vision, or difficulty in passing urine. The phenothiazines may also lower blood pressure, leading to dizziness or fainting.

RISKS AND SPECIAL PRECAUTIONS

Because some antihistamines can make you drowsy, it may be advisable not to drive while taking them. Phenothiazines, butyrophenones, and metoclopramide can produce uncontrolled movements of the face and tongue, so they are used with caution in people with parkinsonism.

COMMON DRUGS

Antihistamines Cinnarizine*, Cyclizine, Meclozine, Promethazine*

Phenothiazines Chlorpromazine*, Levomepromazine, Perphenazine, Prochlorperazine*, Trifluoperazine

5HT3 antagonists Granisetron, Ondansetron*, Palonosetron

Butyrophenones Haloperidol*

Other drugs Aprepitant, Betahistine*, Dexamethasone*, Domperidone*, Hyoscine hydrobromide*, Metoclopramide*, Nabilone

* **See Part 2**

RESPIRATORY SYSTEM

The respiratory system consists of the lungs and the passages, such as the trachea (windpipe) and the bronchi, by which air reaches them. Through the process of inhaling and exhaling air (breathing) the body obtains the oxygen necessary for survival, and expels carbon dioxide, which is the waste product of the basic human biological process.

Air enters the trachea, which branches into two main bronchi, one for each lung. Within the lungs, the air passes into bronchioles, smaller tubes whose muscular walls may contract or dilate in response to drugs and nerve signals. The bronchioles open out into tiny blood-vessel-lined air sacs (alveoli), which allow oxygen to pass into the bloodstream and carbon dioxide to pass from the bloodstream for expiration.

WHAT CAN GO WRONG

Difficulty in breathing may be due to narrowing of the air passages from spasm, as in asthma and bronchitis, or from swelling of the linings of the air passages, as in bronchiolitis and bronchitis. Breathing difficulties may also be due to an infection of the lung tissue, as in pneumonia, or to damage to the small air sacs (alveoli) from emphysema or scarring (fibrosis), or from inhaled dusts or moulds, which cause pneumoconiosis and farmer's lung. Smoking and air pollution can also affect the respiratory system in many ways, leading to diseases such as lung cancer and bronchitis.

Sometimes difficulty in breathing may be due to congestion of the lungs as a result of heart disease, to an inhaled object such as a peanut, or to infection or inflammation of the throat. Symptoms of breathing difficulties often include a cough and a tight feeling in the chest.

WHY DRUGS ARE USED

Drugs with a variety of actions are used to clear the air passages, soothe inflammation, and reduce the production of mucus. Some can be bought without a prescription as single- or combined-ingredient preparations, often with an analgesic (see p.7).

Decongestants (see p.24) reduce swelling inside the nose, thereby making it possible to breathe more freely. If the congestion is due to an allergic response, an antihistamine (see p.56) is often recommended to relieve symptoms or prevent attacks. Bacterial infections of the respiratory tract are usually treated with antibiotics (see p.60), although most respiratory tract infections are viral.

Bronchodilators (see below) are drugs that widen the bronchi. They are used to prevent and relieve asthma attacks. Corticosteroids (see p.78) reduce inflammation in the swollen inner layers of the airways. They are used to prevent asthma attacks. Other drugs, such as sodium cromoglicate, may be used for treating allergies and preventing asthma attacks but are not effective once an asthma attack has begun.

A variety of drugs are used to relieve a cough, depending on the type of cough involved. Some drugs make it easier to eliminate phlegm; others suppress the cough by inhibiting the cough reflex.

MAJOR DRUG GROUPS

- ◆ Bronchodilators
- ◆ Drugs for asthma
- ◆ Decongestants
- ◆ Drugs to treat coughs
- ◆ See also sections on Allergy (p.56) and Infections (p.59)

Bronchodilators

Air entering the lungs passes through narrow tubes called bronchioles. In asthma and bronchitis the bronchioles become narrower, either as a result of contraction of the muscles in their walls, or as a result of mucus congestion. This narrowing of the bronchioles obstructs the flow of air into and out of the lungs and causes breathlessness.

Bronchodilators are prescribed to widen the bronchioles and improve breathing. There are three main groups of bronchodilator drug: sympathomimetics, anticholinergics, and xanthine drugs (which are related to caffeine). They are all used for relief of symptoms, and do not affect the underlying disease process. Anticholinergics are thought to be more effective in, and are used particularly for, bronchitis. In chronic asthma, they are less effective and are usually prescribed as additional therapy when control with other drugs is inadequate. Sympathomimetics are the first choice drugs in the management of asthma, and are frequently used in bronchitis. Xanthines have been used for many years, both for asthma and for bronchitis. They usually need precise adjustment of dosage to be effective while avoiding side effects. This makes them more difficult to use, and they are reserved for people whose condition cannot be controlled by other bronchodilators alone.

WHY THEY ARE USED

Bronchodilator drugs help to dilate the bronchioles of people with asthma or bronchitis. However, they are of little benefit to people who have severe chronic bronchitis.

Bronchodilators are usually taken when they are needed in order to relieve an attack of breathlessness that is in progress. Some people find it helpful to take an extra dose of their bronchodilator immediately before undertaking any activity that is likely to provoke an attack of breathlessness. A patient who requires treatment with a sympathomimetic inhaler more than twice a week or at night should see their doctor about having preventative treatment with an inhaled corticosteroid.

Sympathomimetic drugs are mainly used for the rapid relief of breathlessness; anticholinergic and xanthine drugs are used both for acute attacks and long-term.

HOW THEY WORK

Bronchodilator drugs act by relaxing the muscles surrounding the bronchioles. Sympathomimetic and anticholinergic drugs achieve this effect by interfering with nerve signals that are transmitted to the muscles through the autonomic nervous system (see p.6). Xanthine drugs are thought to relax the muscle in the bronchioles by a direct effect on the muscle fibres, but their precise action is not known.

Bronchodilators usually improve breathing within a few minutes of administration. Corticosteroid drugs act more slowly; it may be several days before the capacity for exercise increases substantially. Eventually the corticosteroids should reduce the need for bronchodilators.

Because sympathomimetic drugs stimulate a branch of the autonomic nervous system that controls the heart rate, they may sometimes cause palpitations and trembling. Typical side effects of anticholinergic drugs include dry mouth, blurred vision, and difficulty in passing urine. Xanthine drugs may cause headaches and nausea.

RISKS AND SPECIAL PRECAUTIONS

Since most bronchodilators are not taken by mouth but inhaled, they do not commonly cause serious side effects. However, because of their possible effect on heart rate, xanthine and sympathomimetic drugs need to be prescribed with caution to people with heart problems, high blood pressure, or an overactive thyroid gland. Smoking tobacco and drinking alcohol increase excretion of xanthines from the body, reducing their effects. Stopping smoking after being stabilized on a xanthine drug may result in a rise in blood concentration and an increased risk of side effects. It is advisable to stop smoking before starting treatment. The anticholinergic drugs may not be suitable for people with urinary retention or those who have a tendency to glaucoma.

COMMON DRUGS

Sympathomimetics Bambuterol, Ephedrine*, Epinephrine*, Fenoterol, Formoterol, Indacaterol, Salbutamol*, Salmeterol*, Terbutaline*, Vilanterol
Anticholinergics Aclidinium, Glycopyrronium, Ipratropium bromide*, Tiotropium*, Umeclidinium
Xanthines Theophylline/aminophylline*
* **See Part 2**

Drugs for asthma

Asthma is a chronic lung disease characterized by episodes (attacks) in which the bronchioles constrict due to oversensitivity. The attacks are usually, but not always, reversible;

asthma is also known as reversible airways obstruction. It often starts in childhood, although it may also first develop in adulthood, and can affect people of any age. Sometimes the inflammation causing the constriction is due to an identifiable allergen in the atmosphere, such as house dust mites, but often there is no obvious trigger. Breathlessness is the main symptom, and wheezing, coughing, and chest tightness are common. People with asthma often have attacks during the night and wake up with breathing difficulty. The illness varies in severity; at its most severe, it can even be life threatening.

A variety of drug types are used in the control of asthma. Where drugs are needed only to control an occasional attack, a sympathomimetic bronchodilator will probably be used in the form of an inhaler. When a person needs continuous preventative treatment there are a number of choices. Often, an inhaled corticosteroid may be used (with a sympathomimetic inhaler if attacks persist). More severe cases may require higher-dose corticosteroids or the addition of a long-acting sympathomimetic bronchodilator. If this is not adequate, the addition of an anticholinergic drug or theophylline, or these in combination with others already tried, may be needed. There are also leukotriene antagonists (see p.58), which may be used alone or with corticosteroids; they are less effective in severe cases when patients are taking high doses of other drugs. Some people with very severe asthma may need such large doses of corticosteroids that they have to take tablets. Antihistamines have been prescribed for asthma in the past, but this has not proved to be a successful treatment.

WHY THEY ARE USED

In asthma, the airways (bronchioles) constrict, which makes it difficult to get air into or out of the lungs. Bronchodilators (sympathomimetics, anticholinergics, and theophylline) (see p.21) relax the constricted muscles around the bronchioles. Short-acting sympathomimetics act within a few minutes when inhaled and are used to provide relief of symptoms during an attack, and in more severe cases the long-acting sympathomimetics may be used to help with continuous protective cover. They are particularly useful for preventing symptoms overnight. Theophylline/aminophylline must be given by mouth or injection; the tablets are used for regular continuous dosing, and the injection is used in hospital to gain control of severe asthma. Drugs that are not bronchodilators, such as corticosteroids and leukotriene receptor antagonists (see p.24), are effective for long-term protection. Corticosteroids are also given orally for severe acute attacks. Although they have a delayed onset of action (12–24 hours), they help to prevent a recurrence of symptoms in the days after an attack.

In some cases, an intravenous injection of magnesium sulfate may be given to treat a severe asthma attack.

HOW THEY WORK

Inhaling a drug directly into the lungs is the best way of obtaining benefit without experiencing excessive side effects. A selection of devices for delivering the drug into the airways is described below.

Inhalers or puffers release a small dose when pressed, but need some skill to use effectively. If you have been given a pressurized metered-dose inhaler, a large, hollow plastic "spacer" fitted to the inhaler can help you to inhale the drug more easily. Some devices are triggered by an inward breath and may be easier to use than a puffer.

To relieve severe attacks, nebulizers pump compressed air through a solution of the drug to produce a fine mist that is inhaled through a face mask. Nebulizers deliver large doses of the drug to the lungs, rapidly relieving breathing difficulty.

Bronchodilators act by relaxing the muscles surrounding the bronchioles. Corticosteroids are used for their anti-inflammatory properties. By suppressing airway inflammation they reduce swelling (oedema) inside the bronchioles; this action complements relaxation of the walls by the bronchodilators, in opening up the airways. Reducing the inflammation also has the effect of reducing the amount of mucus produced in the bronchioles, and this again helps to clear the airways. Corticosteroids usually start to increase the user's capacity for exercise within a few days, and most people find that the frequency of their attacks of breathlessness is greatly reduced.

Leukotrienes, which used to be called "slow reacting substances", occur naturally in the body. They are chemically related to the prostaglandins, but are much more potent in producing an inflammatory reaction; they are also much more potent than histamine at causing bronchoconstriction. Leukotrienes seem to play an important part in asthma. Drugs have been developed that block their receptors (leukotriene receptor antagonists) and therefore reduce the inflammation and bronchoconstriction of asthma. Sodium cromoglicate and nedocromil act by stabilizing mast cells in the lungs, preventing them from releasing histamine, leukotrienes, and other inflammation-causing chemicals.

RISKS AND SPECIAL PRECAUTIONS

The drugs taken by inhalation act locally and are used in much lower doses than would be needed as tablets. They do not commonly cause serious side effects, but the dry powder inhalations can cause a reflex bronchospasm as the powder hits the lining of the airways; this can be avoided by first using a short-acting sympathomimetic.

Inhaled corticosteroids may encourage fungal growth in the mouth and throat (thrush). This can be minimized by using a spacer and by rinsing your mouth out and gargling after each inhalation. High doses of inhaled corticosteroids may suppress adrenal gland function, reduce bone density, cause bruising, increase the risk of glaucoma, and retard growth in children.

Sympathomimetics and theophylline by mouth may affect heart rate, and should be prescribed with caution to people with heart problems, high blood pressure, or an overactive thyroid gland. The effects of theophylline may last longer if you have a viral infection, heart failure, or liver cirrhosis. The drugs also interact with many other drugs.

Anticholinergics must be used with caution in patients who have prostate problems or urinary retention. Leukotriene receptor antagonists may rarely produce a syndrome with several potentially serious effects, including worsening of lung function and heart complications.

COMMON DRUGS

Sympathomimetics Bambuterol, Ephedrine*, Epinephrine*, Fenoterol, Formoterol, Salbutamol*, Salmeterol*, Terbutaline*
Anticholinergics Ipratropium bromide*, Tiotropium*
Leukotriene antagonists Montelukast*, Zafirlukast
Corticosteroids Beclometasone*, Budesonide*, Ciclesonide, Fluticasone*, Mometasone*, Prednisolone*
Xanthines Theophylline/aminophylline*
Other drugs Nedocromil, Sodium cromoglicate*
* **See Part 2**

Decongestants

The usual cause of a blocked nose is swelling of the delicate mucous membrane that lines the nasal passages and excessive production of mucus as a result of inflammation. This may result from an infection (for example, a common cold) or from an allergy (for example, to pollen – a condition known as allergic rhinitis or hay fever). Congestion can also occur in the sinuses (the air spaces in the skull), resulting in sinusitis. Decongestant drugs reduce swelling of the mucous membrane and suppress the production of mucus, helping to clear blocked nasal passages and sinuses. Antihistamines (see p.56) counter the allergic response in allergy-related conditions. If the symptoms are persistent, either topical corticosteroids (see p.78) or sodium cromoglicate (see p.403) may be preferred.

WHY THEY ARE USED

Most common colds and blocked noses do not need to be treated with decongestants. Simple home remedies such as steam inhalation, possibly with the addition of an aromatic oil such as menthol or eucalyptus, are often effective. Decongestants are used when such measures are ineffective or when there is a particular risk from untreated congestion (for example, in people who have recurrent middle-ear or sinus infections).

Decongestants are available in the form of drops or sprays applied directly into the nose (topical decongestants), or they can be taken by mouth. Small quantities of decongestant drugs are added to many over-the-counter cold remedies (see Cold cures, p.26).

HOW THEY WORK

When the mucous membrane lining the nose is irritated by infection or allergy, the blood vessels that supply the membrane become enlarged. This leads to fluid accumulation in the surrounding tissue and encourages the production of larger-than-normal amounts of mucus.

Most decongestants belong to the sympathomimetic group of drugs, which stimulate the sympathetic branch of the autonomic nervous system (see p.6). One effect of this action is to constrict the blood vessels, thereby reducing swelling of the lining of the nose and sinuses.

HOW THEY AFFECT YOU

When applied topically in the form of drops or sprays, these drugs start to relieve congestion within a few minutes. Decongestants by mouth take a little longer to act, but their effect may also last longer.

Used in moderation, topical decongestants have few adverse effects, because they are not absorbed by the body in large amounts. Used for too long or in excess, however, topical decongestants can, after giving initial relief, do more harm than good, causing "rebound congestion". This is a sudden increase in congestion due to widening of the blood vessels in the nasal lining because the blood vessels are no longer constricted by the decongestant. Rebound congestion can be prevented by taking the minimum effective dose and by using decongestant preparations only when absolutely necessary. Decongestants taken by mouth do not cause rebound congestion but are more likely to cause other side effects.

COMMON DRUGS

Used topically Ephedrine*, Ipratropium bromide*, Oxymetazoline, Phenylephrine, Xylometazoline

Taken by mouth Ephedrine*, Phenylephrine, Pseudoephedrine

* **See Part 2**

Drugs to treat coughs

Coughing is a natural response to irritation of the lungs and air passages, designed to expel harmful substances from the respiratory tract. Common causes of coughing include infection of the respiratory tract (for example, bronchitis or pneumonia), inflammation of the airways caused by asthma, reflux of stomach acid, or exposure to certain irritant substances such as smoke or chemical fumes. Depending on their cause, coughs may be productive – that is, phlegm-producing – or they may be dry.

In most cases, coughing is a helpful reaction that assists the body in ridding itself of excess phlegm and substances that irritate the respiratory system; suppressing the cough may actually delay recovery. However, repeated bouts of coughing can be distressing, and may increase irritation of the air passages. In such cases, medication to ease the cough may be recommended.

There are two main groups of cough remedies, according to whether the cough is productive or dry.

PRODUCTIVE COUGHS

Mucolytics and expectorants are sometimes recommended for productive coughs when simple home remedies such as steam inhalation have failed to "loosen" the cough and make it easier to cough up phlegm. Mucolytics alter the consistency of the phlegm, making it less sticky and thus easier to cough up. These drugs are often given by inhalation. However, there is little evidence that they are effective. Dornase alfa may be given to people who have cystic fibrosis; the drug, given by inhalation via a nebulizer, is an enzyme that improves lung function by thinning the mucus. Expectorant drugs are taken by mouth to loosen a cough. There is some evidence that guaifenesin is effective but, overall, evidence of benefit is poor. Expectorants are included in many over-the-counter cough remedies.

DRY COUGHS

In dry coughs, no advantage is gained from promoting the expulsion of phlegm. Drugs used for dry coughs are given to suppress the coughing mechanism by calming the part of the brain that governs the coughing reflex. Antihistamines are often given for mild coughs, particularly in children. A demulcent, such as a simple linctus, can be used to soothe a dry, irritating cough. For persistent coughs, mild opioid drugs such as codeine may be prescribed (see also Analgesics, p.7). All cough suppressants have a generally sedating effect on the brain and nervous system and commonly cause drowsiness and other side effects.

SELECTING A COUGH MEDICATION

There is a bewildering variety of over-the-counter medications available for the treatment of coughs. Most preparations consist of a syrupy base to which active ingredients and flavourings are added. Many contain a number of different active ingredients, sometimes with contradictory effects: it is not uncommon to find an expectorant (for a productive cough) and a decongestant included in the same preparation.

It is important to select the correct type of medication for your cough to avoid the risk of making your condition worse. For example, using a cough suppressant for a productive cough may prevent you from getting rid of excess infected phlegm and may delay your recovery. It is best to choose a preparation with a single active ingredient that is appropriate for your type of cough. People with diabetes may need to select a sugar-free product. If you are in any doubt about which product to choose, ask your doctor or pharmacist for advice. Since there is a danger that use of over-the-counter cough remedies to alleviate symptoms may delay the diagnosis of a more serious underlying disorder, it is important to seek medical advice for any cough that persists for longer than a few days or if a cough is accompanied by additional symptoms such as fever or blood in the phlegm.

COLD CURES

Many preparations are available over the counter to treat different symptoms of the common cold. The main ingredient in most of these preparations is a mild analgesic, such as aspirin or paracetamol, accompanied by a decongestant (see p.24), an antihistamine (see p.56), and sometimes caffeine. In some cases, the dose of each added ingredient is too low to provide any benefit. There is no evidence to suggest that vitamin C (see p.88) speeds recovery. However, zinc supplements (see p.91) may be effective in shortening the duration of a cold.

While some people find these drugs help to relieve symptoms, over-the-counter cold cures do not alter the course of the illness. Most doctors recommend using a product with a single analgesic as the best way of alleviating symptoms. Other decongestants or antihistamines may be taken if needed, although antihistamines may cause sedation. These medicines are not harmless, and care should be taken to avoid overdose if different brands are used.

COMMON DRUGS

Expectorants Ammonium chloride, Guaifenesin
Mucolytics Carbocysteine, Dornase alfa, Mecysteine
Steam inhalation Eucalyptus, Menthol
Opioid cough suppressants Codeine*, Dextromethorphan, Methadone*, Pholcodine
Non-opioid cough suppressants Antihistamines (see p.56)
* **See Part 2**

HEART AND CIRCULATION

The circulatory system comprises the heart, blood vessels, and blood. The blood transports oxygen, nutrients, and heat, contains chemical messages in the form of drugs and hormones, and carries away waste products for excretion by the kidneys. Blood is pumped by the heart to and from the lungs, and then in a separate circuit to the rest of the body, including the brain, digestive organs, muscles, kidneys, and skin.

The heart is a pump with four chambers – two atria and two ventricles. The atrium and ventricle on the left side pump oxygenated blood to the body, while the atrium and ventricle on the right pump deoxygenated blood to the lungs. Backflow of blood is stopped by one-way valves at the chamber exits. Arteries carry blood away from the heart. Their muscle walls are elastic, contracting and dilating in response to nerve signals. Veins carry blood back to the heart. Their walls are thinner and less elastic than those of arteries.

WHAT CAN GO WRONG

The efficiency of the circulation may be impaired by weakening of the heart's pumping action (heart failure) or by irregularity of the heart rate (arrhythmia). In addition, the blood vessels may become narrowed and clogged by fatty deposits (a condition called atherosclerosis). This may reduce blood supply to the brain, the extremities (peripheral vascular disease), or the heart muscle (coronary heart disease), causing angina. These last disorders can be complicated by the formation of clots that may block a blood vessel. A clot in the arteries supplying the heart muscle is known as coronary thrombosis; a clot in an artery inside the brain is the most frequent cause of stroke.

One common circulatory disorder is abnormally high blood pressure (hypertension), in which the pressure of circulating blood on the vessel walls is increased for reasons not fully understood. One factor may be loss of elasticity of the vessel walls (arteriosclerosis). Several other conditions, such as migraine and Raynaud's disease, are caused by temporary alterations to blood vessel size.

WHY DRUGS ARE USED

Because people with heart disease often have more than one problem, several drugs may be prescribed at once. Many act directly on the heart to alter the rate and rhythm of the heart beat. These drugs are known as anti-arrhythmics and include beta blockers, calcium channel blockers, and digoxin.

Other drug types affect the diameter of the blood vessels, either by dilating them (vasodilators) to improve blood flow and reduce blood pressure, or by constricting them (vasoconstrictors).

Drugs may also reduce blood volume and fat levels, and alter clotting ability. Diuretics (used in the treatment of hypertension and heart failure) increase the body's excretion of salt and water. Lipid-lowering drugs reduce blood cholesterol levels, thereby minimizing the risk of atherosclerosis. Drugs to reduce blood clotting are administered if there is a risk of abnormal blood clots forming in the heart, veins, or arteries. Drugs that increase clotting are given when the body's natural clotting mechanism is defective.

MAJOR DRUG GROUPS

- Digitalis drugs
- Beta blockers
- Vasodilators
- Diuretics
- Anti-arrhythmics
- Anti-angina drugs
- Antihypertensive drugs
- Lipid-lowering drugs
- Drugs that affect blood clotting

Digitalis drugs

Digitalis is the collective term for naturally occurring substances (also called cardiac glycosides) that are found in the leaves of plants of the foxglove family and used to treat certain heart disorders. The principal drugs in this group are digoxin and digitoxin. Digoxin is more commonly used because it is shorter acting and dosage is easier to adjust (see also Risks and special precautions, p.28).

WHY THEY ARE USED

Digitalis drugs do not cure heart disease, but they improve the heart's pumping action and thereby relieve many of the symptoms that result from poor heart function. They are useful for treating conditions in which the heart beats irregularly or too rapidly (notably in atrial fibrillation; see Antiarrhythmics, p.32), when it pumps too weakly (in congestive heart failure), or when the heart muscle is damaged and weakened following a heart attack.

Digitalis drugs can be used for a short period when the heart is working poorly, but in many cases they have to be taken indefinitely. Their effect does not diminish with time. In heart failure, digitalis drugs are often given together with a vasodilator or a diuretic drug (see p.30).

HOW THEY WORK

The normal heart beat results from electrical impulses generated in nerve tissue within the heart. These cause the heart muscle to contract and pump blood. By reducing the flow of electrical impulses in the heart, digitalis makes the heart beat more slowly.

The force with which the heart muscle contracts depends on chemical changes in the heart muscle. By promoting these chemical changes, digitalis increases the force of muscle contraction each time the heart is stimulated. This compensates for the loss of power that occurs when some of the muscle is damaged following a heart attack. The stronger heart beat increases blood flow to the kidneys. This increases urine production and helps to remove the excess fluid that often accumulates as a result of heart failure.

HOW THEY AFFECT YOU

Digitalis relieves the symptoms of heart failure – fatigue, breathlessness, and swelling of the legs – and increases your capacity for exercise. The frequency with which you need to pass urine may also be increased initially.

RISKS AND SPECIAL PRECAUTIONS

Digitalis drugs can be toxic; if blood levels of these drugs rise too high, symptoms of digitalis poisoning (excessive tiredness, confusion, loss of appetite, nausea, vomiting, visual disturbances, and diarrhoea) may occur. It is important to report such symptoms to your doctor promptly.

Digoxin is normally removed from the body by the kidneys; if kidney function is impaired, the drug is more likely to accumulate in the body and cause toxic effects. Digitoxin, which is broken down in the liver, is sometimes preferred in such cases. Digitoxin can accumulate after repeated dosage if liver function is severely impaired.

Both digoxin and digitoxin are more toxic when blood potassium levels are low. Potassium deficiency is commonly caused by diuretic drugs (see p.30), so people taking these with digitalis drugs need to have the effects of both drugs and blood potassium levels carefully monitored. Potassium supplements may be required.

COMMON DRUGS

Digitoxin, Digoxin*

*** See Part 2**

Beta blockers

Beta blockers are drugs that interrupt the transmission of stimuli through the beta receptors of the body (see Autonomic nervous system, p.6). Since the actions that they block originate in the adrenal glands (and elsewhere) they are also sometimes called beta adrenergic blocking agents. There are two types of beta receptor in the body: beta 1 and beta 2. Beta 1 receptors are located mainly in the heart muscle; beta 2 receptors, in the airways and blood vessels. Cardioselective drugs act mainly on beta 1 receptors; non-cardioselective drugs on both types. Used mainly in heart disorders, beta blockers are also occasionally prescribed for other conditions.

WHY THEY ARE USED

Beta blockers are used for treating angina (see p.33) and irregular heart rhythms (see p.32). They may also be used for treating hypertension (see p.34) but are not usually used to initiate treatment. They are often given after a heart attack to reduce the likelihood of abnormal heart rhythms or further damage to the heart muscle. They are also prescribed to improve heart function in heart muscle disorders (cardiomyopathies).

Beta blockers may also be given to prevent migraine headaches (see p.18), or to reduce the physical symptoms of anxiety (see p.11). These drugs may be given to control symptoms of an overactive thyroid gland. A beta blocker is sometimes given in the form of eye drops in glaucoma (see p.112) to lower the fluid pressure inside the eye.

HOW THEY WORK

By occupying the beta receptors in different parts of the body, beta blocker drugs nullify the stimulating action of norepinephrine (noradrenaline), the main "fight or flight" hormone. As a result, they reduce the force and speed of the heart beat and prevent the dilation of the blood vessels surrounding the brain and leading to the extremities.

Heart Slowing of the heart rate and reduction of the force of the heart beat reduces the workload of the heart, helping to prevent angina and abnormal heart rhythms. This action may worsen heart failure, however.

Lungs Constriction of the airways may provoke breathlessness in people with asthma or those with chronic bronchitis.

Brain Dilation of the blood vessels that surround the brain is inhibited, thereby preventing migraine.

Blood vessels Constriction of the blood vessels may cause cold hands and feet.

Blood pressure The pressure is lowered due to reduction in the rate and force at which the heart pumps blood around the body.

Eye Beta blocker eye drops reduce fluid production, lowering pressure inside the eye.

Muscles Muscle tremor caused by anxiety or overactivity of the thyroid gland is reduced.

HOW THEY AFFECT YOU

Beta blockers are taken to treat angina. They reduce the frequency and severity of attacks. As part of the treatment for hypertension, beta blockers help to lower blood pressure and thus reduce the health risks that are associated with this condition. Beta blockers also help to prevent severe attacks of arrhythmia, in which the heart beat becomes wild and uncontrolled.

Because beta blockers affect many parts of the body, they often produce minor side effects. By reducing the heart rate and air flow to the lungs, they may reduce the capacity for strenuous exercise, although this is unlikely to be noticed by somebody whose physical activity was previously limited by heart problems. Many people experience cold hands and feet while taking these drugs as a result of the reduction in the blood supply to the limbs. Reduced circulation can also lead to temporary erectile dysfunction during treatment.

RISKS AND SPECIAL PRECAUTIONS

The main risk of beta blockers is that of provoking breathing difficulties as a result of their blocking effect on beta receptors in the lungs. Cardioselective beta blockers, which act principally on the heart, are thought less likely than non-cardioselective ones to cause such problems. Nevertheless, all beta blockers are prescribed with caution for people who have asthma, bronchitis, or other forms of respiratory disease.

Beta blockers are not commonly prescribed to people who have poor circulation in the limbs because they reduce blood flow and may aggravate such conditions. They are of definite benefit in heart failure, but treatment is usually initiated by specialists. People with diabetes who need to take beta blockers should be aware that they may notice a change in the warning signs of low blood sugar; in particular, they may find that symptoms such as palpitations and tremor are suppressed.

Beta blockers should not be stopped suddenly after prolonged use; this may provoke a sudden and severe recurrence of symptoms of the original disorder, or even a heart attack. The blood pressure may also rise markedly. When treatment with beta blockers needs to be stopped, it should be withdrawn gradually under medical supervision.

COMMON DRUGS

Cardioselective Acebutolol, Atenolol*, Betaxolol, Bisoprolol*, Celiprolol, Esmolol, Metoprolol*, Nebivolol

Non-cardioselective Carvedilol, Labetalol, Nadolol, Oxprenolol, Pindolol, Propranolol*, Sotalol*, Timolol*

* **See Part 2**

Vasodilators

Vasodilators are drugs that widen blood vessels. Their most obvious use is to reverse narrowing of the blood vessels when this leads to reduced blood flow and a lower oxygen supply to parts of the body. This problem occurs in angina, when narrowing of the coronary arteries reduces blood supply to the heart muscle. Vasodilators are often used to treat high blood pressure (hypertension).

WHY THEY ARE USED

Vasodilators improve the blood flow and thus the oxygen supply to areas of the body where they are most needed. In angina, dilation of blood vessels throughout the body reduces the force with which the heart needs to pump and thereby eases its workload (see also Anti-angina drugs, p.33). This may also be helpful in treating congestive heart failure when other treatments are not effective.

Because blood pressure partly depends on the diameter of blood vessels, vasodilators are often helpful for hypertension (see p.34).

In peripheral vascular disease, narrowed blood vessels in the legs cannot supply sufficient blood to the extremities, often leading to pain in the legs during exercise. However, because the narrowing is due to atherosclerosis, vasodilators have little effect.

HOW THEY WORK

Vasodilators widen blood vessels by relaxing the muscles surrounding them, either by affecting the action of the muscles directly (nitrates, hydralazine, and calcium channel blockers), or by interfering with the nerve signals that govern contraction of the blood vessels (alpha blockers). ACE (angiotensin-converting enzyme) inhibitors block the activity of an enzyme in the blood that is responsible for producing angiotensin II, a powerful vasoconstrictor. Angiotensin II blockers prevent angiotensin II from constricting the blood vessels by blocking its receptors within the vessels. Sacubitril blocks another enzyme that degrades natriuretic peptides, thus prolonging the vasodilating effects of these peptides. Sacubitril is often given combined with the angiotensin II blocker valsartan.

HOW THEY AFFECT YOU

Vasodilators can have many minor side effects related to their action on the circulation. Flushing and headaches are common at the start of treatment. Dizziness and fainting may result from lowered blood pressure, which is often worse on standing. Dilation of the blood vessels can cause fluid build-up, leading to swelling, particularly of the ankles.

RISKS AND SPECIAL PRECAUTIONS

The major risk with vasodilators is blood pressure falling too low; the drugs are therefore used with caution in people with unstable blood pressure. It is also advisable to sit or lie down after taking the first dose.

COMMON DRUGS

ACE inhibitors Captopril*, Cilazapril, Enalapril*, Fosinopril, Lisinopril*, Perindopril*, Quinapril, Ramipril*, Trandolapril

Angiotensin II blockers Candesartan*, Irbesartan*, Losartan*, Telmisartan

Alpha blockers Doxazosin*, Indoramin, Prazosin, Terazosin

Potassium channel activators Nicorandil*

Nitrates Glyceryl trinitrate*, Isosorbide dinitrate/mononitrate*

Calcium channel blockers Amlodipine*, Diltiazem*, Felodipine*, Lacidipine, Lercanidipine, Nicardipine, Nifedipine*, Verapamil*

Peripheral vasodilators Cilastazol, Naftidrofuryl*, Pentoxifylline

Other drugs Hydralazine, Minoxidil*, Sacubitril/valsartan*

* **See Part 2**

Diuretics

Diuretic drugs help to turn excess body water into urine. As the urine is expelled, two disorders are relieved: excess water in body tissues (oedema) is lessened, and the heart's action improves because it has to pump a smaller volume of blood. There are several classes of diuretic, each of which has different uses, modes of action, and effects (see Types of diuretic, opposite). But all diuretics act on the kidneys, the organs that govern the water content of the body.

WHY THEY ARE USED

Diuretics are most commonly used in the treatment of high blood pressure (hypertension). By removing a larger amount of water than usual from the bloodstream, the kidneys reduce the total volume of blood circulating. This drop in volume causes a reduction of the pressure within the blood vessels (see Antihypertensive drugs, p.34).

Diuretics are also widely used to treat heart failure in which the heart's pumping mechanism has become weak. In the treatment of this disorder, they remove fluid that has accumulated in the tissues and lungs. The resulting drop in blood volume reduces the work of the heart.

Other conditions for which diuretics are often prescribed include nephrotic syndrome (a kidney disorder that causes oedema), liver cirrhosis (in which fluid may accumulate in the abdominal cavity), and premenstrual syndrome (when hormonal activity can lead to fluid retention and bloating).

Less commonly, diuretics are used to treat glaucoma (see p.112) and Ménière's disease (see Anti-emetics, p.19).

TYPES OF DIURETIC

Thiazides The most commonly prescribed diuretics, thiazides may lead to potassium deficiency. For this reason they are sometimes given with potassium supplements, or in conjunction with a potassium-sparing diuretic (see below).

Loop diuretics These fast-acting, powerful drugs increase urine output for a few hours and are therefore sometimes used in emergencies. They can cause excessive potassium loss, which may need to be prevented as for thiazides. Large doses given into a vein may lead to disturbances in hearing.

Potassium-sparing diuretics These mild diuretics are usually used in conjunction with a thiazide or a loop diuretic to prevent excessive loss of potassium.

Osmotic diuretics Prescribed only rarely, osmotics are used to maintain the urine flow through the kidneys after surgery or injury, and to reduce pressure rapidly within fluid-filled body cavities.

Acetazolamide This mild diuretic is used mainly to treat acute glaucoma (see p.112).

HOW THEY WORK

The kidneys' normal filtration process takes water, salts (mainly potassium and sodium), and waste products out of the bloodstream. Most of the salts and water are returned to the bloodstream, but some are expelled from the body together with the waste products in the urine. Diuretics interfere with this filtration process by reducing the amounts of sodium and water taken back into the bloodstream, thus increasing the volume of urine produced. Modifying the filtration process in this way means that the water content of the blood is reduced; less water in the blood causes excess water present in the tissues to be drawn out and eliminated in urine.

HOW THEY AFFECT YOU

All diuretics increase the frequency with which you need to pass urine. This is most noticeable at the start of treatment. People who have had oedema may notice that swelling – particularly of the ankles – is reduced, and those with heart failure may find that breathlessness is relieved.

RISKS AND SPECIAL PRECAUTIONS

Diuretics can cause imbalances in blood chemicals, of which a fall in potassium levels (hypokalaemia) is the most common. This can cause confusion and weakness, and trigger abnormal heart rhythms (especially in people taking digitalis drugs; see also p.27). Potassium supplements or a potassium-sparing diuretic usually corrects the imbalance. A potassium-rich diet (containing plenty of fresh fruits and vegetables) may be helpful.

Some diuretics may raise blood levels of uric acid, increasing the risk of gout. They may also raise blood sugar levels, causing problems for people with diabetes.

COMMON DRUGS

Loop diuretics Bumetanide*, Furosemide/frusemide*, Torasemide

Potassium-sparing diuretics Amiloride*, Eplerenone, Spironolactone*, Triamterene*

Thiazides Bendroflumethiazide*, Chlortalidone, Cyclopenthiazide, Hydrochlorothiazide*, Hydroflumethiazide, Indapamide*, Metolazone, Xipamide

* **See Part 2**

Anti-arrhythmics

The heart contains two upper and two lower chambers, which are known as the atria and the ventricles (see p.27). The pumping actions of these two sets of chambers are normally coordinated by electrical impulses that originate in the heart's pacemaker and then travel along conducting pathways so that the heart beats with a regular rhythm. If this coordination breaks down, the heart will beat abnormally, either irregularly or faster or slower than usual. The general term for abnormal heart rhythm is arrhythmia.

Arrhythmias may occur as a result of a birth defect, coronary heart disease, or other less common heart disorders. A variety of more general conditions, including overactivity of the thyroid gland, and certain drugs, such as caffeine and anticholinergic drugs, can also disturb heart rhythm.

Arrhythmias can be divided into two groups: tachycardias (such as atrial fibrillation), in which the heart rate is faster than normal; and bradycardias (such as heart block), in which the rate is slower.

Atrial fibrillation In this common type of arrhythmia, the atria contract irregularly at such a high rate that the ventricles cannot keep pace with them. Atrial fibrillation is treated with digoxin, verapamil, amiodarone, or a beta blocker.

Ventricular tachycardia This condition arises from abnormal electrical activity in the ventricles that causes them to contract rapidly. Treatment with disopyramide, procainamide, or amiodarone may be effective, although implanted defibrillators are replacing drug treatment for this condition.

Supraventricular tachycardia This condition occurs when extra electrical impulses arise in the pacemaker or atria, stimulating the ventricles to contract rapidly. Attacks may disappear on their own without treatment, but drugs such as adenosine, digoxin, verapamil, or a beta blocker may be given.

Heart block When electrical impulses are not conducted from the atria to the ventricles, the ventricles start to beat at a slower rate. Some cases of heart block do not require treatment. For more severe heart block accompanied by dizziness and fainting, it is usually necessary to fit the patient with an artificial pacemaker.

A wide range of drugs is used to regulate heart rhythm, including beta blockers, digitalis drugs, and calcium channel blockers. Other drugs used are disopyramide, lidocaine, and procainamide.

WHY THEY ARE USED

Minor disturbances of heart rhythm are common and do not usually require drug treatment. However, if the heart's pumping action is seriously affected, the circulation of blood throughout the body may become inefficient, and treatment may be necessary.

Drugs may be taken to treat individual attacks of arrhythmia, or they may be taken on a regular basis to prevent or control abnormal heart rhythms. The particular drug prescribed depends on the type of arrhythmia to be treated, but because people differ in their response, it may be necessary to try several in order to find the most effective one. When the arrhythmia is sudden and severe, it may be necessary to inject an anti-arrhythmic drug immediately to restore normal heart function.

HOW THEY WORK

The heart's pumping action is governed by electrical impulses under the control of the sympathetic nervous system (see Autonomic nervous system, p.6). These signals pass through the heart muscle, causing the two pairs of chambers – the atria and ventricles – to contract in turn.

All anti-arrhythmic drugs alter the conduction of electrical signals in the heart. However, each drug or drug group has a different effect on the sequence of events that controls the pumping action. Some drugs block the transmission of electrical signals to the heart (beta blockers); some affect the way in which signals are conducted within the heart (digitalis drugs); others affect the response of the heart muscle to the signals received (calcium channel blockers, disopyramide, and procainamide).

HOW THEY AFFECT YOU

These drugs usually prevent symptoms of arrhythmia and may restore a regular heart rhythm. Although they do not prevent all arrhythmias, they usually reduce the frequency and severity of any symptoms.

Unfortunately, as well as suppressing arrhythmias, many of these drugs tend to depress normal heart function, and may produce dizziness on standing up, or increased breathlessness on exertion. Mild nausea and visual disturbances are also fairly frequent. Verapamil can cause constipation, especially when it is prescribed in high doses. Disopyramide may interfere with the parasympathetic nervous system (see Autonomic nervous system, p.6), resulting in a number of anticholinergic effects.

RISKS AND SPECIAL PRECAUTIONS

These drugs, in certain circumstances, may further disrupt heart rhythm, and therefore they are used only when the likely benefit outweighs the risks.

Amiodarone may accumulate in the body tissues over time, and may lead to light-sensitive rashes, changes in thyroid function, and lung problems.

COMMON DRUGS

Beta blockers (see also p.28), Sotalol*
Calcium channel blockers Felodipine*, Verapamil*
Digitalis drugs (see also p.27), Digitoxin, Digoxin*
Other drugs Adenosine, Amiodarone*, Disopyramide, Flecainide, Lidocaine, Mexiletine, Moracizine, Procainamide, Propafenone
* **See Part 2**

Anti-angina drugs

Angina is chest pain that occurs when insufficient oxygen reaches the heart muscle. This is usually caused by a narrowing of the blood vessels (coronary arteries) that carry blood and oxygen to the heart muscle. In the most common type (classic angina), pain usually occurs during physical exertion or emotional stress. In variant angina, pain may also occur at rest. In classic angina, the narrowing of the coronary arteries results from deposits of fat, known as atheroma, on the walls of the arteries. In the variant type, however, angina is caused by contraction (spasm) of the muscle fibres in the artery walls.

Atheroma deposits build up more rapidly in the arteries of smokers and people who eat a high-fat diet. This is why, as a basic component of angina treatment, doctors recommend that smoking should be given up and the diet changed. Overweight people are also advised to lose weight in order to reduce the demands on the heart. While such changes in lifestyle often produce an improvement in symptoms, drug treatment to relieve angina is also frequently necessary.

The drugs used to treat angina include beta blockers, nitrates, calcium channel blockers, and potassium channel openers.

WHY THEY ARE USED

Frequent episodes of angina can be disabling and, if left untreated, can lead to an increased risk of a heart attack. Drugs can be used both to relieve angina attacks and to reduce their frequency. People who experience only occasional episodes are usually prescribed a rapid-acting drug to take at the first signs of an attack, or before an activity that is known to bring on an attack. Glyceryl trinitrate, a rapid-acting nitrate drug, is usually prescribed for this purpose.

If attacks become more frequent or more severe, regular preventative treatment may be advised. Beta blockers, long-acting nitrates, and calcium channel blockers are used as regular medication to prevent attacks. The introduction of adhesive patches to administer nitrates through the patient's skin has extended the duration of action of glyceryl trinitrate, making treatment easier.

Drugs can often control angina for many years, but they cannot cure the disorder. When severe angina cannot be controlled by drugs, then surgery to increase the blood flow to the heart may be recommended.

HOW THEY WORK

Nitrates and calcium channel blockers dilate blood vessels by relaxing the muscle layer in the blood vessel walls (see also Vasodilators, p.30). As a result, blood is more easily pumped through the dilated vessels, reducing the strain on the heart.

Beta blockers reduce heart muscle stimulation during exercise or stress by interrupting signal transmission in the heart.

Decreased heart muscle stimulation means that less oxygen is required, reducing the risk of angina attacks. For further information on beta blockers, see p.28.

HOW THEY AFFECT YOU

Treatment with one or more of these drugs usually effectively controls angina. Drugs to prevent attacks allow people with angina to undertake more strenuous activities without provoking pain, and if an attack does occur, nitrates usually provide effective relief.

These drugs do not usually cause serious adverse effects but can produce a variety of minor symptoms. By dilating blood vessels throughout the body, nitrates and calcium channel blockers can cause dizziness (especially on standing) and may cause fainting. Other possible side effects are headaches at the start of treatment, flushing of the skin (especially of the face), and ankle swelling. Beta blockers often cause cold hands and feet, and sometimes they may produce tiredness and a feeling of heaviness in the legs.

COMMON DRUGS

Calcium channel blockers Amlodipine*, Diltiazem*, Felodipine*, Nicardipine, Nifedipine*, Verapamil*
Beta blockers (see p.28)
Nitrates Glyceryl trinitrate*, Isosorbide dinitrate/mononitrate*
Potassium channel opener Nicorandil*
Heparin/low molecular weight heparins * Dalteparin, Enoxaparin
Other drugs Aspirin*, Ezetimibe*, Ivabradine, Ranolazine, Simvastatin*
* **See Part 2**

Antihypertensive drugs

Blood pressure is the force exerted by the blood against the artery walls. Two measurements are taken: the higher figure indicates force while the heart's ventricles are contracting (systolic pressure); the lower figure is pressure during ventricle relaxation (diastolic pressure). Blood pressure varies among individuals and normally increases with age. If blood pressure is higher than normal on at least three separate occasions, a doctor may diagnose the condition as hypertension.

Blood pressure may be elevated as a result of an underlying disorder, which the doctor will try to identify. Usually, however, it is not possible to determine a cause. This condition is referred to as essential hypertension.

Although hypertension does not usually cause any symptoms, severely raised blood pressure may produce headaches, palpitations, and general feelings of ill-health. It is important to reduce high blood pressure because hypertension can have serious consequences, including stroke, heart attack, heart failure, and kidney damage. Certain groups are particularly at risk from high blood pressure. These risk groups include people with diabetes, smokers, people with pre-existing heart damage, and those whose blood contains a high level of fat. High blood pressure is more common among people of Black African or Caribbean descent, and in countries where the diet is high in salt.

A small reduction in blood pressure may be brought about by lifestyle changes, including regular exercise, reducing weight, and lowering salt intake. However, for more severely raised blood pressure, one or more antihypertensive drugs may be prescribed. Several classes of drug have antihypertensive properties, including centrally acting antihypertensives, diuretics (see p.30), beta blockers (see p.28), calcium channel blockers (see p.33), ACE (angiotensin-converting enzyme) inhibitors (see Vasodilators, p.30), angiotensin II blockers, and alpha blockers.

WHY THEY ARE USED

Antihypertensive drugs are prescribed when lifestyle changes have not brought about an adequate reduction in blood pressure, and your doctor sees a risk of serious consequences if hypertension is left untreated. These drugs do not cure hypertension and may have to be taken indefinitely.

HOW THEY WORK

Blood pressure depends not only on the force with which the heart pumps blood, but also on the diameter of blood vessels and the volume of blood in circulation: blood pressure is increased either if the vessels are narrow or if the volume of blood is high. Antihypertensives lower the blood pressure either by dilating the blood vessels or by reducing blood volume. Each type of antihypertensive drug acts in a different way to lower blood pressure.

Centrally acting drugs act on the mechanism in the brain that controls the diameter of the blood vessels.

Beta blockers reduce the force of the heart beat.

Diuretics act on the kidneys to reduce the blood volume.

ACE inhibitors act on enzymes in the blood to dilate blood vessels.

Vasodilators and calcium channel blockers act on the arterial wall muscles to prevent constriction.

Alpha blockers block nerve signals that trigger constriction of blood vessels.

CHOICE OF DRUG

Drug treatment depends on the severity of the hypertension. At the beginning of treatment for mild or moderately high blood pressure, a single drug is used. A thiazide diuretic is often chosen for initial treatment, but it is increasingly common to use a calcium channel blocker or an ACE inhibitor. For those over 50 or of Black African or Caribbean descent, a calcium channel blocker is usually the first-line treatment. If a single drug does not reduce the blood pressure sufficiently, a combination of these drugs may be used. Some people with more severe hypertension require an additional drug, in which case an alpha blocker, beta blocker, or aldosterone blocking drug may be added.

Severe hypertension is usually controlled with a combination of drugs, which may need to be given in high doses. Your doctor may need to try a number of drugs before finding a combination that controls blood pressure without unacceptable side effects.

HOW THEY AFFECT YOU

Treatment with antihypertensive drugs relieves symptoms such as headache and palpitations. However, since most people with hypertension have few, if any, symptoms, side effects may be more noticeable than any immediate beneficial effect. Some antihypertensive drugs may cause dizziness and fainting at the start of treatment because they can sometimes cause an excessive fall in blood pressure. It may take a while for your doctor to determine a dosage that avoids such effects. For detailed information on the adverse effects of drugs for hypertension, consult the individual drug profiles in Part 2.

RISKS AND SPECIAL PRECAUTIONS

Because your doctor needs to know exactly how treatment with a particular drug affects your hypertension – the benefits as well as the side effects – it is important for you to keep using the antihypertensive medication as prescribed, even though you may feel that the problem is under control. Sudden withdrawal of some of these drugs may cause a potentially dangerous rebound increase in blood pressure; when stopping treatment, the dose needs to be reduced gradually under medical supervision.

COMMON DRUGS

ACE inhibitors (see p.30)
Angiotensin II blockers Candesartan*, Irbesartan*, Losartan*, Olmesartan
Beta blockers (see p.28)
Calcium channel blockers (see p.33), Amlodipine*, Diltiazem*, Felodipine*, Isradipine, Lacidipine, Lercanidipine, Nicardipine, Nifedipine*, Verapamil*
Centrally acting antihypertensives Clonidine, Methyldopa, Moxonidine*
Diuretics (see p.30)
Alpha blockers Doxazosin*, Indoramin, Prazosin, Terazosin
Vasodilators (see p.30)
Aldosterone blockers Eplerenone, Spironolactone*
* **See Part 2**

Lipid-lowering drugs

The blood contains several types of fats, or lipids. These fats are necessary for normal body function but can be damaging in excess, particularly saturated fats such as cholesterol. The main risk is atherosclerosis, in which fatty deposits (atheroma) build up in the arteries, restricting and disrupting blood flow. This can increase the likelihood of abnormal blood clots forming, leading to potentially fatal disorders such as stroke and heart attack.

For most people, reducing their fat intake reduces the risk of atherosclerosis; but for those with an inherited tendency to high blood levels of fat (hyperlipidaemia), lipid-lowering drugs may also be recommended.

WHY THEY ARE USED

Lipid-lowering drugs are generally used only when dietary measures have failed to control hyperlipidaemia. They may be prescribed at an earlier stage to people at increased risk of atherosclerosis – such as people with diabetes and those who already have circulatory disorders. The drugs may help the body to remove existing atheroma in the blood vessels and prevent accumulation of new deposits. Low-dose simvastatin is available over the counter to help lower cholesterol levels in certain people.

For maximum benefit, lipid-lowering drugs are used in conjunction with a low-fat diet and a reduction in other risk factors such as obesity and smoking. The choice of drug depends on the type of lipid that is causing problems, so a full medical history, examination, and laboratory analysis of blood samples are needed before drug treatment is prescribed.

HOW THEY WORK

Cholesterol and triglycerides are two of the major fats in the blood. One or both may be raised, influencing the choice of lipid-lowering drug. Bile salts contain a large amount of cholesterol and are normally released into the bowel to aid digestion before being reabsorbed into the blood. Drugs that bind to bile salts reduce cholesterol levels by blocking their reabsorption, allowing them to be lost from the body.

Other drugs act on the liver. Fibrates can reduce the level of both cholesterol and triglycerides in the blood. Statins block cholesterol synthesis in the liver. This causes increased uptake of harmful LDL cholesterol from the blood, thereby lowering blood cholesterol levels. The uptake of LDL cholesterol is also stimulated by the newer anti-PCSK9 drugs, such as evolocumab and alirocumab.

Lipid-lowering drugs do not correct the underlying cause of raised levels of fat in the blood, so it is usually necessary to continue with diet and drug treatment indefinitely. Stopping treatment usually leads to a return of high blood lipid levels.

HOW THEY AFFECT YOU

Because hyperlipidaemia and atherosclerosis are usually without symptoms, you are unlikely to notice any short-term benefits from these drugs. Rather, the aim of treatment is to reduce long-term complications. There may be minor side effects from some of these drugs.

The statin drugs appear to be well tolerated and are widely used to lower cholesterol levels when diet alone is not effective.

RISKS AND SPECIAL PRECAUTIONS

Drugs that bind to bile salts can limit the absorption of some fat-soluble vitamins, and vitamin supplements may therefore be needed. The fibrates can increase susceptibility to gallstones and occasionally upset the balance of fats in the blood. Statins are used with caution in people who have reduced kidney or liver function, and monitoring of blood samples is often advised. You should consult your doctor or pharmacist before taking simvastatin.

COMMON DRUGS

Statins Atorvastatin*, Pravastatin*, Rosuvastatin*, Simvastatin*

Drugs that bind to or reduce bile salts Colestipol, Colestyramine*, Ezetimibe*, Ispaghula

Fibrates Bezafibrate*, Fenofibrate, Gemfibrozil

Other drugs acting on the liver Alirocumab, Evolocumab*, Omega-3 acid ethyl esters

* **See Part 2**

Drugs that affect blood clotting

When bleeding occurs as a result of injury or surgery, the body normally acts swiftly to stem the flow by sealing the breaks in the blood vessels. This occurs in two stages – first when cells called platelets accumulate as a plug at the opening in the blood vessel wall, and then when these platelets produce chemicals that activate clotting factors in the blood to form a protein called fibrin. Vitamin K plays an important role in this process. An enzyme in the blood called plasmin ensures that clots are broken down when the injury has been repaired.

Some disorders interfere with this process, either preventing clot formation or creating clots uncontrollably. If the blood does not clot, there is a danger of excessive blood loss. Inappropriate development of clots may block the supply of blood to a vital organ.

DRUGS USED TO PROMOTE BLOOD CLOTTING

Fibrin formation depends on the presence in the blood of several clotting-factor proteins. When Factor VIII is absent or at low levels, the condition is known as haemophilia A. Factor IX deficiency causes another bleeding condition, haemophilia B (previously known as Christmas disease). Both conditions are inherited and almost always affect only males. Lack of these clotting factors can lead to uncontrolled bleeding or excessive bruising following even minor injuries.

Regular drug treatment for haemophilia is not normally required. However, if severe bleeding or bruising occurs, a concentrated form of the missing factor, extracted from normal blood, may be injected in order to promote clotting and thereby halt bleeding. The injections may need to be repeated for several days after injury.

It is sometimes useful to promote blood clotting in people who do not have haemophilia when bleeding is difficult to stop (for example, following surgery). In such cases, blood clots are sometimes stabilized by reducing the action of plasmin with an antifibrinolytic (or haemostatic) drug such as tranexamic acid; this is also occasionally given to people with haemophilia before minor surgery such as tooth extraction.

A tendency to bleed may also occur with deficiency of vitamin K, which is required for the production of several blood clotting factors. Vitamin K is absorbed from the intestine in fats, but some diseases of the small intestine or pancreas cause fat to be poorly absorbed. As a result, the level of vitamin K in the circulation is low, causing impaired blood clotting. A similar problem sometimes occurs in newborn babies due to absence of vitamin K. Injections of phytomenadione, a vitamin K preparation, are used to restore levels to normal.

DRUGS USED TO PREVENT ABNORMAL BLOOD CLOTTING

Blood clots normally form only as a response to injury. In some people, however, there is a tendency for clots to form in the blood vessels without apparent cause. Disturbed blood flow resulting from the presence of fatty deposits (atheroma) inside the blood vessels increases the risk of formation of this type of abnormal clot (or thrombus). In addition, a portion of a blood clot formed in response to injury or surgery may sometimes break off and be removed in the bloodstream; this kind of fragment is known as an embolus. The likelihood of this happening is increased by long periods of little or no activity. When an abnormal clot forms, there is a risk that an embolus may become lodged in a blood vessel, thereby blocking the blood supply to a vital organ such as the brain or heart.

Three main types of drug are used to prevent and disperse clots: antiplatelet drugs, anticoagulants, and thrombolytics.

ANTIPLATELET DRUGS

Taken regularly by people with a tendency to form clots in the fast-flowing blood of the heart and arteries, these drugs are also given to prevent clots from forming after heart surgery. They reduce the tendency of platelets to stick together when blood flow is disrupted.

The most widely used antiplatelet drug is aspirin (see also Analgesics, p.7), which has an antiplatelet action even when given in much lower doses than would be needed to reduce pain. In such low doses, the adverse effects that may occur with pain-relieving doses are unlikely. Other antiplatelet drugs are clopidogrel and dipyridamole.

ANTICOAGULANTS

Anticoagulants help to maintain normal blood flow in people at risk from clot formation. They can either prevent the formation of blood clots in the veins or stabilize an existing clot so that it does not break away to become a circulation-stopping embolism. All anticoagulants reduce the activity of certain blood clotting factors, but each drug's mode of action differs. They do not dissolve clots that have already formed, however: these are treated with thrombolytic drugs (see right).

Anticoagulants fall into two groups: those that are given by intravenous injection and act immediately, and those that are given by mouth and take effect after a few days.

INJECTED ANTICOAGULANTS

Heparin is the most widely used drug of this type, and it is used mainly in hospital during or after surgery. It is also given during kidney dialysis to prevent clots from forming in the dialysis equipment. Because heparin cannot be taken by mouth, it is less suitable for long-term treatment in the home.

A number of synthetic injected anticoagulants have recently been developed. Some act for a longer time than heparin, and others are alternatives for people who react adversely to heparin.

ORAL ANTICOAGULANTS

Warfarin is the most widely used of the oral anticoagulants. These drugs are mainly prescribed to prevent the formation of clots in veins and in the chambers of the heart (they are less likely to prevent clot formation in arteries). Oral anticoagulants may be given following injury or surgery (in particular, heart valve replacement) when there is a high risk of embolism. They are also given long term as preventative treatment to people at risk of strokes.

A common problem with these drugs is that overdosage may lead to bleeding from the nose or gums, or in the urinary tract. For this reason, the dosage needs to be carefully calculated; regular blood tests are performed to ensure that the clotting mechanism is correctly adjusted, although this is not necessary with new oral anticoagulants such as dabigatran and rivaroxaban.

The action of oral anticoagulants may be affected by many other drugs, and it may therefore be necessary to alter the dosage of anticoagulant when other drugs also need to be given. In particular, no anticoagulant should be taken together with aspirin except on the direction of a doctor.

THROMBOLYTICS

Also known as fibrinolytics, these drugs are used to dissolve clots that have already formed. They are usually given intravenously in hospital to clear a blocked blood vessel (in coronary thrombosis, for example). The sooner they are given after the start of symptoms, the more likely they are to reduce the size and severity of a heart attack. Thrombolytic drugs may be administered either intravenously or directly into the blocked blood vessel. The main thrombolytics are streptokinase and alteplase, which act by increasing the blood level of plasmin, the enzyme that breaks down fibrin. When given promptly, alteplase appears to be tolerated better than streptokinase.

The most common problems with these drugs are increased susceptibility to bleeding and bruising, and allergic reactions to streptokinase, such as rashes or breathing difficulty. Once streptokinase has been given, patients are given a card indicating this, because further treatment with the same drug may be less effective, and an alternative (such as alteplase) used instead.

COMMON DRUGS

Blood clotting factors Factor VIIa, Factor VIII, Factor IX, Fresh frozen plasma

Antifibrinolytic drugs Tranexamic acid

Vitamin K Phytomenadione

Antiplatelet drugs Abciximab, Aspirin*, Clopidogrel*, Dipyridamole*, Eptifibatide, Prasugrel, Tirofiban

Injected anticoagulants Danaparoid, Epoprostenol, Fondaparinux, Heparin*, Lepirudin

Thrombolytic drugs Alteplase*, Reteplase, Streptokinase, Tenecteplase

Oral anticoagulants Acenocoumarol/nicoumalone, Apixaban, Dabigatran*, Rivaroxaban*, Warfarin*

Heparin/low molecular weight heparins * Dalteparin, Enoxaparin, Tinzaparin

* **See Part 2.**

GASTROINTESTINAL TRACT

The gastrointestinal tract, also known as the digestive or alimentary tract, is the pathway through which food passes as it is processed to enable the nutrients it contains to be absorbed for use by the body. It consists of the mouth, oesophagus, stomach, duodenum, small intestine, large intestine (including the colon and rectum), and anus. In addition, a number of other organs are involved in the digestion of food: the salivary glands in the mouth, the liver, pancreas, and gallbladder. These organs, together with the gastrointestinal tract, form the digestive system.

The digestive system breaks down the large, complex chemicals – proteins, carbohydrates, and fats – present in the food we eat into simpler molecules that can be used by the body (see also Nutrition, p.88).

The stomach holds food and passes it into the intestine. The lining of the stomach releases gastric juice that partly digests food. The stomach wall continually produces thick mucus that forms a protective coating.

The duodenum is the tube that connects the stomach to the intestine. Its lining may be damaged by excess acid from the stomach.

The pancreas produces enzymes that digest proteins, fats, and carbohydrates into simpler substances. Pancreatic juices neutralize the acidity of the food passing from the stomach.

The gallbladder stores bile, which is produced by the liver, and releases it into the duodenum. Bile assists the digestion of fats by reducing them to smaller units that are more easily acted upon by digestive enzymes.

The small intestine (small bowel) is a long tube in which food is broken down by digestive juices from the gallbladder and pancreas. The mucous lining of the small intestine consists of tiny, fingerlike projections called villi; these provide a large surface area through which the products of digestion are absorbed into the bloodstream.

The large intestine (large bowel) receives undigested food and indigestible material from the small intestine. Water and mineral salts pass through the lining into the bloodstream.

When a sufficient mass of undigested material, together with some of the body's waste products, has accumulated, it is expelled from the body as faeces.

MOVEMENT OF FOOD THROUGH THE GASTROINTESTINAL TRACT

Food is propelled through the gastrointestinal tract by rhythmic waves of muscular contraction called peristalsis.

Muscle contraction in the gastrointestinal tract is controlled by the autonomic nervous system (p.6) and is therefore easily disrupted by drugs that either stimulate or inhibit the activity of the autonomic nervous system. Excessive peristaltic action may cause diarrhoea, while constipation may result from slowed peristalsis.

WHAT CAN GO WRONG

Inflammation of the lining of the stomach or intestine (gastroenteritis) is usually the result of an infection or parasitic infestation. Damage may also occur through the inappropriate production of digestive juices, leading to minor complaints such as acidity and major disorders like peptic ulcers. The lining of the intestine can be damaged by abnormal functioning of the immune system (inflammatory bowel disease). The rectum and anus can become painful and irritated by damage to the lining, tears in the skin at the opening of the anus (anal fissure), or enlarged veins (haemorrhoids).

Constipation, diarrhoea, and irritable bowel syndrome are the most frequently experienced gastrointestinal disorders. They usually occur when something disrupts the normal muscle contractions that propel food residue through the bowel.

WHY DRUGS ARE USED

Many drugs for gastrointestinal disorders are taken by mouth and act directly on the digestive tract without first entering the bloodstream. They include certain antibiotics and other drugs used to treat infestations. Some antacids for peptic ulcers and excess stomach acidity, and the bulk-forming agents for constipation and diarrhoea, also pass through the system unabsorbed.

However, for many disorders, drugs with a systemic effect are required. These agents include anti-ulcer drugs, opioid antidiarrhoeal drugs, and some of the drugs for inflammatory bowel disease.

MAJOR DRUG GROUPS

- Antacids
- Anti-ulcer drugs
- Antidiarrhoeal drugs
- Drugs for irritable bowel syndrome
- Laxatives
- Drugs for inflammatory bowel disease
- Drugs for rectal and anal disorders
- Drug treatment for gallstones
- Drug treatment for pancreatic disorders

Antacids

Digestive juices in the stomach contain acid and enzymes that break down food before it passes into the intestine. The wall of the stomach is normally protected from the action of digestive acid by a layer of mucus that is constantly secreted by the stomach lining. Problems arise when the stomach lining is damaged or too much acid is produced and eats away at the mucous layer, resulting in pain and inflammation or even ulcers.

Excess acid that leads to discomfort, commonly referred to as indigestion, may be due to anxiety, overeating or eating certain foods, coffee, alcohol, or smoking. Some drugs, notably aspirin and non-steroidal anti-inflammatory drugs, can irritate the stomach lining and even cause ulcers to develop.

Antacids are used to neutralize acid and so relieve pain. They are simple chemical compounds that are mildly alkaline, and some also act as chemical buffers. Their chalky taste is often disguised with flavourings.

WHY THEY ARE USED

Antacids may be needed when simple remedies (such as a change in diet or a glass of milk) fail to relieve indigestion. They are especially useful if taken following a meal to neutralize the acid surge that sometimes occurs after a meal.

Doctors prescribe these drugs in order to relieve dyspepsia (pain in the chest or upper abdomen caused by or aggravated by acid) in disorders such as inflammation or ulceration of the oesophagus, stomach lining, and duodenum. Antacids usually relieve pain resulting from ulcers in the oesophagus, stomach, or duodenum within a few minutes. Regular treatment with antacids reduces the acidity of the stomach, thereby encouraging the healing of any ulcers that may have formed.

TYPES OF ANTACID

Aluminium compounds These drugs have a prolonged action and are widely used, especially for indigestion and dyspepsia. They may cause constipation, but this is often countered by combining this type of antacid with one containing magnesium. Aluminium compounds can interfere with the absorption of phosphate from the diet, causing muscle weakness and bone damage if taken in high doses over a long period. A high blood level of aluminium may build up in people with kidney failure, causing an illness similar to dementia.

Magnesium compounds Like the aluminium compounds, these have a prolonged action. In large doses magnesium compounds can cause diarrhoea, and in people who have impaired kidney function a high blood magnesium level may build up, causing weakness, lethargy, and drowsiness.

Sodium bicarbonate This antacid acts quickly, but its effect soon passes. It reacts with stomach acids to produce gas, which may cause bloating and belching. Sodium bicarbonate is not advised for people who have heart or kidney disease, because it can lead to accumulation of water (oedema) in the legs and lungs or serious changes in the acid-base balance of the blood.

Combined preparations Antacids may be combined with other substances called alginates and antifoaming agents. Alginates are intended to float on the contents of the stomach and produce a neutralizing layer to subdue acid that can otherwise rise into the oesophagus, causing heartburn. Antifoaming agents are used to relieve flatulence. In some preparations, a local anaesthetic is combined with the antacid to relieve discomfort in oesophagitis (inflamed oesophagus). The value of these additives is dubious.

HOW THEY WORK

By neutralizing stomach acid, antacids prevent inflammation, relieve pain, and allow the mucous layer and lining to mend. When used in the treatment of ulcers, they prevent acid from attacking damaged stomach lining and so allow the ulcer to heal.

HOW THEY AFFECT YOU

If antacids are taken according to the instructions, they are usually effective in relieving abdominal discomfort caused by acid. The speed of action, dependent on the ability to neutralize acid, varies. Their duration of action also varies; the short-acting drugs may have to be taken quite frequently.

Although most antacids have few serious side effects when used only occasionally, some types of antacid may cause diarrhoea, and others may cause constipation (see Types of antacid, opposite).

RISKS AND SPECIAL PRECAUTIONS

Antacids should not be taken to prevent abdominal pain on a regular basis except under medical supervision, as they may suppress the symptoms of stomach cancer. Your doctor is likely to want to arrange tests such as endoscopy or barium X-rays before prescribing long-term treatment.

Antacids can interfere with the absorption of other drugs. Therefore, if you are taking a prescription medicine, you should check with your doctor or pharmacist before starting to take an antacid.

COMMON DRUGS

Antacids Aluminium hydroxide*, Calcium carbonate, Hydrotalcite, Magnesium carbonate, Magnesium hydroxide*, Magnesium trisilicate, Sodium bicarbonate
Antifoaming agents Dimeticone, Simeticone
Other drugs Alginates*
* **See Part 2**

Anti-ulcer drugs

Normally, the linings of the oesophagus, stomach, and duodenum are protected from the irritant action of stomach acids or bile by a thin covering layer of mucus. If this lining is damaged, or if large amounts of stomach acid are produced, the underlying tissue may become eroded, causing a peptic ulcer (break in the gut lining). An ulcer often leads to abdominal pain, vomiting, and changes in appetite. The most common type of ulcer occurs just beyond the stomach, in the duodenum. The exact cause of peptic ulcers is not understood, but a number of risk factors have been identified, including heavy smoking, the regular use of aspirin or similar drugs, and family history. An organism found in almost all patients who have peptic ulcers, *Helicobacter pylori*, is believed to be the main causative agent.

The symptoms caused by ulcers may be relieved by an antacid (see opposite), but healing is slow. The usual treatment is with an anti-ulcer drug, such as a proton pump inhibitor, bismuth, or sucralfate, although an H2 blocker may be used. The anti-ulcer drug is usually combined with antibiotics to eradicate *Helicobacter pylori* infection.

WHY THEY ARE USED

Anti-ulcer drugs are used to relieve symptoms and heal the ulcer. Untreated ulcers may erode blood vessel walls or perforate (puncture) the stomach or duodenum.

Eradication of *Helicobacter pylori* by an antisecretory drug (such as a proton pump inhibitor) combined with two antibiotics (known as "triple therapy") may provide a cure in 1 to 2 weeks. Surgery is reserved for complications such as obstruction, perforation, haemorrhage, and when there is a possibility of cancer.

HOW THEY WORK

Drugs protect ulcers from the action of stomach acid, allowing the tissue to heal. H2 blockers, misoprostol, and proton pump inhibitors reduce the amount of acid that is released; bismuth and sucralfate form a protective coating over the ulcer. Bismuth also has an antibacterial effect.

HOW THEY AFFECT YOU

These drugs begin to reduce pain in a few hours and usually allow the ulcer to heal in 4 to 8 weeks. They produce few side effects, although H2 blockers such as cimetidine can cause confusion in older people. Bismuth may cause blackening of the faeces; sucralfate may cause constipation; misoprostol may produce diarrhoea; and proton pump inhibitors may cause either constipation or diarrhoea. Triple therapy is given for 1 or 2 weeks. If *Helicobacter pylori* is eradicated, maintenance therapy should not be necessary. Sucralfate is usually prescribed for up to 12 weeks, and bismuth and misoprostol for 4 to 8 weeks.

Because they may mask symptoms of stomach cancer, H2 blockers and proton pump inhibitors are normally prescribed only when tests have ruled out this disorder.

COMMON DRUGS

Proton pump inhibitors Esomeprazole, Lansoprazole*, Omeprazole*, Pantoprazole, Rabeprazole*
H2 blockers Cimetidine*, Famotidine, Nizatidine, Ranitidine*
Other drugs Antacids (see p.40), Antibiotics (see p.60), Carbenoxolone, Misoprostol*, Sucralfate*, Tripotassium dicitratobismuthate (bismuth chelate)
* **See Part 2**

Antidiarrhoeal drugs

Diarrhoea is an increase in the fluidity and frequency of bowel movements. In some cases diarrhoea protects the body from harmful substances in the intestine by hastening their removal. The most common causes of diarrhoea are viral infection, food poisoning, and parasites, but it also occurs as a symptom of other illnesses. In addition, it can be a side effect of some drugs and may follow radiotherapy for cancer. Diarrhoea may also be caused by anxiety.

An attack of diarrhoea usually clears up quickly without medical attention. The best treatment is to abstain from food and to drink plenty of clear fluids. Oral rehydration solutions containing sugar as well as potassium and sodium salts are widely recommended for preventing dehydration and chemical imbalances, particularly in children. You should consult your doctor if the condition does not improve within 48 hours; the diarrhoea contains blood; there is severe abdominal pain and vomiting; you have recently returned from a foreign country; or diarrhoea occurs in a small child or older adult.

Severe diarrhoea can impair absorption of drugs, and anyone taking a prescribed drug should seek advice from a doctor or pharmacist. Women taking oral contraceptives may require additional contraceptives (see p.103).

The main types of drug used to relieve non-specific diarrhoea are opioids, and bulk-forming and adsorbent agents. Antispasmodic drugs may also be used to relieve accompanying pain (see Drugs for irritable bowel syndrome, opposite).

WHY THEY ARE USED

An antidiarrhoeal drug may be prescribed to provide relief when simple remedies are not effective, and once it is certain the diarrhoea is neither infectious nor toxic.

Opioids are the most effective antidiarrhoeals. They are used when the diarrhoea is severe and debilitating. Bulking and adsorbent agents have a milder effect and are often used when it is necessary to regulate bowel action over a prolonged period (for example, in people with colostomies or ileostomies).

HOW THEY WORK

Opioids decrease the muscles' propulsive activity so that faecal matter passes more slowly through the bowel.

Bulk-forming agents and adsorbents absorb water and irritants in the bowel, resulting in the production of larger, firmer stools at less frequent intervals.

HOW THEY AFFECT YOU

Drugs that are used to treat diarrhoea reduce the urge to move the bowels. Opioids and antispasmodics may relieve abdominal pain. All antidiarrhoeal drugs may cause constipation if used in excess.

RISKS AND SPECIAL PRECAUTIONS

Used in relatively low doses for a limited period of time, opioid drugs are unlikely to produce adverse effects. However, these drugs are not recommended for acute diarrhoea in children and should be used with caution when diarrhoea is caused by an infection, since they may slow the elimination of microorganisms from the intestine. All antidiarrhoeals should be taken with plenty of water. It is important not to take a bulk-forming agent together with an opioid or antispasmodic drug, because a bulky mass could form and obstruct the bowel.

COMMON DRUGS

Antispasmodics Alverine, Atropine*, Dicycloverine (dicyclomine)*, Hyoscine butylbromide*, Mebeverine*, Peppermint oil, Propantheline
Opioids Codeine*, Co-phenotrope*, Loperamide*, Morphine/diamorphine*
Antibacterials Ciprofloxacin*
Bulk-forming agents and adsorbents Ispaghula, Kaolin, Methylcellulose*, Sterculia
Other drugs Aluminium hydroxide*, Colestyramine*
* **See Part 2**

Drugs for irritable bowel syndrome

Irritable bowel syndrome is a common, often stress-related, condition in which the waves of co-ordinated muscular contraction that normally move the bowel contents smoothly through the intestines become strong and irregular. This disruption in muscle activity often causes pain, and may be associated with diarrhoea or constipation.

Symptoms are often relieved by adjusting the amount of fibre in the diet, but medication may also be needed. Bulk-forming agents may be given to regulate consistency of the bowel contents. If the pain is severe, an antispasmodic drug may be prescribed. These drugs are anticholinergics (see Drugs that act on the parasympathetic nervous system, p.7), which reduce the transmission of nerve signals to the bowel wall, thus preventing spasm. Tricyclic antidepressants are sometimes used because their anticholinergic action has a calming effect on the bowel.

COMMON DRUGS

Antispasmodics Atropine*, Dicycloverine (dicyclomine)*, Hyoscine butylbromide*, Mebeverine*
Opioids Loperamide*
Other drugs Peppermint oil
* **See Part 2**

Laxatives

When your bowels do not move as frequently as usual and the faeces are hard and difficult to pass, you have constipation. The most common cause is lack of sufficient fibre in your diet; fibre supplies the bulk that makes the faeces soft and easy to pass. The simplest remedy is more fluid and a diet that contains plenty of foods that are high in fibre, but laxative drugs may also be used.

Ignoring the urge to defecate can also cause constipation, because the faeces will become dry, hard to pass, and too small to stimulate the muscles that propel them through the intestine.

Certain drugs may be constipating: examples include opioid analgesics, tricyclic antidepressants, and antacids that contain aluminium. Some diseases, such as hypothyroidism (an underactive thyroid gland) and scleroderma (a rare disorder of connective tissue characterized by the hardening of the skin), can also lead to constipation.

The onset of constipation in a middle-aged or older person may be an early symptom of bowel cancer. Consult your doctor about any persistent change in bowel habit.

TYPES OF LAXATIVE

Bulk-forming agents These are relatively slow-acting but are less likely than other laxatives to interfere with normal bowel action. For constipation accompanied by abdominal pain they should be taken only after consultation with your doctor, because there is a risk of intestinal obstruction.

Stimulant (contact) laxatives These laxatives are for occasional use when other treatments have failed or when rapid onset of action is needed. They should not normally be used for longer than a week at a time, because they can cause abdominal cramps and diarrhoea.

Softening agents These treatments are often used when hard faeces cause pain as the bowels are opened – especially after surgery, when straining must be avoided, or if you have haemorrhoids (see p.45). Liquid paraffin was once used to relieve faecal impaction (blockage of the intestine by faeces) but, because of its side effects, it has largely been replaced by docusate sodium.

Osmotic laxatives Preparations that contain magnesium carbonate or citrate may be used to evacuate the bowel before surgery or investigative procedures. They are not normally used for the long-term relief of constipation, however, because they can cause chemical imbalances in the blood.

Lactulose is an alternative to bulk-forming laxatives for long-term treatment of chronic constipation. It may cause stomach cramps and flatulence but is usually well tolerated.

WHY THEY ARE USED

Since prolonged use is harmful, laxatives should be used for very short periods only. They may prevent pain and straining in people with either hernias or haemorrhoids (see opposite). Doctors may prescribe them for the same reason after abdominal surgery or childbirth. Laxatives are also used to clear the bowel before investigative procedures such as colonoscopy. In addition, they may be prescribed for older people or those who are confined to bed, because lack of exercise can often lead to constipation.

HOW THEY WORK

Laxatives act on the large intestine by increasing the speed with which faecal matter passes through the bowel, or increasing its bulk and/or water content.

Stimulants encourage the bowel muscles to contract, increasing the speed at which faecal matter passes through the intestine. Bulk-forming laxatives absorb water in the bowel, thereby increasing the volume of faeces, making them softer and easier to pass. Lactulose also causes fluid to accumulate in the intestine. Osmotic laxatives act by keeping water in the bowel, thereby making the bowel movements softer. This also increases the bulk of the faeces and enables them to be passed more easily. Lubricant liquid paraffin preparations make bowel movements softer and easier to pass without increasing their bulk, but prolonged use can interfere with the absorption of some essential vitamins.

RISKS AND SPECIAL PRECAUTIONS

Laxatives can cause diarrhoea if taken in overdose, and constipation if overused. The most serious risk with prolonged use of most laxatives is developing dependence on the drug for normal bowel action. Use of any laxative should therefore be discontinued as soon as normal bowel movements have been re-established. Children should not be given laxatives except in special circumstances on the advice of a doctor.

COMMON DRUGS

Stimulant laxatives Bisacodyl, Dantron, Docusate, Glycerol, Senna, Sodium picosulfate

Bulk-forming agents Bran, Ispaghula, Methylcellulose*, Sterculia

Softening agents Arachis oil, Liquid paraffin

Osmotic laxatives Lactulose*, Macrogols, Magnesium citrate, Magnesium hydroxide*, Magnesium sulfate, Sodium acid phosphate

* **See Part 2**

Drugs for inflammatory bowel disease

Inflammatory bowel disease is the term used for disorders in which inflammation of the intestinal wall causes recurrent attacks of abdominal pain, general feelings of ill-health, and frequently diarrhoea, with blood and mucus present in the faeces. Loss of appetite and poor absorption of food may often result in weight loss.

There are two main types of inflammatory bowel disease: Crohn's disease and ulcerative colitis. In Crohn's disease (also called regional enteritis), any part of the digestive tract may become inflamed, although the small intestine is the most commonly affected site. In ulcerative colitis, it is the large intestine (colon) that becomes inflamed and ulcerated, often producing bloodstained diarrhoea.

The exact cause of Crohn's disease and of ulcerative colitis is not known, although stress-related, dietary, infectious, and genetic factors may all be important.

Establishing a proper diet and a less stressful lifestyle may help to alleviate both of these conditions. Bed rest during attacks is also advisable. However, these simple measures alone do not usually relieve or prevent attacks, and drug treatment is often necessary as well.

Three drug types are used to treat inflammatory bowel disease: corticosteroids (see p.78), immunosuppressants (see p.97), and aminosalicylate anti-inflammatory drugs such as sulfasalazine (see p.410). Nutritional supplements (used especially for Crohn's disease) and antidiarrhoeal drugs (see p.42) may also be used. Surgery to remove damaged areas of the intestine may be needed in severe cases. Newer drugs include infliximab (see p.277), a monoclonal antibody that modifies the action of the immune system.

WHY THEY ARE USED

Drugs cannot cure inflammatory bowel disease, but treatment is needed, not only to control symptoms but also to prevent complications, especially severe anaemia and perforation of the intestinal wall.

Aminosalicylates are used to treat acute attacks of ulcerative colitis and Crohn's disease, and they may be continued as maintenance therapy. People who have severe bowel inflammation are usually prescribed a course of corticosteroids, particularly during a sudden flare-up. Once the disease is under control, an immunosuppressant may be prescribed to prevent a relapse. Therapeutic antibodies that block a molecule called tumour necrosis factor (TNF) are used increasingly for this purpose.

HOW THEY WORK

Corticosteroids and sulfasalazine damp down the inflammatory process, allowing the damaged tissue to recover. They act in different ways to prevent migration of white blood cells into the intestinal wall, which may be responsible in part for the inflammation of the bowel.

HOW THEY AFFECT YOU

Taken to treat attacks, these drugs relieve symptoms within a few days, and general health improves gradually over a period of a few weeks. Aminosalicylates usually provide long-term relief from symptoms.

Immunosuppressants may take several months to produce an improvement, and regular blood tests to monitor possible drug side effects are often required.

RISKS AND SPECIAL PRECAUTIONS

Immunosuppressant drugs and corticosteroids can cause serious adverse effects and are prescribed only when potential benefits outweigh the risks involved.

The side effects of corticosteroids can be reduced by the use of budesonide in a topical preparation (enema) that releases the drug at the site of inflammation.

It is important to continue taking these drugs as instructed because stopping them abruptly may cause a sudden flare-up of the disorder. Doctors usually supervise a gradual reduction in dosage when such drugs are stopped, even when they are given as a short course for an attack. Antidiarrhoeal drugs should not be taken on a routine basis because they may mask signs of deterioration or cause sudden bowel dilation or rupture.

HOW THEY ARE ADMINISTERED

Antidiarrhoeals are usually taken in the form of tablets, although mild ulcerative colitis in the last part of the large intestine may be treated with suppositories or an enema containing a corticosteroid or aminosalicylate.

COMMON DRUGS

Corticosteroids Budesonide*, Hydrocortisone*, Prednisolone*
Immunosuppressants Azathioprine*, Mercaptopurine*, Methotrexate*
Aminosalicylates Balsalazide, Mesalazine*, Olsalazine, Sulfasalazine*
Other drugs Adalimumab, Colestyramine*, Etanercept, Infliximab*, Metronidazole*
* **See Part 2**

Drugs for rectal and anal disorders

The most common disorder affecting the rectum (the last part of the large intestine) and the anus (the opening from the rectum) is haemorrhoids, commonly known as piles. They occur when haemorrhoidal veins become swollen or irritated, often due to prolonged pressure on the area – for example, from pregnancy or long hours of sitting. Haemorrhoids may cause irritation and pain, especially on defecation, and they are aggravated by constipation and straining during defecation. In some cases haemorrhoids may bleed, and occasionally clots form in the swollen veins, leading to severe pain, a condition called thrombosed haemorrhoids.

Other common disorders include anal fissure (painful cracks in the anus) and pruritus ani (itching around the anus). Anal disorders of all kinds occur less frequently in people who have soft, bulky stools.

A number of both over-the-counter and prescription-only preparations are available for the relief of such disorders.

WHY THEY ARE USED

Preparations for the relief of haemorrhoids and anal discomfort fall into three main groups: creams or suppositories that act locally to relieve inflammation and irritation; glyceryl trinitrate ointment, which reduces pain by relieving anal pressure and increasing blood flow; and measures designed to relieve constipation, which contributes to the formation of, and discomfort from, haemorrhoids and anal fissures.

Locally acting treatments often contain a soothing agent that has antiseptic, astringent, or vasoconstrictor properties. Such ingredients include zinc oxide, bismuth, hamamelis (witch hazel), and Peru balsam. Some of these products also include a mild local anaesthetic (see p.9) such as lidocaine. In some cases a doctor may prescribe an ointment containing a corticosteroid to relieve inflammation around the anus (see Topical corticosteroids, p.118).

People who have haemorrhoids or anal fissure are generally advised to include in their diets plenty of fluids and fibre-rich foods, such as fresh fruits, vegetables, and whole grain products, both to prevent constipation and to ease defecation. A mild bulk-forming or softening laxative (see p.43) may also be prescribed.

Neither of these treatments can shrink large haemorrhoids, although they may provide relief while anal fissures heal naturally. Severe, persistently painful haemorrhoids that continue to be troublesome in spite of these measures may need to be removed surgically or, more commonly, by banding. This is a procedure in which a small rubber band is applied tightly to a haemorrhoid, thereby blocking off its blood supply; the haemorrhoid will eventually wither away.

HOW THEY AFFECT YOU

The treatments described above usually relieve discomfort, especially during defecation. Most people experience no adverse effects, although preparations containing local anaesthetics may cause irritation or even a rash in the anal area. It is rare for ingredients in locally acting preparations to be absorbed into the body in sufficient quantities to cause generalized side effects.

The main risk is that self-treatment of haemorrhoids may delay diagnosis of bowel cancer. It is therefore always wise to consult your doctor if symptoms of haemorrhoids are present, especially if you have noticed bleeding from the rectum or a change in your bowel habits.

COMMON DRUGS

Soothing and astringent agents Aluminium acetate, Bismuth, Peru balsam, Zinc oxide
Topical corticosteroids Hydrocortisone*
Local anaesthetics (see p.9)
Laxatives (see p.43)
Other drugs Glyceryl trinitrate*
* **See Part 2**

Drug treatment for gallstones

The formation of gallstones is the most common disorder of the gallbladder. This structure is the storage and concentrating unit for bile, a digestive juice produced by the liver. During digestion, bile passes from the gallbladder via the bile duct into the small intestine, where it assists in the digestion of fats.

Bile is composed of several ingredients, including bile acids, bile salts, and bile pigments. It also contains a significant amount of cholesterol, which is dissolved in bile acid. If the amount of cholesterol in the bile increases, or if the amount of bile acid is reduced, a proportion of the cholesterol cannot remain dissolved, and under certain circumstances this excess accumulates in the gallbladder as gallstones.

Gallstones may be present in the gallbladder for years without causing symptoms. However, if they become lodged in the bile duct they cause pain and block the flow of bile. If the bile accumulates in the blood, it may cause an attack of jaundice, or the gallbladder may become infected and inflamed.

Drug treatment with ursodeoxycholic acid is only effective against stones made principally of cholesterol (some contain other substances), and even these stones take many months to dissolve. Therefore, surgery and ultrasound have become widely used, especially laparoscopic ("keyhole") surgery. Surgery and ultrasound treatments are always used to remove stones blocking the bile duct.

WHY THEY ARE USED

Even if you have not experienced any symptoms, once gallstones have been diagnosed your doctor may advise treatment because of the risk of blockage of the bile duct. Drug treatment is usually preferred to surgery for small cholesterol stones or when there is a possibility that surgery may be risky.

HOW THEY WORK

Ursodeoxycholic acid is a substance that is naturally present in bile. It acts on chemical processes in the liver to regulate the amount of cholesterol in the blood by controlling the amount that passes into the bile. Once the cholesterol level in the bile is reduced, the bile acids are able to start dissolving the stones in the gallbladder. To achieve maximum effect, ursodeoxycholic acid treatment usually needs to be accompanied by adherence to a low-cholesterol, high-fibre diet.

HOW THEY AFFECT YOU

Drug treatment may often take years to dissolve gallstones completely. You will not, therefore, feel any immediate benefit from the drug, but you may have some minor side effects, the most usual of which is diarrhoea. If this occurs, your doctor may adjust the dosage. The effect of drug treatment on the gallstones is usually monitored at regular intervals by means of ultrasound or X-ray examinations.

Even after successful treatment with drugs, gallstones often recur when the drug is stopped. In some cases drug treatment and dietary restrictions may need to be continued even after the gallstones have dissolved, to prevent a recurrence.

Although ursodeoxycholic acid reduces cholesterol in the gallbladder, it increases the level in the blood because it reduces the excretion of cholesterol in the bile. Doctors therefore prescribe it with caution to people who have atherosclerosis (fatty deposits in the blood vessels). The drug is not usually given to people who have liver disorders because it can interfere with normal liver function. Surgical or ultrasound treatment is used for people with liver problems.

COMMON DRUGS

Drugs for gallstones Ursodeoxycholic acid
Other drugs Colestyramine*
* **See Part 2**

Drug treatment for pancreatic disorders

The pancreas releases certain enzymes into the small intestine that are necessary for digestion of a range of foods. If the release of pancreatic enzymes is impaired (by chronic pancreatitis or cystic fibrosis, for example), enzyme replacement therapy may be necessary. Replacement of enzymes does not cure the underlying disorder, but it restores normal digestion. Pancreatic enzymes should be taken just before or with meals, and usually take effect immediately. Your doctor will probably advise you to eat a diet that is high in protein and carbohydrates and low in fat.

Pancreatin, the generic name for those preparations containing pancreatic enzymes, is extracted from pig pancreas. Treatment must be continued indefinitely as long as the pancreatic disorder persists.

COMMON DRUGS

Pancreatic enzymes Amylase, Lipase, Pancreatin, Protease

MUSCLES, BONES, AND JOINTS

The basic architecture of the human body comprises 206 bones, over 600 muscles, and a complex assortment of other tissues that enable the body to move efficiently.

Bones support the body, provide protection for organs, and enable movement.

Tendons attach the muscles that control body movement to the bones.

Muscles work bones so that they act as levers: when the muscle contracts, movement occurs at the joint.

Ligaments are bands of tough fibrous tissue that hold joints together.

Cartilage covers each bone end, reducing friction between the ends of two bones.

WHAT CAN GO WRONG

Although tough, these structures often suffer damage. Muscles, tendons, and ligaments can be strained or torn by violent movement, which may cause inflammation, making the affected tissue swollen and painful. Joints, especially those that bear the body's weight – hips, knees, ankles, and vertebrae – are prone to wear and tear. The cartilage covering the bone ends may tear, causing pain and inflammation. Joint damage also occurs in rheumatoid arthritis, which is thought to be a form of autoimmune disorder. Gout, in which uric acid crystals form in some joints, may also cause inflammation, a condition known as gouty arthritis.

Another problem affecting the muscles and joints includes nerve injury or degeneration, which alters nerve control over muscle contraction. Myasthenia gravis, in which transmission of signals between nerves and muscles is reduced, affects muscle control as a result. Bones may also be weakened by vitamin, mineral, or hormone deficiencies.

WHY DRUGS ARE USED

A simple analgesic drug or one with an anti-inflammatory effect will provide pain relief in most of the conditions described above. For severe inflammation, a doctor may inject a drug with a more powerful anti-inflammatory effect, such as a corticosteroid, into the affected site. In cases of severe progressive rheumatoid arthritis, antirheumatic drugs may halt the progression of the disease and relieve symptoms.

Drugs that reduce the production of uric acid or speed its elimination are often prescribed to treat gout. Relaxants that inhibit transmission of nerve signals to the muscles are used to treat muscle spasm. Drugs that increase nervous stimulation of the muscle are prescribed for myasthenia gravis. Bone disorders in which the mineral content of bone is reduced are treated with supplements of minerals, vitamins, and hormones.

MAJOR DRUG GROUPS

- Non-steroidal anti-inflammatory drugs
- Antirheumatic drugs
- Corticosteroids for rheumatic disorders
- Drugs for gout
- Muscle relaxants
- Drugs used for myasthenia gravis
- Drugs for bone disorders

Non-steroidal anti-inflammatory drugs

Drugs in this group, often referred to as NSAIDs, are used to relieve the pain, stiffness, and inflammation of conditions affecting the muscles, bones, and joints. NSAIDs are called "non-steroidal" to distinguish them from corticosteroid drugs (see p.78), which also damp down inflammation.

WHY THEY ARE USED

NSAIDs are widely prescribed for the treatment of osteoarthritis, rheumatoid arthritis, and other rheumatic conditions. They reduce pain and inflammation in the joints, but they do not alter the progress of these diseases.

The response to the various drugs in this group varies between individuals. It is sometimes necessary to try several different NSAIDs before finding the one that best suits a particular individual.

Because NSAIDs do not change the progress of a disease, additional treatment is often necessary, particularly for rheumatoid arthritis (see below).

NSAIDs are also commonly prescribed to relieve back pain, headaches, gout (see p.51), menstrual pain (see p.102), mild pain following surgery, and pain from soft tissue injuries, such as sprains and strains (see also Analgesics, p.7).

HOW THEY WORK

Prostaglandins are chemicals released by the body at the site of injury. They are responsible for producing inflammation and pain following tissue damage. NSAIDs block an enzyme, cyclo-oxygenase (COX), which is involved in the production of prostaglandins, and thus reduce pain and inflammation (see Analgesics, p.7).

HOW THEY AFFECT YOU

NSAIDs are rapidly absorbed from the digestive system, and most start to relieve pain within an hour. When used regularly they reduce pain, inflammation, and stiffness and may restore or improve the function of a damaged or painful joint.

Most NSAIDs are short acting and need to be taken a few times a day for optimal pain relief. Some need to be taken only twice daily. Others, such as piroxicam, are very slowly eliminated from the body and are effective when taken once a day.

RISKS AND SPECIAL PRECAUTIONS

Most NSAIDs carry a low risk of serious adverse effects, although nausea, indigestion, and altered bowel action are common. The main risk from use of NSAIDs is that, occasionally, they can cause bleeding in the stomach or duodenum; to prevent this problem, the lowest effective dose is given for the shortest possible duration. NSAIDs should be avoided altogether by people who have had peptic ulcers.

Most NSAIDs are not recommended during pregnancy or for breast-feeding mothers. Caution is also advised for people with kidney or liver abnormalities or heart disease, or for those people with a history of hypersensitivity to other drugs.

NSAIDs may impair blood clotting and are, therefore, prescribed with caution to people with bleeding disorders or who are taking drugs that reduce blood clotting.

MISOPROSTOL

An NSAID may cause bleeding if its antiprostaglandin action occurs where it is not wanted, such as in the digestive tract. To protect against this side effect, a prostaglandin-like drug called misoprostol is sometimes prescribed with the NSAID. Preparations are available that incorporate both misoprostol and an NSAID. Misoprostol is also used to help heal peptic ulcers (see p.41).

COX-2 INHIBITORS

NSAIDs block two types of COX, COX-1 and COX-2, at different sites in the body; blocking COX-1 leads to the upper gastrointestinal tract irritation of NSAIDs, while blocking COX-2 gives rise to the anti-inflammatory effect. COX-2 inhibitors block COX-2 but not COX-1. COX-2 inhibitors are not prescribed to anyone who has had a heart attack or stroke, however, because they significantly increase the risk of recurrence, nor are they prescribed to people with peripheral artery disease (poor circulation). They are prescribed with caution to anyone at risk of any of these conditions.

COMMON DRUGS

Aceclofenac, Acemetacin, Aspirin*, Diclofenac*, Felbinac, Fenbufen, Fenoprofen, Flurbiprofen, Ibuprofen*, Indometacin (indomethacin), Ketoprofen*, Mefenamic acid*, Meloxicam, Nabumetone, Naproxen*, Piroxicam*, Sulindac, Tenoxicam, Tiaprofenic acid

COX-2 inhibitors Celecoxib*, Etodolac, Etoricoxib

* **See Part 2**

Antirheumatic drugs

These drugs are used in the treatment of various rheumatic disorders, the most crippling and deforming being rheumatoid arthritis. This is an autoimmune disease in which the body's mechanism for fighting infection contributes to the damage of its own joint tissue. There is pain, stiffness, and swelling of the joints that, over many months, can lead to deformity. Flare-ups of rheumatoid arthritis also cause a general feeling of being unwell, fatigue, and loss of appetite.

The treatments for rheumatoid arthritis include drugs, rest, physiotherapy, changes in diet, and immobilization of joints. The disorder cannot yet be cured, but in many cases it does not progress to permanent disability. It also sometimes subsides spontaneously for prolonged periods.

WHY THEY ARE USED

The aim of drug treatment is to relieve the symptoms of pain and stiffness, maintain mobility, and prevent deformity. Drugs for rheumatoid arthritis fall into two main categories: those that alleviate symptoms, and those that modify, halt, or slow the underlying disease process.

Drugs in the first category include aspirin (p.142) and other NSAIDs (see Non-steroidal anti-inflammatory drugs, p.48). These drugs are usually prescribed as a first treatment.

Drugs in the second category are known collectively as disease-modifying antirheumatic drugs (DMARDs). These drugs may be given if the rheumatoid arthritis is severe or if initial drug treatment has proved to be ineffective. DMARDs may prevent further joint damage and disability, but they are not prescribed routinely because the disease may stop spontaneously and because they have potentially severe adverse effects (see Some types of disease-modifying antirheumatic drug, below, for further information on individual drugs).

Corticosteroids (see p.78) are sometimes used in the treatment of rheumatoid arthritis, but are used only for limited periods because they depress the immune system, increasing susceptibility to infection.

SOME TYPES OF DISEASE-MODIFYING ANTIRHEUMATIC DRUG

Chloroquine Originally developed to treat malaria (see p.73), chloroquine and related drugs are less effective than penicillamine or gold. Prolonged use may cause eye damage, so regular eye tests are needed.

Immunosuppressants These are prescribed if other drugs do not provide relief and if the rheumatoid arthritis is severe and disabling. Regular observation and blood tests must be carried out because immunosuppressants can cause severe complications.

Sulfasalazine Used mainly for ulcerative colitis (p.44), this was originally introduced to treat mild to moderate rheumatoid arthritis. It slows disease progress in some cases and has a low risk of serious adverse effects.

Gold-based drugs These are now seldom used but may be given orally or by injection. Side effects can include a rash and digestive disturbances. Gold may sometimes damage the kidneys, which recover once treatment is stopped; regular urine tests are usually carried out, however. Gold can also suppress blood cell production in the bone marrow, so periodic blood tests are also carried out.

Monoclonal antibodies such as infliximab (see p.277) and adalimumab target a particular body protein responsible for rheumatoid arthritis. These drugs often cause allergy-type reactions, especially at the start of treatment. Infections, particularly of the upper respiratory and urinary tracts, are common.

HOW THEY WORK

It is not known precisely how most DMARDs stop or slow the disease process. Some may reduce the body's immune response, which is thought to be partly responsible for the disease (see also Immunosuppressant drugs, p.97). Monoclonal antibodies such as infliximab combine with a body protein called tumour necrosis factor alpha (TNF), which is overactive in rheumatoid arthritis. By reducing the level of TNF activity, they can improve the arthritis. When effective, DMARDs prevent damage to cartilage and bone, thus reducing progressive deformity and disability. The effectiveness of each drug varies depending on individual response.

HOW THEY AFFECT YOU

DMARDs are generally slow acting; it may be 4 to 6 months before any benefit is noticed. Therefore, treatment with aspirin or other NSAIDs is usually continued until remission occurs. Prolonged treatment with DMARDs can markedly improve symptoms. Arthritic pain is relieved, joint mobility increased, and general symptoms of ill health fade. Side effects (which vary between individual drugs) may be noticed before beneficial effects, so patience is required. Regular monitoring of the kidneys, liver, and bone marrow are needed. Severe adverse effects may require treatment to be abandoned.

COMMON DRUGS

Immunosuppressants Azathioprine*, Ciclosporin*, Cyclophosphamide*, Leflunomide, Methotrexate*
NSAIDs (see p.48)
DMARDs Adalimumab, Chloroquine*, Etanercept*, Hydroxychloroquine, Infliximab*, Penicillamine, Sodium aurothiomalate, Sulfasalazine*
* **See Part 2**

Corticosteroids for rheumatic disorders

The adrenal glands, which lie on the top of the kidneys, produce a number of important hormones. Among these are corticosteroids, so named because they are made in the outer part (cortex) of the glands. The corticosteroids play an important role, influencing the immune system and regulating the carbohydrate and mineral metabolism of the body. A number of drugs that mimic the natural corticosteroids have been developed.

These drugs have many uses and are discussed in detail under Corticosteroids (see p.78). This section concentrates on those corticosteroids injected into an affected site to treat joint disorders.

WHY THEY ARE USED

Corticosteroids given by injection are particularly useful for treating joint disorders – most notably rheumatoid arthritis and osteoarthritis – when one or only a few joints are involved, and when pain and inflammation have not been relieved by other drugs. In such cases, it is possible to relieve symptoms by injecting each of the affected joints individually. Corticosteroids may also be injected to relieve pain and inflammation due to strained or contracted muscles, ligaments, and/or tendons – for example, in frozen shoulder or tennis elbow. In addition, they may be given for bursitis, tendinitis, or swelling that is compressing a nerve. Corticosteroid injections are sometimes used in order to relieve pain and stiffness sufficiently to permit physiotherapy.

HOW THEY WORK

Corticosteroid drugs have two important actions that are believed to account for their effectiveness. They block the production of prostaglandins – body chemicals that are responsible for triggering inflammation and pain – and depress the accumulation and activity of the white blood cells that cause the inflammation. Injection of these drugs concentrates their effects at the site of the problem, thus giving the maximum benefit where it is most needed.

HOW THEY AFFECT YOU

Corticosteroids usually give dramatic relief from symptoms when injected into a joint. Often a single injection is sufficient to relieve pain and swelling, and to improve mobility. When used to treat muscle or tendon pain, they may not always be effective because it is difficult to position the needle so that the drug reaches the right spot. In some cases, repeated injections are necessary.

Because these drugs are concentrated in the affected area, rather than being dispersed in significant amounts in the body, the generalized adverse effects that sometimes occur when corticosteroids are taken by mouth are unlikely. Minor side effects, such as loss of skin pigment at the injection site, are uncommon. Occasionally, a temporary increase in pain (steroid flare) may occur. In such cases, rest, local application of ice, and analgesic medication may relieve the condition. Sterile injection technique is critically important.

COMMON DRUGS

Dexamethasone*, Hydrocortisone*, Methylprednisolone, Prednisolone*, Triamcinolone
* **See Part 2**

Drugs for gout

Gout is a disorder that arises when the blood contains increased levels of uric acid, which is a by-product of normal body metabolism. When its concentration in the blood is excessive, uric acid crystals may form in various parts of the body, especially in the joints of the foot (most often the big toe), the knee, and the hand, causing intense pain and inflammation known as gout. Crystals may form as white masses, known as tophi, in soft tissue, and in the kidneys as stones. Attacks of gout can recur and may lead to damaged joints and deformity, a condition known as gouty arthritis. Kidney stones can cause kidney damage.

An excess of uric acid can be caused either by increased production or by decreased elimination by the kidneys, which normally remove it from the body. The disorder tends to run in families and is far more common in men than women. The risk of attack is increased by high alcohol intake, the consumption of certain foods (red meat, sardines, anchovies, yeast extract, and offal such as liver, brains, and sweetbreads), and obesity. An attack may be triggered by drugs such as thiazide diuretics (see p.30) or anticancer drugs (see p.94), or excessive intake of alcohol, especially beer. Changes in diet and a reduction in alcohol consumption may be important parts of treatment.

Drugs used to treat acute attacks of gout include NSAIDs (see Non-steroidal anti-inflammatory drugs, p.48), and colchicine. Other drugs, which lower the blood level of uric acid, are used for the long-term prevention of gout. These include uricosuric drugs (such as sulfinpyrazone) and allopurinol, which is the drug of choice. Aspirin is not prescribed for pain relief because it slows the excretion of uric acid.

WHY THEY ARE USED

Drugs may be prescribed either to treat an attack of gout or to prevent recurrent attacks that could lead to deformity of affected joints and kidney damage. NSAIDs and colchicine are both used to treat an attack of gout and should be taken as soon as an attack begins. Because colchicine is relatively specific in relieving the pain and inflammation arising from gout, doctors sometimes administer it in order to confirm their diagnosis of the condition before prescribing an NSAID.

If symptoms recur, your doctor may advise long-term treatment with either allopurinol or a uricosuric drug. One of these drugs must usually be taken indefinitely. Since they can trigger attacks of gout at the beginning of treatment, colchicine is sometimes given together with these drugs for a few months.

HOW THEY WORK

Allopurinol and febuxostat reduce the level of uric acid in the blood by interfering with the activity of xanthine oxidase, an enzyme involved in the production of uric acid in the body. Sulfinpyrazone increases the rate at which uric acid is excreted by the kidneys. The process by which colchicine reduces inflammation and relieves pain is poorly understood. The actions of NSAIDs are described on p.49.

HOW THEY AFFECT YOU

Drugs used in the long-term treatment of gout are usually successful in preventing attacks and joint deformity. However, the body's response may be slow. Colchicine can disturb the digestive system, causing diarrhoea, in which case treatment is stopped.

RISKS AND SPECIAL PRECAUTIONS

Since they increase the output of uric acid through the kidneys, uricosuric drugs can cause crystals of uric acid salts (urates) to form in the kidneys. They are not, therefore, usually prescribed for those people who already have impaired kidney function or urate stones. In such cases, allopurinol may be preferred.

It is important to drink plenty of fluids while taking drugs for gout in order to prevent kidney crystals from forming. Regular blood tests to monitor levels of uric acid in the blood may be required.

COMMON DRUGS

Drugs to treat attacks Colchicine*, NSAIDs but not aspirin (see p.48)

Drugs to treat high uric acid caused by cytotoxic drugs Rasburicase

Drugs to prevent attacks Allopurinol*, Febuxostat, Sulfinpyrazone

* **See Part 2**

Muscle relaxants

Several drugs are available to treat muscle spasm – the involuntary, painful contraction of a muscle or a group of muscles that can stiffen an arm or leg, or make it almost impossible to straighten your back. There are various causes. It can follow an injury, or come on without warning. It may also be brought on by a disorder like osteoarthritis, the pain in the affected joint triggering abnormal tension in a nearby muscle.

Spasticity is another form of muscle tightness seen in some neurological disorders, such as multiple sclerosis, stroke, or cerebral palsy. Spasticity can sometimes be helped by physiotherapy, but in severe cases drugs may be used to relieve symptoms.

WHY THEY ARE USED

Muscle spasm resulting from direct injury is usually treated with a non-steroidal anti-inflammatory drug (see p.48) or an analgesic (see p.7). However, if the muscle spasm is severe, a muscle relaxant may also be tried for a short period.

In spasticity, the legs may become so stiff and uncontrollable that walking unaided is impossible. In such cases, a drug may be used to relax the muscles. Relaxation of the muscles often permits physiotherapy to be given for longer-term relief from spasms.

The muscle relaxant botulinum toxin may be injected locally to relieve muscle spasm in small groups of accessible muscles, such as those around the eye or in the neck.

HOW THEY WORK

Muscle-relaxant drugs work in one of several ways. Centrally acting drugs damp down the passage of the nerve signals from the brain and spinal cord that cause muscles to contract, thus reducing excessive stimulation of muscles as well as unwanted muscular contraction. Dantrolene reduces the sensitivity of the muscles to nerve signals. Botulinum toxin injected locally prevents transmission of impulses between nerves and muscles.

HOW THEY AFFECT YOU

Drugs taken regularly for a spastic disorder of the central nervous system usually reduce stiffness and improve mobility. They may restore the use of the arms and legs when this has been impaired by muscle spasm.

Unfortunately, most centrally acting drugs can have a generally depressant effect on nervous activity and produce drowsiness, particularly at the beginning of treatment. Too high a dosage can excessively reduce the muscles' ability to contract and can therefore cause weakness. For this reason, the dosage needs to be carefully adjusted to identify a level that controls the symptoms but which, at the same time, maintains sufficient muscle strength.

RISKS AND SPECIAL PRECAUTIONS

The main long-term risk associated with centrally acting muscle relaxants is that the body becomes dependent on them. If they are withdrawn suddenly, the stiffness may become worse than before drug treatment.

Rarely, dantrolene can cause serious liver damage. Anyone who is taking this drug should have their blood tested regularly to assess liver function.

Unless used very cautiously, botulinum toxin can paralyse unaffected muscles, and might interfere with functions such as speech and swallowing.

COMMON DRUGS

Centrally acting drugs Baclofen*, Diazepam*, Orphenadrine*, Tizanidine
Other drugs Botulinum toxin*, Dantrolene
* **See Part 2**

Drugs used for myasthenia gravis

Myasthenia gravis is a disorder that occurs when the immune system (see p.93) becomes defective and produces antibodies that disrupt the signals being transmitted between the nervous system and muscles that are under voluntary control. As a result, the body's muscular response is progressively weakened. The first muscles to be affected are those controlling the eyes, eyelids, face, pharynx, and larynx, with muscles in the arms and legs becoming involved as the disease progresses. Myasthenia gravis is often linked to a disorder of the thymus gland, which is the source of the destructive antibodies concerned.

Various methods can be used in the treatment of myasthenia gravis, including removal of the thymus gland (called a thymectomy) or temporarily clearing the blood of antibodies (a procedure known as plasmapheresis, or plasma exchange). Drugs that improve muscle function, principally neostigmine and pyridostigmine, may be prescribed. These drugs may be used alone or together with other drugs that depress the immune system – usually azathioprine (see Immunosuppressant drugs, p.97) or corticosteroids (see p.78). Intravenous immunoglobulins may also be used in severe cases in which a person experiences breathing and swallowing problems.

WHY THEY ARE USED

Drugs that improve the muscle response to nerve impulses have several uses. One such drug, edrophonium, acts very quickly, and, once administered intravenously, it brings about a dramatic improvement in the symptoms. This effect is used to confirm the diagnosis of myasthenia gravis. However, because of its short duration of action, edrophonium is not used for long-term treatment. Pyridostigmine and neostigmine are preferred for long-term treatment, especially when removal of the thymus gland is not feasible or does not provide adequate relief.

These drugs may also be given to non-myasthenic patients after surgery to reverse the effects of a muscle-relaxant drug given as part of the general anaesthetic.

HOW THEY WORK

Normal muscle action occurs when a nerve impulse triggers a nerve ending to release a neurotransmitter, which combines with a specialized receptor on the muscle cells and causes the muscles to contract. In myasthenia gravis, the body's immune system destroys many of these receptors, so that the muscle is less responsive to nervous stimulation. Drugs used to treat the disorder increase the amount of neurotransmitter at the nerve ending by blocking the action of an enzyme that normally breaks it down. Increased levels of the neurotransmitter permit the remaining receptors to function more efficiently.

HOW THEY AFFECT YOU

These drugs usually restore the muscle function to a normal or near-normal level, particularly when the disease takes a mild form. Unfortunately, the drugs can produce unwanted muscular activity by enhancing the transmission of nerve impulses elsewhere in the body.

Common side effects include vomiting, nausea, diarrhoea, and muscle cramps in the arms, legs, and abdomen.

RISKS AND SPECIAL PRECAUTIONS

Muscle weakness can suddenly worsen even when it is being treated with drugs. Should this occur, it is important not to take larger doses of the drug to try to relieve the symptoms, because excessive drug levels can interfere with the transmission of nerve impulses to muscles, causing further weakness. Administration of other drugs, including some antibiotics, can also markedly increase the symptoms of myasthenia gravis. If your symptoms suddenly become worse, consult your doctor.

COMMON DRUGS

Azathioprine*, Corticosteroids (see p.78), Distigmine, Edrophonium, Neostigmine, Pyridostigmine*

* **See Part 2**

Drugs for bone disorders

Bone is a living structure. Its hard, mineral quality is created by the action of the bone cells. These cells continually deposit and remove phosphorus and calcium, which are stored in a honeycombed protein framework called the matrix. Because the rates of deposit and removal (the bone metabolism) are about equal in adults, the bone mass remains fairly constant.

Removal and renewal are regulated by hormones and influenced by a number of factors: notably the level of calcium in the blood, which depends on the intake of calcium and vitamin D from the diet, and the actions of various hormones, plus everyday movement and weight-bearing stress. When normal bone metabolism is altered, various bone disorders result.

OSTEOPOROSIS

In osteoporosis, the strength and density of bone are reduced. Such wasting occurs when the rate of removal of mineralized bone exceeds the rate of deposit. In most people, bone density decreases very gradually from the age of 30. But bone loss can dramatically increase when a person is immobilized for a period, and this is an important cause of osteoporosis in older people. Hormone deficiency is another important cause, commonly occurring in women with lowered oestrogen levels after the menopause or removal of the ovaries. Osteoporosis also occurs in disorders in which there is excess production of adrenal or thyroid hormones. In addition, osteoporosis can result from long-term treatment with corticosteroid drugs.

People with osteoporosis often have no symptoms, but if the vertebrae become so weakened that they are unable to bear the body's weight, they may collapse spontaneously or after a minor accident. Subsequently, the affected person develops back pain, reduced height, and a round-shouldered appearance. Osteoporosis also makes a fracture of an arm, leg, or hip more likely.

Most doctors emphasize the need to prevent the disorder by an adequate intake of protein and calcium and by regular exercise throughout adult life. Oestrogen supplements are no longer usually recommended to prevent osteoporosis.

The condition of bones damaged by osteoporosis cannot usually be improved, but drug treatment can help to prevent further deterioration and help fractures to heal. For people whose diet is deficient in calcium or vitamin D, supplements may be prescribed. However, these are of limited value and are often less useful than drugs that inhibit removal of calcium from the bones. In the past, the hormone calcitonin was used, but it has now been largely superseded by drugs such as alendronate. These drugs, known as bisphosphonates, bind very tightly to the bone matrix, preventing its removal by bone cells.

OSTEOMALACIA AND RICKETS

In osteomalacia (called rickets when it affects children), a lack of vitamin D leads to loss of calcium, resulting in softening of the bones. There is pain and tenderness and a risk of fracture and bone deformity. In children, growth is retarded.

Osteomalacia is most commonly caused by a lack of vitamin D. This can result from an inadequate diet, inability to absorb the vitamin, or insufficient exposure of the skin to sunlight (the action of the sun on the skin produces vitamin D inside the body). Individuals who are at special risk include those whose absorption of vitamin D is impaired by an intestinal disorder, such as Crohn's disease or coeliac disease. People with dark skin living in northern Europe or North America are also susceptible. Chronic kidney disease is an important cause of rickets in children and of osteomalacia in adults, since healthy kidneys play an essential role in the body's metabolism of vitamin D.

Long-term relief depends on treating the underlying disorder where possible. In rare cases, treatment may be lifelong.

VITAMIN D

A number of substances that are related to vitamin D may be used in the treatment of bone disorders. These substances include alfacalcidol, calcitriol, and ergocalciferol. The treatment that is prescribed depends on the underlying problem.

COMMON DRUGS

Alendronic acid*, Alfacalcidol, Calcitonin, Calcitriol, Calcium carbonate, Conjugated oestrogens*, Ergocalciferol, Fluoride, Pamidronate, Risedronate*, Salcatonin (salmon calcitonin), Teriparatide, Vitamin D

* **See Part 2**

ALLERGY

Allergy, a hypersensitivity to certain substances, is a reaction of the body's immune system. Through a variety of mechanisms (see Malignant and immune disease, p.93), the system protects the body by eliminating unrecognized foreign substances, such as microorganisms (bacteria or viruses).

One way in which the immune system acts is through the production of antibodies. When the body encounters a particular foreign substance (or allergen) for the first time, one type of white blood cell, the lymphocyte, produces antibodies that attach themselves to another type of white blood cell, the mast cell. If the same substance is encountered again, the allergen binds to the antibodies on the mast cells, causing the release of chemicals known as mediators.

The most important mediator is histamine. Its release can produce a rash, swelling, narrowing of the airways, and a drop in blood pressure. Although these effects are important in protecting the body against infection, they may also be triggered inappropriately in an allergic reaction.

WHAT CAN GO WRONG

One of the most common allergic disorders, hay fever, is caused by an allergic reaction to inhaled pollen leading to allergic rhinitis – swelling and irritation of the nasal passages and watering of the nose and eyes. Other substances, such as house-dust mites, animal fur, and feathers, may cause a similar reaction in susceptible people.

Asthma, another allergic disorder, may result from the action of leukotrienes rather than histamine. Other allergic conditions include urticaria (hives) or other rashes (sometimes in response to a drug), some forms of eczema and dermatitis, and allergic alveolitis (farmer's lung). Anaphylaxis is a serious systemic allergic reaction that occurs when an allergen reaches the bloodstream (see also Epinephrine (adrenaline), p.234).

WHY DRUGS ARE USED

Antihistamines and drugs that inhibit mast cell activity are used to prevent and treat allergic reactions. Other drugs minimizee symptoms; these drugs include decongestants (see p.24) to clear the nose in allergic rhinitis, bronchodilators (see p.21) to widen the airways of people with asthma, and corticosteroids applied to areas of skin affected by eczema (see p.123).

MAJOR DRUG GROUPS

- Antihistamines
- Other allergy treatments
- Corticosteroids (see p.78)
- Drugs for asthma (see p.22)

Antihistamines

Antihistamines are the most widely used drugs in the treatment of allergic reactions of all kinds. They can be subdivided according to their chemical structure, each subgroup having slightly different actions and characteristics (see table on p.58). Their main action is to counter the effects of histamine, one of the chemicals released in the body when there is an allergic reaction.

Histamine is also involved in other body functions, including dilation and constriction of blood vessels, contraction of muscles in the respiratory and gastrointestinal tracts, and the release of digestive juices in the stomach. The antihistamine drugs described here are also known as H1 blockers because they block the action of histamine only on certain receptors, known as H1 receptors. Another group of antihistamines, known as H2 blockers, is used in the treatment of peptic ulcers (see Anti-ulcer drugs, p.41).

Some antihistamines have a significant anticholinergic action (see p.7). This is used to advantage in various conditions, but it also causes certain undesired side effects.

WHY THEY ARE USED

Antihistamines relieve allergy-related symptoms when it is not possible to prevent exposure to the substance that has provoked the reaction. They are most commonly used in the prevention of allergic rhinitis (hay fever), the inflammation of the nose and upper airways that results from an allergic reaction to a substance such as pollen, house dust, or animal fur. Antihistamines are more effective when taken before the start of an attack. If they are taken only after an attack has begun, beneficial effects may be delayed.

Antihistamines are not usually effective in asthma caused by similar allergens because the symptoms of this allergic disorder are not solely caused by the action of histamine, but are likely to result from more complex mechanisms. Antihistamines are usually the first drugs to be tried in treating allergic disorders, but alternatives can be prescribed (see Other allergy treatments, p.58).

Antihistamines are also prescribed for the itching, swelling, and redness of allergic reactions involving the skin, such as urticaria (hives) and dermatitis. Irritation due to chickenpox may be reduced by these drugs. Allergic reactions to insect stings may also be reduced by antihistamines. In such cases the drug may be taken by mouth or applied topically. Applied as drops, antihistamines can reduce inflammation and irritation of the eyes and eyelids in allergic conjunctivitis.

Antihistamines are often included as an ingredient in cough and cold preparations (see p.25); in these products, the anticholinergic effect of drying mucus secretions and their sedative effect on the coughing mechanism may be helpful.

Because most of the antihistamines have a depressant effect on the brain, these drugs are sometimes used to promote sleep, especially when discomfort from itching is disturbing sleep (see also Sleeping drugs, p.9). The depressant effect of antihistamines on the brain also extends to the centres that control nausea and vomiting. Antihistamines are therefore often effective for preventing and controlling these symptoms (see Anti-emetics, p.19).

Occasionally, antihistamines are used to treat fever, rash, and breathing difficulties that may occur in adverse reactions to blood transfusions and allergic reactions to drugs. Promethazine and alimemazine may also be used as premedication to provide sedation and to dry secretions during surgery, particularly in children.

HOW THEY WORK

Antihistamines block the action of histamine on H1 receptors. These are found in various body tissues, particularly the small blood vessels in the skin, nose, and eyes. This helps to prevent the dilation of the vessels, thus reducing the redness, watering, and swelling. In addition, the anticholinergic action of these drugs contributes to this effect by reducing the secretions from tear glands and nasal passages.

Antihistamines pass from the blood into the brain. In the brain, the blocking action of the antihistamines on histamine activity may produce general sedation and depression of various brain functions, including the vomiting and coughing mechanisms.

HOW THEY AFFECT YOU

Antihistamines often cause a degree of drowsiness and may affect coordination, leading to clumsiness. Some newer drugs have little or no sedative effect (see table, p.58).

Anticholinergic side effects, including dry mouth, blurred vision, and difficulty passing urine, are common. Most side effects diminish with continued use and can often be helped by an adjustment in dosage or a change to a different drug.

RISKS AND SPECIAL PRECAUTIONS

It is advisable to avoid driving or operating machinery while taking antihistamines, particularly those that are more likely to cause drowsiness (see table, p.58). Antihistamines can also increase the sedative effects of alcohol, sleeping drugs, opioid analgesics, and anti-anxiety drugs.

In high doses, or in children, some antihistamines can cause excitement, agitation, and even, in extreme cases, hallucinations and seizures. Abnormal heart rhythms have occurred after high doses with some antihistamines (mostly now discontinued) or when drugs that interact with them, such as antifungals and antibiotics, have been taken at the same time. Heart rhythm problems may also affect people with liver disease, electrolyte disturbances, or abnormal heart activity. A person who has these conditions, or who has glaucoma or prostate trouble, should seek medical advice before taking antihistamines because their various drug actions may make such conditions worse.

COMMON DRUGS

Non-sedating Acrivastine, Cetirizine*, Fexofenadine, Levocetirizine, Loratadine/desloratadine*, Mizolastine
Sedating Alimemazine, Chlorphenamine*, Cinnarizine*, Clemastine, Diphenhydramine, Hydroxyzine, Promethazine*
* **See Part 2**

OTHER ALLERGY TREATMENTS

Sodium cromoglicate This drug (see p.403) prevents the release of histamine from mast cells (see p.56) in response to exposure to an allergen, thereby preventing the physical symptoms of allergies. Sodium cromoglicate is commonly given by inhaler for the prevention of allergy-induced rhinitis (hay fever) or asthma attacks and by drops for the treatment of allergic eye disorders.
Leukotriene antagonists Like histamine, leukotrienes are substances that occur naturally in the body and seem to play an important part in asthma. Drugs such as montelukast (see p.331) and zafirlukast (leukotriene antagonists) have been developed to prevent asthma attacks. They are not bronchodilators, however, and will not relieve an existing attack (see Drugs for asthma, p.22).
Corticosteroids These drugs are used to treat allergic rhinitis and asthma. They are usually given by inhaler, which supplies much lower doses to the body than tablets.
Desensitization This treatment may be tried in conditions such as allergic rhinitis due to pollen sensitivity and insect venom hypersensitivity, when avoidance, antihistamines, and other treatments have not been effective and tests have shown one or two specific allergens to be responsible. Desensitization often provides incomplete relief and can be time-consuming.

Treatment involves a series of injections containing increasing doses of an extract of the allergen. The way in which this prevents allergic reactions is poorly understood. Perhaps controlled exposure may trigger the immune system into producing increasing levels of antibodies so that the body no longer responds dramatically when the allergen is encountered naturally.

Desensitization must be carried out under medical supervision because it can provoke a severe allergic response. Therefore, it is important that you remain near emergency medical facilities for at least an hour after each injection.

COMPARISON OF ANTIHISTAMINES

The table below indicates the main uses of some common antihistamines and lists their relative strength of anticholinergic action, sedative effects, and duration of action.

KEY
● Drug used ■ Strong ◩ Medium □ Minimal
▲ Long (over 12 hours) ◭ Medium (6–12 hours)
△ Short (4–6 hours)

	COMMON USES: Allergic rhinitis	Skin allergy	Sedation	Premedication	Nausea/vomiting	Cough/cold remedies	ACTIONS AND EFFECTS: Drowsiness	Anticholinergic action	DURATION OF ACTION
Alimemazine		●	●	●			■	□	◭
Acrivastine	●	●					□	◩	△
Cetirizine	●	●					□	□	▲
Chlorphenamine	●	●	●			●	◩	◩	△
Cyclizine					●		◩	◩	△
Diphenhydramine			●		●	●	◩	◩	△
Hydroxyzine		●	●				■	◩	▲
Loratadine	●	●					□	□	▲
Promethazine	●	●	●	●		●	■	◩	◭

INFECTIONS AND INFESTATIONS

The human body provides a suitable environment for the growth of many types of microorganism, including bacteria, viruses, fungi, yeasts, and protozoa. It may also become the host for animal parasites such as insects, worms, and flukes.

Microorganisms (also known as microbes) exist all around us and can be transmitted from person to person in many ways: direct contact, inhalation of infected air, and consumption of contaminated food or water. Not all microorganisms cause disease; many types of bacteria exist on the skin surface or in the bowel without causing ill effects, while others cannot live either in or on the body.

Normally, the immune system protects the body from infection. Invading microbes are killed before they can multiply in sufficient numbers to cause serious disease. (See also Malignant and immune disease, p.93.)

TYPES OF INFECTING ORGANISM

A typical bacterium consists of a single cell with a protective wall. Some bacteria are aerobic (requiring oxygen) and are therefore more likely to infect surface areas such as the skin or respiratory tract. Others are anaerobic and multiply in oxygen-free surroundings such as the bowel or deep wounds. Bacteria can cause symptoms of disease in two principal ways: by releasing toxins that harm body cells and by provoking an inflammatory response in the infected tissues.

Viruses are smaller than bacteria and consist simply of a core of genetic material surrounded by a protein coat. A virus can multiply only in a living cell, by using the host tissue's replicating material.

Protozoa are single-celled parasites slightly bigger than bacteria. Many protozoa live in the human intestine and are harmless. However, other types cause malaria, sleeping sickness, and dysentery.

INFESTATIONS

Invasion by parasites living on the body (such as lice) or in the body (such as tapeworms) is known as infestation. Since the body lacks strong natural defences against infestation, antiparasitic treatment is necessary. Infestation is often associated with tropical climates and poor standards of hygiene.

WHAT CAN GO WRONG

Infectious diseases occur when the body is invaded by microbes. This may be caused by the body having little or no natural immunity to the invading organism, or the number of invading microbes being too great for the body's immune system to overcome. Serious infections can occur when the immune system does not function properly or when a disease weakens or destroys the immune system, as occurs in AIDS (acquired immune deficiency syndrome).

Infections (such as childhood infectious diseases or those with flulike symptoms) can cause generalized illness, or they may affect a specific part of the body (as in wound infections). Some parts are more susceptible to infection than others – respiratory tract infections are relatively common, whereas bone and muscle infections are rare.

Some symptoms are the result of damage to body tissues by the infection, or by toxins that are released by the microbes. In other cases, the symptoms result from the body's defence mechanisms.

Most bacterial and viral infections cause fever. Bacterial infections may also result in inflammation and pus in the affected area.

WHY DRUGS ARE USED

Treatment of an infection is necessary only when the type or severity of symptoms shows that the immune system has not overcome the infection.

Bacterial infection can be treated with antibiotic or antibacterial drugs. Some of these drugs kill infecting bacteria, while others prevent them from multiplying. Unnecessary use of antibiotics may lead to the development of resistant bacteria (see p.63).

Some antibiotics can be used to treat a broad range of infections, while others are effective against a particular type of bacterium or in a certain part of the body. Antibiotics are most commonly given by mouth, or by injection in severe infections, but they may be applied topically for a local action.

Antiviral drugs are used for severe viral infections that threaten body organs or survival. Antivirals may be used in topical preparations, given by mouth, or administered by injection, usually in hospital.

Other drugs used to fight infection include antiprotozoal drugs for protozoal infections such as malaria; antifungal drugs for infection by fungi and yeasts, including candida (thrush); and anthelmintics to eradicate worm and fluke infestations. Infestation by skin parasites is usually treated with the topical application of insecticides (see p.120).

MAJOR DRUG GROUPS

- Antibiotics
- Drugs for meningitis
- Antibacterial drugs
- Drug treatment for leprosy
- Antituberculous drugs
- Antiviral drugs
- Vaccines and immunization
- Antiprotozoal drugs
- Antimalarial drugs
- Antifungal drugs
- Anthelmintic drugs

Antibiotics

One in six prescriptions that British doctors write every year is for antibiotics. These drugs are usually safe and effective treatments for bacterial disorders ranging from minor infections, such as conjunctivitis, to life-threatening diseases like pneumonia, meningitis, and septicaemia. They are similar in function to the antibacterial drugs (see p.64), but the early antibiotics all had a natural origin in moulds and fungi, although most are now synthesized.

Since the 1940s, when penicillin was introduced, many different classes of antibiotic have been developed. Each one has a different chemical composition and is effective against a particular range of bacteria. None of them is effective against viral infections (see Antiviral drugs, p.67).

Some of the antibiotics have a broad spectrum of activity against a wide variety of bacteria. Others are used in the treatment of infection by only a few specific organisms. For a description of each common class of antibiotic, see Classes of antibiotic, p.62.

WHY THEY ARE USED

We are surrounded by bacteria – in the air we breathe, on the mucous membranes of our mouth and nose, on our skin, and in our intestines – but we are protected, most of the time, by our immunological defences. When these break down, or when bacteria already present migrate to a vulnerable new site, or when harmful bacteria not usually present invade the body, infectious disease sets in.

The bacteria multiply uncontrollably, destroying tissue, releasing toxins, and, in some cases, threatening to spread via the bloodstream to such vital organs as the heart, brain, lungs, and kidneys. The symptoms of infectious disease vary widely, depending on the site of infection and type of bacteria.

Confronted with a sick person and suspecting a bacterial infection, the doctor will need to identify the organism causing the disease before prescribing any drug. However, tests to analyse blood, sputum, urine, stool, or pus usually take 24 hours or more. In the meantime, especially if the person is in discomfort or pain, the doctor usually makes a preliminary drug choice, based on an educated guess as to the causative organism. In starting this empirical treatment, as it is called, the doctor is guided by the site of the infection, the nature and severity of the symptoms, the likely source of infection, and the prevalence of any similar illnesses in the community at that time.

In such circumstances, pending laboratory identification of the trouble-making bacteria, the doctor may initially prescribe a broad-spectrum antibiotic, which is effective against a wide variety of bacteria. As soon as tests provide more exact information, the doctor may switch the person to the recommended antibiotic treatment for the identified bacteria. In some cases, more than one antibiotic is prescribed, to be sure of eliminating all strains of bacteria.

In most cases, antibiotics can be given by mouth. However, in serious infections when high blood levels of the drug are needed

USES OF ANTIBIOTICS

The table below shows common drugs in each antibiotic class, used for infections in different parts of the body. (It is not intended as a guide to prescribing.) For comparison, some antibacterial drugs (p.64) are included under "sulfonamides" and "other drugs".

ANTIBIOTIC / SITE OF INFECTION	Ear, nose, throat, and mouth	Respiratory tract	Skin and soft tissue	Gastrointestinal tract	Eye	Kidney and urinary tract	Brain and nervous system	Heart and blood	Bones and joints	Genital tract
Penicillins										
Amoxicillin	●	●	●			●		●	●	
Ampicillin	●	●	●			●	●		●	
Benzylpenicillin	●	●	●				●	●		●
Co-amoxiclav	●	●	●			●				
Flucloxacillin	●		●					●	●	
Phenoxymethylpenicillin	●	●	●							
Cephalosporins										
Cefaclor	●	●				●				
Cefalexin		●	●			●				
Cefotaxime		●		●			●	●		
Macrolides										
Azithromycin	●	●	●							●
Clarithromycin	●	●	●	●						
Erythromycin	●	●	●	●	●				●	●
Tetracyclines										
Doxycycline	●	●	●			●				●
Oxytetracycline	●	●	●							
Tetracycline	●	●	●		●	●				●
Aminoglycosides										
Amikacin		●	●	●		●	●		●	
Gentamicin		●	●	●	●	●	●	●	●	
Neomycin			●	●						
Streptomycin		●						●		
Tobramycin		●	●	●		●	●		●	
Sulfonamide										
Co-trimoxazole		●				●				
Other drugs										
Chloramphenicol	●				●		●			
Ciprofloxacin		●		●	●	●				●
Clindamycin		●	●	●					●	
Colistin		●								
Dapsone			●							
Fusidic acid			●		●			●	●	
Levofloxacin	●	●	●			●				
Linezolid		●	●							
Metronidazole	●		●	●				●	●	●
Nalidixic acid						●				
Nitrofurantoin						●				
Teicoplanin			●					●	●	
Trimethoprim						●				
Vancomycin			●					●	●	

rapidly, or when a type of antibiotic is needed that cannot be given by mouth, the drug may be given by injection. Antibiotics are also included in topical preparations for localized skin, eye, and ear infections (see also Anti-infective skin preparations, p.119, and Drugs for ear disorders, p.115).

HOW THEY WORK

Depending on the type of drug and the dosage, antibiotics are either bactericidal, killing organisms directly, or bacteriostatic, halting the multiplication of bacteria and enabling the body's natural defences to overcome the remaining infection.

Penicillins and cephalosporins are bactericidal, destroying bacteria by preventing them from making normal cell walls; most other antibiotics act inside the bacteria by interfering with the chemical activities essential to their life cycle.

CLASSES OF ANTIBIOTIC

Penicillins First introduced in the 1940s, penicillins are still widely used to treat many common infections. Some penicillins are not effective when they are taken by mouth and therefore have to be given by injection in hospital. Unfortunately, certain strains of bacteria are resistant to penicillin treatment, and other drugs may have to be substituted.

Cephalosporins These are broad-spectrum antibiotics that are similar to the penicillins. Cephalosporins are often used when penicillin treatment has proved ineffective. Some of the cephalosporins can be given by mouth, but others are given only by injection. About 10 per cent of people who are allergic to penicillins may be allergic to cephalosporins. Some cephalosporins can occasionally damage the kidneys, particularly if they are used with aminoglycosides.

Macrolides Erythromycin is the most common drug in this group. This is a broad-spectrum antibiotic that is often prescribed as an alternative to penicillins or cephalosporins. Erythromycin is also effective against certain diseases, such as Legionnaires' disease (a rare type of pneumonia), that cannot be treated with other antibiotics. The main risk with erythromycin is that it can occasionally impair liver function.

Tetracyclines These have a broader spectrum of activity than other classes of antibiotic. Increasing bacterial resistance (see Antibiotic resistance, opposite) has limited their use, but they are still widely prescribed. As well as being used for the treatment of infections, tetracyclines are also used in the long-term treatment of acne, although this application is probably not entirely due to their antibacterial action. A major drawback to the use of tetracycline antibiotics in pregnant women and young children is that they are deposited in developing bones and teeth.

With the exception of doxycycline, drugs from this group are poorly absorbed through the intestines, and when given by mouth they have to be administered in high doses in order to reach effective levels in the blood. Such high doses increase the likelihood of diarrhoea as a side effect. The absorption of tetracyclines can be further reduced by interaction with calcium and other minerals. Drugs from this group should not therefore be taken with iron tablets or milk products.

Aminoglycosides These potent drugs are effective against a wide range of bacteria. They are not as widely used as some other antibiotics, however, since they have to be given by injection and have potentially serious side effects, especially on the kidneys and middle ear. Their use is therefore limited to hospital treatment of serious infections. They are often given with other antibiotics.

Lincosamides The lincosamide antibiotic clindamycin is not commonly used because it is more likely than other antibiotics to cause serious disruption of bacterial activity in the bowel. This drug is reserved mainly for treating bone, joint, abdominal, and pelvic infections that do not respond well to other antibiotics. It is also used topically for acne and vaginal infections.

Quinolones This group of drugs consists of nalidixic acid and substances chemically related to it, including the fluoroquinolones. Fluoroquinolones have a wide spectrum of activity. They are used to treat urinary infections and acute diarrhoeal diseases, including that caused by *Salmonella*, as well as in the treatment of enteric fever.

The absorption of quinolones is reduced by antacids containing magnesium and aluminium. Fluoroquinolones are generally well tolerated but may cause seizures in some people. These drugs are less frequently used in children because there is a theoretical risk of damage to the developing joints.

HOW THEY AFFECT YOU

Antibiotics stop most common types of infection within days. Because they do not relieve symptoms directly, your doctor may advise additional medication, such as analgesics (see p.7), to relieve pain and fever until the antibiotics take effect.

It is important to complete the course of medication as prescribed, even if all of your symptoms have disappeared. Failure to do this can lead to a resurgence of the infection in an antibiotic-resistant form (see Antibiotic resistance, below).

Most antibiotics used in the home do not cause any adverse effects if taken in the recommended dosage. In people who do experience adverse effects, nausea and diarrhoea are among the more common ones (see also individual drug profiles in Part 2). Some people may be hypersensitive to certain types of antibiotic, which can result in a variety of serious adverse effects.

ANTIBIOTIC RESISTANCE

The increasing use of antibiotics in the treatment of infection has led certain types of bacteria to become resistant to the effects of particular antibiotics. This resistance to the drug usually occurs when bacteria develop mechanisms of growth and reproduction that are not disrupted by the effects of the antibiotics. In other cases, bacteria produce enzymes that neutralize the antibiotics.

Antibiotic resistance may develop in a person during prolonged treatment when a drug has failed to eliminate the infection quickly. The resistant strain of bacteria is able to multiply, thereby prolonging the illness. It may also infect other people and result in the spread of resistant infection.

One particularly important example of a resistant strain of bacteria is methicillin-resistant *Staphylococcus aureus* (MRSA), which resists most antibiotics but can be treated with other drugs such as teicoplanin and vancomycin. Doctors try to prevent the development of antibiotic resistance by selecting the drug that is most likely to eliminate the bacteria present in each individual case as quickly and as thoroughly as possible. Failure to complete a course of antibiotics that has been prescribed by your doctor increases the likelihood that the infection will recur in a resistant form.

RISKS AND SPECIAL PRECAUTIONS

Most antibiotics used for short periods outside a hospital setting are safe for most people. The most common risk, particularly with cephalosporins and penicillins, is an allergic reaction that causes a rash. Very rarely, the reaction may be severe, causing swelling of the throat and face, breathing difficulty, and circulatory collapse – a potentially fatal condition called anaphylactic shock. If you have an allergic reaction, the drug should be stopped and immediate medical advice sought. If you have had a previous allergic reaction to an antibiotic, all other drugs in that class and related classes should be avoided. It is therefore important to tell your doctor if you have previously had an adverse reaction to an antibiotic (with the exception of minor bowel disturbances).

Another risk of antibiotic treatment, especially if prolonged, is that the balance among microorganisms normally inhabiting the body may be disturbed. In particular, antibiotics may destroy the bacteria that normally limit the growth of *Candida*, a yeast that is often present in the body in small amounts. This can lead to overgrowth of *Candida* (thrush) in the mouth, vagina, or bowel, and an antifungal drug (see p.74) may be needed.

A rarer, but more serious, result of disruption of normal bacterial activity in the body is a disorder known as pseudomembranous colitis, in which bacteria (called *Clostridium difficile*) resistant to the antibiotic multiply in the bowel, causing violent, bloody diarrhoea. This potentially fatal disorder can occur with any antibiotic, but is most common with cephalosporins and clindamycin.

COMMON DRUGS

Aminoglycosides Amikacin, Gentamicin*, Neomycin, Streptomycin, Tobramycin

Cephalosporins Cefaclor, Cefadroxil, Cefalexin*, Cefixime, Cefpodoxime, Ceftazidime
Tetracyclines Doxycycline*, Minocycline*, Oxytetracycline, Tetracycline/lymecycline*
Macrolides Azithromycin, Clarithromycin*, Erythromycin*
Penicillins Amoxicillin/co-amoxiclav*, Benzylpenicillin, Co-fluampicil, Flucloxacillin*, Phenoxymethylpenicillin*, Piperacillin/tazobactam
Lincosamides Clindamycin*
Other drugs Aztreonam, Chloramphenicol*, Ciprofloxacin*, Colistin, Fusidic acid, Imipenem, Levofloxacin*, Linezolid, Metronidazole*, Rifampicin*, Teicoplanin, Trimethoprim*, Vancomycin
* **See Part 2**

Drugs for meningitis

Meningitis is inflammation of the meninges (the membranes surrounding the brain and spinal cord). This infection can be caused by both bacteria and viruses. Bacterial meningitis can kill previously well individuals in a matter of hours.

If bacterial meningitis is suspected, intramuscular or intravenous antibiotics will be needed immediately, and admission to hospital is arranged.

In cases of bacterial meningitis caused by *Haemophilus influenzae* or *Neisseria meningitidis*, people who have been in contact with an infected person are advised to have a preventative course of antibiotics, usually rifampicin (see p.386) or ciprofloxacin (see p.183).

Antibacterial drugs

This broad classification of drugs comprises agents that are similar to antibiotics (p.60) in function but dissimilar in origin. The original antibiotics were derived from living organisms such as moulds and fungi. Antibacterial drugs were developed from chemicals. The sulfonamides were the first drugs to be given for the treatment of bacterial infections, and they provided the mainstay of the treatment of infection before penicillin (the first antibiotic) became generally available. Increasing bacterial resistance and the development of antibiotics that are more effective and less toxic have reduced the use of sulfonamides.

WHY THEY ARE USED

Sulfonamides are less commonly used these days; the sulfonamide drug co-trimoxazole is reserved for rare cases of pneumonia in immunocompromised patients.

Trimethoprim is used to treat chest and urinary tract infections. The drug used to be combined with sulfamethoxazole as co-trimoxazole, but because of the side effects of sulfamethoxazole, trimethoprim on its own is usually preferred now.

Antibacterials used for tuberculosis are discussed on p.65. Other types of antibacterial sometimes classified as antimicrobials include metronidazole, which is used for a variety of genital infections and some serious infections of the abdomen, pelvic region, heart, and central nervous system. Other antibacterials are used to treat urinary infections. These include nitrofurantoin and quinolones (see Classes of antibiotic, p.62) such as nalidixic acid, which can be used to cure or prevent recurrent infections.

The quinolones are effective against a broad spectrum of bacteria. More potent relatives of nalidixic acid include norfloxacin, which is used to treat urinary tract infections, and ciprofloxacin, levofloxacin, and ofloxacin. These are all also used to treat many serious bacterial infections.

HOW THEY WORK

Most antibacterials act by preventing growth and multiplication of bacteria. For example, folic acid, a chemical necessary for the growth of bacteria, is produced in bacterial cells by an enzyme that acts on a chemical called para-aminobenzoic acid. Sulfonamides interfere with release of the enzyme, stopping folic acid from being formed, so the bacterium cannot function properly and dies.

HOW THEY AFFECT YOU

Antibacterials usually take several days to eliminate bacteria. During this time your doctor may recommend additional medication to alleviate pain and fever. Possible side effects of sulfonamides include loss of appetite, nausea, a rash, and drowsiness.

RISKS AND SPECIAL PRECAUTIONS

Like antibiotics, most antibacterials can cause allergic reactions in susceptible people. Possible symptoms that should always be brought to a doctor's attention include rashes and fever. If such symptoms occur, a change to another drug is likely to be necessary.

Treatment with sulfonamides carries a number of serious but uncommon risks. Some drugs in this group can cause crystals to form in the kidneys, a risk that can be reduced by drinking adequate amounts of fluid during prolonged treatment. Because sulfonamides may also occasionally damage the liver, they are not usually prescribed for people with impaired liver function. These drugs are also less frequently used in children because there is a theoretical risk of damage to the developing joints.

COMMON DRUGS

Quinolones Ciprofloxacin*, Levofloxacin*, Moxifloxacin, Nalidixic acid, Norfloxacin, Ofloxacin
Sulfonamides Co-trimoxazole*, Sulfadiazine
Other drugs Clofazimine, Dapsone, Daptomycin, Linezolid, Metronidazole*, Nitrofurantoin, Thalidomide*, Tinidazole, Trimethoprim*
* **See Part 2**

Drug treatment for leprosy

Leprosy, also known as Hansen's disease, is a bacterial infection caused by *Mycobacterium leprae*. It is rare in the United Kingdom but relatively common in parts of Africa, Asia, and Latin America.

Hansen's disease progresses slowly, first affecting the peripheral nerves and causing loss of sensation in the hands and feet. This leads to frequent unnoticed injuries and consequent scarring. Later, the nerves of the face may also be affected.

Treatment involves the use of three drugs together to prevent resistance from developing. Usually, dapsone, rifampicin, and clofazimine will be given for at least 2 years. If one of these drugs cannot be used, then a second-line drug (ofloxacin, minocycline, or clarithromycin) might be substituted. Complications during treatment may require the use of prednisolone, aspirin, chloroquine, or even thalidomide.

Antituberculous drugs

Tuberculosis is an infectious bacterial disease acquired, often in childhood, by inhaling the tuberculosis bacilli present in the spray of a sneeze or cough from an actively infected person. It may also, rarely, be acquired from infected unpasteurized cow's milk. The disease usually starts in a lung and takes one of two forms: primary or reactivated infection.

In 90 to 95 per cent of those with a primary infection, the body's immune system suppresses the infection but does not kill the bacilli. The infection is said to be latent and the dormant bacilli can be reactivated. After they are reactivated, the tuberculosis bacilli may spread via the lymphatic system and bloodstream throughout the body.

The first symptoms of primary infection may include a cough, fever, tiredness, night sweats, and weight loss. Tuberculosis is confirmed through clinical investigations, which may include a chest X-ray, isolation of the bacilli from the person's sputum, and a positive reaction – localized inflammation – to a skin test in which tuberculin, a protein extracted from tuberculosis bacilli, is injected into the skin.

In adults, the gradual emergence of the destructive and progressive form of tuberculosis is caused by the reactivated infection. It occurs in 5 to 10 per cent of those who have had a previous primary infection. Another form, reinfection tuberculosis, occurs when someone with the dormant primary form is reinfected. This type of tuberculosis is clinically identical to the reactivated form.

Reactivation tuberculosis is more likely in people whose immune system is suppressed, such as older adults, those taking corticosteroids or other immunosuppressants, patients receiving anti-tumour necrosis factor (anti-TNF) drugs such as infliximab, and those with AIDS. Reactivation may start in any part of the body seeded with the bacilli. It is most often first seen in the upper lobes of the lung, and is frequently diagnosed after a chest X-ray. The early symptoms may be identical to those of the primary infection: a cough, tiredness, night sweats, fever, and weight loss.

If it is left untreated, tuberculosis continues to destroy tissue, spreading throughout the body and eventually causing death. It was one of the most common causes of death in the United Kingdom until the 1940s, but the disease is now on the increase again worldwide. Vulnerable groups are homeless people and those with suppressed immune systems.

WHY THEY ARE USED

A person diagnosed as having tuberculosis is likely to be treated with three or four antituberculous drugs. This helps to overcome the risk of drug-resistant strains of the bacilli emerging (see Antibiotic resistance, p.63).

The standard drug combination comprises rifampicin, isoniazid, pyrazinamide, and ethambutol. However, other drugs may be substituted if the initial treatment fails or if drug sensitivity tests indicate that the bacilli are resistant to these drugs.

The standard duration of treatment for a newly diagnosed tuberculosis infection is a 6-month regimen as follows: isoniazid, rifampicin, pyrazinamide, and ethambutol daily for 2 months, followed by isoniazid and rifampicin daily for 4 months. The duration of treatment can be extended from 9 months to up to 2 years in people at particular risk, such as those with a suppressed immune system or those in whom tuberculosis has infected the central nervous system.

Corticosteroids may be added to the treatment, if the patient does not have a suppressed immune system, to reduce the amount of tissue damage.

Both the number of drugs required and the long duration of treatment may make treatment difficult, particularly for those who are homeless. To help with this problem, supervised administration of treatment is available when required, both in the community and in hospital.

Tuberculosis in patients with HIV infection or AIDS is treated with the standard antituberculous drug regimen; however, lifelong preventative treatment with isoniazid may be necessary.

HOW THEY WORK

Antituberculous drugs act in the same way as other antibiotics, either by killing bacilli or by preventing them from multiplying. (See also Antibiotics, p.60).

HOW THEY AFFECT YOU

The drugs start to combat the disease within days, but benefits are not usually noticeable for a few weeks. As the infection is eradicated, the body repairs the damage caused by the disease. Symptoms gradually subside, and appetite and general health improve.

RISKS AND SPECIAL PRECAUTIONS

Antituberculous drugs may cause nausea, vomiting, and abdominal pain and occasionally lead to serious allergic reactions. When this happens, another drug is substituted.

Rifampicin and isoniazid may affect liver function; isoniazid may adversely affect the nerves as well. Ethambutol can cause changes in colour vision. Dosage is carefully monitored, especially in children, older adults, and people with reduced kidney function.

TUBERCULOSIS PREVENTION

A vaccine prepared from an artificially weakened strain of cattle tuberculosis bacteria can provide immunity from tuberculosis by provoking the development of natural resistance to the disease (see Vaccines and immunization, p.68). The BCG (Bacille Calmette-Guérin) vaccine is a form of tuberculosis bacillus that provokes the body's immune response but does not cause the illness because it is not infectious. The vaccine is no longer given as part of the routine immunization schedule but is offered to certain high-risk groups, for example newborn babies in areas where there is a high rate of tuberculosis.

The vaccine is usually injected into the upper arm. A small pustule usually appears 6 to 12 weeks later, by which time the person can be considered immune.

COMMON DRUGS

Amikacin, Capreomycin, Ciprofloxacin*, Clarithromycin*, Cycloserine, Ethambutol*, Isoniazid*, Pyrazinamide, Rifabutin, Rifampicin*, Streptomycin

* **See Part 2**

Antiviral drugs

Viruses are simpler and smaller organisms than bacteria and are less able to sustain themselves. These organisms can survive and multiply only by penetrating body cells. Because viruses perform few functions independently, medicines that disrupt or halt their life cycle without harming human cells have been difficult to develop.

There are many different types of virus, and viral infections cause illnesses with various symptoms and degrees of severity. Common viral illnesses include colds, influenza and flulike illnesses, cold sores, and childhood diseases such as chickenpox, mumps, and measles. Throat infections, pneumonia, acute bronchitis, gastroenteritis, and meningitis are often, but not always, due to a virus.

Fortunately, the body's natural defences are usually strong enough to overcome infections such as these, with drugs given to ease pain and lower fever. However, more serious viral diseases, such as pneumonia and meningitis, need close medical supervision.

Another difficulty with viral infections is the speed with which the virus multiplies. By the time symptoms appear, the viruses are so numerous that antiviral drugs have little effect. Antiviral agents must be given early in the course of a viral infection. They may also be used prophylactically (as a preventative). Some viral infections can be prevented by vaccination (see p.68).

WHY THEY ARE USED

Antiviral drugs are helpful in the treatment of various conditions caused by the herpes virus: cold sores, encephalitis, genital herpes, chickenpox, and shingles.

Aciclovir and penciclovir are applied topically to treat outbreaks of cold sores, herpes eye infections, and genital herpes. They can reduce the severity and duration of an outbreak, but they do not eliminate the infection permanently.

Aciclovir, famciclovir, and valaciclovir are given by mouth, or in exceptional circumstances by injection, to prevent chickenpox or severe, recurrent attacks of herpes virus infections in those people who are already weakened by other conditions.

Influenza may sometimes be prevented or treated using oseltamivir or zanamivir. Oseltamivir may also be used to treat the symptoms of influenza in at-risk people, such as those over 65 or people with respiratory diseases such as chronic obstructive pulmonary disease (COPD) or asthma, cardiovascular disease, kidney disease, immunosuppression, or diabetes mellitus.

Interferons are proteins produced by the body and involved in the immune response. Interferon is effective in reducing the activity of hepatitis B and hepatitis C. Hepatitis B replication can be controlled with tenofovir, and hepatitis C can be cured in most cases by antivirals such as ledipasvir and sofosbuvir.

Ganciclovir is sometimes used for cytomegalovirus (CMV). Respiratory syncytial virus (RSV) has been treated with ribavirin, and prevented by palivizumab. Drug treatment for AIDS is discussed on p.98.

HOW THEY WORK

Some antiviral drugs act by altering the building blocks for the cells' genetic material (DNA), so that the virus cannot multiply. Others stop viruses multiplying by blocking enzyme activity within the host cell. Halting multiplication prevents the virus from spreading to uninfected cells and improves symptoms rapidly. However, in herpes infections, it does not eradicate the virus from the body. Infection may therefore flare up again in the future.

HOW THEY AFFECT YOU

Topical antiviral drugs usually start to act immediately. Provided that the treatment is applied early enough, an outbreak of herpes can be cut short. Symptoms usually clear up within 2 to 4 days.

Antiviral ointments may cause irritation and redness. Antiviral drugs given by mouth or injection can occasionally cause nausea and dizziness.

RISKS AND SPECIAL PRECAUTIONS

Because some of these drugs may affect the kidneys adversely, they are prescribed with caution to people with reduced kidney function. Some antivirals can adversely affect the activity of normal body cells, particularly in the bone marrow. For this reason, the drug idoxuridine is available only for topical use.

COMMON DRUGS

Aciclovir*, Amantadine, Cidofovir, Daclatasvir, Famciclovir, Foscarnet, Ganciclovir, Inosine pranobex, Ledipasvir, Oseltamivir*, Palivizumab, Peginterferon alfa, Penciclovir, Ribavirin, Sofosbuvir, Tenofovir*, Valaciclovir, Valganciclovir, Zanamivir, Zidovudine/ lamivudine*

* **See Part 2**

See also Drugs for HIV, p.98

Vaccines and immunization

Many infectious diseases, including most common viral infections, occur only once during a person's lifetime. This is because the antibodies produced in response to the disease remain in the body afterwards, prepared to combat any future invasion by the infectious organisms. The duration of such immunity varies, but it can last a lifetime.

Protection against many infections can be provided artificially by using vaccines derived from altered forms of the infecting organism. These vaccines stimulate the immune system in the same way as a genuine infection, and provide lasting, active immunity. Because each type of microbe stimulates the production of a specific antibody, a different vaccine must be given for each disease.

Another type of immunization, called passive immunization, relies on giving antibodies (see Immunoglobulins, p.70).

WHY THEY ARE USED

Some infectious diseases cannot be treated effectively or are potentially so serious that prevention is the best course of action. Routine immunization not only protects the individual but may gradually eradicate the disease completely from a population, as has been the case with smallpox.

Newborn babies receive antibodies for many diseases from their mothers, but this protection lasts only for about 3 months. Most children are vaccinated against a range of common childhood infectious diseases. Additionally, travellers are advised to be vaccinated against diseases common in the areas they are visiting.

Effective lifelong immunization can sometimes be achieved by a single dose of the vaccine. However, in many cases, reinforcing doses (boosters) are needed later to maintain reliable immunity.

Vaccines do not provide immediate protection, and it may be up to 4 weeks before full immunity develops. When immediate protection is needed, it may be necessary to establish passive immunity with immunoglobulins (see p.70).

HOW THEY WORK

Vaccines provoke the immune system into creating antibodies that help the body to resist specific infectious diseases. Some vaccines (live vaccines) are made from artificially weakened forms of the disease-causing organism. Others rely on inactive (or killed) disease-causing organisms, or inactive derivatives of those organisms. Whatever their type, all vaccines stimulate antibody production and establish active immunity.

HOW THEY AFFECT YOU

The degree of protection varies among different vaccines. Some provide reliable lifelong immunity; others may not give full protection against a disease, or the effects may last for as little as 6 months. Influenza vaccines usually protect only against the strains of virus causing the latest outbreaks of flu.

Any vaccine may cause side effects, but they are usually mild and soon disappear. The most common reactions are a red, slightly raised, tender area at the site of injection, and a slight fever or a flulike illness lasting for 1 or 2 days.

RISKS AND SPECIAL PRECAUTIONS

Serious reactions are rare, and for most people the risk is far outweighed by the protection given. A family or personal history of seizures is not necessarily a contraindication to immunization, but immunization may be delayed if the condition is unstable. Children with any infection more severe than a common cold will not be given any routine vaccination until they have recovered.

COMMON VACCINATIONS

INFECTION	HOW GIVEN	AGE/TO WHOM GIVEN
Diphtheria/tetanus/pertussis/polio/ *Haemophilus influenzae* type b (Hib), hepatitis B (DTaP/IPV/Hib HepB) **Pneumococcal infection (PCV – pneumococcal conjugate vaccine)** **Rotavirus infection** **Meningitis B (MenB)**	1 injection 1 injection 1 oral dose 1 injection	8 weeks.
Diphtheria/tetanus/pertussis/polio/ Hib/hepatitis B (DTaP/IPV/Hib/HepB) **Rotavirus infection**	1 injection 1 oral dose	12 weeks.
Diphtheria/tetanus/pertussis/polio/ Hib/hepatitis B (DTaP/IPV/Hib/HepB) **Pneumococcal infection (PCV)** **Meningitis B (MenB)**	1 injection 1 injection 1 injection	16 weeks.
Hib/meningitis C (Hib/MenC) **Measles/mumps/rubella (MMR)** **Pneumococcal infection (PCV)** **Meningitis B (MenB)**	1 injection 1 injection 1 injection 1 injection	1 year.
Childhood influenza	1 dose of nasal spray	2–8 years (annually). Also offered annually to those aged 2–17 years who are at risk due to long-term health conditions.
Diphtheria/tetanus/pertussis/ polio (DTaP/IPV or dTaP/IPV) **Measles/mumps/rubella (MMR)**	1 injection 1 injection	3 years 4 months or soon after.
Human papillomavirus (HPV)	2 injections, 6–24 months apart	12–13 years (girls only).
Meningitis A, C, W, and Y (MenACWY) **Diphtheria/tetanus/polio (Td/IPV)**	1 injection 1 injection	14 years.
Influenza	1 injection	Offered routinely from the age of 65. Also offered to pregnant women, at-risk babies aged 6 months to 2 years, and at-risk adults over 18.
Pneumococcal infection (PPV – pneumococcal polysaccharide vaccine)	1 injection	Single dose offered to those aged 65 or over. Also offered to those at risk due to health problems, including children who cannot have the PCV vaccine.
Shingles	1 injection	Single dose offered to those aged 70–79.
Tuberculosis	1 injection	Infants and children at high risk of contracting TB or who have recently arrived from an area with a high level of TB; unimmunized people under 35 in certain high-risk groups (e.g. some health-care workers).
Chickenpox	2 injections, 4–8 weeks apart	Recommended for non-immune people in close contact with those at risk of serious illness from chickenpox.

Live vaccines should not be given during pregnancy, because they may affect a developing baby, nor should they be given to people whose immune systems are weakened. Those taking high doses of corticosteroids are advised to delay vaccinations until the end of drug treatment.

The risk of fever following the DTaP/IPV/Hib/HepB (diphtheria, tetanus, acellular pertussis, inactivated polio, *Haemophilus influenzae* type b, and hepatitis B) vaccine can be reduced by giving paracetamol at the time of the vaccination. The pertussis vaccine may rarely cause a mild seizure, which is brief, usually associated with fever, and stops without treatment. Children who have experienced such seizures recover completely.

IMMUNOGLOBULINS

Antibodies, which can result from exposure to snake and insect venom as well as infectious disease, are carried around the body in the serum of the blood (the fluid part that remains after the red cells and clotting agents are removed). The concentrated serum of people who have survived diseases or poisonous bites is called immunoglobulin. Given by injection, it creates passive immunity. Immunoglobulins may be obtained from human donors or extracted from horse blood following repeated doses of the toxin.

Because immunoglobulins do not stimulate the body to produce its own antibodies, continued protection requires repeated injections of immunoglobulins.

Adverse effects from immunoglobulins are uncommon. Some people are sensitive to horse globulins, and about a week after the injection they may experience a reaction known as serum sickness, in which they have fever, a rash, joint swelling, and pain. Serum sickness usually ends in a few days but should be reported to your doctor before any further immunization.

TRAVEL VACCINATIONS

Vaccinations are not normally necessary for travel to western Europe, North America, Australia, or New Zealand (although you should make sure that your tetanus and poliomyelitis boosters are up to date). However, you should consult your doctor if you are visiting other destinations. If you are taking children, make sure that they have had the full set of childhood vaccinations as well as any vaccinations needed for the areas in which you will be travelling.

If you are visiting an area where there is yellow fever, you will need an International Certificate of Vaccination. Many countries also require an International Certificate of Vaccination if you have already been to a country where yellow fever is present.

Other infectious diseases are a risk in many parts of the world, and appropriate vaccinations are a wise precaution. For example, visitors to Saudi Arabia, especially for the Hajj or Umrah pilgrimages, may be required to have had the meningitis A, C, W135, and Y (now called the MenACWY) vaccine beforehand.

If you are planning to stay for a long time or you are backpacking, additional vaccinations may be advisable – for example, hepatitis A, hepatitis B, BCG (tuberculosis), and possibly rabies.

All immunizations should be completed well before departure as the vaccinations do not give instant protection, and some need more than one dose to be effective. The NHS website gives travel health advice (www.nhs.uk/conditions/travelvaccinations), including vaccination advice as well as information about specific health hazards such as malaria.

Antiprotozoal drugs

Protozoa are single-celled organisms that are present in soil and water. They may be transmitted to or between humans via contaminated food or water, sexual contact, or insect bites. There are many types of protozoal infection, each of which causes a different disease depending on the organism involved. Trichomoniasis, toxoplasmosis, cryptosporidium, giardiasis, and pneumocystis pneumonia are probably the most common protozoal infections seen in the United Kingdom. The rarer infections are usually contracted as a result of exposure to infection in another part of the world.

Many types of protozoa infect the bowel, causing diarrhoea and generalized symptoms of ill-health. Others may infect the

TRAVEL IMMUNIZATIONS

Recommended immunizations depend on the part of the world you plan to visit. Wherever you intend to go, make sure that you have been immunized against diphtheria, tetanus, and polio and have had boosters if necessary. Advice on immunization may change; ask your doctor or travel clinic for up-to-date information. The recommendations here are for adults; consult your doctor about travel immunizations for children.

DISEASE	NUMBER OF DOSES	WHEN EFFECTIVE	PERIOD OF PROTECTION	WHO SHOULD BE IMMUNIZED
Cholera	2 oral doses, 1–6 weeks apart	1 week after 2nd dose	Up to 2 years	People travelling to areas where cholera is endemic or epidemic. Vaccination does not provide complete protection; it is also crucial to pay scrupulous attention to food, water, and personal hygiene.
Hepatitis A	2 injections 6–12 months apart	2 weeks after 1st dose	1st dose protects for 1 year; 2nd for at least 20 years	Travellers to high-risk areas outside northern and western Europe, North America, Australia, New Zealand, and Japan.
Hepatitis B	3 injections, over a period of 3 weeks to 6 months	After 3rd dose	At least 5 years	People travelling to countries in which hepatitis B is prevalent and who might need medical or dental treatment and/or are likely to have unprotected sex.
Japanese encephalitis	2 injections 28 days apart	About 1 week after 2nd dose	1–2 years	People staying for an extended period in rural areas where the disease is prevalent, including the Indian subcontinent, China, Southeast Asia, and the Far East.
Meningitis A, C, W135, and Y (MenACWY)	1 injection	After 2–3 weeks	About 5 years	People travelling to sub-Saharan Africa and parts of Saudi Arabia. Immunization certificate needed if travelling to Saudi Arabia for the Hajj and Umrah pilgramages.
Rabies	3 injections. 1 week between 1st and 2nd doses, 2 or 3 weeks between 2nd and 3rd doses	After 3rd dose	Those at continued risk: 1 year; boosters protect for 3–5 years. Travellers: about 10 years	Travellers to areas where rabies is endemic, particularly those at high risk (e.g. veterinary surgeons) and/or those travelling to areas with limited medical facilities. The vaccine may also be given after rabies exposure.
Typhoid	1 injection or 3 oral doses, each dose on an alternate day	2 weeks after injection, or 7–10 days after last oral dose	Injection: about 3 years. Oral vaccine: about 1 year	People travelling to areas with poor sanitation and hygiene, especially those at high risk of infection (e.g. aid workers in disaster areas). Scrupulous attention to personal hygiene is also important.
Yellow fever	1 injection	After 10 days	At least 10 years	Yellow fever vaccination is compulsory for entry to some countries and advisable for others within yellow fever zones. May also be needed when travelling from yellow fever zones.

genital tract or skin. Some protozoa may penetrate vital organs such as the lungs, brain, and liver. Prompt diagnosis and treatment are important in order to limit the spread of the infection within the body and, in some cases, prevent it from spreading to other people. Increased attention to hygiene is an important factor in controlling the spread of the disease.

A variety of medicines is used in the treatment of these diseases. Some, such as metronidazole and tetracycline, are also commonly used for their antibacterial action (see p.64). Others, such as pentamidine, are rarely used except to treat specific protozoal infections.

HOW THEY AFFECT YOU

Protozoa are often difficult to eradicate from the body. Drug treatment may therefore need to be continued for several months in order to eliminate the infecting organisms completely and thus prevent recurrence of the disease. In addition, unpleasant side effects such as nausea, diarrhoea, and abdominal cramps are often unavoidable because of the limited choice of drugs and the need to maintain dosage levels that will effectively cure the disease. For detailed information on the risks and adverse effects of individual antiprotozoals, consult the appropriate drug profile in Part 2.

TYPES OF PROTOZOAL DISEASE

Amoebiasis *(Entamoeba histolytica)*, or amoebic dysentery, is an infection of the bowel (and sometimes the liver and other organs) usually transmitted in contaminated food or water. Its major symptom is violent, sometimes bloody, diarrhoea. Treatment is with diloxanide, metronidazole, or tinidazole.

Balantidiasis *(Balantidium coli)* is an infection of the bowel, specifically the colon, that is usually transmitted through contact with infected pigs. Possible symptoms include diarrhoea and abdominal pain. Treatment of the infection is with tetracycline, metronidazole, or di-iodohydroxyquinoline.

Cryptosporidiosis *(Cryptosporidium)* affects the bowel (and occasionally the respiratory tract and bile ducts). Cryptosporidiosis is spread through contaminated food or water or by contact with animals or other humans. Symptoms include diarrhoea and abdominal pain. There are no specific drugs to treat it, but paromomycin, azithromycin, or eflornithine may be effective.

Giardiasis *(Giardia lamblia)*, or lambliasis, affects the bowel. It is usually transmitted in contaminated food or water, but it may also be spread by some types of sexual contact. Major symptoms are general ill-health, diarrhoea, flatulence, and abdominal pain. Treatment is with metronidazole or tinidazole.

Leishmaniasis *(Leishmania)* is a mainly tropical and subtropical disease caused by organisms spread through sandfly bites. It affects the mucous membranes of the mouth, nose, and throat and may, in its severe form, invade organs such as the liver. Treatment is with paromomycin, sodium stibogluconate, pentamidine, or amphotericin.

Pneumocystis pneumonia *(Pneumocystis jirovecii)* is a potentially fatal lung infection usually affecting only people with reduced resistance to infection, such as those who are HIV positive. Symptoms include fever, cough, breathlessness, and chest pain. Treatment is with drugs such as atovaquone, co-trimoxazole, pentamidine, and dapsone with trimethoprim.

Toxoplasmosis *(Toxoplasma gondii)* is usually spread via cat faeces or by eating undercooked meat. Although usually symptomless, toxoplasmosis may cause generalized ill-health, mild fever, and eye inflammation. Treatment is necessary only if the eyes are involved or the patient is immunosuppressed (as in HIV). It may also pass from mother to baby during pregnancy, leading to severe disease in the fetus. Treatment is usually with pyrimethamine with sulfadiazine, or with azithromycin, clarithromycin, or clindamycin/spiramycin (during pregnancy).

Trichomoniasis *(Trichomonas vaginalis)* most often affects the vagina, causing irritation and an offensive discharge. In men, it may occur in the urethra. It is usually sexually transmitted. Treatment is with metronidazole or tinidazole.

Trypanosomiasis *(Trypanosoma)*, also known as African trypanosomiasis (sleeping sickness), is spread by the tsetse fly and causes fever, swollen glands, and drowsiness. South American trypanosomiasis (Chagas' disease) is spread by assassin bugs and causes inflammation, enlargement of internal organs, and infection of the brain. Sleeping sickness is treated with pentamidine, suramin, eflornithine, or melarsoprol. Chagas' disease is treated with primaquine or nifurtimox.

Antimalarial drugs

Malaria is one of the main killing diseases in the tropics. It is most likely to affect people who live in or travel to such places.

The disease is caused by protozoa (see p.70) whose life cycle is far from simple. The malaria parasite, called *Plasmodium*, lives in and depends on the female *Anopheles* mosquito during one part of its life cycle. It lives in and depends on human beings during other parts of its life cycle.

Transferred to humans in the saliva of the female mosquito as she penetrates ("bites") the skin, the malaria parasite enters the bloodstream and settles in the liver, where it multiplies asexually.

Following its stay in the liver, the parasite (or plasmodium) enters another phase of its life cycle, circulating in the bloodstream, penetrating and destroying red blood cells, and reproducing again. If the plasmodia then transfer back to a female *Anopheles* mosquito via another "bite", they breed sexually, and are again ready to start a human infection.

Following the emergence of plasmodia from the liver, the symptoms of malaria occur: episodes of high fever and profuse sweating alternate with equally agonizing episodes of shivering and chills. One of the four strains of malaria (*Plasmodium falciparum*) can produce a single severe attack that can be fatal unless treated. The others cause recurrent attacks, sometimes extending over many years.

A number of drugs are available for prevention of malaria; the choice depends on the region in which the disease can be contracted and the resistance to the commonly used drugs (see below). In most areas, *Plasmodium falciparum* is resistant to chloroquine. In all regions, four drugs are commonly used for treating malaria: quinine, mefloquine, Malarone (a brand-name drug containing the antimalarials proguanil with atovaquone), and Riamet (a brand-name drug containing the antimalarials artemether with lumefantrine).

PREVENTION OF MALARIA

Malaria is found in more than 100 countries across the world, mainly in tropical and subtropical regions. The vast majority of cases (over 90%) occur in Africa, but the disease also occurs in Southeast Asia and the eastern Mediterranean countries, as well as in India, China, Central America, and northern South America. Babies, children under 5 years, pregnant women, and immunocompromised people (particularly those with HIV/AIDS) are most at risk of infection with malaria and of developing severe symptoms. The incidence of malaria is declining, but drug resistance has become a problem. Such resistance may be countered by giving combinations of drugs, such as proguanil with atovaquone.

There are two preventative regimens, which differ according to the area to be visited (low risk or high risk). However, prevalent strains of malaria change very rapidly, and the risk may vary in different areas and/or countries. Consequently, recommendations for prevention change frequently and **you must always seek specific medical advice before travelling.**

Low risk Preventative drugs not usually advised but mosquito bites should be avoided.
High risk Proguanil with atovaquone (Malarone), or doxycycline, or mefloquine.

In addition, these websites also provide information about malaria prevention:
www.fitfortravel.nhs.uk/advice/malaria
bnf.nice.org.uk/treatment-summary/malaria-prophylaxis.html
www.cdc.gov/malaria/travelers/country_table/a.html
www.who.int/malaria/travellers/en

WHY THEY ARE USED

The medical response to malaria takes three forms: prevention, treatment of attacks, and the complete eradication of the plasmodia (radical cure).

For someone planning a trip to an area where malaria is prevalent, drugs are given that destroy the parasites as they enter the liver. This preventative treatment needs to start up to 3 weeks before departure and continue for 1 to 4 weeks after returning from the area (the exact timings depend on the drugs taken).

Drugs such as mefloquine and Riamet can produce a radical cure, but chloroquine does not. After chloroquine treatment of non-falciparum malaria, a 14- to 21-day course of primaquine is administered. The drug is highly effective in destroying plasmodia in the liver but is weak against plasmodia in the blood. Primaquine is recommended only after a person has left the malarial area because of the high risk of re-infection.

HOW THEY WORK

When taken to prevent the disease, the drugs kill the plasmodia in the liver, preventing them from multiplying. Once the plasmodia have multiplied, the same drugs may be used in higher doses to kill plasmodia that re-enter the bloodstream. If these drugs are not effective, primaquine may be used to destroy any plasmodia that are still present in the liver.

HOW THEY AFFECT YOU

The low doses of antimalarial drugs taken for prevention rarely produce noticeable effects. Drugs taken for an attack usually begin to relieve symptoms within a few hours. Most of them can cause nausea, vomiting, and diarrhoea. Quinine can cause disturbances in vision and hearing. Mefloquine can cause sleep disturbance, dizziness, and difficulties in coordination.

RISKS AND SPECIAL PRECAUTIONS

When drugs are given for malaria, the full course must be taken. No drugs give long-term protection; a new course of treatment is needed for each journey.

Most of these drugs do not produce severe adverse effects, but primaquine can cause the blood disorder haemolytic anaemia, particularly in people with glucose-6-phosphate dehydrogenase (G6PD) deficiency. Blood tests are taken before treatment to identify susceptible individuals. Mefloquine is not prescribed for those who have had psychological disorders or seizures.

OTHER PROTECTIVE MEASURES

Because *Plasmodium* strains continually develop resistance to the available drugs, prevention using drugs is not absolutely reliable. Protection from mosquito bites is of the highest priority. Such protection includes the use of insect repellents and mosquito nets impregnated with permethrin insecticide, as well as covering any exposed skin after dark.

COMMON DRUGS

Drugs for prevention Chloroquine*, Doxycycline*, Mefloquine*, Proguanil, Proguanil with atovaquone (Malarone)*

Drugs for treatment Artemether with lumefantrine (Riamet), Chloroquine*, Mefloquine*, Primaquine, Proguanil with atovaquone (Malarone)*, Pyrimethamine with sulfadoxine*, Quinine*

* **See Part 2**

Antifungal drugs

We are continually exposed to fungi in the air and in food and water. Most species cannot live in the body, and few are harmful. However, some can grow in the mouth, skin, hair, or nails, causing irritating or unsightly changes, and a few can cause serious and possibly fatal disease. The most common fungal infections are caused by the tinea group. They include tinea pedis (athlete's foot), tinea cruris (jock itch), tinea corporis (ringworm), and tinea capitis (scalp ringworm). Caused by a variety of organisms, they are spread by direct or indirect contact with infected humans or animals. Infection is encouraged by warm, moist conditions.

Problems may also result from the proliferation of a fungus normally present in the body; the most common example is excessive growth of *Candida*, a yeast that causes thrush infection of the mouth, vagina, and bowel. It can also infect other organs if it spreads through the body via the bloodstream. Overgrowth of *Candida* may occur in people taking antibiotics (see p.60) or oral contraceptives (see p.103), in pregnant women, or in those with diabetes or immune system disorders such as HIV.

Superficial fungal infections (those that attack only the outer layer of the skin and mucous membranes) are relatively common and, although irritating, do not usually present a threat to general health. Internal fungal infections (for example, of the lungs, heart, or other organs) are very rare, but may be serious and prolonged.

Because antibiotics and other antibacterial drugs have no effect on fungi and yeasts, a different type of drug is needed. Drugs for fungal infections are either applied topically to treat minor infections of the skin, nails, and mucous membranes or given by mouth or injection to eliminate serious fungal infections of the internal organs and nails.

WHY THEY ARE USED

Drug treatment is necessary for most fungal infections since they rarely improve alone. Measures such as careful washing and drying of affected areas may help but are not a substitute for antifungal drugs. The use of over-the-counter preparations to increase the acidity of the vagina is not usually effective except if accompanied by drug treatment.

Fungal infections of the skin and scalp are usually treated with a cream or shampoo. Drugs for vaginal thrush are most often applied in the form of vaginal pessaries or cream applied with a special applicator. For very severe or persistent vaginal infections, a short course of fluconazole or itraconazole may be given by mouth. Mouth infections are usually eliminated by lozenges dissolved in the mouth or an antifungal solution or gel applied to the affected areas. For severe or persistent nail infections, griseofulvin or terbinafine are given by mouth until the infected nails have grown out.

In the rare cases of fungal infections of internal organs, such as the blood, the heart, or the brain, potent drugs such as fluconazole and itraconazole are given by mouth, or amphotericin and flucytosine are given by injection. These drugs pass into the bloodstream to fight the fungi.

HOW THEY WORK

Most antifungals alter the permeability of the fungal cell's walls. Chemicals needed for cell life leak out and the fungal cell dies.

HOW THEY AFFECT YOU

The speed with which antifungals provide benefit varies with the type of infection. Most fungal or yeast infections of the skin, mouth, and vagina improve within a week. The condition of nails affected by fungal infections improves only when new nail growth occurs,

CHOICE OF ANTIFUNGAL DRUG

The table below shows the range of uses for some antifungal drugs. The particular drug chosen in each case depends on the precise nature and site of the infection. The usual route of administration for each drug is also indicated.

DRUG	INFECTION									ADMINISTRATION		
	Oesophageal thrush	Cryptococcal meningitis	Skin ringworm	Scalp ringworm	Nail infection	Mouth thrush	Vaginal thrush	Candida of the skin	Systemic candida	Topical	Injection	Oral
Amphotericin B	●	●				●			●		●	●
Caspofungin	●								●		●	
Clotrimazole			●	●			●	●		●		
Fluconazole	●	●					●	●	●		●	●
Flucytosine	●	●							●		●	●
Griseofulvin			●	●	●							●
Ketoconazole			●	●	●		●	●		●		
Miconazole			●			●	●	●		●		●
Nystatin	●					●	●	●		●		●
Terbinafine			●	●	●							●
Voriconazole	●						●		●		●	●

which takes months. Systemic infections of the internal organs can take weeks to cure.

Antifungals applied topically rarely cause side effects, although they may irritate the skin. However, treatment by mouth or injection for systemic and nail infections may produce more serious side effects. Amphotericin B, injected in cases of life-threatening systemic infections, can cause potentially dangerous effects, including kidney damage.

COMMON DRUGS

Amorolfine, Amphotericin B*, Caspofungin, Clotrimazole*, Econazole, Fluconazole*, Flucytosine, Griseofulvin, Itraconazole, Ketoconazole*, Miconazole*, Nystatin*, Terbinafine*, Tioconazole, Voriconazole

* **See Part 2**

Anthelmintic drugs

Anthelmintics are drugs that are used to eliminate the many types of worm (helminths) that can enter the body and live there as parasites, producing a general weakness in some cases and serious harm in others. The body may be host to many different worms (see Types of infestation, right). Most species spend part of their life cycle in another animal, and the infestation is often passed on to humans in food contaminated with the eggs or larvae. In some cases, such as hookworm, larvae enter the body through the skin. Larvae or adults may attach themselves to the intestinal wall and feed on the bowel contents; others feed off the intestinal blood supply, causing anaemia. Worms can also infest the bloodstream or lodge in the muscles or internal organs.

Many people have worms at some time during their life, especially during childhood; most worms can be effectively eliminated with anthelmintic drugs.

WHY THEY ARE USED

Most worms common in the United Kingdom cause only mild symptoms and usually do not pose a serious threat to general health. Anthelmintic drugs are usually necessary, however, because the body's natural defences against infection are not effective against most worm infestations. Certain types of infestation must always be treated since they can cause serious complications. In some cases, such as threadworm infestation, doctors may recommend anthelmintic treatment for the whole family to prevent reinfection. If worms have invaded tissues and formed cysts, they may have to be removed surgically. Laxatives are given with some anthelmintics to hasten expulsion of worms from the bowel. Other drugs may be prescribed to ease symptoms or compensate for any blood loss or nutritional deficiency.

TYPES OF INFESTATION

Threadworm (enterobiasis) The most common worm infection in the UK, especially among young children. The worm lives in the intestine but travels to the anus at night to lay eggs, causing itching; scratching leaves eggs on the fingers, usually under the fingernails. Sucking the fingers or eating food with unwashed hands often transfers these eggs to the mouth. Keeping the nails short; good hygiene, including washing the hands after using the toilet and before each meal; and an early morning bath to remove the eggs are important in eradicating the infection.
Drugs Mebendazole
All members of the household should be treated simultaneously.

Common roundworm (ascariasis) The most common worm infection worldwide. It is transmitted to humans in contaminated raw food or in soil. The worms are large, and they infect the intestine, which can be blocked by dense clusters of them.
Drugs Levamisole, mebendazole

Tropical threadworm (strongyloidiasis) Occurs in the tropics and southern Europe. Larvae from contaminated soil penetrate the skin, pass into the lungs, are swallowed, and pass into the gut.
Drugs Albendazole, tiabendazole, ivermectin

Whipworm (trichuriasis) Mainly occurs in tropical areas of the world as a result of eating contaminated raw vegetables. The worms infest the intestines.
Drug Mebendazole

Hookworm (uncinariasis) Mainly found in tropical areas. The worm larvae penetrate the skin and pass via the lymphatic system and

bloodstream to the lungs. They then travel up the airways, are swallowed, and attach themselves to the intestinal wall, where they feed off the intestinal blood supply.
Drug Mebendazole

Pork roundworm (trichinosis) Transmitted in infected undercooked pork. Initially, the worms lodge in the intestines, but larvae may invade muscle to form cysts that are often resistant to drug treatment and may require surgery.
Drugs Mebendazole, tiabendazole

Toxocariasis (visceral larva migrans) Usually occurs as a result of eating soil or eating with fingers contaminated with dog or cat faeces. The eggs hatch in the intestine and may travel to the lungs, liver, kidney, brain, and eyes. Treatment is not always effective.
Drugs Mebendazole, tiabendazole, diethylcarbamazine

Creeping eruption (cutaneous larva migrans) Mainly occurs in tropical areas and coastal areas of the southeastern US following skin contact with larvae from cat and dog faeces. Infestation is usually confined to the skin.
Drugs Tiabendazole, ivermectin, albendazole

Filariasis (including onchocerciasis and loiasis) Occurs in tropical areas only. Infection is spread by the bites of insects that are carriers of worm larvae or eggs. It may affect the lymphatic system, blood, eyes, and skin.
Drugs Diethylcarbamazine, ivermectin

Flukes Sheep liver fluke (fascioliasis) is indigenous to the UK. Infestation usually results from eating watercress grown in contaminated water. It mainly affects the liver and biliary tract. Other flukes only found abroad may infect the lungs, intestines, or blood.
Drug Praziquantel

Tapeworms (including beef, pork, fish, and dwarf tapeworms) Depending on the type, worms may be carried by cattle, pigs, or fish and transmitted to humans in undercooked meat. Most types affect the intestines. Larvae of the pork tapeworm may form cysts in muscle and other tissues.
Drugs Niclosamide, praziquantel

Hydatid disease (echinococciasis) The eggs are transmitted in dog faeces. Larvae may form cysts over many years, commonly in the liver. Surgery is the usual treatment for cysts.
Drug Albendazole

Bilharzia (schistosomiasis) Occurs in polluted water in tropical areas. The larvae may be swallowed or penetrate the skin. Once inside the body, they migrate to the liver; adult worms live in the bladder.
Drug Praziquantel

HOW THEY WORK

The anthelmintic drugs act in several ways. Many of them kill or paralyse the worms, which pass out of the body in the faeces. Others, which act systemically, are used to treat infection in the tissues.

Many anthelmintics are specific for particular worms, and the doctor must identify the nature of the infection before selecting the most appropriate treatment (see Types of infestation). Most of the common intestinal infestations are easily treated, often with only one or two doses of the drug. However, tissue infections may require more prolonged treatment.

HOW THEY AFFECT YOU

Once the drug has eliminated the worms, symptoms caused by infestation rapidly disappear. Taken as a single dose or a short course, anthelmintics do not usually produce side effects. However, treatment can disturb the digestive system, causing abdominal pain, nausea, and vomiting.

COMMON DRUGS

Albendazole, Diethylcarbamazine, Ivermectin, Levamisole, Mebendazole*, Niclosamide, Praziquantel, Tiabendazole

* **See Part 2**

HORMONES AND ENDOCRINE SYSTEM

The endocrine system is a collection of glands located throughout the body that produce hormones and release them into the bloodstream. Each endocrine gland produces one or more hormones, each of which governs a particular body function, including growth and repair of tissues, sexual development and reproductive function, and the body's response to stress.

The pituitary gland produces hormones that regulate growth and sexual and reproductive development, and also stimulate other endocrine glands (see p.83).

The thyroid gland regulates metabolism. If it does not function well, hyperthyroidism or hypothyroidism may occur (see p.82).

The adrenal glands produce hormones that regulate the body's mineral and water content and reduce inflammation (see Corticosteroids, below right). They also produce stress hormones and male sex hormones.

The pancreas produces insulin, to regulate blood glucose levels, and glucagon, to help the liver and muscles store glucose (see p.80).

The kidneys produce a hormone, erythropoietin (see p.237), needed for red blood cell production. Patients with kidney failure lack this hormone and become anaemic; they may be given epoetin, a version of the hormone.

The ovaries (in women) secrete oestrogen and progesterone, responsible for female sexual and physical development (see p.86).

The testes (in men) produce testosterone, which controls the development of male sexual and physical characteristics (see p.85).

Most hormones are released continuously from birth, but the amount produced fluctuates with the body's needs. Others are produced mainly at certain times – for example, growth hormone is released mainly during childhood and adolescence. Sex hormones are produced by the testes and ovaries from puberty onwards (see p.101).

Many endocrine glands release their hormones in response to triggering hormones produced by the pituitary gland. This gland releases a variety of pituitary hormones, each of which, in turn, stimulates the appropriate endocrine gland to produce its hormone.

A feedback system usually regulates blood hormone levels: if the blood level rises too high, the pituitary responds by reducing the amount of stimulating hormone produced, so allowing the blood level to return to normal.

WHAT CAN GO WRONG

Endocrine disorders, usually resulting in too much or too little of a particular hormone, have a variety of causes. Some are congenital in origin; others may be caused by autoimmune disease (including some forms of diabetes mellitus), malignant or benign tumours, injury, or certain drugs.

WHY DRUGS ARE USED

Natural hormone preparations or their synthetic versions are often prescribed to treat deficiency. Sometimes drugs are given to stimulate increased hormone production in a particular endocrine gland, such as oral antidiabetic drugs, which act on the insulin-producing cells of the pancreas. When too much hormone is produced, drug treatment may reduce the activity of the gland.

Hormones or related drugs are also used to treat certain other conditions. Corticosteroids related to adrenal hormones are prescribed to relieve inflammation and to suppress immune system activity (see p.97). Several types of cancer are treated with sex hormones (see p.94). Female sex hormones are used as contraceptives (see p.103) and to treat menstrual disorders (see p.102).

MAJOR DRUG GROUPS

- Corticosteroids
- Drugs used in diabetes
- Drugs for thyroid disorders
- Drugs for pituitary disorders
- Male sex hormones
- Female sex hormones

Corticosteroids

Corticosteroid drugs – often just called steroids – are derived from, or are synthetic variants of, the natural corticosteroid hormones formed in the outer part (cortex) of the adrenal glands on top of each kidney.

Corticosteroids produced by the body may have either mainly glucocorticoid or mainly mineralocorticoid effects. The main mineralocorticoid effects are the regulation of the balance of mineral salts and of the water content in the body. Glucocorticoid effects include the maintenance of normal levels of sugar in the blood and the promotion of recovery from injury and stress. Release of these hormones is governed by the pituitary gland (see p.83). When present in large amounts, glucocorticoids act to reduce inflammation and suppress allergic reactions and immune system activity. They are distinct from another group of steroid hormones, the anabolic steroids (see p.86).

Although corticosteroid drugs have broadly similar actions, they vary in their relative strength and duration of action. Their mineralocorticoid effects also vary in strength.

WHY THEY ARE USED

Glucocorticoid-type corticosteroids are used primarily for their effect in controlling inflammation, whatever its cause. Topical preparations containing corticosteroids are often used to treat many inflammatory skin disorders (see p.118). These drugs may also be injected directly into a joint or around a tendon to relieve inflammation caused by injury or disease (see p.51). However, if these local treatments are not possible or not effective, corticosteroids may be given systemically by mouth or by intravenous injection.

Corticosteroids are commonly used in many disorders in which inflammation is thought to be due to excessive or inappropriate immune system activity. These disorders include inflammatory bowel disease (see p.44), rheumatoid arthritis (see p.49), glomerulonephritis (a kidney disease), and some rare connective tissue disorders, such as systemic lupus erythematosus. In these conditions corticosteroids relieve symptoms and may also temporarily halt the disease.

Corticosteroids may be given regularly by mouth or inhaler to treat asthma, although their effect on relieving acute asthma attacks is delayed by a few hours (see Bronchodilators, p.21 and Drugs for asthma, p.22).

An important use of oral corticosteroids is to correct the deficiency of natural hormones resulting from reduced adrenal gland function, as in Addison's disease. In these cases, the drugs most closely resembling the actions of the natural hormones are selected and a combination of these may be used.

Some cancers of the lymphatic system (lymphomas) and of the blood (leukaemias) may also respond to corticosteroid treatment. In addition, these drugs are widely used to prevent or treat rejection of organ transplants, usually in conjunction with other drugs, such as azathioprine (see Immunosuppressants, p.97).

HOW THEY WORK

Given in high doses, corticosteroids reduce inflammation by blocking the action of chemicals such as prostaglandins that trigger the inflammatory response. These drugs also temporarily depress the immune system by reducing the activity of certain types of white blood cell. In addition, they may be used to treat severe allergic reactions or anaphylaxis.

HOW THEY AFFECT YOU

Corticosteroid drugs often produce a dramatic improvement in symptoms. Given systemically, they may also act on the brain to produce a heightened sense of well-being and, in some people, a sense of euphoria. Troublesome day-to-day side effects are rare. Long-term treatment, however, carries a number of serious risks for the patient.

RISKS AND SPECIAL PRECAUTIONS

In the treatment of Addison's disease, corticosteroids can be considered as "hormone replacement therapy", with the drugs replacing the natural hormone hydrocortisone. This physiological replacement means that adverse effects are rarely seen.

Drugs with strong mineralocorticoid effects, such as fludrocortisone, may cause water retention, swelling (especially of the ankles), and an increase in blood pressure. Because corticosteroids reduce the effect of insulin (among their other effects), they may create problems in people with diabetes and may even give rise to diabetes in susceptible people. They can also cause peptic ulcers.

Because corticosteroids suppress immune system activity, they increase susceptibility to infection. They also suppress symptoms of infectious disease. People taking the drugs should avoid exposure to chickenpox or shingles; if they catch either disease, drugs such as aciclovir tablets may be prescribed.

With long-term use, corticosteroids may cause various adverse effects, such as mood changes, acne, a moon-shaped face, increased blood pressure and fluid retention, peptic ulcers, a fat pad on the top of the back, thin skin, and easy bruising. Doctors try to avoid long-term use of corticosteroids for children because it may retard growth.

Long-term corticosteroid use suppresses production of the body's own corticosteroid hormones. For this reason, treatment lasting for more than a few weeks should be withdrawn gradually to give the body time to adjust. If stopped abruptly, the lack of corticosteroid hormones may lead to fatigue, nausea, vomiting, or even sudden collapse.

People taking corticosteroids by mouth for longer than 1 month are advised to carry a warning card. If someone who is taking steroids long term has a serious accident or surgery, their defences against shock may need to be supported with extra hydrocortisone, administered intravenously.

COMMON DRUGS

Alclometastone, Beclometasone*, Betamethasone*, Budesonide*, Clobetasol*, Clobetasone, Deflazacort, Dexamethasone*, Diflucortolone, Fludrocortisone, Fludroxycortide, Flumetasone, Flunisolide, Fluocinolone, Fluocinonide, Fluocortolone, Fluticasone*, Hydrocortisone*, Methylprednisolone, Mometasone*, Prednisolone*, Triamcinolone

* **See Part 2**

Drugs used in diabetes

The body obtains most of its energy from glucose, a simple form of sugar formed in the gut from the breakdown of starch and other sugars or by metabolic processes in the liver, fat, and muscle. Insulin, one of the hormones produced in the pancreas, enables body tissues to take up glucose from the blood, either to use it for energy or to store it. In diabetes mellitus, there is either a complete lack of insulin or too little is produced. This results in reduced uptake of glucose by the tissues and thus an abnormal rise in the blood glucose level. A high blood glucose level is known medically as hyperglycaemia.

There are two main types of diabetes mellitus. Type 1 (insulin-dependent) diabetes usually appears in young people, with 50 per cent of cases occurring around the time of puberty. The insulin-secreting cells in the pancreas are gradually destroyed. An autoimmune condition (where the body misidentifies its pancreas as "foreign" and tries to eliminate it) or a childhood viral infection is the most likely cause. Although the decline in insulin production is slow, the condition often appears suddenly, brought on by periods of stress (for example, infection or puberty) when the body's insulin requirements are high. Symptoms of Type 1 diabetes include extreme thirst, increased urination, lethargy, and weight loss. This type of diabetes is fatal if it is left untreated.

In Type 1 diabetes, insulin treatment is the only treatment option. It has to be continued for the rest of the patient's life. Several types of insulin are available, which are broadly classified by their duration of action (short-, medium-, and long-acting).

Type 2, formerly known as non-insulin-dependent diabetes mellitus (NIDDM) or maturity-onset diabetes, tends to appear at an older age (usually over 40, although it has become increasingly common in younger age groups) and to come on much more gradually – there may be a delay in its diagnosis for several years because of the gradual onset of symptoms. In this type of diabetes, the levels of insulin in the blood are usually high. However, the body cells are resistant to the effects of insulin and have a reduced glucose uptake despite the high insulin levels. This results in hyperglycaemia. Obesity is the most common cause of Type 2 diabetes.

In both types of diabetes, an alteration in diet is vital. A healthy diet that is low in fats and simple sugars (cakes, sweets) and high in fibre and foods with complex sugars and a low glycaemic index (brown rice, wholewheat pasta), is advised. In Type 2 diabetes, a reduction in weight alone may be sufficient to lower the body's energy requirements and restore blood glucose to normal levels. If an alteration in diet fails, oral antidiabetic drugs, such as metformin, acarbose, or sulfonylureas, are prescribed. Insulin may need to be given to people with Type 2 diabetes if the above treatments fail, or in pregnancy, during severe illness, and before any surgery requiring a general anaesthetic.

IMPORTANCE OF TREATING DIABETES

If diabetes is left untreated, the continual high blood glucose levels damage various parts of the body. The major problems are caused by atherosclerosis, in which a build-up of fatty deposits in the arteries narrows them, reducing the flow of blood. This can result in heart attacks, blindness, stroke, kidney failure, reduced circulation in the legs, and even gangrene. The risk of these conditions is greatly reduced with treatment. Careful control of diabetes in young people, during puberty and afterwards, is essential in reducing the risk of possible long-term complications. Good diabetic control before conception reduces the chance of miscarriage or abnormalities in the baby.

HOW ANTIDIABETIC DRUGS WORK

Insulin treatment directly replaces the natural hormone that is deficient in diabetes mellitus. Synthetic human insulins are now the preferred forms. Insulin cannot be taken by mouth because it is broken down in the digestive tract before it reaches the bloodstream; regular injections are therefore necessary (see Administration of insulin, below).

Sulfonylurea oral antidiabetics encourage the pancreas to produce insulin. They are therefore effective only when some insulin-secreting cells remain active; this is why they are ineffective in the treatment of Type 1 diabetes. Metformin alters the way in which the body metabolizes sugar. Acarbose slows digestion of starch and sugar. Both slow the increase in blood sugar that occurs after a meal. Nateglinide and repaglinide stimulate insulin release. Pioglitazone reduces the body's resistance to insulin. Exenatide and sitagliptin stimulate insulin release and block the release of glucagon (a substance that raises blood glucose), thereby helping to prevent the rise in blood sugar after a meal. The new gliflozin drugs (such as dapagliflozin) block reabsorption of sugar by the kidneys, so it is lost in the urine.

ADMINISTRATION OF INSULIN

A healthy pancreas produces a background level of insulin, with additional insulin being produced as required in response to meals. The insulin delivery systems currently available cannot mimic this process precisely. In people with Type 1 diabetes, short-acting insulin is usually given before meals, and medium-acting either before the evening meal or at bedtime. Insulin pen injectors are useful for daytime administration because they are discreet and easy to use. In people with Type 2 diabetes who need insulin, a mixture of short- and medium-acting insulin may be given twice a day. Pumps that deliver continuous subcutaneous insulin are now used in some people with Type 1 diabetes and some who find it difficult to control their insulin levels with injections. Some new insulin types called insulin analogues (e.g. insulin lispro) act very rapidly and may be better at mimicking the insulin-producing behaviour of a healthy pancreas.

INSULIN TREATMENT AND YOU

The insulin requirements in diabetes vary greatly between individuals and also depend on physical activity and calorie intake. Hence, insulin regimens are tailored to particular needs, and the person is encouraged to take an active role in their own management.

A regular record of home blood glucose monitoring should be kept. This is the basis on which insulin doses are adjusted, preferably by the person with diabetes.

A person with diabetes should learn to recognize the warning signs of a "hypo", or attack of hypoglycaemia (low blood sugar): hunger, anxiety, slurred speech, tremor, cold sweats, blurred vision, and headache. The symptoms disappear when glucose is administered, so anyone with diabetes should always carry glucose tablets or sweets with them. Recurrent "hypos" at specific times may require a reduction of insulin dose. Rarely, undetected low glucose levels may lead to coma. The injection of glucagon rapidly reverses this, so a carer or relative should be shown how to give the injection.

Repeated injection at the same site may disturb the fat layer beneath the skin, producing swelling or dimpling. This alters the rate of insulin absorption. However, it can be avoided by regularly rotating injection sites.

Insulin requirements are increased during illness and pregnancy. During an illness, the urine or blood should be checked for ketones, substances that are produced in the body when there is insufficient insulin to permit the normal uptake of glucose by the tissues. If high ketone levels occur in the urine during an illness, urgent medical advice should be sought. The combination of high blood glucose, high urinary ketones, and vomiting is a diabetic emergency, and the person should be taken to an Accident and Emergency department without delay.

Exercise increases the body's need for glucose, so extra calories may be needed before and during exertion. The effects of vigorous exercise on blood glucose may last up to 18–24 hours, and the subsequent (post-exercise) doses of insulin may need to be reduced by 10–25 per cent to avoid hypoglycaemia.

People with diabetes are advised to carry a card or bracelet detailing their condition and treatment in case of medical emergency.

ANTIDIABETIC DRUGS AND YOU

The sulfonylureas may lower the blood glucose too much. This can be avoided by starting treatment with low doses and ensuring a regular food intake. Rarely, these drugs cause a decrease in the blood cell count, a rash, or intestinal or liver disturbances. Interactions may occur with other drugs, so your doctor should be informed of your treatment before prescribing any medicines for you.

Unlike the sulfonylureas, metformin does not cause hypoglycaemia. Its most common side effects are nausea, weight loss, abdominal distension, and diarrhoea. It should not be used in people with liver, kidney, or heart problems. Acarbose does not cause hypoglycaemia if used on its own. The tablets must either be chewed with the first mouthful of food at meal times or swallowed whole with a little liquid immediately before food. Sitagliptin is taken orally once a day, either with or without food. Exetanide, used mainly in obese patients, is given by injection twice a day before meals.

COMMON DRUGS

Sulfonylurea drugs Glibenclamide*, Gliclazide*, Glimepiride, Glipizide, Tolbutamide*

Other drugs Acarbose, Dapagliflozin*, Dulaglutide*, Exenatide*, Glucagon*, Insulin*, Insulin aspart, Insulin glargine, Insulin glulisine, Insulin lispro, Liraglutide, Metformin*, Nateglinide, Pioglitazone*, Repaglinide*, Sitagliptin*

* **See Part 2**

Drugs for thyroid disorders

The thyroid gland produces thyroxine, which regulates the body's metabolism. Thyroxine is essential during childhood for normal physical and mental development. Calcitonin, also produced by the thyroid, regulates calcium metabolism and is used as a drug for certain bone disorders (see p.54).

HYPERTHYROIDISM

In this condition (also called thyrotoxicosis), the thyroid is overactive and produces too much thyroxine. Women are more commonly affected than men. Symptoms include anxiety, palpitations, weight loss, increased appetite, heat intolerance, diarrhoea, and menstrual disturbances. Graves' disease is the most common form of hyperthyroidism. This is an autoimmune disease in which the body produces antibodies that stimulate the thyroid to make excess thyroxine. Affected people may develop abnormally protuberant eyes (exophthalmos) or a swelling involving the skin over the shins (pretibial myxoedema). Hyperthyroidism can be caused by a benign tumour of the thyroid (an adenoma) or a pre-existing multinodular goitre. Rarely, an overactive thyroid may follow a viral infection, a condition called thyroiditis, or use of certain medications (such as amiodarone or alemtuzumab). Inflammation of the gland leads to the release of stored thyroxine. **Goitre** is a swelling of the thyroid gland. It may occur only temporarily, during puberty or pregnancy, or may be due to abnormal growth of thyroid tissue that requires surgical removal. Goitre may also, rarely, result from iodine deficiency, which can be prevented or treated with iodine supplements.

MANAGEMENT OF HYPERTHYROIDISM

There are three possible treatments: antithyroid drugs, radioactive iodine (radio-iodine), and surgery. The most commonly used antithyroid drug is carbimazole, which inhibits the formation of thyroid hormones and reduces their levels to normal over about 4–8 weeks. In the early stage of treatment, a beta blocker (see p.28) may be prescribed to control symptoms. This should be stopped once thyroid function returns to normal. Long-term carbimazole is usually given for 12–18 months to prevent relapse. A "block and replace" regimen may also be used. In this treatment, the thyroid gland is blocked by high doses of carbimazole and thyroxine is added when the blood level of thyroid hormone falls below normal.

Carbimazole may cause minor side effects such as nausea, vomiting, skin rashes, or headaches. Rarely, the drug may reduce the white blood cell count. Propylthiouracil may be used as an alternative antithyroid drug.

Radio-iodine is often used as a first-line therapy, especially in older adults, or as a second choice if hyperthyroidism recurs following use of carbimazole. It acts by destroying thyroid tissue. Hypothyroidism occurs in up to 80 per cent of people within 20 years after treatment. Long-term studies show radio-iodine to be safe, but it should be avoided during pregnancy and breast-feeding, and in patients with thyroid eye disease.

Surgery is a third-line therapy. Its use may be favoured for patients with a large goitre, particularly one that causes difficulty in swallowing or breathing. Thyroid eye disease may require corticosteroids (see p.78) or other immunomodulatory drugs.

HYPOTHYROIDISM

This is a condition resulting from too little thyroxine. Sometimes it may be caused by an autoimmune disorder, in which the immune system attacks the thyroid gland. Other cases may follow treatment for hyperthyroidism. In newborn babies, hypothyroidism may be the result of an inborn enzyme disorder. In the past, it also arose from a deficiency of iodine in the diet.

The symptoms of adult hypothyroidism develop slowly and include weight gain, mental slowness, dry skin, hair loss, increased sensitivity to cold, and heavy menstrual periods. In babies, low levels of thyroxine cause permanent mental and physical retardation and, for this reason, babies are tested for hypothyroidism shortly after birth.

MANAGEMENT OF HYPOTHYROIDISM

Lifelong oral treatment with synthetic thyroid hormones (thyroxine (levothyroxine), or rarely liothyronine) is the only option. Blood tests are done regularly to monitor treatment and permit dosage adjustments. In older people and those with heart disease, thyroxine is introduced gradually to prevent strain on the heart.

In severely ill patients, thyroid hormone may be given by injection. Hormone injections may also be used to treat newborn infants with low levels of thyroxine.

Symptoms of thyrotoxicosis may appear if excess thyroxine replacement is given. Otherwise, no adverse events occur since treatment is adjusted to replace the hormone that the body should normally produce itself.

COMMON DRUGS

Drugs for hypothyroidism Levothyroxine (thyroxine)*, Liothyronine

Drugs for hyperthyroidism Carbimazole*, Iodine, Nadolol, Propranolol*, Propylthiouracil*, Radioactive iodine (radio-iodine)

* **See Part 2**

Drugs for pituitary disorders

The pituitary gland, which lies at the base of the brain, produces a number of hormones that regulate physical growth, metabolism, sexual development, and reproductive function. Many of these hormones act indirectly by stimulating other glands, such as the thyroid, adrenal glands, ovaries, and testes, to release their own hormones.

Thyroid-stimulating hormone stimulates production and release of thyroid hormones.

Prolactin stimulates glands in the breast to produce milk in women and helps sperm production in men.

Corticotrophin (ACTH) controls production and release of adrenal corticosteroid hormones.

Gonadotrophins known as follicle-stimulating hormone (FSH) and luteinizing hormone (LH) act on the sex glands to stimulate egg production and release in females, and sperm production in males. They also control the output of the sex hormones oestrogen, progesterone, and testosterone.

Growth hormone promotes normal growth and development.

Melanocyte-stimulating hormone controls skin pigmentation.

Antidiuretic hormone (ADH or vasopressin) regulates the output of water in the urine.

An excess or a lack of one of the pituitary hormones may produce serious effects, the nature of which depends on the hormone involved. Abnormal levels of a particular hormone may be caused by a pituitary tumour, which may be treated with surgery, radiotherapy, or drugs. In other cases, drugs may be used to correct the imbalance.

The more common pituitary disorders that can be treated with drugs are those involving growth hormone, antidiuretic hormone, prolactin, adrenal hormones, and the gonadotrophins. The first three are discussed below. For information on the use of drugs to treat infertility arising from inadequate levels of gonadotrophins, see p.107. Lack of corticotrophin, leading to inadequate production of adrenal hormones, is usually treated with corticosteroids (see p.78).

DRUGS FOR GROWTH HORMONE DISORDERS

Growth hormone (somatotropin) is the principal hormone required for normal growth in childhood and adolescence. Lack of growth hormone impairs normal physical growth. Doctors administer hormone treatment only after tests have proven that a lack of this hormone is the cause of the disorder. If treatment is started at an early age, regular injections of somatropin, a synthetic form of natural growth hormone, administered until the end of adolescence, usually allow normal growth and development to take place.

Growth hormone deficiency in adults is rare but may cause loss of strength and stamina, reduced bone mass, weight gain, and psychological symptoms such as poor memory and depression. In some cases, it may be treated with somatotropin.

Less often, the pituitary produces an excess of growth hormone. In children this can result in pituitary gigantism; in adults, it can produce a disorder known as acromegaly. This disorder, which is usually the result of a pituitary tumour, is characterized by thickening of the skull, face, hands, and feet, and enlargement of some internal organs.

The pituitary tumour may either be surgically removed or destroyed by radiotherapy. In frail or older people, drugs are used to reduce growth hormone levels. Drugs may also be administered as an adjunctive treatment before surgery and in people with increased growth hormone levels occurring after surgery. People who have undergone surgery and/or radiotherapy may require long-term replacement of other hormones (such as sex hormones, thyroid hormone, or corticosteroids).

DRUGS FOR DIABETES INSIPIDUS

Antidiuretic hormone (also called ADH or vasopressin) acts on the kidneys to control the amount of water retained in the body and returned to the blood. Defective ADH function can be caused by pituitary damage reducing production, or by defects in the kidneys' response to ADH. Both cause the rare condition of diabetes insipidus, in which the kidneys cannot retain water and large quantities pass into the urine. The chief symptoms are constant thirst and the production of large volumes of urine.

Diabetes insipidus due to pituitary damage is treated with ADH or a related synthetic drug, desmopressin. These replace naturally produced ADH. If it is due to the kidneys not responding to ADH (nephrogenic diabetes insipidus), other drugs such as thiazide diuretics (p.30) or non-steroidal anti-inflammatory drugs (p.48) may be used. These drugs usually increase urine production, but in diabetes insipidus they have the opposite effect.

DRUGS TO REDUCE PROLACTIN LEVELS

Prolactin, also called lactogenic hormone, is produced in both men and women. In women, it controls the secretion of breast milk following childbirth. Its function in men is not understood, although it seems to be necessary for sperm production.

The disorders associated with prolactin are all to do with overproduction. High levels in women can cause galactorrhoea (lactation that is not associated with pregnancy and birth), amenorrhoea (lack of menstruation), and infertility. Excess levels in men may cause galactorrhoea, gynaecomastia (growth of breast tissue), erectile dysfunction, or infertility.

Some drugs, notably methyldopa, oestrogen, metoclopramide, domperidone, and antipsychotics, can raise the prolactin level in the blood. More often, however, an increase in prolactin results from a pituitary tumour and is usually treated with a dopamine mimetic such as cabergoline to inhibit prolactin production.

COMMON DRUGS

Drugs for growth hormone disorders
Bromocriptine*, Lanreotide, Octreotide, Pegvisomant, Somatropin

Drugs for diabetes insipidus Carbamazepine*, Chlortalidone, Desmopressin*, Vasopressin (ADH)

Drugs to reduce prolactin levels Bromocriptine*, Cabergoline, Quinagolide

* **See Part 2**

Male sex hormones

Male sex hormones (androgens) are responsible for the development of male sexual characteristics. The principal androgens are testosterone, produced by the testes, and its more active conversion product dihydrotestosterone, produced in other tissues. Women produce small amounts of testosterone in their adrenal glands and ovaries. In both sexes, androgens stimulate libido (sex drive).

Testosterone has two major effects: an androgenic effect and an anabolic effect. Its androgenic effect is to stimulate the development of the secondary sexual characteristics at puberty, such as growth of body hair, deepening of the voice, and an increase in genital size. Its anabolic effects are to increase muscle mass, bone density, and growth rate in adolescents.

There are several synthetic derivatives of testosterone that produce varying degrees of the androgenic and anabolic effects mentioned above. Those with a mainly anabolic effect are called anabolic steroids (see p.86).

Testosterone and its derivatives have been used medically in both men and women to treat a number of conditions.

WHY THEY ARE USED

Male sex hormones are mainly given to men to promote the development of, or maintain, male sexual characteristics when hormone production is deficient. Such deficiency may result from abnormality or absence of the testes or inadequate production of the pituitary hormones that stimulate the testes to release testosterone.

Androgens are sometimes given to adolescent boys if the onset of puberty is delayed by pituitary problems. The treatment may also help to stimulate development of secondary male sexual characteristics and to increase libido in men with inadequate testosterone levels. This has been found to reduce sperm production, however. (For information on drug treatment of male infertility, see p.107.) An anti-androgen (a substance that inhibits the effects of androgens) may be used to treat prostate cancer or benign prostatic hyperplasia, or BPH (an enlarged prostate gland).

Androgens may also be prescribed for women to treat certain cancers of the breast and uterus (see Anticancer drugs, p.94). Testosterone can be given by injection, as a gel to rub into the skin, or as a nasal spray.

HOW THEY WORK

Taken in low doses as part of replacement therapy when natural production is low, male sex hormones act in the same way as the natural hormones. In adolescents experiencing delayed puberty, hormone treatment produces both androgenic and anabolic effects, initiating the development of secondary sexual characteristics over a few months; full sexual development usually takes place over 3 to 4 years. When male sex hormones are given to adult men, the effects on physical appearance and libido may begin to be felt within a few weeks.

RISKS AND SPECIAL PRECAUTIONS

The main risks with these drugs occur when they are given to boys with delayed puberty and to women with breast cancer. Given to initiate the onset of puberty, they may stunt growth by prematurely sealing the growing ends of the long bones. Doctors normally try to avoid prescribing hormones in these circumstances until growth is complete. High doses given to women have various masculinizing effects, including increased facial and body hair, and a deeper voice. The drugs may also produce enlargement of the clitoris, changes in libido, and acne.

ANABOLIC STEROIDS

These drugs are synthetic variants that mimic the anabolic effects of natural steroids. They increase muscle bulk and body growth.

Doctors very occasionally prescribe anabolic steroids and a high-protein diet to promote recovery after serious illness or major surgery. The steroids may also help to increase the production of blood cells in some forms of anaemia and to reduce itching in chronic obstructive jaundice.

Anabolic steroids have been widely misused in sports such as weight-lifting, athletics, and body-building, because they are perceived by some users to enhance athletic performance, especially with regard to muscle power and overall endurance. The use of anabolic steroids by sportspeople to improve their performance is condemned by doctors and banned by many athletic organizations because of the risks to health, particularly for women. Side effects include acne, baldness, psychological changes, fluid retention, reduced fertility in men and women, hardening of the arteries, a long-term risk of liver disease, and certain forms of cancer.

COMMON DRUGS

Primarily androgenic Mesterolone, Testosterone*
Primarily anabolic Nandrolone
Anti-androgens Cyproterone*, Dutasteride, Finasteride*
* **See Part 2**

Female sex hormones

There are two types of female sex hormone: oestrogen and progesterone. In women, these hormones are secreted by the ovaries from puberty until the menopause and by the placenta during pregnancy. Production of oestrogen and progesterone is regulated by the two gonadotrophin hormones (FSH and LH), which are produced by the pituitary gland (see p.83). Each month (in non-pregnant women) the levels of oestrogen and progesterone fluctuate, giving rise to the menstrual cycle (see p.102).

In girls, oestrogen is responsible for the development of secondary sexual characteristics at puberty, including breast development and widening of the pelvis. During the menstrual cycle, progesterone prepares the lining of the uterus for implantation of a fertilized egg. Progesterone is also important for the maintenance of pregnancy.

Synthetic forms of these hormones, known as oestrogens and progestogens, are used medically to treat a number of conditions. They can be given as tablets, patches, gels, implants, and intravaginal creams, pessaries, and rings.

WHY THEY ARE USED

The best-known use of oestrogens and progestogens is in oral contraceptives (see p.103). Other uses include the treatment of menstrual disorders (see p.102) and certain hormone-sensitive cancers (see p.94), and the management of gender reassignment. This article discusses the drug treatments that are used for natural hormone deficiency.

HORMONE DEFICIENCY

Deficiency of female sex hormones may result from deficiency of gonadotrophins, which in turn may be due to a pituitary disorder or to abnormal development of the ovaries (ovarian failure). This may lead to the absence of menstruation and lack of sexual development.

If tests show a deficiency of gonadotrophins, preparations of these hormones may be prescribed (see p.107). These trigger the release of oestrogen and progesterone from the ovaries. If pituitary function is normal and ovarian failure is diagnosed as the cause of hormone deficiency, oestrogens and progestogens may be given as supplements. In this situation, supplements ensure development of normal female sexual characteristics but cannot stimulate ovulation.

MENOPAUSE

A decline in the levels of oestrogen and progesterone occurs naturally following the menopause, when the ovaries stop functioning and the menstrual cycle ceases. The sudden reduction in levels of oestrogen can cause various symptoms, often including hot flushes, sweating, and palpitations. Many doctors suggest that hormone replacement therapy (HRT) be used around the time of the menopause (see Effects of hormone replacement therapy (HRT), right). HRT may also be prescribed for women who have undergone early or premature menopause: for example, due to surgical removal of the ovaries or radiotherapy for ovarian cancer.

HRT helps to reduce menopausal symptoms, including hot flushes and vaginal dryness. It is not normally recommended for long-term use or to treat osteoporosis (see p.55), however, because of the increased risk of disorders such as breast cancer, stroke, and thromboembolism. In HRT, oestrogen is used together with a progestogen unless the woman has had a hysterectomy, in which case oestrogen alone is used. If dryness of the vagina is a particular problem, a cream containing an oestrogen drug may be prescribed for short-term use.

HOW THEY AFFECT YOU

Hormones that are given to treat ovarian failure or delayed puberty take 3 to 6 months to produce a noticeable effect on sexual development. Taken for menopausal symptoms, they can dramatically reduce the number of hot flushes within a week.

Both oestrogens and progestogens can cause fluid retention, and oestrogens may cause nausea, vomiting, breast tenderness, headache, dizziness, and depression. Progestogens may cause breakthrough bleeding between menstrual periods. In the comparatively low doses used to treat these disorders, however, side effects are unlikely.

RISKS AND SPECIAL PRECAUTIONS

Because oestrogens increase the risk of hypertension (raised blood pressure), thrombosis (abnormal blood clotting), and breast cancer, there are risks associated with long-term HRT. Treatment is used with caution in women who have heart or circulatory disorders and in those who are overweight or who smoke. HRT given via patches or gels does not carry an increased risk of blood clots. Tibolone has both oestrogenic and progestogenic properties and may be used on its own.

The use of oestrogens and progestogens as replacement therapy in ovarian failure has few risks for otherwise healthy young women.

EFFECTS OF HORMONE REPLACEMENT THERAPY (HRT)

HRT is primarily used to alleviate symptoms related to menopause, such as hot flushes, mood swings, night sweats, and vaginal dryness. It may also be used to prevent or treat osteoporosis (p.55). However, the benefits must be weighed against increased health risks associated with its use, such as breast cancer, stroke, and thromboembolism.

Breasts There is a slightly increased risk of breast cancer with HRT (apart from vaginal oestrogen). The increase is related to the length of time for which HRT is used. If HRT is stopped, however, the risk reduces to its pre-treatment level within about 5 years.

Heart and circulation HRT increases the risk of thromboembolism and does not prevent coronary artery disease.

Bones For women who go through premature menopause, HRT reduces the thinning of bone that occurs in osteoporosis and thus protects against fractures.

Brain HRT increases the risk of stroke.

Reproductive organs HRT can prevent thinning and dryness of the vaginal tissues leading to painful intercourse.

COMMON DRUGS

Oestrogens Conjugated oestrogens*, Estradiol*, Estriol, Estrone, Ethinylestradiol*

Progestogens Desogestrel*, Dydrogesterone*, Levonorgestrel*, Medroxyprogesterone*, Norethisterone*, Norgestrel, Progesterone

Other drugs Raloxifene*

* **See Part 2**

NUTRITION

Food provides energy (as calories) and nutrients needed for growth and renewal of tissues. Protein, carbohydrate, and fat are the three major nutrient components of food. Vitamins and minerals are also required to maintain health. Fibre, found only in foods from plants, is needed for the digestive system to work efficiently.

Proteins in moderate amounts are vital for tissue growth and repair. They are found in meat and dairy products, cereals, and pulses.

Carbohydrates are a major energy source, and are stored as fat when taken in excess. They can be found in cereals, sugar, and vegetables. Starchy foods are preferable to sugar.

Fats are a concentrated energy form needed only in small quantities. They are contained in animal products such as butter and in the oils of plants such as corn and nuts.

Vitamins and minerals are found only in small amounts in food but are very important for the normal functioning of the body.

Fibre (non-starch polysaccharides) is the indigestible part of any fruit, vegetable, or food or product derived from plants. Fibre contains no nutrients but adds bulk to faeces.

During digestion, large molecules of food are broken down into smaller molecules, releasing nutrients that are absorbed into the bloodstream. Carbohydrate and fat are then metabolized by body cells to produce energy. They may also be incorporated with protein into the cell structure. Each metabolic process is promoted by a specific enzyme and often requires the presence of a particular vitamin or mineral.

WHY DRUGS ARE USED

Dietary deficiency of essential nutrients can lead to illness. In poorer countries where there is a shortage of food, marasmus (resulting from lack of food energy) and kwashiorkor (from lack of protein) are common. In rich countries, however, excessive food intake leading to obesity is more common. Nutritional deficiencies in developed countries result from poor food choices and usually stem from a lack of a specific vitamin or mineral, such as in iron-deficiency anaemia.

Some nutritional deficiencies may be caused by an inability of the body to absorb nutrients from food (malabsorption) or to utilize them once they have been absorbed. Malabsorption may be caused by lack of an enzyme or an abnormality of the digestive tract. Errors of metabolism are often inborn and are not yet fully understood. They may be caused by failure of the body to produce the chemicals required to process nutrients.

WHY SUPPLEMENTS ARE USED

Deficiencies such as kwashiorkor or marasmus are usually treated by dietary improvement and, in some cases, food supplements rather than drugs. Vitamin and mineral deficiencies are usually treated with appropriate supplements. Malabsorption disorders may require changes in diet or long-term use of supplements. Metabolic errors are not easily treated with supplements or drugs, and a special diet may be the main treatment.

The preferred treatments of obesity are reduced food intake, altered eating patterns, and increased exercise. If these steps are not effective and the body mass index (BMI) is 30 or more, anti-obesity drugs may be used.

MAJOR DRUG GROUPS

- Vitamins
- Minerals

Vitamins

Vitamins are complex chemicals that are vital for a variety of body functions. With the exception of vitamin D, the body cannot manufacture these substances and therefore we need to include them in our diet.

There are 13 major vitamins: A, C, D, E, K; the B complex vitamins – thiamine (B1), riboflavin (B2), niacin (B3), pantothenic acid (B5), pyridoxine (B6), and cobalamin (B12); folic acid; and biotin. Most are required in very small amounts, and each is found in one or more foods (see Main food sources of vitamins, p.90). Vitamin D is also made in the body when the skin is exposed to sunlight.

Vitamins fall into two groups: water-soluble and fat-soluble (see below).

Water-soluble vitamins Vitamin C and the B vitamins dissolve in water. Most are stored in the body for only a short period and are excreted rapidly by the kidneys if taken in higher amounts than the body needs. Vitamin B12 is the exception; it is stored in the liver, which may hold up to 6 years' supply. For these reasons, foods containing water-soluble vitamins need to be eaten daily. These vitamins are easily lost in cooking, so uncooked foods containing them should be eaten regularly. An overdose does not usually cause toxic effects, but adverse reactions to large dosages of vitamin C and pyridoxine (vitamin B6) have been reported.

Fat-soluble vitamins Vitamins A, D, E, and K are absorbed from the intestine into the bloodstream together with fat. Deficiency of these vitamins may result from any disorder that affects fat absorption (such as coeliac disease). They are stored in the liver, and reserves of some of them may last for several years. Taking an excess of a fat-soluble vitamin for a long period may cause it to build up to a harmful level in the body. Ensuring that foods rich in these vitamins are regularly included in the diet usually provides a sufficient supply without risking overdosage.

A number of vitamins (such as vitamins A, C, and E) have now been recognized as having strong antioxidant properties. Antioxidants neutralize the effect of free radicals, substances produced during the body's normal processes that may be potentially harmful if they are not neutralized. Free radicals are believed to play a role in cardiovascular disease, ageing, and cancer.

A balanced, varied diet is likely to contain adequate amounts of all the vitamins. Inadequate intake of any vitamin over an extended period can lead to symptoms of deficiency.

A doctor may recommend vitamin supplements to prevent deficiency in people considered at risk, to treat symptoms of deficiency, and for certain medical conditions.

WHY THEY ARE USED

Preventing deficiency Most people in the UK obtain sufficient quantities of vitamins in their diet and therefore do not need to take additional vitamins in the form of supplements. People who are unsure if their present diet is adequate are advised to look at the table on p.90 to check that vitamin-rich foods are eaten regularly. Vitamin intake can often be boosted simply by increasing the quantities of fresh foods and raw fruit and vegetables in the diet. Certain groups in the population are, however, at increased risk of vitamin deficiency. These include people who have an increased need for certain vitamins that may not be met from dietary sources – in particular, pregnant or breast-feeding women, and infants and young children. Older people who may not be eating a varied diet may also be at risk. Strict vegetarians, vegans, and others on restricted diets may not receive adequate amounts of all vitamins.

In addition, people who have disorders in which absorption of nutrients from the bowel is impaired, or who need to take drugs that reduce the absorption of vitamins (such as some types of lipid-lowering drugs), are usually given additional vitamins.

In these cases, the doctor is likely to advise supplements of one or more vitamins. Although most preparations are available without prescription, it is important to seek specialist advice before starting a course of vitamin supplements, to obtain a proper assessment of your individual requirements.

Vitamin supplements should not be used as a general tonic to improve wellbeing (they are not effective for this purpose) nor as a substitute for a balanced diet.

Treating deficiency It is rare for a diet to completely lack a particular vitamin, but if intake of a particular vitamin is regularly lower than the body's requirements, over time the body's stores of that vitamin may become depleted and symptoms of deficiency may appear. In the UK, vitamin deficiency disorders are most common among homeless people, those who misuse alcohol, and those on low incomes who do not eat an adequate diet. Deficiencies of water-soluble vitamins are more likely since most are not stored in large quantities in the body.

Dosages prescribed to treat vitamin deficiency are likely to be larger than those used to prevent deficiency. Medical supervision is required when correcting vitamin deficiency.

MAIN FOOD SOURCES OF VITAMINS

The table below indicates which foods are especially good sources of particular vitamins. Ensuring that you regularly select foods from a variety of categories helps to maintain adequate intake for most people, without the need for supplements. Processed and overcooked foods are likely to contain fewer vitamins than fresh, raw, or lightly cooked foods.

Vitamins	Red meat	Poultry	Liver	Milk	Cheese	Butter/margarine	Eggs	Fish	Cereals and bread	Green vegetables	Root vegetables	Pulses/legumes	Nuts	Fruit
Biotin			●				●					●	●	
Folic acid			●				●			●				●
Niacin as nicotinic acid	●	●	●					●	●			●	●	
Pantothenic acid			●					●	●					
Pyridoxine	●	●	●				●	●	●					
Riboflavin			●	●	●		●		●			●	●	●
Thiamine	●		●						●			●	●	
Vitamin A			●	●	●	●	●			●	●			●
Vitamin B12	●		●	●	●		●	●						
Vitamin C										●	●			●
Vitamin D				●		●	●	●						
Vitamin E						●	●		●	●		●	●	
Vitamin K										●	●			

Other medical uses of vitamins Various claims have been made for the value of vitamins in treating disorders other than vitamin deficiency. High doses of vitamin C have been said to be effective in preventing and treating the common cold, but such claims are not yet proved; zinc, however, may be helpful for this purpose. Vitamin and mineral supplements do not improve IQ in well-nourished children, but quite small dietary deficiencies can cause poor academic performance.

Certain vitamins have recognized medical uses apart from their nutritional role. Vitamin D has been used to treat bone-wasting disorders (see p.54). Niacin is sometimes used (in the form of nicotinic acid) as a lipid-lowering drug (see p.35). Derivatives of vitamin A (retinoids) are part of the treatment for severe acne (see p.121). Many women with premenstrual syndrome take pyridoxine (vitamin B6) to relieve symptoms (see Drugs used to treat menstrual disorders, p.102).

VITAMIN REQUIREMENTS

Normal daily vitamin requirements are usually given as Reference Nutrient Intakes (RNIs), sometimes called Reference Intakes (RIs). These figures are based on how much of a nutrient is enough to meet the needs of 97 per cent of people in a particular group. Those having much less than the RNI on a daily basis may be at risk of getting less than their minimum needs. Treating deficiency usually needs doses much higher than the RNI and requires medical supervision.

Biotin No RNI established; 10–200mcg is considered safe.

Folic acid (as folate) 50mcg (birth–1 year); 70mcg (1–3 years); 100mcg (4–6 years); 150mcg (7–10 years); 200mcg (11 years and over). For a woman planning a pregnancy who is at low risk of having a baby with a neural tube defect: 400mcg per day before conception and during the first 12 weeks of pregnancy. Couples are considered to be at high risk of having a baby with a neural tube defect if either partner has a personal or family history of the condition (including a previous pregnancy); if the woman has a malabsorption disorder such as coeliac disease; if she has diabetes or sickle cell disease; or if she is taking anticonvulsant medication. Women at high risk should take 5mg per day before conception and during the first 12 weeks of pregnancy; women with sickle cell disease should continue taking 5mg per day throughout pregnancy. Daily requirements increase by 60mcg during breast-feeding.

Niacin 3mg (birth–6 months); 4mg (7–9 months); 5mg (10–12 months); 8mg (1–3 years); 11mg (4–6 years); 12mg (7–10 years and females aged 11–14 years); 15mg (males aged 11–14 years); 18mg (males aged 15–18 years); 14mg (females aged 15–18 years); 17mg (males aged 19–50 years); 13mg (females aged 19–50 years); 16mg (males 51 years and over); 12mg (females 51 years and over); 2mg extra during breast-feeding.

Pantothenic acid No RNI established; adults require 3–7mg daily.

Pyridoxine 0.2mg (birth–6 months); 0.3mg (7–9 months); 0.4mg (10 months–1 year); 0.7mg (1–3 years); 0.9mg (4–6 years); 1mg (7–10 years and females aged 11–14 years); 1.2mg (males aged 11–14 years); 1.5mg (males aged 15–18 years); 1.2mg (females 15 and over); 1.4mg (males 19 and over).

Riboflavin 0.4mg (birth–1 year); 0.6mg (1–3 years); 0.8mg (4–6 years); 1mg (7–10 years); 1.2mg (males aged 11–14 years); 1.1mg (females aged 11 and over); 1.3mg (males aged 15 and over); extra 0.3mg in pregnancy and 0.5mg during breast-feeding.

Thiamine 0.2mg (birth–9 months); 0.3mg (10–12 months); 0.5mg (1–3 years); 0.7mg (4–10 years and females aged 11–14 years); 0.9mg (males aged 11–14 years); 1.1mg (males aged 15–18 years); 0.8mg (females aged 15 and over); 1mg (males aged 19–50 years); 0.9mg (males aged 51 and over). Extra 0.1mg in last 3 months of pregnancy and 0.2mg during breast-feeding.

Vitamin A 350mcg (up to 1 year); 400mcg (1–6 years); 500mcg (7–10 years); 600mcg (males aged 11–14 years, females 11 years and over); 700mcg (males 15 and over, and pregnant women); 950mcg (breast-feeding).

Vitamin B12 Only minute quantities required. 0.3mcg (birth–6 months); 0.4mcg (7–12 months); 0.5mcg (1–3 years); 0.8mcg (4–6 years); 1mcg (7–10 years); 1.2mcg (11–14 years); and 1.5mcg (15 years and over); extra 0.5mcg per day during breast-feeding.

Vitamin C 25mg (birth–1 year); 30mg (1–10 years); 35mg (11–14 years); 40mg (15 years and over); 50mg in pregnancy; 70mg during breast-feeding.

Vitamin D 8.5–10mcg (birth–1 year); 10mcg (all those over 1 year old, including women who are pregnant or breast-feeding). 1mcg of vitamin D equals 40 international units (IU).

Vitamin E No official UK RNI. Requirement depends on intake of polyunsaturated fatty acid, which varies widely; approximate recommended requirement 3–15mg per day.

Vitamin K Newborn infants may be given 1mg by single injection or may receive it orally; 2 doses of 2mg are given in the first week and a third dose at 1 month for breast-fed babies (omitted in formula-fed babies). No UK RNI has been set for other groups.

RISKS AND SPECIAL PRECAUTIONS

Vitamins are essential for health. Most people can take supplements without risk, but it is important not to exceed the recommended dosage, particularly for fat-soluble vitamins, which may accumulate in the body. Dosage needs to be carefully calculated, taking into account degree of deficiency, dietary intake, and duration of treatment. Overdosage has no therapeutic value and may even be harmful. Multivitamin preparations do not usually contain large amounts of each vitamin and are not likely to be harmful unless the dose is greatly exceeded. Single vitamin supplements can be harmful (excess of one vitamin may increase requirements for others) so should be used only on medical advice.

Minerals

Minerals are chemical elements (the simplest form of substance). Many are vital in trace amounts for normal body processes. A balanced diet usually contains all the minerals needed; deficiency diseases are uncommon, except for iron-deficiency anaemia.

Dietary supplements are necessary only when a doctor has diagnosed a specific deficiency, or in preventing or treating a disorder. Doctors often prescribe minerals for people with intestinal diseases that reduce absorption of minerals from the diet. Iron supplements are often advised for pregnant or breast-feeding women, and iron-rich foods for infants over 6 months.

Taking mineral supplements, unless under medical direction, is not advisable. Exceeding the body's daily requirements is not beneficial, and large doses may be harmful.

MINERAL REQUIREMENTS

As with vitamins, normal daily mineral requirements are usually based on the Reference Nutrient Intake (RNI).

Calcium 525mg (birth–1 year); 350mg (1–3 years); 450mg (4–6 years); 550mg (7–10 years); 1,000mg (males 11–18 years); 800mg (females 11–18 years); 700mg (19 years and older); 1,250mg during breast-feeding.

Chromium Only minute quantities needed. RNI not established; about 25mcg is considered safe for adults.

Copper 0.2mg (birth–3 months); 0.3mg (4 months–1 year); 0.4mg (1–3 years); 0.6mg (4–6 years); 0.7mg (7–10 years); 0.8mg (11–14 years); 1.0mg (15–18 years); 1.2mg (19 years and over); 0.3mg extra required during breast-feeding.

Fluoride No RNI established.

Iodine 50mcg (birth–3 months); 60mcg (4–12 months); 70mcg (1–3 years); 100mcg (4–6 years); 110mcg (7–10 years); 130mcg (11–14 years); 140mcg (15 years and over).

Iron 1.7mg (birth–3 months); 4.3mg (4–6 months); 7.8mg (7–12 months); 6.9mg (1–3 years); 6.1mg (4–6 years); 8.7mg (7–10 years); 11.3mg (males aged 11–18 years); 14.8mg (females aged 11–50 years); 8.7mg (males aged 19 and over, and females 51 and over). Requirements may be increased during pregnancy and after childbirth.

Magnesium 55mg (birth–3 months); 60mg (4–6 months); 75mg (7–9 months); 80mg (10–12 months); 85mg (1–3 years); 120mg (4–6 years); 200mg (7–10 years); 280mg (11–14 years); 300mg (males aged 15 and over, and females aged 15–18 years); 270mg (females aged 19 and over); 50mg extra during breast-feeding.

Potassium 0.8g (birth–3 months); 0.85g (4–6 months); 0.7g (7–12 months); 0.8g (1–3 years); 1.1g (4–6 years), 2g (7–10 years), 3.1g (11–14 years); 3.5g (15 years and over).

Selenium 10mcg (birth–3 months); 13mcg (4–6 months); 10mcg (7–12 months); 15mcg (1–3 years); 20mcg (4–6 years); 30mcg (7–10 years); 45mcg (11–14 years); 70mcg (males aged 15–18 years); 60mcg (females aged 15 and over); 75mcg (males aged 19 and over); 15mcg extra during breast-feeding.

Sodium 0.21g (birth–3 months); 0.28g (4–6 months); 0.32g (7–9 months); 0.35g (10–12 months); 0.5g (1–3 years); 0.7g (4–6 years); 1.2g (7–10 years); 1.6g (11 years and over). (1 teaspoon, or 6g, of table salt contains about 2g of sodium.)

Zinc 4mg (birth–6 months); 5mg (7 months–3 years); 6.5mg (4–6 years); 7mg (7–10 years); 9mg (11–14 years); 9.5mg (males aged 15 years and over); 7mg (females aged 15 years and over); 13mg for first 4 months of breast-feeding and 9.5mg thereafter.

MAIN FOOD SOURCES OF MINERALS

The table below shows foods that are especially good sources of particular minerals. A balanced diet usually contains all the minerals required by the body without the need for supplements. Some, known as trace elements, are required only in minute amounts.

Minerals	Red meat	Poultry	Liver	Milk	Cheese	Butter/margarine	Eggs	Fish	Cereals and bread	Green vegetables	Root vegetables	Pulses/legumes	Nuts	Fruit
Calcium				●	●					●		●	●	
Chromium	●				●				●	●				
Copper	●	●	●					●	●	●		●	●	
Fluoride								●						
Iodine				●	●			●	●					
Iron	●	●	●				●	●	●	●				
Magnesium				●				●	●	●		●	●	
Phosphorus	●	●	●	●	●		●	●	●	●	●	●	●	●
Potassium									●	●		●		●
Selenium	●		●	●				●	●					
Sodium	●	●	●	●	●	●	●	●	●	●	●	●	●	●
Zinc	●				●			●	●			●		

MALIGNANT AND IMMUNE DISEASE

The body constantly needs to produce new cells to replace those that wear out and die naturally and to repair injured tissue. Normally, the rate at which cells are created is carefully regulated. However, sometimes abnormal cells are formed that multiply uncontrollably. These cells may form lumps of abnormal tissue, or tumours.

Usually, tumours are confined to one place and cause few problems; these are benign growths, such as warts. In other types of tumour, cells may invade or destroy the structures around the tumour, and abnormal cells may spread to other parts of the body, forming satellite or metastatic tumours. These are malignant growths, also called cancers.

Opposing the development of tumours is the immune system. This can recognize as foreign not only invading bacteria and viruses but also transplanted tissue and cells that have become cancerous. The system relies on different types of white blood cell, produced in the lymph glands and bone marrow, which respond to foreign cells in a variety of ways.

TYPES OF CANCER

Inappropriate multiplication of cells leads to the formation of tumours that may be benign or malignant. Benign tumours do not spread to other tissues; malignant (cancerous) tumours do, however.

Carcinomas affect the skin and cells in glandular tissue lining internal organs.

Sarcomas affect muscles, bones, and fibrous tissues and lining cells of blood vessels.

Leukaemia affects white blood cells.

Lymphomas affect the lymph glands.

WHAT CAN GO WRONG

No single cause for cancer has been identified. An individual's risk of developing cancer may depend both upon genetic predisposition (some families seem prone to cancers of one or more types) and upon exposure to external risk factors, known as carcinogens. These include tobacco smoke, which increases the risk of lung cancer, and ultraviolet light, which makes skin cancer more likely in those who spend long periods in the sun. Long-term suppression of the immune system by disease (as in AIDS) or by drugs – for example, those given to prevent rejection of transplanted organs – increases the risk of developing infections and also certain cancers. This demonstrates the importance of the immune system in removing abnormal cells that have the potential to give rise to a tumour.

Overactivity of the immune system may also cause problems. The system may respond excessively to an innocuous stimulus, as in hay fever (see Allergy, p.56), or may mount a reaction against normal tissues (autoimmunity), leading to disorders known as autoimmune diseases. These include rheumatoid arthritis, systemic lupus erythematosus, pernicious anaemia, and some forms of hypothyroidism. Immune system activity can also be troublesome following a transplant, when it may lead to rejection of the foreign tissue. Medication is then needed to damp down the immune system and enable the body to accept the foreign tissue.

WHY DRUGS ARE USED

In cancer treatment, conventional chemotherapy involves using cytotoxic (cell-killing) drugs to eliminate abnormally dividing cells. These slow the growth rate of tumours and sometimes lead to their complete disappearance. However, because the drugs act against all rapidly dividing cells, they also reduce the number of normal cells, including blood cells, being produced from bone marrow. This can produce serious adverse effects such as anaemia and neutropenia in cancer patients. On the other hand, this action can be useful in limiting white cell activity in autoimmune disorders. Newer anticancer drugs are more selective in the cells they target. For example, trastuzumab (Herceptin) targets a specific protein produced by certain types of breast cancer cell.

Other drugs that have immunosuppressant effects include corticosteroids, azathioprine, and ciclosporin, which are used after transplant surgery. No drugs are yet available to stimulate the entire immune system directly.

However, growth factors may be used to increase the number and activity of some white blood cells, and antibody infusions may help those with deficient production or be used against specific targets in organ transplantation and cancer.

MAJOR DRUG GROUPS

- Anticancer drugs
- Immunosuppressant drugs
- Drugs for HIV and AIDS

Anticancer drugs

Cancer is a general term that covers a wide range of disorders, ranging from the leukaemias (blood cancers) to solid tumours of the lung, breast, and other organs. In all cancers, a group of cells escape from the normal controls on cell growth and multiplication. As a result, the cancerous (malignant) cells begin to crowd out the normal cells, and a tumour develops. Cancerous cells are often unable to perform their usual functions, and this may lead to progressively impaired function of the organ or area concerned. Cancers may develop from cells of the blood, skin, muscle, or any other tissue.

Malignant tumours spread into nearby structures, blocking blood vessels and compressing nerves and other structures. Fragments of the tumour may become detached and carried in the bloodstream to other parts of the body, where they form secondary growths (metastases).

Many different factors, or a combination of them, can provoke cancerous changes in cells. These factors include an individual's genetic background, impairment or failure of the immune system, and exposure to cancer-causing agents (carcinogens). Known carcinogens include ultraviolet light, tobacco smoke, radiation, certain chemicals, viruses, and dietary factors.

Treating cancer is a complicated process that depends on the type of cancer, its stage of development, and the patient's condition and wishes. Any of the following treatments may be used either alone or in combination with the others: surgery, radiotherapy, and drug therapy.

Until recently, drug treatment of cancer relied heavily on hormonal and cytotoxic agents (usually referred to as chemotherapy). Hormone treatments are suitable for only a few types of cancer and cytotoxic drugs, although valuable, can have severe side effects because of the damage that they do to normal tissues. However, as understanding of cancer biology has increased, new anticancer drugs have been developed. These targeted agents predominantly take the forms of small molecule inhibitors, which target growth and survival signals arising within cancer cells, and monoclonal antibodies, which affect growth and survival signals arising outside the cancer cells. In addition, immunomodulatory drugs (immunotherapies), pioneered by agents such as interleukin-2, are now entering the mainstream.

WHY THEY ARE USED

Cytotoxic drugs can cure rapidly growing cancers and are the treatment of choice for leukaemias, lymphomas, and certain cancers of the testis. They are less effective against slow-growing solid tumours, such as those of the breast and bowel, but they can relieve symptoms and prolong life when given as palliative chemotherapy (treatment that relieves symptoms but does not cure the disease). Adjuvant chemotherapy is increasingly being used following surgery, especially for breast and bowel tumours, to prevent regrowth of the cancer from cells left behind after the surgery. Neoadjuvant or primary chemotherapy is sometimes used before surgery to reduce the size of the tumour.

Hormone treatment is offered in cases of hormone-sensitive cancer, such as breast, uterine, and prostatic cancers, where it can be used to relieve disease symptoms or provide palliative treatment in advanced disease.

Targeted agents such as small molecule inhibitors and monoclonal antibodies are increasingly useful when used alone or in combination with other therapies to induce disease responses or maintain remission. There is gathering data that immunotherapies may give prolonged responses akin to cure even in cases of metastatic cancer.

Most anticancer drugs, especially cytotoxic drugs, have side effects that can be severe; treatment decisions have to balance possible benefits against side effects. Often a combination of several drugs is used. Special regimes of different drugs used together and in succession have been devised to maximize their activity and minimize the side effects.

HOW THEY WORK

Anticancer drugs work in many different ways. The main groups of drugs and how they work are described below.

Cytotoxic drugs There are several classes of cytotoxic drugs, including the alkylating agents, antimetabolites, taxanes, and cytotoxic antibiotics. Each class has a different mechanism of action, but all act by interfering with basic processes of cell replication and division. They are particularly potent against rapidly dividing cells. These include cancer cells but also certain normal cells, especially those in the hair follicles, gut lining, and bone marrow. This action explains their side effects and why treatment needs careful scheduling.

Hormone therapies These treatments counteract the effects of the hormone that is promoting growth of the cancer. For example, some breast cancers are stimulated by the female sex hormone oestrogen; the action of oestrogen is opposed by the drug tamoxifen. Other cancers, by contrast, are damaged by very high doses of a particular sex hormone. One example is medroxyprogesterone, a progesterone that is often used to halt the spread of endometrial cancer.

Monoclonal antibodies Antibodies are a fundamental building block of the immune system. These are proteins that recognize and bind very specifically to foreign proteins on the surface of bacteria, viruses, and parasites, marking them out for destruction by other parts of the immune system. Monoclonal antibodies are produced in tissue culture using cells that have been genetically engineered to make antibodies against a particular target protein. If the target is carefully selected, the antibodies can be used to identify cancer cells for destruction. If the target is found only on cancer cells, or on the cancer cells and the normal tissue from which it arose, the damage to healthy tissues during treatment is limited.

Monoclonal antibodies are being used increasingly in cancer treatment. Examples include trastuzumab (Herceptin), which binds to a protein produced by certain types of breast cancer cell, and alemtuzumab and rituximab, which recognize different types of protein on white blood cells and are used to treat leukaemias and lymphomas. These antibodies are very specific for certain types of cancer, and they cause little of the toxicity of conventional chemotherapy. They can, however, cause allergy-type reactions, especially at the beginning of treatment.

Growth factor inhibitors The growth of cells is controlled by a complex network of growth factors that bind very specifically to receptor sites on the cell surface. This triggers a complex series of chemical reactions that transmit the "grow" message to the nucleus, triggering cell growth and replication. In many cancers, this system is faulty and there are either too many receptors on the cell surface or other abnormalities that result in inappropriate "grow" messages. The extra or abnormal cell surface receptors can be used as targets for monoclonal antibodies.

Other defects in this system are being used as the basis for further new drugs. For example, imatinib very selectively interferes with an abnormal version of an enzyme found in certain leukaemic cells. This abnormal enzyme causes the cell nucleus to receive a "grow" signal continually, resulting in the uncontrolled growth of cancer. By stopping the enzyme working, it is possible to selectively "turn off" the growth of the abnormal cells. Imatinib is proving successful in treating certain types of leukaemia, with few serious side effects.

Another new area of cancer treatment is the use of drugs that inhibit growth of new blood vessels to tumours (anti-angiogenesis agents), thereby depriving the tumours of the nutrients and oxygen they need to grow. One example is bevacizumab, a monoclonal antibody that blocks vascular endothelial growth factor (VEGF), a protein produced by certain tumours that promotes blood vessel growth. Bevacizumab is used to treat advanced cancer of the bowel, breast, lung, or kidney. Other new drugs are being developed that work in similar ways.

HOW THEY AFFECT YOU

Cytotoxic drugs are generally associated with more side effects than other types of anticancer drug. At the start of treatment, adverse effects of the drugs may be more noticeable than benefits. The most common side effect is nausea and vomiting, for which an anti-emetic drug (see p.19) will usually be prescribed. Effects on the blood are also common. Many cytotoxic drugs cause hair loss due to the effect of their activity on the hair follicle cells, but the hair usually starts to grow back after chemotherapy has been completed. Individual drugs may produce other side effects.

Cytotoxic drugs are, in most cases, administered in the highest doses that can be tolerated in order to kill as many cancer cells as quickly as possible.

The unpleasant side effects of intensive chemotherapy, combined with a delay of several weeks before any benefits are seen and the seriousness of the disease, often lead to depression in those who are receiving anticancer drugs. Specialist counselling, support from family and friends, and, in some cases, treatment with antidepressant drugs may be helpful.

SUCCESSFUL CHEMOTHERAPY

Not all types of cancer respond to treatment with anticancer drugs, but some cancers can be cured by drug treatment, and in other cancers, drug treatment can slow or temporarily halt the progress of the disease. In certain cases, drug treatment has no beneficial effect but other treatments, such as surgery, often produce significant benefits. The main cancers that fall into each of the first two groups are listed below.

Cancers that can often be cured by drugs

- Some cancers of the lymphatic system (including Hodgkin's disease)
- Acute leukaemias (forms of blood cancer)
- Choriocarcinoma (cancer of the placenta)
- Germ cell tumours (cancers affecting sperm and egg cells)
- Wilms' tumour (a rare form of kidney cancer that affects children)
- Cancer of the testis

Cancers in which drugs may produce worthwhile benefits

- Breast cancer
- Ovarian cancer
- Some leukaemias
- Multiple myeloma (a bone marrow cancer)
- Many types of lung cancer
- Head and neck cancers
- Cancer of the stomach
- Cancer of the prostate
- Some cancers of the lymphatic system
- Bladder cancer
- Endometrial cancer (cancer affecting the lining of the uterus)
- Cancer of the large intestine
- Cancer of the oesophagus
- Cancer of the pancreas
- Cancer of the cervix

Successful drug treatment of cancer usually requires repeated courses of anticancer drugs because the treatment needs to be halted periodically to allow the blood-producing cells in the bone marrow to recover.

RISKS AND SPECIAL PRECAUTIONS

All cytotoxic anticancer drugs interfere with the activity of non-cancerous cells, and for this reason they often produce serious adverse effects during long-term treatment. In particular, these drugs often adversely affect rapidly dividing cells such as the blood-producing cells in the bone marrow. The numbers of red and white blood cells and of platelets (particles in the blood responsible for clotting) may all be reduced. In some cases, symptoms of anaemia (weakness and fatigue) and an increased risk of abnormal or excessive bleeding may develop as a result of treatment with anticancer drugs.

A reduction in the number of white blood cells may result in increased susceptibility to infection. Even a simple infection such as a sore throat may be a sign of depressed white cell production in a patient taking anticancer drugs, and it must be reported to the doctor without delay. In addition, wounds may take longer to heal, and susceptible people can develop gout as a result of increased uric acid production due to cells being broken down.

Because of these problems, anticancer chemotherapy is often given in hospital, where the adverse effects can be closely monitored. Several short courses of treatment are usually given, thus allowing the bone marrow time to recover in the period between courses (see Successful chemotherapy, opposite). Blood tests are performed regularly. When necessary, blood transfusions, antibiotics, or other forms of treatment are used to overcome the adverse effects. When relevant, contraceptive advice is given early in treatment because most anticancer drugs can damage a developing baby. Eggs or sperm may be harvested before chemotherapy for later in vitro fertilization (IVF) after the chemotherapy is completed.

In addition to these general effects, individual drugs may have adverse effects on particular organs. These are described under individual drug profiles in Part 2.

By contrast, other anticancer drugs, such as hormonal drugs, antibodies, and small molecule inhibitors, are much more selective in their actions and they generally have less serious side effects.

COMMON DRUGS

Alkylating agents Chlorambucil, Cyclophosphamide*, Melphalan
Antimetabolites Azathioprine*, Capecitabine, Cytarabine, Fluorouracil*, Mercaptopurine*, Methotrexate*
Cytotoxic antibiotics Doxorubicin*, Epirubicin
Hormone treatments Anastrozole*, Bicalutamide, Cyproterone*, Flutamide*, Goserelin*, Letrozole, Leuprorelin, Medroxyprogesterone*, Megestrol, Tamoxifen*
Immunotherapies Interferon alfa*, Interleukin-2
Taxanes Docetaxel, Paclitaxel
Monoclonal antibodies Alemtuzumab, Bevacizumab*, Rituximab*, Trastuzumab*
Growth factor inhibitors Erlotinib, Imatinib*
Other drugs Carboplatin, Cisplatin*, Etoposide, Irinotecan
* **See Part 2**

Immunosuppressant drugs

The body is protected against attack from bacteria, fungi, and viruses by specialized cells and proteins in the blood and tissues that make up the immune system. White blood cells called lymphocytes kill invading organisms directly or produce proteins (antibodies) to destroy them. These mechanisms are also responsible for eliminating abnormal or unhealthy cells that could otherwise multiply and develop into a cancer.

In certain conditions, however, it is medically necessary to damp down the activity of the immune system. These include autoimmune disorders, in which the immune system attacks normal body tissue. Autoimmune disorders may affect a single organ – for example, the kidneys in Goodpasture's syndrome or the thyroid gland in Hashimoto's disease – or they may result in widespread damage: for example, in rheumatoid arthritis or systemic lupus erythematosus.

Immune system activity may also need to be reduced following an organ transplant, when the body's defences would otherwise attack and reject the transplanted tissue.

Several drug types are used as immunosuppressants: anticancer drugs (see p.94), corticosteroids (see p.78), ciclosporin (see p.180), and monoclonal antibodies (see p.95).

WHY THEY ARE USED

Immunosuppressant drugs are given to treat autoimmune disorders, such as rheumatoid arthritis, when symptoms are severe and other treatments have not provided adequate relief. Corticosteroids are usually prescribed initially. The pronounced anti-inflammatory effect of these drugs, as well as their immunosuppressant action, helps to promote healing of tissue damaged by abnormal immune system activity. Anticancer drugs such as methotrexate (see p.317) may be used in addition to corticosteroids if these do not produce sufficient improvement or if their effect wanes (see also Antirheumatic drugs, p.49).

Immunosuppressant drugs are given before and after organ and other tissue transplants. Treatment may have to be continued indefinitely to prevent rejection. Various drugs and drug combinations are used, depending on which organ is being transplanted and the underlying condition of the patient. However, ciclosporin, along with the related drug tacrolimus (see p.412), is now the most widely used drug for preventing organ rejection. It is also increasingly used to treat autoimmune disorders. It is often used in combination with a corticosteroid or the more specific drug mycophenolate mofetil.

Monoclonal antibodies, which destroy specific cells of the immune system, are also used to aid transplantation and are increasingly being used to treat autoimmune disorders. For example, infliximab (see p.277) is used to treat certain types of arthritis while rituximab (see p.389) is also used for systemic lupus erythematosus and vasculitis.

HOW THEY WORK

Immunosuppressant drugs reduce the effectiveness of the immune system, either by depressing the production of lymphocytes or by altering their activity.

HOW THEY AFFECT YOU

When immunosuppressants are given to treat an autoimmune disorder, they reduce the severity of symptoms and may temporarily halt the progress of the disease. However, they cannot restore major tissue damage.

Immunosuppressant drugs can produce a variety of unwanted side effects. The side effects of corticosteroids are described in more detail on p.78. Anticancer drugs, when prescribed as immunosuppressants, are given in low doses that produce only mild side effects. They may cause nausea and vomiting, for which an anti-emetic drug (p.19) may be prescribed. Hair loss is rare and regrowth usually occurs when the drug treatment is discontinued. Ciclosporin may cause increased growth of facial hair, swelling of the gums, and tingling in the hands.

RISKS AND SPECIAL PRECAUTIONS

All of these drugs may produce potentially serious adverse effects. By reducing the activity of the immune system, immunosuppressant drugs can affect the body's ability to fight invading microorganisms, thereby increasing the risk of serious infections. Because lymphocyte activity is also important for preventing the multiplication of abnormal cells, there is an increased risk of certain types of cancer. A major drawback of anticancer drugs is that, in addition to their effect on the production of lymphocytes, they interfere with the growth and division of other blood cells in the bone marrow. Reduced production of red blood cells can cause anaemia; when the production of blood platelets is suppressed, blood clotting may be less efficient.

Although ciclosporin is more specific in its action than either corticosteroids or anticancer drugs, it can cause kidney damage and, in too high a dose, may affect the brain, causing hallucinations or seizures. Ciclosporin also tends to raise blood pressure, and another drug may be required to counteract this effect (see Antihypertensive drugs, p.34).

COMMON DRUGS

Anticancer drugs Azathioprine*, Chlorambucil, Cyclophosphamide*, Methotrexate*

Corticosteroids (see p.78)

Antibodies Adalimumab, Anti-lymphocyte globulin, Basiliximab, Infliximab*, Rituximab*

Other drugs Ciclosporin*, Mycophenolate mofetil, Tacrolimus*

* **See Part 2**

Drugs for HIV and AIDS

AIDS (acquired immune deficiency syndrome) is caused by infection with the human immunodeficiency virus (HIV). This virus invades certain cells of the immune system, particularly the white blood cells called T-helper lymphocytes (or CD4 cells), which normally activate other immune cells to fight infection. HIV kills T-helper lymphocytes, so that the body cannot fight the virus or subsequent infections; this results in immune deficiency. In recent years the number of drugs to treat HIV has increased considerably, as well as knowledge about how best to use them in combination.

WHY THEY ARE USED

Drug treatments for HIV and AIDS can be divided into treatment of the initial infection with HIV and treatment of diseases and complications associated with AIDS.

Drugs that act directly against HIV are called antiretrovirals. The two most common groups work by interfering with enzymes that are vital for virus replication. The first group inhibit an enzyme called reverse

ANTIRETROVIRAL DRUGS

Drug name	Formulation	Additional information
Abacavir Ziagen	Tablets (300mg). Oral solution (20mg/ml)	Abacavir can cause a severe allergic-type reaction (see additional product information)
Abacavir, lamivudine Kivexa	Kivexa contains abacavir (600mg) and lamivudine (300mg)	Abacavir can cause a severe allergic-type reaction (see additional product information)
Abacavir, lamivudine, zidovudine (AZT) Trizivir	Trizivir contains abacavir (300mg), lamivudine (150mg), and zidovudine (300mg)	The abacavir contained in Trizivir can cause a severe allergic-type reaction (see additional product information)
Atazanavir Reyataz	Capsules (200mg, 150mg, 100mg)	
Darunavir Prezista	Tablets (400mg, 600mg, 800mg). Oral solution (100mg/ml)	Co-administered with a pharmacokinetic enhancer such as low-dose ritonavir
Dolutegravir Tivicay	Tablets (10mg, 25mg, 50mg)	
Efavirenz Sustiva	Capsules (200mg, 50mg). Tablets (600mg)	Efavirenz can cause a severe allergic-type rash (see additional product information)
Emtricitabine Emtriva	Capsules (200mg). Oral solution (10mg/ml)	
Enfuvirtide Fuzeon	Subcutaneous injection (90mg) powder for reconstitution	Caution in liver impairment, including hepatitis B or C
Indinavir Crixivan	Capsules (400mg, 200mg)	Indinavir should be taken with a low-fat meal, or 1 hour before or 2 hours after any other meal
Lamivudine (3TC) Epivir	Tablets (300mg, 150mg). Oral solution (50mg/5ml)	Lamivudine can also be used to treat hepatitis B
Lopinavir with ritonavir Kaletra	Tablets (200mg lopinavir, 50mg ritonavir). Capsules (133mg, 33mg). Oral solution (400mg, 100mg/5ml)	
Maraviroc Celsentri	Tablets (25mg, 75mg, 150mg, 300mg)	
Nevirapine Viramune	Tablets (200mg). Suspension (50mg/5ml)	Nevirapine can cause a severe allergic-type reaction (see additional product information)
Raltegravir Isentress	Tablets (400mg, 600mg)	
Ritonavir Norvir	Capsules (100mg). Oral solution (400mg/5ml)	Doses should be taken with food
Saquinavir Invirase	Capsules (200mg). Tablets (500mg)	Doses should be taken within 2 hours of a full meal
Stavudine (d4T) Zerit	Capsules (40mg, 30mg, 20mg). Oral solution (1mg/ml)	
Tenofovir disoproxil Viread	Tablets (245mg as disoproxil fumarate = 300mg tenofovir)	Tenofovir should be taken with food
Tenofovir disoproxil, emtricitabine Truvada	Truvada contains tenofovir (245mg) and emtricitabine (200mg)	
Zidovudine (AZT) Retrovir	Capsules (250mg, 100mg). Syrup (50mg/5ml). Injection (10mg/ml)	
Zidovudine (AZT), lamivudine Combivir	Combivir contains zidovudine (300mg) and lamivudine (150mg)	

transcriptase. They are divided into nucleoside inhibitors (also called nucleoside analogues), nucleotide inhibitors (nucleotide analogues), and non-nucleoside inhibitors. The second group interfere with an enzyme called protease.

Integrase inhibitors prevent the virus from injecting its DNA into the cell nucleus and are joining first-line therapy combinations. Entry inhibitors interfere with the entry of the virus into the cell. Further groups are being developed to target the receptor sites that the virus uses for entry into cells.

Antiretrovirals are much more effective in combination. Treatment usually starts with two nucleoside transcriptase inhibitors plus a non-nucleoside drug, integrase inhibitor, or protease inhibitor. If combination antiretroviral therapy (ART) is started before the immune system is too damaged, it can dramatically reduce the level of HIV in the body and improve the outlook for HIV-infected people, although it is not a cure and such people remain infectious.

The mainstays of drug treatment for AIDS-related diseases are antimicrobials for the bacterial, viral, fungal, and protozoal infections to which people with AIDS are particularly susceptible. These include antituberculous drugs (p.65), co-trimoxazole for pneumocystis pneumonia, and ganciclovir to treat cytomegalovirus (CMV) infection.

HOW THEY WORK

The process of infection with HIV involves several stages, in which the virus enters T-helper white blood cells containing the CD4 protein and a co-receptor protein and replicates itself. The major groups of drugs to combat HIV are designed to take effect at different stages of the process.

Stages 1 and 2 The virus binds to a specialized set of receptors on a T-helper cell with CD4 protein, and then enters the cell.

Drugs such as enfuvirtide and dolutegravir block the entry of HIV into T-helper cells. Drugs that block the receptor site on the cell include maraviroc, which blocks the co-receptor.

Stages 3 and 4 The virus loses its protective coat and releases RNA, its genetic material, and the enzyme reverse transcriptase. The reverse transcriptase converts viral RNA into a form that can enter the host cell's nucleus and become integrated with the cell's genetic material.

The reverse transcriptase inhibitors, such as zidovudine, efavirenz, and tenofovir, act at this point.

Stages 5 and 6 The host cell starts to produce new viral RNA and protein from the viral material that has been integrated into its nucleus. The new viral RNA and proteins assemble to produce new viruses. These leave the host cell (which then dies) and are free to attack other cells in the body.

The protease inhibitors prevent formation of viral proteins and viral assembly.

COMMON DRUGS

Nucleoside reverse transcriptase inhibitors (nucleoside analogues) Abacavir, Emtricitabine*, Lamivudine, Stavudine, Zidovudine (AZT)/lamivudine*

Nucleotide reverse transcriptase inhibitor (nucleotide analogue) Tenofovir*

Non-nucleoside reverse transcriptase inhibitors Efavirenz*, Nevirapine

Integrase inhibitors Dolutegravir, Raltegravir

Protease inhibitors Atazanavir, Darunavir, Lopinavir/ritonavir*, Saquinavir

Entry/fusion inhibitors Enfuvirtide, Maraviroc

*** See Part 2**

REPRODUCTIVE & URINARY TRACTS

The reproductive systems of men and women consist of those organs that produce and release sperm (male), or that store and release eggs and then nurture a fertilized egg until it develops into a baby (female).

The urinary system filters wastes and water from the blood, producing urine, which is then expelled from the body.

The reproductive and urinary systems of men are partially linked, but those of women form two physically close but functionally separate systems.

The female reproductive organs comprise the ovaries, the fallopian tubes, and the uterus (womb). The uterus opens via the cervix (neck of the uterus) into the vagina. The principal male reproductive organs are the two sperm-producing glands, the testes (testicles), which lie within the scrotum, and the penis. Other parts of the system in males include the prostate gland and several tubular structures – the tightly coiled epididymides (singular: epididymis), the vas deferens, the seminal vesicles, and the urethra.

The urinary organs in both sexes comprise the kidneys, which filter the blood and excrete urine; the ureters, down which urine passes from the kidneys; and the bladder, where urine is stored until it is released from the body through the urethra.

WHAT CAN GO WRONG

The reproductive and urinary tracts are both subject to infection. Such infections (apart from those transmitted by sexual activity) are relatively uncommon in males because the long urethra prevents bacteria and other organisms from passing easily to the bladder and upper urinary tract, and to the male sex organs. The shorter female urethra does allow urinary tract infections, especially of the bladder (cystitis) and the urethra (urethritis), to occur commonly. The female reproductive tract is also vulnerable to infection, which in some cases is sexually transmitted.

Reproductive function may be disrupted by hormonal disturbances that lead to reduced fertility. Women may also develop symptoms arising from normal activity of the reproductive organs, including menstrual disorders as well as problems associated with childbirth.

The most common urinary problems apart from infection are those related to bladder function. Urine may be released involuntarily (incontinence) or it may be retained in the bladder. Such urinary disorders are usually the result of abnormal nerve signals to the bladder or sphincter muscle. The filtering action of the kidneys may be affected by alteration in the composition of the blood or the hormones that regulate urine production, or by damage to the filtering units themselves from infection or inflammation.

WHY DRUGS ARE USED

Antibiotic drugs (p.60) are used to eliminate infections of the urinary and reproductive tracts (including sexually transmitted infections). In addition, certain infections of the vagina are caused by fungi or yeasts and require antifungal drugs (p.74).

Hormone drugs are used both to reduce fertility deliberately (oral contraceptives) and to increase fertility in certain conditions in which it has not been possible for a couple to conceive. Hormones may also be used to regulate menstruation when it is irregular or excessively painful or heavy. Analgesic drugs (see p.7) are used to treat menstrual period pain and are also widely used for pain relief in labour. Other drugs used in labour include those that increase contraction of the muscles of the uterus and those that limit blood loss after the birth. Drugs may also be employed to halt premature labour.

Drugs that alter the transmission of nerve signals to the bladder muscles have an important role in the treatment of urinary incontinence and retention. Drugs that increase the kidneys' filtering action are commonly used to reduce blood pressure and fluid retention (see Diuretics, p.30). Other drugs may alter the composition of the urine – for example, the uricosuric drugs that are used in the treatment of gout (see p.51) increase the amount of uric acid.

THE MENSTRUAL CYCLE

A monthly cycle of hormone interactions in females allows an egg to be released and, if it is fertilized, creates the correct environment for it to implant in the uterus. Major changes occur in the body, the most obvious of which is monthly vaginal bleeding (menstruation). The menstrual cycle usually starts between the ages of 11 and 14 years and continues until the menopause, which occurs at around the age of 50. After the menopause, child-bearing is no longer possible. The cycle is usually 28 days, but this varies from one individual to another.

Menstruation If no egg is fertilized, the endometrium is shed (days 1–5).

Fertile period Conception may take place in the two days after ovulation (days 14–16).

MAJOR DRUG GROUPS

- Drugs used to treat menstrual disorders
- Oral contraceptives
- Drugs for infertility
- Drugs used in labour
- Drugs used for urinary disorders

Drugs used to treat menstrual disorders

The menstrual cycle results from the actions of female sex hormones that cause ovulation (the release of an egg from an ovary) and thickening of the endometrium (the lining of the uterus) each month in preparation for pregnancy. Unless the egg is fertilized, the endometrium will be shed approximately 2 weeks later during menstruation (see also The menstrual cycle, above).

The main problems associated with menstruation that may require medical treatment are excessive blood loss (menorrhagia), pain during menstruation (dysmenorrhoea), and the distressing physical and psychological symptoms that sometimes occur before menstruation (premenstrual syndrome).

The absence of periods (amenorrhoea) is commonly due to pregnancy in women of childbearing age or to the menopause in older women; other causes are discussed under female sex hormones (see p.86).

The drugs most commonly used to treat the menstrual disorders described in this section include oestrogens, progestogens, and analgesics (painkillers).

WHY THEY ARE USED

Drug treatment for menstrual disorders is undertaken only when the doctor has ruled out the possibility of an underlying gynaecological disorder, such as a pelvic infection or fibroids. In some cases, especially in women over the age of 35, a D and C (dilatation and curettage) may be recommended. When no underlying reason for the problem is found, drug treatment aimed primarily at the relief of symptoms is usually prescribed.

Dysmenorrhoea Painful menstrual periods are usually treated initially with a simple analgesic drug (see p.7). Non-steroidal anti-inflammatory drugs (NSAIDs, see p.48) are often most effective because they counter the effects of prostaglandins, chemicals that are partly responsible for transmission of pain to the brain. The NSAID mefenamic acid has the additional ability to reduce the excessive blood loss of menorrhagia (see below).

When these drugs are not sufficient to provide adequate pain relief, hormonal drug treatment may be recommended. If contraception is also required, treatment may involve an oral contraceptive pill containing both an oestrogen and a progestogen, or a progestogen alone. Non-contraceptive progestogen preparations may also be prescribed. These are usually taken for only a few days during each month.

Menorrhagia Excessive loss of blood during menstruation can sometimes be reduced by some NSAIDs. Tranexamic acid, an antifibrinolytic drug (see p.36), is an effective treatment for menorrhagia. Alternatively, danazol, a drug that reduces production of the female sex hormone oestrogen, may be prescribed to reduce blood loss.

Premenstrual syndrome This is a collection of psychological and physical symptoms that affect many women to some degree in the days before menstruation. Psychological symptoms include mood changes such as increased irritability, depression, and anxiety. Principal physical symptoms are bloating, headache, and breast tenderness.

Combined oral contraceptives may be prescribed, and, for severe premenstrual syndrome, SSRI antidepressants (see p.12) are sometimes given. Other drugs sometimes used include pyridoxine (vitamin B6), diuretics (see p.30) if bloating due to fluid retention is a problem, and bromocriptine when breast tenderness is the major symptom.

Endometriosis is a condition in which fragments of endometrial tissue (uterine lining) occur outside the uterus in the pelvic cavity. It can cause severe pain during menstruation or intercourse, as well as cyclical gastrointestinal or urinary symptoms, and may sometimes lead to infertility. Drugs used for this disorder are similar to those prescribed for heavy periods (menorrhagia). In this case, however, the intention is to suppress endometrial development for an extended period so that the abnormal tissue eventually withers away. Progesterone supplements that suppress endometrial thickening may be prescribed throughout the menstrual cycle. Alternatively, danazol, which suppresses endometrial development by reducing oestrogen production, may be prescribed. Any drug treatment usually needs to be continued for a minimum of 6 months. If drug treatment is unsuccessful, surgical removal of the abnormal tissue is usually necessary.

HOW THEY WORK

Drugs used to treat menstrual disorders act in a variety of ways. Hormonal treatments are aimed at suppressing the pattern of hormonal changes that is causing troublesome symptoms. Contraceptive preparations override the woman's normal menstrual cycle. Ovulation does not occur, and the endometrium does not thicken normally. Bleeding that occurs at the end of a cycle is less likely to be abnormally heavy, to be accompanied by severe discomfort, or to be preceded by distressing symptoms.

Non-contraceptive progestogen preparations taken in the days before menstruation do not suppress ovulation. Increased progesterone during this time reduces premenstrual symptoms and prevents excessive thickening of the endometrium.

Danazol, a potent drug, prevents the thickening of the endometrium, thereby correcting excessively heavy periods. Blood loss is reduced, and in some cases menstruation ceases altogether during treatment.

COMMON DRUGS

Oestrogens and progestogens (see p.86)
NSAID analgesics Aspirin*, Dexibuprofen, Dexketoprofen, Diclofenac*, Flurbiprofen, Ibuprofen*, Indometacin, Ketoprofen*, Mefenamic acid*, Naproxen*
Diuretics (see p.30)
Other drugs Bromocriptine*, Buserelin, Danazol, Gestrinone, Goserelin*, Leuprorelin, Nafarelin, Pyridoxine, Tranexamic acid, Triptorelin
* **See Part 2**

Oral contraceptives

There are various methods of ensuring that conception and pregnancy do not follow sexual intercourse, but for many women oral contraception is the preferred method because it is highly effective (see chart, p.104), convenient, and unobtrusive during sexual intercourse. About 30 per cent of the women who seek contraceptive protection in the UK choose a form of oral contraceptive.

There are three main types of oral contraceptive: the combined pill, the progestogen-only pill (POP), and the phased pill. All three types contain a progestogen (a synthetic form of the female sex hormone progesterone). Both the combined and phased pills also contain a natural or synthetic oestrogen (see also Female sex hormones, p.86).

The following list indicates the number of pregnancies occurring with each method of contraception per 100 women using that method in a year. The figures are for correct usage; if a contraceptive is used incorrectly, the failure rate will be higher. The variation that occurs with some of these methods takes into account pregnancies that occur through incorrect use (e.g. the wide variation in figures for the "morning after" pill reflects the difference in effectiveness depending on how soon it is taken after unprotected sex). Figures for typical use, if different from those for correct use, are given in brackets.

- Combined or phased pill Less than 1 (9)
- IUD (Intrauterine device) Less than 1

- IUS (Intrauterine system) Less than 1
- Contraceptive implant Less than 1
- Contraceptive injection Less than 1
- Progestogen-only pill About 1 (9)
- Male condom About 2 (18)
- Female condom About 5 (21)
- Diaphragm with spermicide 4–8 (12–29)
- Cap with spermicide 4–8 (12–29)
- "Morning after" pill About 2–42 (N/A)

WHY THEY ARE USED

The combined pill This is the most widely prescribed form of oral contraceptive and has the lowest failure rate in terms of unwanted pregnancies. It is referred to as the "pill" and is the type thought most suitable for young women who want to use a hormonal form of contraception. The combined pill is particularly suitable for those women who regularly experience exceptionally painful, heavy, or prolonged periods (see Drugs used to treat menstrual disorders, p.102).

There are many different products available containing a fixed dose of an oestrogen and a progestogen drug. They are divided generally into three groups according to their oestrogen content (see table, below). Low-dose products are chosen when possible to minimize the risk of adverse effects.

Progestogen-only pill (POP) The POP is often recommended for women who react adversely to the oestrogen in the combined pill or for whom the combined pill is not considered suitable because of their age or medical history (see Risks and special precautions, opposite). It is also prescribed for breast-feeding women as it does not reduce milk production. The POP has a higher failure rate than the combined pill and, for maximum contraceptive effect, must be taken at precisely the same time each day. It works by changing the quality of the endometrium (lining of the uterus), making implantation of a fertilized egg less likely. However, Cerazette (a brand of the progestogen desogestrel) also inhibits ovulation, making it more reliable than other POPs.

Phased pills The third form of oral contraceptive is a pack of pills divided into two or three groups or phases. Each phase contains a different proportion of an oestrogen and a progestogen. The aim is to provide a hormonal balance that closely resembles the fluctuations of a normal menstrual cycle. Phased pills provide effective protection for many women who have side effects with other available forms of oral contraceptive.

HOW THEY WORK

In a normal menstrual cycle, the ripening and release of an egg and the preparation of the uterus for implantation of a fertilized egg

HORMONE CONTENT OF COMMON ORAL CONTRACEPTIVES

Oestrogen-containing forms are classified by their oestrogen content as follows: low: 20 micrograms; standard: 30–35 micrograms; high: 50 micrograms; phased pills: 30–40 micrograms. Morning after: 1.5 milligrams (levonorgestrel), 30 milligrams (ulipristal).

TYPE OF PILL (oestrogen content)	BRAND NAMES
Combined (20mcg)	Loestrin 20, Femodette, Gedarel 20/150, Mercilon, Millinette 20/75, Sunya 20/75
(30–35mcg)	Brevinor, Cilest, Femodene, Femodene ED, Gedarel 30/150, Katya 30/75, Levest, Loestrin 30, Marvelon, Microgynon 30, Microgynon 30 ED, Millinette 30/75, Norimin, Ovranette, Rigevidon, Yasmin
(50mcg)	Norinyl-1 (as Mestranol)
Phased (30–40mcg)	Logynon, Logynon ED, Synphase, TriRegol
Progestogen-only (no oestrogen)	Cerazette, Cerelle, Feanolla, Micronor, Norgeston, Noriday
Postcoital (morning after) (no oestrogen)	EllaOne, Levonelle 1500, Levonelle One Step

result from a complex interplay between the natural female sex hormones, oestrogen and progesterone, and the pituitary hormones, follicle-stimulating hormone (FSH) and luteinizing hormone (LH) (see also p.107). The oestrogen and progestogens in oral contraceptives disrupt the menstrual cycle in such a way that conception is less likely.

With combined pills and phased pills, the increased levels of oestrogen and progesterone produce similar effects to the hormonal changes of pregnancy. The actions of the hormones inhibit the production of FSH and LH, thereby preventing the egg from ripening in the ovary and from being released.

The POP has a slightly different effect. It does not always prevent release of an egg; its main contraceptive action may be to thicken the mucus that lines the cervix, preventing sperm from crossing it. This effect occurs to some extent with combined and phased pills. Cerazette, additionally, inhibits ovulation.

HOW THEY AFFECT YOU

Each course of combined and phased pills lasts for 21 days, followed by a pill-free 7 days during which time menstruation occurs. Some brands contain additional inactive pills. With these, the new course directly follows the last so that the habit of taking the pill daily is not broken. Progestogen-only pills are taken for 28 days each month. Menstruation usually occurs during the last few days of the menstrual cycle.

Women taking oral contraceptives, especially drugs that contain oestrogen, usually find that their menstrual periods are lighter and relatively pain-free. Some women cease to menstruate altogether. This is not a cause for concern in itself, provided no pills have been missed, but it may make it difficult to determine if pregnancy has occurred. An apparently missed period probably indicates a light one, rather than pregnancy. However, if you have missed two consecutive periods and you feel that you may be pregnant, it is advisable to have a pregnancy test.

All forms of oral contraceptive may cause spotting of blood in the middle of the menstrual cycle (breakthrough bleeding), especially at first, but this can be a particular problem with the POP.

Oral contraceptives that contain oestrogen may produce any of a large number of mild side effects, depending on the dose. Symptoms similar to those experienced early in pregnancy may occur, particularly in the first few months of pill use: some women complain of nausea and vomiting, weight gain, depression, altered libido, increased appetite, and cramps in the legs and abdomen. The pill may also affect the circulation, producing minor headaches and dizziness. All of these effects usually disappear within a few months, but if they persist it may be advisable to change to a brand containing a lower dose of oestrogen or to some other contraceptive method.

RISKS AND SPECIAL PRECAUTIONS

All oral contraceptives need to be taken regularly for maximum protection against pregnancy. Contraceptive protection can be reduced by missing a pill (see What to do if you miss a pill, p.107). It may also be reduced by vomiting or diarrhoea. If you vomit within 2 hours of taking a pill, take another one. If vomiting and diarrhoea persist, follow the instructions on the packet or consult your doctor or pharmacist. Many drugs may also affect the action of oral contraceptives, and it is essential to tell your doctor that you are taking oral contraceptives before taking additional prescribed medications.

Oral contraceptives, particularly those containing an oestrogen, have been found to carry a number of risks (see Balancing the risks and benefits of oral contraceptives, p.106). One of the most serious potential adverse effects of oestrogen-containing pills is development of a thrombus (blood clot) in a vein or artery. The thrombus may travel to the lungs or cause a stroke or heart attack. The risk of thrombus formation increases with age and other factors, notably obesity, high blood pressure, and smoking. Doctors assess these risk factors for each person when prescribing oral contraceptives. A woman over 35 may be advised against taking a combined pill, especially if she smokes or has an underlying medical condition such as diabetes. Some studies have found that women who take a combined oral contraceptive containing desogestrel or gestodene are at greater risk of developing a venous thromboembolism. The risk is still very small, however, and is lower than the risk of developing a venous thromboembolism during pregnancy. The combined oral contraceptive pills that contain desogestrel include Marvelon and Mercilon; those that contain gestodene include Femodene, Femodette, Katya 30/75, Millinette 20/75 and 30/75, and Sunya 20/75.

High blood pressure is a possible complication of oral contraceptives for some women. Measurement of blood pressure before the pill is prescribed and every 6 months after the woman starts taking oral contraceptives is advised for all women taking oral contraceptives.

Some very rare liver cancers have occurred in women using the pill, and breast cancer and cervical cancer may be slightly more common, but cancers of the ovaries and uterus are less common.

Although there is no evidence that oral contraceptives reduce a woman's fertility or damage babies conceived after they are discontinued, doctors recommend waiting for at least one normal menstrual period before you attempt to conceive.

BALANCING THE RISKS AND BENEFITS OF ORAL CONTRACEPTIVES

Oral contraceptives are safe for the vast majority of young women. However, every woman who is considering oral contraception should discuss with her doctor the risks and possible adverse effects of the drugs before deciding whether or not hormonal contraception is the most suitable method in her case.

A variety of factors must be taken into account, including the woman's age, her own medical history and that of her close relatives, and factors such as whether or not she is a smoker. The importance of such factors varies depending on the type of oral contraceptive under consideration.

The principal advantages and disadvantages of oestrogen-containing and progestogen-only pills are listed below.

Advantages of oestrogen-containing combined and phased pills Very reliable; convenient and unobtrusive; regularize menstruation; reduce menstrual pain and blood loss; reduce risks of benign breast disease, endometriosis, ectopic pregnancy, ovarian cysts, pelvic infection, ovarian and endometrial cancer.

Advantages of progestogen-only pill Very reliable; convenient and unobtrusive, although the timing of doses is more critical than in the case of combined and phased pills; suitable for use during breast-feeding; avoids any oestrogen-related side effects and risks; allows rapid return to fertility; suitable for women in whom use of oestrogen-containing contraception is not possible.

Side effects of oestrogen-containing combined and phased pills Weight gain; depression; breast swelling; reduced sex drive; headaches; increased vaginal discharge; nausea.

Side effects of progestogen-only pill Irregular menstruation; nausea; headaches; breast discomfort; depression; changes in libido; weight changes.

Risks of oestrogen-containing combined and phased pills Thromboembolism; heart disease; high blood pressure; liver impairment/ cancer of the liver (rare); gallstones; breast and/or cervical cancer (although risk is low).

Risks of progestogen-only pill Ectopic pregnancy; ovarian cysts; breast cancer (although risk is low).

Factors that may prohibit use of oestrogen-containing combined and phased pills Previous thrombosis*; heart disease; high levels of lipid in blood; liver disease; blood disorders; high blood pressure; unexplained vaginal bleeding; migraine; otosclerosis; presence of several risk factors (see below).

Factors that may prohibit use of progestogen-only pill Previous ectopic pregnancy; heart or circulatory disease; unexplained vaginal bleeding; history of breast cancer.

Factors that increase risks of oestrogen-containing combined and phased pills Smoking*; obesity*; increasing age; diabetes mellitus; family history of heart or circulatory disease*; current treatment with other drugs.

Factors that increase risks of progestogen-only pill As for oestrogen-containing pills, but to a lesser degree.

*Products containing desogestrel or gestodene have a higher excess risk with these factors than other progestogens.

HOW TO MINIMIZE YOUR HEALTH RISKS WHILE TAKING THE PILL

- Do not smoke.
- Maintain a healthy weight and diet.
- Have regular blood pressure and blood lipid checks.
- Have regular cervical screening tests.
- Remind your doctor that you are taking oral contraceptives before taking other prescription drugs.
- Stop taking oestrogen-containing oral contraceptives 4 weeks before any planned major surgery (use alternative method of contraception).

WHAT TO DO IF YOU MISS A PILL

Contraceptive protection may be reduced if blood levels of the hormones in the body fall due to missing a pill. It is particularly important to ensure that progestogen-only pills are taken punctually. If you miss a pill, the action you take depends on the degree of lateness and type of pill being used (see below).

Combined and phased pills* If you are less than 24 hours late, take the missed pill now and the next on time. If you are over 24 hours late, the pill may not work. Take the missed pill now and the next on time. If more than one pill has been missed, just take one, then take the next on time (even if on the same day). Take additional precautions for the next 7 days. If the 7 days extends into the pill-free (or inactive pill) period, start the next packet without a break (or without taking inactive pills).

* Except Qlaira, Zoely, Eloine, and Daylette; refer to patient information leaflet.

Progestogen-only pills If you are less than 3 hours late (12 for Cerazette), take the missed pill now and the next on time. If you are over 3 hours late (12 for Cerazette), take the missed pill now and the next on time. If more than one pill has been missed, just take one, then take the next on time (even if on the same day). In either case, you are not protected and will need to take additional precautions for the next 7 days.

POSTCOITAL CONTRACEPTION

Pregnancy following intercourse without contraception may be avoided by taking a postcoital (morning after) pill. The drugs in this pill (levonorgestrel and ulipristal) are synthetic progestogens that work by inhibiting ovulation and also by changing the endometrium (uterine lining) to reduce the likelihood of a fertilized egg implanting.

The drugs should be taken as soon as possible after unprotected intercourse; levonorgestrel is only effective if taken within 72 hours, ulipristal if taken within 120 hours. The high progestogen dose required makes this method unsuitable for regular use. It also has a higher failure rate than the usual oral contraceptives. Having a coil (IUD) inserted within 120 hours of unprotected intercourse can also prevent pregnancy.

COMMON DRUGS

Progestogens Desogestrel*, Dienogest, Drospirenone, Gestodene, Levonorgestrel*, Nomegestrol, Norethisterone*, Norgestimate, Ulipristal*

Oestrogens Estradiol*, Ethinylestradiol*, Mestranol

* **See Part 2**

Drugs for infertility

Conception and the establishment of pregnancy require a healthy reproductive system in both partners. The man must be able to produce sufficient numbers of healthy sperm; the woman must be able to produce a healthy egg that is able to pass freely down the fallopian tube to the uterus. The lining of the uterus must be in a condition that allows the implantation of the fertilized egg.

The cause of infertility may sometimes remain undiscovered, but in the majority of cases it is due to one of the following factors: intercourse taking place at the wrong time during the menstrual cycle; the man producing too few or unhealthy sperm; the woman either failing to ovulate (release an egg) or having blocked fallopian tubes, perhaps as a result of previous pelvic infection. Alternatively, production of gonadotrophin hormones – follicle-stimulating hormone (FSH) and luteinizing hormone (LH) – needed for ovulation and implantation of the egg may be affected by illness or psychological stress.

If no simple explanation can be found, the man's semen will be analysed. If these tests show that abnormally low numbers of sperm are being produced, or if a large proportion of the sperm produced are unhealthy, drug treatment may be tried.

If no abnormality of sperm production is discovered, the woman will be given a thorough medical examination. Ovulation is monitored and blood tests may be performed to assess hormone levels. If ovulation does not occur, the woman may be offered drug treatment.

WHY THEY ARE USED

In men, the evidence is poor for treating low sperm production with gonadotrophins – FSH or human chorionic gonadotrophin (hCG) – or a pituitary-stimulating drug (for example, clomifene) and corticosteroids.

In women, drugs are useful in helping to achieve pregnancy only if a hormone defect inhibiting ovulation has been diagnosed. Treatment may continue for months and does not always result in pregnancy. Women in whom the pituitary gland is producing some FSH and LH may be given courses of clomifene for several days during each month. Usually, up to three courses may be tried. An effective dose produces ovulation 5 to 10 days after the last tablet is taken.

Clomifene may thicken cervical mucus, impeding the passage of sperm, but the advantage of achieving ovulation outweighs the risk of this side effect. If treatment with clomifene fails to produce ovulation, or if a disorder of the pituitary gland prevents the production of FSH and LH, treatment with FSH and LH together, FSH alone, or hCG may be given. In menstruating women, FSH is started within the first 7 days of the menstrual cycle.

HOW THEY WORK

Ovulation (release of an egg) and implantation are governed by hormones produced by the pituitary gland. FSH stimulates ripening of the egg follicle. LH triggers ovulation and ensures that progesterone is produced to prepare the uterus for the implantation of the egg. Drugs for female infertility raise the chance of ovulation by boosting levels of LH and FSH. Clomifene stimulates the pituitary gland to increase its output of these two hormones. Artificially produced FSH and hCG mimic the action of naturally produced FSH and LH, respectively. Both treatments, when successful, stimulate ovulation and implantation of the fertilized egg.

HOW THEY AFFECT YOU

Clomifene may produce hot flushes, nausea, headaches, and, rarely, ovarian cysts and visual disturbance, while hCG can cause tiredness, headaches, and mood changes. FSH can cause the ovaries to enlarge, resulting in abdominal discomfort. The drugs increase the likelihood of multiple births, usually twins.

DRUGS FOR ERECTILE DYSFUNCTION

Erectile dysfunction (also known as impotence) is a male disorder defined as inability to achieve or maintain an erection. The penis contains three cylinders of erectile tissue: the two corpora cavernosa and the corpus spongiosum. Normally, when a man is sexually aroused, the arteries in the penis relax and widen, allowing more blood than usual to flow into the organ, filling the corpora cavernosa and corpus spongiosum. As these tissues expand and harden, the veins that carry blood out of the penis are compressed, reducing outflow and resulting in an erection. In some forms of erectile dysfunction, this does not happen. Drugs can be used to increase blood flow into the penis and thus produce an erection.

Sildenafil and tadalafil not only increase the blood flow into the penis but also prevent the muscle wall from relaxing, so the blood does not drain out of the blood vessels and the penis remains erect.

Alprostadil is a prostaglandin drug that helps men achieve an erection by widening the blood vessels, but it must be injected directly into the penis, or applied into the urethra using a special syringe.

COMMON DRUGS

Bromocriptine*, Buserelin, Cetrorelix, Chorionic gonadotrophin (hCG), Clomifene*, Follitropin (FSH), Ganirelix, Goserelin*, Lutropin (LH), Menopausal gonadotrophins (Menotrophin), Nafarelin, Tamoxifen*

Drugs for erectile dysfunction

Alprostadil, Sildenafil/tadalafil*, Vardenafil

* **See Part 2**

Drugs used in labour

Normal labour has three stages. In the first stage, the uterus begins to contract, initially irregularly and then gradually more regularly and powerfully, while the cervix dilates until it is fully stretched. During the second stage, powerful contractions of the uterus push the baby down the mother's birth canal and out of her body. The third stage involves the delivery of the placenta.

Drugs may be required during one or more stages of labour for any of the following reasons: to induce or augment labour; to delay premature labour (see Uterine muscle relaxants, right); and to relieve pain. The administration of some drugs may be viewed as part of normal obstetric care; for example, the uterine stimulants ergometrine and oxytocin may be injected routinely before the third stage of labour to prevent excessive bleeding. Other drugs are administered only when the condition of the mother or baby requires intervention. The possible adverse effects on both mother and baby are always carefully balanced against the benefits.

DRUGS TO INDUCE OR AUGMENT LABOUR

Induction of labour may be advised when a doctor considers it risky for the health of the mother or baby for the pregnancy to continue – for example, if natural labour does not occur within 2 weeks of the due date or when a woman has pre-eclampsia. Other common reasons for inducing labour include premature rupture of the membrane surrounding the baby (breaking of the waters), slow growth of the baby due to poor nourishment by the placenta, or death of the fetus in the uterus.

When labour needs to be induced, oxytocin may be administered intravenously. Alternatively, a prostaglandin pessary may be given to soften and dilate the cervix. If these methods are ineffective or cannot be used because of potential adverse effects (see Risks and special precautions, below), a caesarean delivery may have to be performed.

Oxytocin may also be used to strengthen the force of the contractions in labour that has started spontaneously but has not continued normally.

A combination of oxytocin and another uterine stimulant, ergometrine, is given to most women as the baby is being born or immediately following birth to prevent excessive bleeding after the delivery of the placenta. This drug combination encourages the uterus to contract after delivery, which restricts the flow of blood.

RISKS AND SPECIAL PRECAUTIONS

When oxytocin is used to induce labour, the dosage is carefully monitored throughout to prevent the possibility of excessively violent contractions. It is administered to women who have had surgery on the uterus only with careful monitoring. The drug is not known to affect the baby adversely. Ergometrine is not given to women who have had high blood pressure during pregnancy or those who have cardiovascular disease.

DRUGS USED FOR PAIN RELIEF

Opioid analgesics Pethidine, morphine, or other opioids may be given once active labour has been established (see Analgesics, p.7). Possible side effects in the mother include drowsiness, nausea, and vomiting. Opioid drugs may cause breathing difficulties for the new baby, but these problems may be reversed by the antidote naloxone.

Epidural anaesthesia This provides pain relief during labour and birth by numbing the nerves leading to the uterus and pelvic area. It is often used during a planned caesarean delivery, thus enabling the mother to be fully conscious for the birth.

An epidural involves the injection of a local anaesthetic drug (see p.9) into the epidural space between the spinal cord and the vertebrae. An epidural may block the mother's urge to push during the second stage, and a forceps delivery may be necessary. Headaches may occasionally occur following epidural anaesthesia.

Oxygen and nitrous oxide These gases are combined to produce a mixture that reduces the pain caused by contractions. During the first and second stages of labour, gas is self-administered by inhalation through a mouthpiece or mask. If it is used over too long a period, it may produce nausea, confusion, and dehydration in the mother.

Local anaesthetics These drugs are injected inside the vagina or near the vaginal opening and are used to numb sensation during forceps delivery, before an episiotomy (an incision that is made to enlarge the vaginal opening), and when stitches are necessary. Side effects are rare.

UTERINE MUSCLE RELAXANTS

When contractions of the uterus start before the 34th week of pregnancy, doctors usually advise bed rest and may also administer a drug that relaxes the muscles of the uterus, and thus halts labour. Initially, the drug is given in hospital by injection, but it may be continued orally at home. These drugs work by stimulating the sympathetic nervous system (see Autonomic nervous system, p.6) and may cause palpitations and anxiety in the mother. They have not been shown to have adverse effects on the baby.

DRUGS USED TO TERMINATE PREGNANCY

Drugs may be used to terminate pregnancy or to empty the uterus after the death of the baby. The principal drugs used are mifepristone and a prostaglandin (usually gemeprost or misoprostol). The effect of these drugs is to stimulate a miscarriage. Mifepristone blocks the action of progesterone, which is necessary for continuation of pregnancy, and ripens the cervix. The prostaglandin causes the uterine lining to break down and be shed from the body, causing bleeding. Surgical methods, such as suction termination or dilation and evacuation, can be used either instead of drugs or when a drug-induced termination is unsuccessful; these may be carried out under local or general anaesthesia.

COMMON DRUGS

Prostaglandins Carboprost, Dinoprostone, Gemeprost, Misoprostol*
Pain relief Entonox® (oxygen and nitrous oxide), Fentanyl, Morphine*, Pethidine
Antiprogestogen Mifepristone
Uterine muscle relaxants Atosiban, Salbutamol*, Terbutaline*
Uterine stimulants Ergometrine, Oxytocin
Local anaesthetics Bupivacaine, Lidocaine (lignocaine)
* **See Part 2**

Drugs used for urinary disorders

Urine is produced by the kidneys and stored in the bladder. As the urine accumulates, the bladder walls stretch and pressure within the bladder increases. Eventually, the stretching stimulates nerve endings that produce the urge to urinate. The ring of muscle (sphincter) around the bladder neck normally keeps the bladder closed until it is consciously relaxed, allowing urine to pass via the urethra out of the body.

A number of disorders can affect the urinary tract. The most common of these disorders are infection in the bladder (cystitis) or the urethra (urethritis), and loss of reliable control over urination (urinary incontinence). A less common problem is inability to expel urine (urinary retention). Drugs used to treat these problems include antibiotics (see p.60) and antibacterial drugs (see p.64), analgesics (see p.7), drugs to increase the acidity of the urine, and drugs that act on nerve control over the muscles of the bladder and sphincter.

DRUGS FOR URINARY INFECTION

Nearly all infections of the bladder are caused by bacteria. Symptoms include a continual urge to urinate, although often nothing is passed; pain on urinating; and pain in the lower abdomen.

Many antibiotics and antibacterials are used to treat urinary tract infections. Among the most widely used, because of their effectiveness, are cephalosporins, amoxicillin, and trimethoprim (see Antibiotics, p.60, and Antibacterial drugs, p.64).

Measures are also sometimes taken to increase the acidity of the urine, thereby making it hostile to bacteria. Ascorbic acid (vitamin C) and acid fruit juices have this effect, although making the urine less acidic with potassium or sodium citrate during an attack of cystitis helps to relieve the discomfort. Symptoms are commonly relieved within a few hours of the start of treatment.

For maximum effect, all drug treatments prescribed for urinary tract infections need to be accompanied by increased fluid intake.

DRUGS FOR URINARY INCONTINENCE

Urinary incontinence can occur for several reasons. A weak sphincter muscle allows the involuntary passage of urine from the bladder when abdominal pressure is raised by coughing or physical exertion. This is known as stress incontinence and commonly affects women who have had children. Urgency – the sudden need to urinate – stems from oversensitivity of the bladder muscle; small quantities of urine in the bladder stimulate the urge to urinate frequently.

Incontinence can also occur due to loss of nerve control in neurological disorders such as multiple sclerosis. In children, the inability to control urination at night (a condition called nocturnal enuresis) is also a form of urinary incontinence.

Drug treatment is not necessary or appropriate for all forms of incontinence. In stress incontinence, exercises to strengthen the pelvic floor muscles or surgery to tighten stretched ligaments may be effective. In urgency, regular emptying of the bladder can often avoid the need for medical intervention. Incontinence caused by loss of nerve control is unlikely to be helped by drug treatment. However, frequency of urination in urgency may be reduced by anticholinergic and antispasmodic drugs. These drugs reduce nerve signals from the muscles in the bladder, thereby allowing greater volumes of urine to accumulate without stimulating the urge to pass urine.

Tricyclic antidepressants, such as imipramine (see p.275), have a strong anticholinergic action and have been prescribed for nocturnal enuresis in children, but many doctors believe that the risk of overdosage is unacceptable. Desmopressin, a synthetic derivative of antidiuretic hormone (see p.84), is also used to treat nocturnal enuresis.

DRUGS FOR URINARY RETENTION

Urinary retention is the inability to empty the bladder completely. This usually results from the failure of the bladder muscle to contract sufficiently to expel the accumulated urine. Possible causes include an enlarged prostate gland or tumour, or a longstanding neurological disorder. Some drugs can also cause urinary retention.

Most cases of urinary retention need to be relieved by inserting a tube (catheter) into the urethra. Surgery may be needed to prevent a recurrence of the problem.

Drugs that relax the sphincter or stimulate bladder contraction are now rarely used in the treatment of urinary retention, but two types of drug are used in the long-term management of prostatic enlargement: finasteride and alpha blockers. Finasteride prevents production of male hormones that stimulate prostate growth, and alpha blockers, such as prazosin, tamsulosin, and terazosin, relax prostatic and urethral smooth muscle, thereby improving urine outflow. Long-term drug treatment of urinary retention can relieve symptoms and delay the need for surgery.

COMMON DRUGS

Antibiotics and antibacterials (see pp.60–64)
Anticholinergics Flavoxate, Imipramine*, Oxybutynin*, Propantheline, Propiverine, Solifenacin, Tolterodine*, Trospium
Parasympathomimetics Bethanechol, Distigmine
Alpha blockers Alfuzosin, Doxazosin*, Indoramin, Prazosin, Tamsulosin*, Terazosin
Other drugs Desmopressin*, Dimethyl sulfoxide, Duloxetine, Finasteride*, Potassium citrate, Sodium bicarbonate/citrate, Vitamin C
* **See Part 2**

EYES AND EARS

The eye and the ear are the two sense organs that provide us with the most information about the world around us. The eye is the organ of vision that converts light into nerve signals, which are transmitted to the brain for interpretation into images. The ear not only provides the means by which sound is detected and communicated to the brain, but it also contains the organ of balance that tells the brain about the position and movement of the body. It is divided into three parts: the outer, middle, and inner ear.

WHAT CAN GO WRONG

The most common eye and ear disorders are infection and inflammation (sometimes caused by allergy). Many parts of the eye may be affected, notably the conjunctiva (the membrane that covers the front of the eye and lines the eyelids) and the iris. The middle and outer ear are more commonly affected by infection than the inner ear.

The eye may also be damaged by glaucoma, a disorder in which the optic nerve, which connects the eye to the brain, becomes damaged. Glaucoma is usually caused by fluid building up in the front part of the eye and may eventually threaten the vision. Eye problems such as retinopathy (disease of the retina) or cataract (clouding of the lens) may result from diabetes or other causes, but both of these eye problems are now treatable.

Other disorders affecting the ear include build-up of wax (cerumen) in the outer ear canal and disturbances to the balance mechanism within the ear (vertigo and Ménière's disease, see Anti-emetics, p.19).

WHY DRUGS ARE USED

Doctors usually prescribe antibiotics (see p.60) to clear ear and eye infections. These drugs may be given by mouth or topically. Topical eye and ear preparations may contain a corticosteroid (see p.78) to reduce inflammation. When inflammation has been caused by allergy, antihistamines (see p.56) may also be taken. Decongestant drugs (see p.24) are often prescribed to help clear the eustachian tube in middle-ear infections.

Various drugs are used to reduce fluid pressure in glaucoma. These include diuretics (see p.30), beta blockers (see p.28), and miotics (drugs to narrow the pupil). In other cases, the pupil may need to be widened by mydriatic drugs. (See also Drugs affecting the pupil, p.114.)

MAJOR DRUG GROUPS

- ◆ Drugs for glaucoma
- ◆ Drugs affecting the pupil
- ◆ Drugs for ear disorders

Drugs for glaucoma

Glaucoma is the name for a group of conditions that damage the optic nerve, which transmits vision signals from the eye to the brain. One of the main modifiable risk factors for glaucoma is abnormally high fluid pressure inside the eye, which compresses the blood vessels that supply the optic nerve. This problem may result in irreversible nerve damage and permanent loss of vision.

In the most common form, chronic (or open-angle) glaucoma, reduced drainage of fluid from the eye causes pressure in the eye to build up slowly. Progressive reduction in the peripheral field of vision may take months or years to be noticed. Acute (closed-angle) glaucoma occurs when the drainage angle between the iris and cornea is suddenly blocked by the iris. Fluid pressure usually builds up quite suddenly, blurring vision in that eye. The eye becomes red and painful, and there may be a headache and sometimes vomiting. The main attack is often preceded by milder warning attacks, such as seeing haloes around lights, in the previous weeks or months. Older, long-sighted people are particularly at risk of developing acute glaucoma. The angle may also narrow suddenly following injury or after taking certain drugs, such as anticholinergic drugs. Closed-angle glaucoma may develop more slowly (chronic closed-angle glaucoma).

Drugs are used to treat both types of glaucoma. These include miotics (see Drugs affecting the pupil, p.114), beta blockers (see p.28), and carbonic anhydrase inhibitors and osmotics (see Diuretics, p.30).

WHY THEY ARE USED

Chronic (open-angle) glaucoma In this condition, drugs are used to reduce pressure inside the eye. They will prevent further deterioration of vision, but cannot repair damage that has already occurred and may therefore be required for life. In most patients, treatment starts with eye drops containing a beta blocker to reduce fluid production in the eye. Miotic eye drops to constrict the pupil and improve fluid drainage may be given. Prostaglandin analogues, such as latanoprost (see p.291), are also used to increase fluid outflow. If none of these drugs is effective, dipivefrine, apraclonidine, or brimonidine (see p.159) may be tried to reduce secretion and help outflow. Sometimes a carbonic anhydrase inhibitor such as acetazolamide or dorzolamide may be given to reduce fluid production. Laser treatment and surgery may also be used to improve fluid drainage.

Acute (closed-angle) glaucoma Immediate medical treatment is needed to prevent total loss of vision. Drugs are used initially to bring down the pressure within the eye. Laser treatment or surgery is then carried out to prevent a recurrence so that long-term drug treatment is seldom required.

Acetazolamide is often the first drug used when the condition is diagnosed. It may be injected into a vein for rapid effect and thereafter given by mouth. Frequent applications of eye drops containing pilocarpine or carbachol are given. An osmotic diuretic such as mannitol may be administered. This draws fluid out of all body tissues, including the eye, and reduces pressure within the eye.

HOW THEY WORK

Drugs for glaucoma act in various ways to reduce fluid pressure inside the eye. Miotics improve fluid drainage. In chronic glaucoma, this is achieved by increasing the outflow of aqueous humour through a drainage channel called the trabecular meshwork. In acute glaucoma, the pupil-constricting effect of miotics pulls the iris away from the drainage channel, allowing the aqueous humour to flow out. Prostaglandin analogues increase fluid flow from the eye. Beta blockers and carbonic anhydrase inhibitors act on fluid-producing cells inside the eye to reduce the production of aqueous humour. Sympathomimetics such as brimonidine and apraclonidine are also thought to act partly in this way and partly by improving fluid drainage.

HOW THEY AFFECT YOU

Drugs for acute glaucoma relieve pain and other symptoms within a few hours of being used. The benefits of treatment in chronic glaucoma, however, may not be immediately apparent since treatment is only able to halt a further deterioration of vision.

People receiving miotic eye drops are likely to notice darkening of vision and difficulty in seeing in the dark. Increased shortsightedness may be noticeable. Some miotics also cause irritation and redness of the eyes.

Beta blocker eye drops have few day-to-day side effects but carry risks for a few people (see below). Oral acetazolamide usually causes an increase in frequency of urination and thirst. Nausea and a pins-and-needles sensation are also common.

RISKS AND SPECIAL PRECAUTIONS

Miotics can cause alteration in vision. Beta blockers are absorbed into the body and can affect the lungs, heart, and circulation. For this reason, cardioselective beta blockers, such as betaxolol, are prescribed with caution to people with asthma or certain circulatory disorders, or withheld altogether. The amount of the drug absorbed into the body can be reduced by pressing on the lacrimal (tear) duct in the corner of the eye while applying the number of drops prescribed by your doctor. Acetazolamide may cause troublesome adverse effects, including tingling hands and feet, kidney stones, and, rarely, kidney damage. People with existing kidney problems are not usually given this drug.

COMMON DRUGS

Miotics Carbachol, Pilocarpine*

Carbonic anhydrase inhibitors Acetazolamide, Brinzolamide*, Dorzolamide*

Prostaglandin analogues Bimatoprost, Latanoprost*, Travoprost

Beta blockers Betaxolol, Carteolol, Levobunolol, Metipranolol, Timolol*

Sympathomimetics Apraclonidine, Brimonidine*, Dipivefrine

* **See Part 2**

Drugs affecting the pupil

The pupil of the eye is the circular opening in the centre of the iris (the coloured part of the eye) through which light enters. It continually changes in size to adjust to variations in the intensity of light; in bright light it becomes quite small (constricts), but in dim light the pupil enlarges (dilates).

Eye drops containing drugs that act on the pupil are widely used by specialists. There are two categories: mydriatics, which dilate the pupil, and miotics, which constrict it.

WHY THEY ARE USED

Mydriatic drugs are most often used to allow the doctor to view the inside of the eye – particularly the retina, the optic nerve head, and the blood vessels that supply the retina. Many of these drugs cause a temporary paralysis of the eye's focusing mechanism, a state called cycloplegia. This state is sometimes induced to help identify any focusing errors, especially in babies and young children. By producing cycloplegia, it is possible for the doctor to determine the precise optical prescription required for a child, especially in the case of a squint.

Dilation of the pupil is part of the treatment for uveitis, an inflammatory disease of the iris and focusing muscle. In uveitis, the inflamed iris may stick to the lens, causing severe damage to the eye. This complication can be prevented by early dilation of the pupil so that the iris is no longer in contact with the lens.

Constriction of the pupil with miotic drugs is often required in the treatment of glaucoma (see p.112). Miotics can also be used to restore the pupil to a normal size after dilation is induced by mydriatics.

HOW THEY WORK

Pupil size is controlled by two separate sets of muscles in the iris: the circular muscle and the radial muscle. The two sets are governed by separate branches of the autonomic nervous system (see p.6): the radial muscle is controlled by the sympathetic nervous system, and the circular muscle is controlled by the parasympathetic nervous system.

Individual mydriatic and miotic drugs affect different branches of the autonomic nervous system, and cause the pupil to dilate or contract, depending on the type of drug.

HOW THEY AFFECT YOU

Mydriatic drugs – especially the long-acting types – impair the ability to focus the eye(s) for several hours or even days after use. This interferes particularly with close activities such as reading. Bright light may cause discomfort. Miotics often interfere with night vision and may cause temporary short sight.

Normally, these eye drops produce few serious adverse effects. Sympathomimetic mydriatics may raise blood pressure and are used with caution in people with hypertension or heart disease. Miotics may irritate the eyes, but rarely cause generalized effects.

ARTIFICIAL TEAR PREPARATIONS

Tears are continually produced to keep the front of the eye covered with a thin, moist film. This is essential for clear vision and for keeping the front of the eye free from dirt and other irritants. In some conditions, known collectively as dry eye syndromes (for example, Sjögren's syndrome), inadequate tear production may make the eyes feel dry and sore. Sore eyes can also occur in disorders where the eyelids do not close properly, causing the eye to become dry.

Why they are used Since prolonged deficiency of natural tears can damage the cornea, regular application of artificial tears in the form of eye drops is recommended for all of the conditions described above. Artificial tears may also be used to provide temporary relief from any feeling of discomfort and dryness in the eye caused by irritants or exposure to wind or sun, or following the initial wearing of contact lenses.

Although artificial tears are non-irritating, they often contain a preservative (such as thiomersal or benzalkonium chloride) that may cause irritation. This risk of irritation is increased for wearers of soft contact lenses, who should ask their optician for advice before using any type of eye drops.

COMMON DRUGS

Sympathomimetic mydriatics Phenylephrine
Miotics Carbachol, Pilocarpine*
Anticholinergic mydriatics Atropine*, Cyclopentolate, Homatropine, Tropicamide
* **See Part 2**

Drugs for ear disorders

Inflammation and infection of the outer and middle ear are the most common ear disorders treated with drugs. Drug treatment for Ménière's disease, which affects the inner ear, is described under Anti-emetics, p.19.

The type of drug treatment given for ear inflammation depends on the cause of the trouble and the site affected.

INFLAMMATION OF THE OUTER EAR

Inflammation of the external ear canal (otitis externa) can be caused by eczema or by a bacterial or fungal infection. The risk of inflammation in the ear canal is increased by swimming in dirty water, an accumulation of wax in the ear, or scratching or poking too frequently at the ear.

Symptoms vary, but in many cases there is itching, pain (which may be severe if there is a boil in the ear canal), tenderness, and possibly some loss of hearing. If the ear is infected there will probably be a discharge.

Drug treatment A corticosteroid (see p.78) in the form of ear drops may be used to treat inflammation of the outer ear when there is no infection. Aluminium acetate solution, as drops or applied on a piece of gauze, may also be used. Relief is usually obtained within a day or two. Prolonged use of corticosteroids is not advisable because they may reduce the ear's resistance to infection.

If there is both inflammation and infection, your doctor may prescribe ear drops containing an antibiotic (see p.60) combined with a corticosteroid to relieve the inflammation. Usually, a combination of antibiotics is prescribed to make the treatment effective against a wide range of bacteria. Commonly used antibiotics include framycetin, neomycin, and polymyxin B. These are not used if the eardrum is perforated and are not usually applied for long periods because they can irritate the skin that lines the ear canal.

Sometimes an antibiotic given as drops is not effective, and another type of antibiotic may also have to be taken by mouth.

INFECTION OF THE MIDDLE EAR

Infection of the middle ear (otitis media) often causes severe pain and hearing loss. It is particularly common in young children, in whom infecting organisms are able to spread easily into the middle ear from the nose or throat via the eustachian tube.

Viral infections of the middle ear usually cure themselves and are less serious than those caused by bacteria. Bacterial infections often cause the eustachian tube to swell and become blocked. When a blockage occurs, pus builds up in the middle ear and puts pressure on the eardrum, which may perforate as a result.

Drug treatment For bacterial infections, doctors usually prescribe a decongestant (see p.24) or antihistamine (see p.56) to reduce swelling in the eustachian tube, thus allowing the pus to drain out of the middle ear. Usually, an antibiotic is also given by mouth or injection to clear the infection.

Although antibiotics are not effective against viral infections, it is often difficult to distinguish between a viral and a bacterial infection of the middle ear, so your doctor may prescribe an antibiotic as a precautionary measure. Paracetamol, an analgesic (see p.7), may be given to relieve pain.

COMMON DRUGS

Antibiotic and antibacterial ear drops
Chloramphenicol*, Clioquinol, Clotrimazole*, Framycetin, Gentamicin*, Neomycin
Decongestants Ephedrine*, Oxymetazoline, Xylometazoline
Corticosteroids Betamethasone*, Dexamethasone*, Flumetasone, Hydrocortisone*, Prednisolone*, Triamcinolone
Other drugs Aluminium acetate, Antihistamines (see p.56), Choline salicylate
* **See Part 2**

SKIN

The skin waterproofs, cushions, and protects the rest of the body and is, in fact, its largest organ. It provides a barrier against innumerable infections and infestations, it helps the body to retain its vital fluids, it plays a major role in temperature control, and it houses the sensory nerves of touch.

The skin consists of two main layers: a thin, tough top layer, called the epidermis, and below it a thicker layer, the dermis. The epidermis also has two layers: the skin surface, or stratum corneum (horny layer) consisting of dead cells, and below, a layer of active cells. The cells in the active layer divide and eventually die, maintaining the horny layer. Living cells produce keratin, which toughens the epidermis and is the basic substance of hair and nails. Some living cells in the epidermis produce melanin, a pigment released in increased amounts following exposure to sunlight.

The dermis contains different nerve endings to sense pain, pressure, and temperature; sweat glands to cool the body; sebaceous glands that secrete oil to lubricate and waterproof the skin; and white blood cells to help keep the skin clear of infection.

WHAT CAN GO WRONG

Most skin disorders are not serious, but they may be distressing if they are visible. They include infection, inflammation and irritation, infestation by skin parasites, and changes in skin structure and texture (such as psoriasis, eczema, and acne).

WHY DRUGS ARE USED

Skin problems often resolve themselves without drug treatment. Over-the-counter preparations containing drugs are available, but doctors generally advise against their use because they could aggravate some skin conditions if used inappropriately.

Prescribed drugs, including antibiotics (see p.60) for bacterial infections, antifungals (see p.74) for fungal infections, agents for skin parasites (see p.120), and topical corticosteroids (see p.118) for inflammatory conditions, are often highly effective, however. Specialized drugs are available for conditions such as psoriasis and acne.

Many drugs are topical medications, but they must be used carefully because, like oral drugs, they can cause adverse effects.

MAJOR DRUG GROUPS

- Antipruritics
- Topical corticosteroids
- Anti-infective skin preparations
- Drugs to treat skin parasites
- Drugs used to treat acne
- Drugs for psoriasis
- Treatments for eczema
- Drugs for dandruff
- Drugs for hair loss
- Sunscreens

Antipruritics

Itching (irritation of the skin that creates the urge to scratch), also known as pruritus, most often occurs as a result of minor physical irritation or chemical changes in the skin caused by disease, inflammation, allergy, or exposure to irritant substances. People differ in their tolerance to itch, and a person's threshold can be altered by stress and other psychological factors.

Itching is a common symptom of many skin disorders, including eczema and psoriasis and allergic conditions such as urticaria (hives). It is sometimes caused by a localized fungal infection or parasitic infestation. Diseases such as chickenpox may also cause itching. Less commonly, itching may occur as a symptom of diabetes mellitus, jaundice, kidney failure, or drug reactions.

In many cases, generalized itching is caused by dry skin. Itching in particular parts of the body is often caused by a specific problem. For example, itching around the anus (pruritus ani) may result from haemorrhoids or worm infestation, while genital itching in women (pruritus vulvae) may be caused by vaginal infection or, in post-menopausal women, may be the result of a hormone deficiency.

Although scratching frequently provides temporary relief, it can often increase skin inflammation and make the condition worse. Continued scratching of an area of irritated skin may occasionally lead to a vicious "itch-scratch" cycle that continues long after the original cause has been removed.

Many types of medicine, including soothing topical preparations and drugs taken by mouth, relieve irritation. The main drugs in antipruritic products are local anaesthetics (see p.9), topical corticosteroids (see p.118), and antihistamines (see p.56). Simple emollient or cooling creams or ointments, with no active ingredients, are often recommended, especially if there is associated dry skin.

WHY THEY ARE USED

For mild itching arising from sunburn, urticaria, or insect bites, a cooling lotion such as calamine, perhaps containing menthol, phenol, or camphor, may be the most appropriate treatment. Local anaesthetic creams are sometimes helpful for small areas of irritation, such as insect bites, but are unsuitable for widespread itching. The itching caused by dry skin is often soothed by a simple emollient. Avoiding excessive bathing and using moisturizing bath oils may also help.

Severe itching in eczema or other inflammatory skin conditions may be treated with a topical corticosteroid preparation. When the irritation prevents sleep, a doctor may prescribe a sedating antihistamine drug, such as hydroxyzine, to promote sleep as well as to relieve itching (see also Sleeping drugs, p.9). Antihistamines are also sometimes included in topical preparations to relieve skin irritation, but their effectiveness when administered in this way is doubtful.

For the treatment of pruritus ani, see Drugs for rectal and anal disorders (p.45). Postmenopausal pruritus vulvae may be helped by vaginal creams containing oestrogen (see Female sex hormones, p.86). Itching due to an underlying systemic illness cannot be helped by skin creams and requires treatment for the principal disorder.

HOW THEY WORK

Irritation of the skin prompts the release of substances such as histamine, which cause blood vessels to dilate and fluid to accumulate under the skin; this results in itching and inflammation. Antipruritic drugs act either by reducing inflammation and thus irritation, or by numbing the nerve impulses that transmit sensation to the brain.

Corticosteroids applied to the skin surface reduce itching caused by allergy within a few days, and the soothing effect of the cream may produce an immediate improvement. The drugs pass into the underlying tissues and blood vessels and reduce the release of histamine, the chemical that causes itching and inflammation.

Antihistamines act within a few hours to reduce allergy-related skin inflammation. Applied to the skin, they pass into the underlying tissue and block the effects of histamine on the blood vessels beneath the skin. Taken by mouth, they also act on the brain to reduce the perception of irritation.

Local anaesthetics absorbed through the skin numb the transmission of signals from the nerves in the skin to the brain.

Soothing and emollient creams such as calamine lotion, applied to the skin surface, reduce inflammation and itching by cooling the skin. Emollient creams lubricate the skin surface and prevent dryness.

RISKS AND SPECIAL PRECAUTIONS

The main risk from any antipruritic, except simple emollient and soothing preparations, is skin irritation, and therefore aggravated itching, caused by prolonged or heavy use. Antihistamine and local anaesthetic creams are especially likely to cause a reaction, and must be stopped if they do so. Antihistamines taken by mouth to relieve itching may cause drowsiness. The special risks of topical corticosteroids are discussed on p.118.

Because itching can be a symptom of many underlying conditions, self-treatment should be continued for no longer than a week before seeking medical advice.

COMMON DRUGS

Antihistamines (see also p.56), Cetirizine*, Chlorphenamine*, Diphenhydramine, Fexofenadine, Hydroxyzine

Corticosteroids (see also p.78), Betamethasone*, Hydrocortisone*

Local anaesthetics Benzocaine, Lidocaine, Tetracaine
Emollient and cooling preparations Aqueous cream, Calamine lotion, Cold cream, Emulsifying ointment
Other drugs Colestyramine*, Crotamiton, Doxepin
* **See Part 2**

Topical corticosteroids

Corticosteroid drugs (which are often simply referred to as steroids) are related to the hormones that are produced by the adrenal glands. For a full description of these drugs, see p.78. Topical preparations containing a corticosteroid drug are often used to treat skin conditions in which inflammation is a prominent feature.

WHY THEY ARE USED

Corticosteroid creams and ointments are most commonly given to relieve the itching and inflammation that are associated with skin diseases such as eczema and dermatitis. Corticosteroid preparations may also be prescribed for a number of other skin conditions, including psoriasis (see p.122).

Corticosteroids do not affect the underlying cause of skin irritation, and the condition is therefore likely to recur unless the substance (allergen or irritant) that has provoked the irritation is removed, or the underlying condition is treated.

In most cases, treatment is started with a preparation containing a low concentration of a mild corticosteroid drug. A stronger preparation may be prescribed subsequently if the first product is ineffective.

HOW THEY WORK

Irritation of the skin, caused by exposure to allergens or irritant factors, provokes white blood cells to release substances that dilate the blood vessels. This reaction makes the skin hot, red, and swollen.

Applied to the skin surface, corticosteroids are absorbed into the underlying tissue. There, they inhibit the action of the substances that cause inflammation, allowing the blood vessels to return to normal and reducing the swelling.

HOW THEY AFFECT YOU

Corticosteroids prevent the release of substances that trigger inflammation, and conditions that are treated with these drugs typically improve within a few days of starting the drug. Applied topically, corticosteroids rarely cause side effects, although there are certain risks associated with the stronger drugs used in high concentrations.

RISKS AND SPECIAL PRECAUTIONS

Prolonged use of potent corticosteroids in high concentrations can lead to permanent skin changes. Applying them sparingly and only to the affected area minimizes the risk.

The most common change is thinning of the skin, sometimes resulting in permanent stretch marks. Fine blood vessels under the skin surface may become prominent (a condition known as telangiectasia). Because the skin on the face is especially vulnerable to such damage, only milder corticosteroids should be prescribed for use on the face. Dark-skinned people may sometimes experience a temporary reduction in pigmentation at the site of application.

When topical corticosteroids have been used for a prolonged period, abrupt discontinuation may cause a reddening of the skin called rebound erythema. This may be avoided by gradual dosage reduction.

Corticosteroids suppress the immune system (see p.97), thereby increasing the risk of infection. For this reason, they are never used alone to treat skin inflammation that is caused by bacterial or fungal infection. However, corticosteroids are sometimes included in topical preparations that also contain an antibiotic or antifungal agent (see Anti-infective skin preparations, opposite).

COMMON DRUGS

Very potent Clobetasol*
Potent Beclometasone*, Betamethasone*, Fluocinolone, Fluocinonide, Fluticasone*, Mometasone*, Triamcinolone
Moderate Alclometasone, Clobetasone, Fludroxycortide, Fluocortolone
Mild Hydrocortisone*
* **See Part 2**

Anti-infective skin preparations

The skin is the body's first line of defence against infection. Yet skin can also become infected itself, especially if the outer layer (epidermis) is damaged by a burn, cut, scrape, insect bite, or an inflammatory skin condition such as eczema or dermatitis.

Several different types of organism may infect the skin, including bacteria, viruses, fungi, and yeasts. This section focuses on drugs applied topically for bacterial infections, including antiseptics, antibiotics, and other antibacterial agents. Infection by other organisms is covered elsewhere (see Antiviral drugs, p.67, Antifungal drugs, p.74, and Drugs used to treat skin parasites, p.120).

WHY THEY ARE USED

Bacterial infection of a skin wound can usually be prevented by thorough cleansing of the damaged area and the application of antiseptic creams or lotions. If infection does occur, the wound usually becomes inflamed and swollen, and pus may form. If you develop these signs, you should see your doctor. The usual treatment for a wound infection is an antibiotic taken orally, although often an antibiotic cream is also prescribed.

An antibiotic or antibacterial skin cream may also be used to prevent infection when your doctor considers this to be a particular risk (for example, in the case of severe burns).

Other skin disorders for which topical antibiotic treatment may be prescribed include impetigo and infected eczema, bedsores, and nappy rash.

Often, a preparation containing two or more antibiotics is prescribed to ensure that all of the bactería are eradicated. The antibiotics selected for inclusion in topical preparations are usually drugs that are poorly absorbed through the skin, such as aminoglycosides. Thus the drug remains concentrated on the surface and in the skin's upper layers, where it is intended to have its effect. However, if the infection is deep under the skin surface, or is causing fever and general malaise, antibiotics may need to be given by mouth or injection.

RISKS AND SPECIAL PRECAUTIONS

Any topical antibiotic product can irritate the skin or cause an allergic reaction. Irritation is sometimes provoked by another ingredient of the preparation rather than the active drug, such as a preservative contained in the product. An allergic reaction causing swelling and reddening of the skin is more likely to be caused by the antibiotic itself. Any adverse reaction of this kind should be reported to your doctor, who may substitute another drug, or a different preparation.

Always follow your doctor's instructions on how long the treatment with antibiotics should be continued. Stopping too soon may cause the infection to flare up again.

Never use a skin preparation that has been prescribed for someone else, because it may aggravate your condition. Always throw away any unused medication.

BASES FOR SKIN PREPARATIONS

Drugs that are applied to the skin are usually contained in a preparation known as a base (or vehicle), such as a cream, lotion, ointment, gel, or paste. Many bases are beneficial on their own.

Creams These have an emollient effect. They are usually composed of an oil-in-water emulsion and are used in the treatment of dry skin disorders, such as psoriasis and eczema. They may also contain other ingredients, such as camphor or menthol.

Ointments These are usually greasy. Ointments are suitable for treating eczema and very dry chronic lesions.

Gels These preparations are jellylike in consistency and are often water-based. They are used increasingly for a wide variety of topical skin treatments because they are easy to apply, usually non-greasy, and more rapidly absorbed than ointments.

Barrier preparations These may be creams or ointments. They protect skin against water and irritating substances, and may be used for nappy rash or to protect the skin around an open sore. They may contain powders and water-repellent substances, such as silicones.

Lotions These thin, semi-liquid preparations are often used to cool and soothe inflamed skin. They are most suitable for use on large, hairy areas. Preparations called shake lotions contain fine powder that remains on the skin surface when the liquid has evaporated. They encourage scabs to form.

Pastes These are ointments containing large amounts of finely powdered solids such as starch or zinc oxide. Pastes protect the skin and absorb unwanted moisture. They are used for skin conditions that affect clearly defined areas, such as psoriasis.

Collodions These preparations, when applied to damaged areas of the skin such as ulcers and minor wounds, dry to form a protective film. They are sometimes used to keep a dissolved drug in contact with the skin.

COMMON DRUGS

Antibiotics Bacitracin, Colistin, Framycetin, Fusidic acid, Gramicidin, Metronidazole*, Mupirocin, Neomycin, Oxytetracycline, Polymyxin B

Antiseptics and other antibacterials Cetrimide, Chlorhexidine, Povidone iodine, Silver sulfadiazine, Triclosan

* **See Part 2**

Drugs to treat skin parasites

Mites and lice are the most common parasites that live on the skin. One common mite causes the skin disease scabies. The mite burrows into the skin and lays eggs, causing intense itching. Scratching the affected area results in bleeding and scab formation, as well as increasing the risk of infection.

There are three types of lice, each of which infests a different part of the human body: the head louse, the body (or clothes) louse, and the crab louse, which often infests the pubic areas but is also sometimes found on other hairy areas such as the eyebrows. All of these lice cause itching and lay eggs (nits) that look like white grains attached to hairs.

Both mites and lice are passed on by direct contact with an infected person (during sexual intercourse in the case of pubic lice) or, particularly in the case of body lice, by contact with infected bedding or clothing.

The drugs most often used to eliminate skin parasites are insecticides that kill both the adult insects and their eggs. The most effective drugs for scabies are malathion and permethrin; benzyl benzoate is occasionally used. Very severe scabies may require oral ivermectin as well. For lice infestation, malathion, permethrin, and phenothrin are used.

WHY THEY ARE USED

Skin parasites do not represent a serious threat to health, but their prompt eradication is needed since they can cause severe irritation and spread rapidly if left untreated. Drugs are used to eradicate them from the body, but bedding, clothing and other items should also be disinfected to avoid the possibility of reinfestation.

ELIMINATING PARASITES FROM BEDDING AND CLOTHING

Most skin parasites may also infest bedding and clothing that has been next to an infected person's skin. To avoid re-infestation following treatment of the body, any insects and eggs lodged in the bedding or clothing must also be eradicated.

Washing Because all skin parasites are killed by heat, washing any affected items of clothing and bedding in hot water and drying them in a hot tumble dryer is an effective and convenient way to deal with the problem.

Non-washable items Items that cannot be washed should be isolated in plastic bags. The insects and their eggs cannot survive for long without their human hosts and die within days. The length of time they can survive, and therefore the period of isolation, varies depending on the type of parasite.

HOW THEY ARE USED

Lotions for treating scabies are applied to the whole body, apart from the head and neck, after a bath or shower. Many people find these lotions messy to use, but they should not be washed off for 8–12 hours (permethrin), 24 hours (malathion) or 48 hours (benzyl benzoate), otherwise they will not be effective. It is probably most convenient to apply permethrin or malathion before going to bed. The lotion may then be washed off the following morning.

Two treatments 1 week apart are normally sufficient to remove the scabies mites. However, the itch associated with scabies may persist after the mite has been removed, so it may be necessary to use a soothing cream or medication containing an antipruritic drug (see p.116) to ease this discomfort. People who have direct skin-to-skin contact with someone who has scabies, such as family members and sexual partners, should also be treated with antiparasitic preparations at the same time. Head and pubic lice infestations are usually treated by applying a preparation of one of the products and washing it off with water when and as instructed by the leaflet given with the preparation. If the skin has become infected as a result of scratching, a topical antibiotic (see Anti-infective skin preparations, p.119) may also be prescribed.

RISKS AND SPECIAL PRECAUTIONS

Lotions prescribed to control parasites can cause irritation and stinging that may be intense if they come into contact with the eyes, mouth, or other moist membranes. Therefore, lotions and shampoos should be applied carefully, following the instructions of your doctor or the manufacturer.

Because antiparasitic drugs are applied topically, they do not usually have generalized effects. Nevertheless, it is important not to apply them more often than directed.

COMMON DRUGS

Benzyl benzoate, Crotamiton, Dimeticone, Ivermectin, Malathion*, Permethrin*, Phenothrin

* **See Part 2**

Drugs used to treat acne

Acne, known medically as acne vulgaris, is a common condition caused by excess production of the skin's natural oil (sebum), leading to blockage of hair follicles. The condition chiefly affects adolescents, but it may occur at any age, due to certain drugs, exposure to industrial chemicals, oily cosmetics, or hot, humid conditions.

Acne primarily affects the face, neck, back, and chest. The primary skin signs are blackheads, papules (inflamed spots), and pustules (raised pus-filled spots with a white centre). Mild acne may produce only blackheads and an occasional papule or pustule. Moderate cases are characterized by larger numbers of pustules and papules. In severe cases of acne, painful, inflamed cysts also develop. These cysts can lead to permanent pitting and scarring.

Medication for acne can be divided into two groups: topical preparations applied directly to the skin and systemic treatments taken by mouth.

WHY THEY ARE USED

Mild acne usually does not need medical treatment; instead, it can be controlled by regular washing. Over-the-counter antibacterial soaps and lotions are limited in use and may cause irritation.

When a doctor or dermatologist thinks acne is severe enough to need medical treatment, they usually recommend a topical preparation containing benzoyl peroxide or salicylic acid. If this does not produce an improvement, preparations containing tretinoin (a drug related to vitamin A), azelaic acid, or the antibiotics clindamycin, erythromycin, or tetracycline may be prescribed.

If the acne is severe or does not respond to topical treatments, a doctor may prescribe antibiotics by mouth (usually a tetracycline). If these are unsuccessful, the more powerful vitamin A-like drug isotretinoin, taken by mouth, may be prescribed.

Oestrogen-containing drugs may have a beneficial effect on acne. A woman with acne who also needs contraception may be given an oestrogen-containing oral contraceptive (see p.103). In severe cases, a preparation that contains an oestrogen and cyproterone (a drug that opposes male sex hormones) may be prescribed.

HOW THEY WORK

Drugs to treat acne act in different ways. Some have a keratolytic effect – that is, they loosen the dead cells on the skin surface. Others work by countering bacterial activity in the skin or reducing sebum production.

Topical preparations, such as benzoyl peroxide, salicylic acid, and tretinoin, have a keratolytic effect. Benzoyl peroxide also has an antibacterial effect. Topical or systemic tetracyclines reduce bacteria but may also have a direct anti-inflammatory effect on the skin. Isotretinoin reduces sebum production, soothes inflammation, and helps to unblock hair follicles.

HOW THEY AFFECT YOU

Keratolytic preparations often make the skin sore, especially at the start of treatment. If this persists, a change to a milder preparation may be recommended. Day-to-day side effects are rare with antibiotics. Treatment with isotretinoin often causes dry and scaly skin, particularly on the lips. The skin may become itchy and some hair loss may occur.

RISKS AND SPECIAL PRECAUTIONS

Antibiotics in skin ointments may, in rare cases, provoke an allergic reaction requiring discontinuation of treatment. The tetracyclines, some of the most commonly used antibiotics for acne, have the advantage of being effective both topically and systemically. However, they are not suitable for use by mouth in pregnancy since they can affect the bones and teeth of the developing baby.

Isotretinoin sometimes increases blood lipid levels. More seriously, it is known to damage a developing baby if taken during pregnancy. Women taking this drug must use effective contraception for at least 1 month before treatment, during treatment, and for at least 1 month after stopping.

COMMON DRUGS

Topical treatments Adapalene, Azelaic acid, Benzoyl peroxide*, Isotretinoin*, Nicotinamide (niacin), Salicylic acid, Tretinoin

Oral and topical antibiotics Clindamycin, Doxycycline*, Erythromycin*, Tetracycline*, Trimethoprim*

Other oral drugs Co-cyprindiol (women only), Isotretinoin*

* **See Part 2**

Drugs for psoriasis

The skin is constantly being renewed; as fast as dead cells in the outer layer (epidermis) are shed, they are replaced by cells from the base of the epidermis. Psoriasis occurs when the production of new cells increases while shedding of old cells remains normal. As a result, the live skin cells accumulate and produce patches of inflamed, thickened skin covered by silvery scales. In some cases, the affected area is extensive and causes severe embarrassment and physical discomfort. Psoriasis may occasionally be accompanied by arthritis, in which the joints become swollen and painful.

The underlying cause of psoriasis is not well understood. The disorder usually first occurs between the ages of 15 and 30, with a second peak between 50 and 60 years, and may recur throughout life. Flares of the disorder may be triggered by stress, skin damage, drugs, and physical illness. Psoriasis can also recur as a result of the withdrawal of corticosteroid drugs.

There is no complete cure for psoriasis. Simple measures, such as avoiding trigger factors and regular use of an emollient cream (see Antipruritics, p.116) may relieve symptoms and improve the condition. However, often drug therapy is needed.

WHY THEY ARE USED

Drugs are used to decrease the size of affected skin areas and to reduce scaling and inflammation. Mild and moderate psoriasis are usually treated with a topical preparation. Coal tar preparations, which are available as creams, pastes, or bath additives, are often helpful. Dithranol is also occasionally used. Once it has been applied to the affected areas, the preparation is left for a few minutes or overnight (depending on the product), before being washed off. Both dithranol and coal tar can stain clothes and bed linen. If these agents alone do not produce adequate benefit, ultraviolet light therapy in the form of regulated exposure to natural sunlight or specialist phototherapy with UVB light or PUVA may be advised. Salicylic acid may be applied to help remove thick scale and crusts, especially from the scalp.

Topical corticosteroids (see p.118) may be used as a treatment for psoriasis. This is often in combination with other agents, such as vitamin D analogues like calcitriol or calcipotriol (p.166).

If psoriasis is severe and other treatments have not been effective, specialist treatment may involve the use of more potent drugs.

These may include vitamin A derivatives (e.g. acitretin), methotrexate (see p.317), ciclosporin (see p.180), apremilast (a drug that modulates the inflammatory process in cells), or monoclonal antibodies (see p.95).

PUVA

PUVA is the combined use of a psoralen drug (e.g. methoxsalen) and ultraviolet A light (UVA). The drug is applied topically or taken by mouth; then, some hours later, the skin is exposed to UVA, which enhances the effect of the drug on skin cells. The drug is activated by exposure of the skin to the UVA; the light acts on the cell's genetic material (DNA) to regulate its rate of division.

This therapy is given two to three times a week and produces an improvement within about 4 to 6 weeks. Possible adverse effects include nausea, itching, and painful reddening of normal areas of skin. More seriously, there is a risk of premature skin ageing and a long-term risk of skin cancer, particularly in people with fair skins. For these reasons, PUVA therapy is generally recommended only for severe psoriasis, when other treatments have failed.

HOW THEY WORK

Dithranol and methotrexate slow down the rapid rate of cell division that causes skin thickening. Acitretin and calcipotriol also reduce production of keratin, the hard protein that forms in the outer layer of skin. Salicylic acid and coal tar remove the layers of dead skin cells. Corticosteroids, ciclosporin, apremilast, and monoclonal antibodies reduce inflammation of underlying skin.

HOW THEY AFFECT YOU

Appropriate treatment of psoriasis usually improves the skin's appearance. However, since drugs cannot cure the underlying cause of the disorder, psoriasis tends to recur, even following successful treatment.

Individual drugs may cause side effects. Topical preparations can cause stinging and inflammation, especially if applied to normal skin. Coal tar increases the skin's sensitivity to sunlight; excessive sunbathing or overexposure to artificial ultraviolet light may damage skin and worsen the condition.

Acitretin, ciclosporin, and methotrexate can have several serious side effects, including gastrointestinal upsets, liver damage (acitretin and methotrexate), kidney damage (ciclosporin), and bone marrow damage (methotrexate). Acitretin, apremilast, and methotrexate are contraindicated in pregnancy; women are advised not to become pregnant for 3 years after completing treatment with acitretin. Topical corticosteroids may cause rebound worsening of psoriasis when treatment is stopped.

COMMON DRUGS

Acitretin, Adalimumab, Calcipotriol*, Calcitriol, Ciclosporin*, Coal tar, Dithranol, Etanercept*, Hydroxycarbamide, Infliximab*, Methotrexate*, Methoxsalen, Salicylic acid, Secukinumab, Topical corticosteroids (see p.118), Ustekinumab

* **See Part 2**

Treatments for eczema

Eczema is a condition causing a dry, itchy rash that may be inflamed and blistered. There are several types, some of which are called dermatitis. Eczema can be triggered by allergy but often occurs for no known reason. In the long term, it can thicken (lichenify) the skin due to persistent scratching.

The most common type, atopic eczema, may appear in infancy, but many children grow out of it. There is often a family history of eczema, asthma, or allergic rhinitis. Atopic eczema commonly appears on the hands, due to detergents, and the feet, due to warm, moist conditions in enclosed footwear.

Irritant contact dermatitis, another common form of eczema, is caused by chemicals, detergents, or soap. It may appear only after repeated exposure to the substance, but strong acids or alkalis can cause a reaction within minutes. It can also result from irritation of the skin by traces of detergent on clothes and bedding.

Allergic contact dermatitis can appear days or even years after initial contact with triggers such as nickel, hair dyes, rubber, elastic, or drugs (e.g. antibiotics, antihistamines, antiseptics, or local anaesthetics). Sunlight can also trigger contact dermatitis following use of perfumes or some components of sunscreens.

Nummular (or discoid) eczema causes round, dry, scaly, itchy patches to appear anywhere on the body, with bacteria often found in these areas. The cause is unknown.

Seborrhoeic dermatitis mainly affects the scalp and the face (see Drugs for dandruff, facing page). A species of yeast called *Malassezia* is thought to play a role in its development.

WHY THEY ARE USED

Emollients soften and moisten the skin. Oral antihistamines (see p.56) may be prescribed for a particularly itchy rash (topical antihistamines make the skin more sensitive and should not be used). Coal tar or ichthammol may be used for chronic atopic eczema, but topical corticosteroids (see p.118) may be needed to help control a flare. Rarely, severe cases that are resistant to other treatments may need to be treated with the immunosuppressant ciclosporin (see p.180). A short course of oral corticosteroids (see p.78) may be used to treat severe contact dermatitis. Nummular eczema requires treatment with topical corticosteroids and a thick moisturizing ointment.

HOW THEY WORK

Emollients make the skin less dry and itchy. They are available as ointments, creams, lotions, soap substitutes, or bath oils. The effect is not long-lasting, so they need to be applied frequently. Emollients do not usually contain an active drug.

Antihistamines block the action of histamine (see p.56). Histamine dilates the blood vessels in the skin, causing redness and swelling of the surrounding tissue due to fluid leaking from the circulation. The drugs also prevent histamine from irritating the nerve fibres to cause itching.

Topical corticosteroids are absorbed into the tissues to relieve itching and inflammation. The least potent drug that is effective will be prescribed. Hydrocortisone 1 per cent is often used in 1- to 2-week courses.

Oral or topical antibiotics destroy the bacteria that are sometimes present in broken, oozing, or blistered skin.

Ciclosporin blocks the action of white blood cells, which are involved in the immune response. The drug is given in short courses to gain control of severe eczema. Other oral medications for chronic eczema include methotrexate and azathioprine. An injectable drug called dupilumab has been approved for severe treatment-resistant eczema.

RISKS AND SPECIAL PRECAUTIONS

All types of eczema can become infected, and antibiotics may be necessary. Herpes virus may infect atopic eczema. Therefore, direct contact with infected people, such as those with a cold sore, should be avoided. Ciclosporin and other oral drugs may produce some adverse effects.

PREVENTING ECZEMA

Triggers identified by patch testing (see below) should be avoided. PVC gloves should be worn to protect the hands from detergents. Cotton clothing should be worn next to the skin. Moisturizers containing perfumes and other sensitizers should be avoided.

PATCH TESTING

Low concentrations of suspected substances are applied as spots to the skin of the back and held in place with non-absorbent adhesive tape. This procedure allows a number of potential allergens (substances that can cause an allergic reaction) to be tested at the same time. After 48 hours, the adhesive tape is removed and the skin inspected for any redness, swelling, or blistering that has developed. The skin is then assessed again after a further 48 hours. Reactions present at the second assessment usually indicate a true contact allergy.

COMMON DRUGS

Emollient and cooling preparations Aqueous cream, Calamine lotion, Cold cream, Emulsifying ointment

Antihistamines (see also p.56) Cetirizine*, Chlorphenamine*, Clemastine, Fexofenadine

Corticosteroids (see also p.78) Betamethasone*, Hydrocortisone*

Other drugs Azathioprine*, Ciclosporin*, Coal tar, Ichthammol, Mycophenolate mofetil, Pimecrolimus, Tacrolimus*

* **See Part 2**

Drugs for dandruff

Dandruff is an irritating, but harmless, condition that involves an acceleration in the normal shedding of skin cells from the scalp. Extensive dandruff is considered to be a mild form of a type of dermatitis known as seborrhoeic dermatitis, which is caused by an overgrowth of a yeast called *Malassezia* that lives in the scalp. In severe cases, a rash and reddish-yellow, scaly pimples appear along the hairline and on the face.

WHY THEY ARE USED

Frequent washing with a detergent shampoo usually keeps the scalp free of dandruff, but more persistent dandruff can be treated with a shampoo containing the antifungal drug ketoconazole (see p.286), medicated shampoos containing zinc pyrithione or selenium sulfide, or shampoos containing coal tar or salicylic acid. Ointments containing coal tar and salicylic acid are also available. Corticosteroid gels and lotions may be needed to treat an itchy rash, especially in cases of severe seborrhoeic dermatitis.

HOW THEY WORK

Coal tar and salicylic acid preparations reduce the overproduction of new skin cells and break down flakes and scales, which can then be washed off while shampooing. Antifungal drugs (see p.74) reduce the overgrowth of yeast on the scalp by altering the permeability of the fungal cell walls. Corticosteroid drugs (see p.78) help to relieve an itchy rash by reducing inflammation of the underlying skin.

COMMON DRUGS

Antifungals Ketoconazole*, Pyrithione zinc
Other drugs Arachis oil, Coal tar, Corticosteroids, Salicylic acid, Selenium sulfide
* **See Part 2**

Drugs for hair loss

Hair loss (alopecia) is the result of greater than normal shedding of hairs or reduced hair production. Hair loss can be caused by a number of skin conditions, including autoimmune disorders such as lupus erythematosus and alopecia areata. Other forms of hair loss are caused by a disorder of the follicles themselves and may be a response to illness, malnutrition, or a reaction to some drugs, such as anticancer drugs or anticoagulants. The hair loss may be diffuse or in a pattern, as in male-pattern baldness, which is caused by oversensitivity to the male hormone testosterone.

WHY THEY ARE USED

If the hair loss is due to a skin disorder such as scalp ringworm, an antifungal drug will be used as treatment. If male-pattern baldness is a response to testosterone, finasteride may be used to reduce the effect of the hormone. The antihypertensive drug minoxidil (see p.326) can also be applied to the scalp to promote hair growth.

HOW THEY WORK

Some forms of hair loss are reversible, but this depends on the underlying cause. Finasteride by mouth inhibits conversion of testosterone to its more active form and reduces sensitivity to androgens. The role of minoxidil in hair growth is not fully understood, but it is thought to stimulate the hair follicles.

RISKS AND SPECIAL PRECAUTIONS

Finasteride can lead to loss of libido or erectile dysfunction. For minoxidil, anyone with a history of heart disease or high blood pressure should consult their doctor before using the drug.

COMMON DRUGS

Antifungals Griseofulvin, Ketoconazole*, Terbinafine*
Other drugs Finasteride*, Minoxidil*
* **See Part 2**

Sunscreens

Sunscreens and sunblocks are chemicals, usually formulated as creams or oils, that protect the skin from the damaging effects of ultraviolet (UV) radiation from the sun.

People vary in their sensitivity to sunlight. Fair-skinned people generally have the least tolerance and tend to burn easily when exposed to the sun, while those with darker skin can withstand exposure to the sun for longer periods.

In a few cases, the skin's sensitivity to sunlight is increased by a disease such as pellagra or herpes simplex infection. Some drugs, such as thiazide diuretics, phenothiazine antipsychotics, psoralens, sulfonamide antibacterials, tetracycline antibiotics, and nalidixic acid, can also increase sensitivity.

Apart from sunburn and premature ageing of the skin, the most serious health risk from sunlight is skin cancer. Reducing the skin's exposure to sunlight (and avoiding the use of sunbeds) can help to prevent cancers.

HOW THEY WORK

Sunlight consists of different wavelengths of radiation. Of these, ultraviolet (UV) radiation is particularly harmful to the skin, causing ageing and burning. Excessive exposure to UV radiation also increases the risk of developing skin cancer. UV radiation is mainly composed of UVA and UVB rays, both of which age the skin. In addition, UVA rays cause tanning and UVB rays cause burning. People with fair skins and those being treated with immunosuppressant drugs are especially vulnerable to skin damage.

Sunscreens absorb some of the UVB radiation, ensuring that less of it reaches the skin. Sunscreens are graded using the Sun Protection Factor (SPF) – the degree of protection that a sunscreen gives against sunburn. The SPF is a measure of the amount of UVB radiation that a sunscreen absorbs; the higher the number, the greater the protection.

Some sunscreens protect against UVA radiation as well; these are often called sunblocks. The term "broad spectrum" is used to describe sunscreens that offer both UVA and UVB protection.

Some sunscreens use a "star" classification. The stars indicate a ratio of UVA to UVB protection. A rating of 4 stars means that the product gives balanced protection against both UVA and UVB. Sunscreens with a rating of 1, 2, or 3 give more protection against UVB than UVA.

A sunscreen is particularly advisable for people who are visiting tropical, subtropical, and mountainous areas, and for those who wish to sunbathe, because sunscreens can prevent burning while allowing the skin to tan. Sunscreens must be applied before exposure to the sun and re-applied every 2 hours. People who have fair skin should use a sunscreen with a higher SPF than people who have darker skin.

RISKS AND SPECIAL PRECAUTIONS

Sunscreens only form a physical barrier to the passage of UV radiation. They do not alter the skin to make it more resistant to sunlight. Sunscreen lotions must therefore be applied thickly and frequently during exposure to the sun for protection to be maintained. People who have very fair skin or who are known to be very sensitive to sunlight should never expose their skin to direct sunlight, even if they are using a sunscreen, because not even sunscreens with high SPF values can give complete protection.

Sunscreens can irritate the skin, and some preparations may cause an allergic rash. People who are sensitive to some drugs, such as procaine and benzocaine, and to some hair dyes, might develop a rash after applying any sunscreen containing aminobenzoic acid or a benzophenone derivative such as oxybenzone.

COMMON DRUGS

Ingredients in sunscreens and sunblocks Aminobenzoic acid, Benzones, Dibenzoylmethanes, Drometizole trisiloxane, Ethylhexyl methoxycinnamate, Methylbenzylidene camphor, Octocrylene, Oxybenzone, Padimate-O, Titanium dioxide, Zinc oxide

PART 2

A-Z OF DRUGS

This part of the book contains 285 generic drugs, individually profiled, and written to a standard format to help you find specific information quickly and easily; cross-references to the relevant major drug groups are provided.

ACICLOVIR

Brand names Action Cold Sore Cream, Boots Avert, Cymex Ultra, Lypsyl Aciclovir 5%, Virasorb, Zovirax

Used in the following combined preparations None

QUICK REFERENCE

Drug group Antiviral drug (p.67)

Overdose danger rating Low

Dependence rating Low

Prescription needed No (cold sore cream); Yes (other preparations)

Available as generic Yes

GENERAL INFORMATION

Aciclovir is an antiviral drug used in the treatment of herpes infections, which can cause cold sores and genital herpes. It is available as tablets, a liquid, a cream, eye ointment, and injection. The cream is commonly used to treat cold sores, and can speed up the healing of the lesions, provided it is started as soon as symptoms occur and as the lesions appear. The tablets and injection are used to treat severe herpes infections, shingles, chickenpox, and genital herpes. The tablets can also be used to prevent the development of herpes infection in people who have reduced immunity. Herpes infection affecting the eye can be treated with an eye ointment.

INFORMATION FOR USERS

Follow the instructions on the label. Call your doctor if symptoms worsen.

How taken/used Tablets, liquid, injection, cream, eye ointment.

Frequency and timing of doses 2–5 x daily. Start as soon as possible.

Adult dosage range *Tablets, liquid* 1–4g daily (treatment); 800mg–1.6g daily (prevention). *Injection* 5–10mg per kg body weight 3 x daily. *Cream, eye ointment* 5 x daily.

Onset of effect Within 24 hours.

Duration of action Up to 8 hours.

Diet advice Drink plenty of water when taking high doses by mouth or injection.

Storage Keep in original container at room temperature out of the reach of children. Protect from light.

Missed dose *Tablets/liquid* Take as soon as you remember. *Cream, eye ointment* Do not apply the missed dose. Apply next dose as usual.

Stopping the drug Complete the full course as directed.

Exceeding the dose An occasional unintentional extra dose is unlikely to be a cause for concern. But if you notice any unusual symptoms, or if a large overdose has been taken, notify your doctor.

POSSIBLE ADVERSE EFFECTS

Serious adverse effects are rare. Topical applications commonly cause burning, stinging, and itching at the site of application, or, rarely, a rash; if a rash occurs, stop taking the drug and consult your doctor. Taken by mouth, aciclovir may occasionally cause nausea, vomiting, dizziness, confusion, hallucinations, or a rash. Tell your doctor if nausea and/or vomiting are severe. If a rash develops, stop taking the drug and consult your doctor. If confusion or hallucinations occur, stop taking the drug and call your doctor immediately. Given by injection, aciclovir may rarely cause inflammation at the injection site, confusion, or hallucinations. If any of these effects occur, stop the drug and call your doctor immediately.

INTERACTIONS (by mouth or injection only)

General note Any drug that affects the kidneys increases the risk of side effects with aciclovir.

Probenecid and cimetidine These drugs may increase the level of aciclovir in the blood.

Mycophenolate mofetil Aciclovir may increase levels of this drug in the blood and vice versa.

Ciclosporin Aciclovir may increase the levels of this drug in the blood and increase the risk of kidney problems.

SPECIAL PRECAUTIONS

Be sure to consult your doctor or pharmacist before taking this drug if:

- You have a long-term kidney problem.
- You have reduced immunity.
- You are taking other medicines.

Pregnancy Topical preparations carry negligible risk. Oral and injectable forms may be prescribed if the benefits outweigh the risks. Discuss with your doctor.

Breast-feeding No evidence of risk with topical forms but avoid using on the breast area. The drug passes into the breast milk following injection or oral administration. Discuss with your doctor.

Infants and children Reduced dose necessary in young children.

Over 60 Reduced dose may be necessary.

Driving and hazardous work No known problems. High doses of oral and injectable forms may cause drowsiness; if so, avoid driving and hazardous activities.
Alcohol No known problems.

PROLONGED USE
Aciclovir is usually given as single courses of treatment and is not given long term, except for people with reduced immunity.

ALENDRONIC ACID

Brand names Binosto, Fosamax, Fosamax Once Weekly
Used in the following combined preparation Fosavance

QUICK REFERENCE
Drug group Drug for bone disorders (p.54)
Overdose danger rating Medium
Dependence rating Low
Prescription needed Yes
Available as generic Yes

GENERAL INFORMATION
Alendronic acid is used to treat osteoporosis, treat or prevent corticosteroid-induced osteoporosis, and prevent post-menopausal osteoporosis in women at risk of developing it. A calcium supplement and vitamin D may be prescribed if dietary intake is inadequate, but calcium should not be taken at the same time as alendronic acid because calcium reduces its absorption. Combined use with HRT (p.87) in post-menopausal women is more effective than either treatment alone. The drug should be taken first thing in the morning, swallowed whole with a full glass of tap water (not even mineral water is acceptable due to the minerals' possible effect on absorption). Stay upright for at least 30 minutes afterwards to prevent the tablets from sticking in the oesophagus, where they could cause ulcers or irritation. Those with poor dental health should have a dental check before starting alendronic acid.

INFORMATION FOR USERS
Your drug prescription is tailored for you. Do not alter the dosage without checking with your doctor.
How taken/used Tablets. Take with water.
Frequency and timing of doses Once daily, first thing in the morning. Once weekly, first thing in the morning (post-menopausal women).
Adult dosage range *Treatment*: 10mg daily (for all indications) or 70mg taken once weekly.
Onset of effect It may take some months before you notice any improvement.
Duration of action Some effects may persist for months or years.
Diet advice Do not eat or take other medicines for at least 30 minutes after doses.
Storage Keep in original container at room temperature out of the reach of children.
Missed dose Take the next dose at the usual time next morning.
Stopping the drug Do not stop the drug without consulting your doctor. Stopping may lead to worsening of the underlying condition.
Exceeding the dose An occasional unintentional extra dose is unlikely to cause problems. However, large overdoses may cause stomach problems including heartburn, irritation, and ulcers. If you have taken a large overdose, tell your doctor at once, and try to remain upright.

POSSIBLE ADVERSE EFFECTS
The most frequent adverse effect is abdominal pain, distension, or indigestion resulting from irritation to the oesophagus, stomach, or small intestine. Discuss with your doctor if the pain is severe. Other adverse effects include diarrhoea or constipation; muscle, joint, or bone pain; headache; and nausea or vomiting. Discuss with your doctor if any of these are severe. If the drug causes a rash, abnormal sensitivity to light, eye inflammation, jaw pain, or ear pain, consult your doctor. Rarely, it can cause severe irritation and inflammation of the oesophagus that may lead to pain or difficulty in swallowing, or new or worsening heartburn. If any of these occur, stop taking the drug and consult your doctor.

INTERACTIONS
Antacids and products containing calcium or iron These reduce absorption of alendronic acid and should be taken at a different time of day.

SPECIAL PRECAUTIONS
Be sure to tell your doctor if:
- You have pain or difficulty in swallowing, or problems with your oesophagus.
- You have significant dental health problems.
- You have a history of peptic ulcers or stomach problems.
- You have long-term kidney problems.

◆ You have low calcium levels in your blood.
◆ You are/may be pregnant or are planning pregnancy.
◆ You are unable to sit or stand upright for at least 30 minutes.
◆ You are taking other medicines.

Pregnancy Not recommended.
Breast-feeding Not recommended.
Infants and children Not recommended.
Over 60 No special problems.
Driving and hazardous work No special problems.
Alcohol Avoid. The drug may cause further stomach irritation.

PROLONGED USE

Alendronic acid is usually prescribed long term, but the need for continued treatment should be reassessed periodically (especially after 5 years) to ensure the benefits continue to outweigh the risks in each individual case. Inappropriate prolonged use may lead to complications such as atypical bone fractures.

Monitoring Blood and urine tests may be carried out at intervals.

ALGINATES

Brand names [dressings] Algisite M, Kaltostat, Kendall, Melgisorb, Sorbalgon, Sorbsan; [oral] Gaviscon Infant
Used in the following combined preparations Acidex, Gastrocote, Gaviscon, Peptac liquid aniseed, Rennie heartburn relief

QUICK REFERENCE

Drug group Antacid (p.40)
Overdose danger rating Low
Dependence rating Low
Prescription needed No
Available as generic Yes

GENERAL INFORMATION

"Alginates" is a group term for a mixture of compounds extracted from brown algae (seaweeds). When the powdered extract is mixed with water, alginates become a thick, viscous fluid or gel depending on the chemicals used. Alginates combined with antacids form a "raft" that floats on the surface of the stomach contents, which reduces reflux and protects the lining of the oesophagus from attack by acid regurgitated from the stomach. Many of these combined preparations of alginates are used to treat mild gastro-oesophageal reflux disease. A number of indigestion remedies on sale to the public also contain alginates.

Alginates are also used in wound dressings, where they absorb fluids from the wound, keeping it moist and allowing it to heal.

INFORMATION FOR USERS

Follow instructions on the label. Inform your doctor if you have no relief after 7 days of intake or if symptoms worsen.

How taken/used Chewable tablets, liquid, powder.
Frequency and timing of doses 4 x daily after meals and at bedtime (as oral solution).
Adult dosage range 800–2,000mg daily.
Onset of effect 10–20 minutes.
Duration of action 3–4 hours.
Diet advice None.
Storage Keep in original container at room temperature out of the reach of children.
Missed dose Take as soon as you remember, if you need it.
Stopping the drug Alginates can be safely stopped as soon as you no longer need them.
Exceeding the dose Overdose is likely to cause abdominal distension without any other symptoms. Tell your doctor if symptoms are severe.

POSSIBLE ADVERSE EFFECTS

The antacid salts used in combined oral preparations may cause abdominal discomfort and distension, and, rarely, nausea. Notify your doctor if any of these symptoms are severe.

INTERACTIONS

Other medications A time interval of 2 hours should be considered between alginate antacid medication and any other medicinal products, especially tetracyclines, digoxin, fluoroquinolone, iron salt, ketoconazole, antipsychotics, thyroid hormones, penicillamine, beta blockers (atenolol, metoprolol, propanolol), glucocorticoid, chloroquine, and bisphosphonates.
Sodium bicarbonate Due to effects at the renal level, may reduce plasma lithium levels and increase plasma quinidine levels.

SPECIAL PRECAUTIONS

Be sure to consult your doctor or pharmacist before taking this drug if:
◆ You are on a salt-restricted diet.
◆ You are taking other medicines.
◆ You have renal failure.

Pregnancy No evidence of risk to fetus. Some products can be used in pregnancy.
Breast-feeding No evidence of risk.
Infants and children Reduced dose necessary.
Over 60 No special problems.
Driving and hazardous work No known problems.
Alcohol No known problems.

PROLONGED USE

Alginates should not be taken as an antacid for more than 2 weeks. If symptoms persist after this time, discuss them with your doctor, to rule out more serious possible problems such as cancer of the oesophagus or stomach.

ALLOPURINOL

Brand names Caplenal, Cosuric, Rimapurinol, Zyloric
Used in the following combined preparations None

QUICK REFERENCE

Drug group Drug for gout (p.51)
Overdose danger rating Medium
Dependence rating Low
Prescription needed Yes
Available as generic Yes

GENERAL INFORMATION

Allopurinol is used to prevent gout, which is caused by deposits of uric acid crystals in joints. The drug blocks an enzyme called xanthine oxidase that is involved in forming uric acid. It is also used to lower high uric acid levels (hyperuricaemia) caused by other drugs and sometimes for preventing uric acid kidney stones. Allopurinol should never be started until several weeks after an acute attack has subsided because it may cause a further episode. Treatment should continue indefinitely to prevent further attacks. At the start, an acute attack may occur and colchicine or an anti-inflammatory drug may also be given until uric acid levels fall. If an acute attack occurs while on allopurinol, treatment should continue along with an anti-inflammatory drug.

INFORMATION FOR USERS

Your drug prescription is tailored for you. Do not alter dosage without checking with your doctor.
How taken/used Tablets.
Frequency and timing of doses 1–3 x daily after food.
Adult dosage range 100–900mg daily.
Onset of effect Within 24–48 hours. Full effect may not be felt for several weeks.
Duration of action Up to 30 hours. Some effect may last for 1–2 weeks after drug is stopped.
Diet advice A high fluid intake (2 litres of fluid daily) is recommended.
Storage Keep in original container at room temperature out of the reach of children.
Missed dose If your next dose is not due for another 12 hours or more, take a dose as soon as you remember and take the next one as usual. Otherwise skip the missed dose and take your next dose on schedule.
Stopping the drug Do not stop the drug without consulting your doctor; symptoms may recur.
Exceeding the dose An occasional unintentional extra dose is unlikely to cause problems. Large overdoses may cause nausea, vomiting, abdominal pain, diarrhoea, and dizziness. Notify your doctor.

POSSIBLE ADVERSE EFFECTS

Adverse effects are not very common. The most serious are an allergic rash, sore throat, fever, and chills. If you experience any of these symptoms, report them to your doctor and stop taking the drug; an alternative drug may need to be substituted. Nausea can be avoided by taking allopurinol after food. The drug may also cause drowsiness, dizziness, headache, and taste or visual disturbances. Discuss with your doctor if these problems occur.

INTERACTIONS

ACE inhibitors Allopurinol may increase the risk of toxicity from these drugs.
Anticoagulant drug Allopurinol may increase the effects of these drugs.
Ciclosporin Allopurinol may increase the effects of this drug.
Didanosine Allopurinol increases levels of drug.
Mercaptopurine and azathioprine Allopurinol blocks the breakdown of these drugs, requiring a reduction in their dosage.
Theophylline Allopurinol may increase levels of this drug.

SPECIAL PRECAUTIONS

Be sure to tell your doctor if:
- You have long-term liver or kidney problems.
- You have had a previous sensitivity reaction to allopurinol.

◆ You have a current attack of gout.
◆ You are taking other medicines.

Pregnancy Safety in pregnancy not established. Discuss with your doctor.
Breast-feeding The drug passes into the breast milk but is not known to be harmful to the baby. Discuss with your doctor.
Infants and children Reduced dose necessary.
Over 60 Reduced dose may be necessary.
Driving and hazardous work Avoid until you have learned how allopurinol affects you because the drug can cause drowsiness.
Alcohol Avoid. Alcohol may worsen gout.

PROLONGED USE

Apart from an increased risk of gout in the first weeks or months, no problems are expected.
Monitoring Periodic checks on uric acid levels in the blood are usually performed, and the dose of allopurinol adjusted if necessary.

ALTEPLASE

Brand name Actilyse
Used in the following combined preparations None

QUICK REFERENCE

Drug group Thrombolytic drug (p.38)
Overdose danger rating Medium
Dependence rating Low
Prescription needed Yes
Available as generic No

GENERAL INFORMATION

Alteplase belongs to a group of drugs called thrombolytics, which act by dissolving blood clots that have formed in blood vessels. Synthesized by genetically modified bacteria, alteplase works by dissolving fibrin (see p.37) in blood clots. It is used to treat a number of conditions caused by clots in blood vessels, including heart attacks due to clots in the arteries of the heart, pulmonary embolism due to clots in the lungs' blood vessels, and acute stroke from a clot in an artery of the brain.

Alteplase is administered via a catheter inserted into an artery or vein and works rapidly. It is given within a few hours of a heart attack or stroke to reduce damage to the heart or brain. As with other thrombolytic agents, alteplase is associated with a risk of bleeding, which may occasionally be life-threatening, so treatment is closely supervised.

INFORMATION FOR USERS

This drug is given only under medical supervision and is not for self-administration.
How taken/used Injection, infusion.
Frequency and timing of doses Usually given as a single intravenous injection followed by continuous intravenous infusion over several hours.
Adult dosage range Dosage is determined individually based on the condition being treated and the patient's body weight.
Onset of effect 30 minutes.
Duration of action 60 minutes.
Diet advice None.
Storage Not applicable. The drug is not normally kept at home.
Missed dose Not applicable. The drug is given only in hospital under close supervision.
Stopping the drug The drug is usually given over several hours and then stopped.
Exceeding the dose Overdose unlikely as treatment is closely monitored by medical staff.

POSSIBLE ADVERSE EFFECTS

Alteplase is given under strict medical supervision and adverse effects are closely monitored. The main adverse effect is bleeding, which is common where the catheter is inserted but may occur anywhere in the body. Nausea and vomiting are also common. Other, more rare adverse effects include collapse, rash, wheezing, and swelling of the lips and/or face. Any adverse effects should be reported to medical staff immediately.

INTERACTIONS

Anticoagulant drugs (e.g. warfarin, heparin) There is an increased risk of bleeding when these are taken before, during, or soon after alteplase is used.
Antiplatelet drugs (e.g. aspirin, clopidogrel) There is an increased risk of bleeding when these are taken before, during, or soon after alteplase.

SPECIAL PRECAUTIONS

Alteplase is only prescribed under close medical supervision, usually in life-threatening circumstances. The doctor will usually go through a checklist of questions before administering the drug to assess your risk of bleeding.
Pregnancy Safety not established. Alteplase carries a risk of bleeding for the mother and baby and may damage the placenta. Discuss with your doctor.

Breast-feeding Safety not established. Breast milk should not be used for 24 hours after treatment with alteplase. Discuss with doctor.
Infants and children Not recommended.
Over 60 Increased risk of bleeding. Close observation required.
Driving and hazardous work Not applicable.
Alcohol Not applicable.

PROLONGED USE

Alteplase is never used long term.

ALUMINIUM HYDROXIDE

Brand name Alu-Cap, Alu-Tab, Amphojel, Dialume
Used in the following combined preparations Algicon, Aludrox, Asilone, Co-magaldrox, Maalox, Mucogel, Topal, and others

QUICK REFERENCE

Drug group Antacid (p.40)
Overdose danger rating Low
Dependence rating Low
Prescription needed No
Available as generic Yes

GENERAL INFORMATION

Aluminium hydroxide is a common ingredient of many over-the-counter indigestion and heartburn remedies. Because it is constipating (it is sometimes used to treat diarrhoea), it is usually combined with a magnesium-containing antacid with a balancing laxative effect. The combination is sometimes referred to by the generic name of co-magaldrox.

The prolonged action of aluminium hydroxide makes it useful in preventing the pain of stomach and duodenal ulcers or heartburn. It can also promote the healing of ulcers.

The drug may be more effective as an antacid in liquid form rather than as tablets. Some antacid preparations include large amounts of sodium; these should be used with caution by those on low-sodium diets.

In the intestine, aluminium hydroxide binds with, and thereby reduces the absorption of, phosphate. This makes the drug helpful in treating high blood phosphate (hyperphosphataemia), which occurs in some people who have impaired kidney function. However, prolonged heavy use can lead to phosphate deficiency and a consequent weakening of the bones.

INFORMATION FOR USERS

Follow instructions on the label. Call your doctor if symptoms worsen.
How taken/used Capsules, chewable tablets, liquid (suspension). The tablets should be well chewed.
Frequency and timing of doses *As antacid* 4 x daily as needed, or 1 hour before and after meals. *Peptic ulcer* 4 x daily. *Hyperphosphataemia* 3–4 x daily with meals.
Dosage range *Adults* Up to 70ml daily (liquid), 2–10g daily (tablets or capsules). *Children over 6 years* Reduced dose according to age and weight.
Onset of effect Within 15 minutes.
Duration of action 2–4 hours.
Diet advice For hyperphosphataemia, a low-phosphate diet may be advised in addition to aluminium hydroxide treatment.
Storage Keep in original container at room temperature out of the reach of children.
Missed dose Do not take the missed dose. Take your next dose as usual.
Stopping the drug Can be safely stopped as soon as you no longer need it (indigestion). When taken as ulcer treatment or for hyperphosphataemia resulting from kidney failure, do not stop without consulting your doctor.
Exceeding the dose An occasional unintentional extra dose is unlikely to be a cause for concern. If you notice any unusual symptoms, or if a large overdose has been taken, tell your doctor.

POSSIBLE ADVERSE EFFECTS

Constipation is common; nausea and vomiting may occur because of the granular, powdery nature of the drug. Bone pain may also occur, but usually only when large doses have been taken regularly for months or years. Vomiting or severe constipation or nausea should be reported to your doctor.

INTERACTIONS

General note Aluminium hydroxide may interfere with the absorption or excretion of many drugs, including oral anticoagulants, digoxin, many antibiotics, penicillamine, corticosteroids, antipsychotics, and phenytoin. It should only be taken at least 2 hours before or after other drugs.
Enteric-coated tablets Aluminium hydroxide may lead to the break-up of the enteric coating of tablets (e.g. bisacodyl, or enteric-coated

prednisolone) before they leave the stomach, leading to stomach irritation.

SPECIAL PRECAUTIONS

Be sure to consult your doctor or pharmacist before taking this drug if:

- You have a long-term kidney problem.
- You have heart problems.
- You have high blood pressure.
- You have constipation.
- You have a bone disease.
- You have porphyria.
- You are taking other medicines.

Pregnancy Safety in pregnancy not established. Discuss with your doctor.
Breast-feeding No evidence of risk.
Infants and children Not recommended under 6 years except on the advice of a doctor.
Over 60 No special problems.
Driving and hazardous work No known problems.
Alcohol No known problems.

PROLONGED USE

Aluminium hydroxide should not be used for longer than 4 weeks without consulting your doctor. Prolonged use of high doses in people with normal kidney function may deplete blood phosphate and calcium levels, leading to weakening of the bones and fractures. In people with kidney disease, long-term treatment may lead to accumulation of aluminium in the brain, causing dementia.

AMILORIDE

Brand name None
Used in the following combined preparations
Co-amilofruse, Co-amilozide, Frumil, Moduretic, Navispare, and others

QUICK REFERENCE

Drug group Potassium-sparing diuretic (p.31)
Overdose danger rating Low
Dependence rating Low
Prescription needed Yes
Available as generic Yes

GENERAL INFORMATION

Amiloride is a mild diuretic. It acts on the kidneys to increase the amount of urine passed. It is used for oedema (fluid retention), which can result from heart failure or liver disease, and for hypertension (high blood pressure). The effect on urine flow may last for several hours, so amiloride should be taken in the morning. The drug causes the kidneys to conserve potassium (it is a potassium-sparing diuretic) and should not be used when there is a high blood level of potassium. It is prescribed with caution in people taking potassium supplements or those with kidney disease. Amiloride is often combined with other diuretics such as furosemide (co-amilofruse) and hydrochlorothiazide (co-amilozide).

INFORMATION FOR USERS

Your drug prescription is tailored for you. Do not alter dosage without checking with your doctor.
How taken/used Tablets, liquid.
Frequency and timing of doses Once or twice daily, usually in the morning.
Adult dosage range 5–20mg daily.
Onset of effect Within 2–4 hours.
Duration of action 12 hours.
Diet advice Avoid foods that are high in potassium – for example, dried fruit, bananas, tomatoes, and "low salt" salt substitutes.
Storage Keep in original container at room temperature out of the reach of children.
Missed dose Take as soon as you remember. However, if it is late in the day, do not take the dose, or you may need to get up at night to pass urine. Take the next scheduled dose as usual.
Stopping the drug Do not stop the drug without consulting your doctor; symptoms may recur.
Exceeding the dose An occasional unintentional extra dose is unlikely to be a cause for concern. But if you notice unusual symptoms, or if a large overdose has been taken, tell your doctor.

POSSIBLE ADVERSE EFFECTS

Amiloride has few adverse effects. The main risk is that potassium may be retained by the body or excessive sodium lost in the urine, causing muscle weakness or heart rhythm problems. Rarely, there may be digestive disturbance, confusion, muscle cramps, dry mouth and thirst, or dizziness; tell your doctor if any of these occur. If a rash develops, stop taking the drug and consult your doctor.

INTERACTIONS

Lithium Amiloride may increase the blood levels of lithium, leading to an increased risk of lithium toxicity.

ACE inhibitors, angiotensin II blockers, renin inhibitors (e.g. aliskiren), ciclosporin, drosperinone, tacrolimus, and NSAIDs These drugs may increase the risk of potassium retention if taken with amiloride.

SPECIAL PRECAUTIONS

Be sure to tell your doctor if:

- You have long-term liver or kidney problems.
- You are taking other medicines.

Pregnancy Not usually prescribed. The drug may cause a reduction in the blood supply to the developing baby. Discuss with your doctor.

Breast-feeding Not usually prescribed during breast-feeding. Discuss with your doctor.

Infants and children Not recommended.

Over 60 Increased likelihood of adverse effects. Reduced dose may be necessary.

Driving and hazardous work No known problems.

Alcohol No special problems.

PROLONGED USE

Monitoring Blood tests may be carried out to monitor levels of body salts.

AMIODARONE

Brand name Cordarone X

Used in the following combined preparations None

QUICK REFERENCE

Drug group Anti-arrhythmic drug (p.32)

Overdose danger rating High

Dependence rating Low

Prescription needed Yes

Available as generic Yes (tablets)

GENERAL INFORMATION

Amiodarone is used for a variety of abnormal heart rhythms (arrhythmias). It acts by slowing nerve impulses in the heart muscle. The drug is given to prevent recurrent atrial and ventricular fibrillation (irregular heart beat) and to treat ventricular and supraventricular tachycardias (overly fast heart beat) and Wolff-Parkinson-White syndrome (persistent tachycardia due to an abnormal extra electrical connection in the heart). Often the last choice when other treatments have failed, especially for long-term use, it has serious adverse effects including liver damage, thyroid problems, and eye and lung damage. Treatment should be started only under specialist supervision or in hospital.

INFORMATION FOR USERS

Your drug prescription is tailored for you. Do not alter dosage without checking with your doctor.

How taken/used Tablets, injection.

Frequency and timing of doses 3 x daily or by injection initially; reduced to twice daily, then once daily or every other day (maintenance).

Adult dosage range 600mg daily, reduced to 400mg, then 100–200mg daily.

Onset of effect By mouth, some effects may occur in 72 hours; full benefits may take some weeks to show. By injection, effects may occur within 30 minutes.

Duration of action 3–12 months.

Diet advice Grapefruit juice should be avoided.

Storage Keep in original container at room temperature out of the reach of children. Protect from light.

Missed dose Take as soon as you remember. If the next dose is due within 12 hours, do not take the missed dose. Take the next scheduled dose as usual.

Stopping the drug Do not stop the drug without consulting your doctor; symptoms may recur.

OVERDOSE ACTION

Seek immediate medical advice in all cases. Take emergency action if collapse or loss of consciousness occur.

POSSIBLE ADVERSE EFFECTS

Amiodarone has a number of unusual side effects, including a metallic taste in the mouth, a greyish skin colour (on prolonged use), and increased sensitivity of the skin to sunlight. It can also cause nausea and vomiting; liver damage; visual disturbances; thyroid problems; heart rate disturbances; numbness and tingling in the extremities; shortness of breath; cough; headache; weakness; and fatigue. Discuss with your doctor if nausea and vomiting are severe or if any other adverse effects occur.

INTERACTIONS

General note Consult your doctor or pharmacist before taking other medications.

Diuretics Some cause potassium loss and increase the toxic effects of amiodarone.

Other anti-arrhythmic drugs Amiodarone may increase the effects of these drugs.

Warfarin Amiodarone may increase the anticoagulant effect of warfarin.
Anti-hepatitis C drugs Use with amiodarone raises the risk of bradycardia or heart block.

SPECIAL PRECAUTIONS

Be sure to tell your doctor if:
- You have long-term liver problems.
- You have heart problems.
- You have eye disease.
- You have a lung disorder such as asthma or bronchitis.
- You have a thyroid disorder.
- You are sensitive to iodine.
- You are taking other medicines.

Pregnancy Not recommended. Discuss with your doctor.
Breast-feeding The drug passes into the breast milk and may affect the baby. Safety not established. Discuss with your doctor.
Infants and children Not recommended.
Over 60 Increased likelihood of adverse effects. Reduced dose may therefore be necessary.
Driving and hazardous work Avoid until you know how the drug affects you because it can cause the eyes to be dazzled by bright light.
Alcohol No known problems.

PROLONGED USE

Prolonged use may cause a number of adverse effects on the eyes, heart, skin, nervous system, lungs, thyroid gland, and liver.
Monitoring A chest X-ray may be taken before treatment starts. Blood tests are done before treatment starts and then every 6 months to check thyroid and liver function. Regular eye examinations are required.

AMISULPRIDE/SULPIRIDE

Brand names [amisulpride] Solian; [sulpiride] Dolmatil
Used in the following combined preparations None

QUICK REFERENCE

Drug group Antipsychotic drug (p.13)
Overdose danger rating Medium
Dependence rating Low
Prescription needed Yes
Available as generic Yes

GENERAL INFORMATION

Amisulpride and sulpiride are antipsychotic drugs for acute and chronic schizophrenia, in which a person has "positive" symptoms such as delusions, hallucinations, and thought disorders, and/or "negative" symptoms such as emotional and social withdrawal. People with mainly positive symptoms are given higher doses; those with mainly negative symptoms are given lower doses. Sulpiride has also been used in the treatment of Tourette's syndrome.

An advantage of amisulpride, an "atypical" antipsychotic, is that it is less likely than older antipsychotics to cause the movement disorders parkinsonism or tardive dyskinesia.

INFORMATION FOR USERS

Your drug prescription is tailored for you. Do not alter dosage without checking with your doctor.
How taken/used Tablets, liquid.
Frequency and timing of doses 1–2 x daily (doses of up to 300mg amisulpride may be 1 x daily).
Dosage range *Amisulpride* 50–300mg daily (mainly negative symptoms); 400–1,200mg daily (mainly positive symptoms). *Sulpiride* 400–800mg daily (mainly negative symptoms); 400–2,400mg daily (mainly positive symptoms).
Onset of effect 1 hour.
Duration of action 12–24 hours.
Diet advice None.
Storage Keep in original container at room temperature out of the reach of children.
Missed dose Take as soon as you remember. If your next dose is due within 2 hours, take a single dose now and skip the next dose.
Stopping the drug Do not stop without consulting your doctor; symptoms may recur.
Exceeding the dose An occasional unintentional extra dose is unlikely to cause problems. Large overdoses may cause drowsiness and low blood pressure. Tell your doctor immediately.

POSSIBLE ADVERSE EFFECTS

Most of the side effects of antipsychotics such as amisulpride and sulpiride are mild. Insomnia is the most common problem, although drowsiness and anxiety or agitation are also fairly common. More rarely, there may be weight gain, nausea, or vomiting. Consult your doctor if any of these symptoms become severe. Other rare side effects include breast swelling; parkinsonism; loss of libido; and, in women, menstrual irregularities. Consult your doctor if you develop any of these symptoms.

INTERACTIONS

Amiodarone, disopyramide, diuretics, droperidol, erythromycin, methadone, sotalol These drugs increase the risk of abnormal heart rhythms when taken with amisulpride or sulpiride.

Antihypertensive drugs Amisulpride and sulpiride may reduce the blood-pressure-lowering effect of certain of these drugs.

Central nervous system depressants These drugs may all increase the sedative effects of amisulpride and sulpiride.

SPECIAL PRECAUTIONS

Be sure to tell your doctor if:

- You have liver or kidney problems.
- You have heart problems or hypertension.
- You have epilepsy.
- You have Parkinson's disease.
- You have a pituitary tumour or breast cancer.
- You have phaeochromocytoma.
- You have had blood problems.
- You are taking other medicines.

Pregnancy Short-term nervous system problems may occur in babies if the drug is taken in the third trimester. Discuss with your doctor.

Breast-feeding Safety not established. Discuss with your doctor.

Infants and children Not recommended.

Over 60 Reduced dose may be necessary.

Driving and hazardous work Avoid such activities until you have learned how amisulpride and sulpiride affect you; the drugs can slow reaction times and may occasionally cause drowsiness or loss of concentration.

Alcohol Avoid. Alcohol increases the sedative effects of these drugs.

PROLONGED USE

An adverse effect called tardive dyskinesia (involuntary movements of the tongue and face) may rarely occur during long-term use.

AMITRIPTYLINE

Brand names None

Used in the following combined preparation Triptafen

QUICK REFERENCE

Drug group Tricyclic antidepressant drug (p.12)

Overdose danger rating High

Dependence rating Low

Prescription needed Yes

Available as generic Yes

GENERAL INFORMATION

Amitriptyline belongs to the tricyclic group of antidepressants. These drugs are effective for long-term depression but are poorly tolerated and dangerous in overdose so they are second-line choices after SSRI antidepressants (p.12). The sedative effect of amitriptyline is useful if depression is accompanied by anxiety or insomnia. Taken at night, the drug encourages sleep and reduces the need for additional sleeping drugs. Amitriptyline is sometimes used to treat nocturnal enuresis (bedwetting) in children. It may also be used to treat neuropathic pain such as postherpetic neuralgia after shingles and to prevent tension headache and migraine. In overdose, the drug may cause abnormal heart rhythms, seizures, and coma.

INFORMATION FOR USERS

Your drug prescription is tailored for you. Do not alter dosage without checking with your doctor.

How taken/used Tablets, liquid.

Frequency and timing of doses 1–3 x daily, usually as a single dose at night.

Adult dosage range 10–150mg daily.

Onset of effect Sedation can appear within hours, although full antidepressant effect may not be felt for 2–4 weeks.

Duration of action Antidepressant effect may last for 6 weeks; common adverse effects gone within 1 week.

Diet advice None.

Storage Keep in original container at room temperature out of the reach of children. Protect from light.

Missed dose Take as soon as you remember. If your next dose is due within 3 hours, take a single dose now and skip the next.

Stopping the drug An abrupt stop can cause withdrawal symptoms and recurrence of the original trouble. Consult your doctor, who may supervise a gradual reduction in dosage over at least 4 weeks.

OVERDOSE ACTION

Seek immediate medical advice in all cases. Take emergency action if palpitations are noted or consciousness is lost.

POSSIBLE ADVERSE EFFECTS

The possible adverse effects of this drug are mainly the result of its anticholinergic action and its blocking action on the transmission of signals through the heart. Common adverse effects include drowsiness, sweating, dry mouth, and constipation. Discuss with your doctor if any of these are severe or if you have blurred vision or difficulty in passing urine. If you experience dizziness, fainting, or confusion, stop taking the drug and consult your doctor. If you have palpitations, stop taking the drug and consult your doctor immediately.

INTERACTIONS

Monoamine oxidase inhibitors (MAOIs) In the rare cases where these are given with amitriptyline, there is a risk of serious interactions.
Anticonvulsants The effects of these drugs are reduced by amitriptyline as it lowers the threshold for seizures.
Sedatives All drugs that have sedative effects intensify those of amitriptyline.
Anti-arrhythmic drugs There is an increased risk of abnormal heart rhythms when these drugs are taken with amitriptyline.

SPECIAL PRECAUTIONS

Be sure to tell your doctor if:

- You have heart problems.
- You have had epileptic seizures.
- You have long-term liver or kidney problems.
- You have glaucoma.
- You have prostate trouble.
- You have thyroid disease.
- You have had mania or a psychotic illness.
- You are taking other medicines.

Pregnancy Avoid if possible. Discuss with your doctor.
Breast-feeding The drug passes into the breast milk, but at normal doses adverse effects are unlikely. Discuss with your doctor.
Infants and children Not recommended under 16 years for depression, or under 6 years for enuresis.
Over 60 Reduced dose may be necessary because older people are more sensitive to adverse reactions.
Driving and hazardous work Avoid such activities until you have learned how amitriptyline affects you because the drug may cause blurred vision and reduced alertness.
Alcohol Avoid. Alcohol may increase the sedative effects of this drug.
Surgery and general anaesthetics Amitriptyline treatment may need to be stopped before you have a general anaesthetic. Discuss this with your doctor or dentist before any operation.

PROLONGED USE

No problems expected.

AMLODIPINE

Brand name Istin
Used in the following combined preparations Exforge, Sevikar

QUICK REFERENCE

Drug group Anti-angina drug (p.33) and antihypertensive drug (p.34)
Overdose danger rating Medium
Dependence rating Low
Prescription needed Yes
Available as generic Yes

GENERAL INFORMATION

Amlodipine belongs to a group of drugs called calcium channel blockers, which interfere with the conduction of signals in the muscles of the heart and blood vessels.

The drug is used in the treatment of angina, to help prevent attacks of chest pain. Unlike some other anti-angina drugs (such as beta blockers), it can be used safely by people with asthma and those with diabetes who require insulin. Amlodipine is also used to reduce raised blood pressure (hypertension).

Like other drugs of its class, amlodipine may cause blood pressure to fall too low at the start of treatment. In rare cases, angina may become worse at the start of treatment.

INFORMATION FOR USERS

Your drug prescription is tailored for you. Do not alter dosage without checking with your doctor.
How taken/used Tablets, liquid (oral solution).
Frequency and timing of doses Once daily.
Adult dosage range 5–10mg daily.
Onset of effect 6–12 hours.
Duration of action 24 hours.
Diet advice Avoid grapefruit juice, because it may interact with amlodipine and increase the drug's effects.
Storage Keep in original container at room temperature out of the reach of children.
Missed dose If you miss a dose and you remember it within 12 hours, take it as soon as you

remember. However, if you do not remember until later, do not take the missed dose and do not double up the next one. Instead, go back to your regular schedule.

Stopping the drug Do not stop taking the drug without consulting your doctor; stopping the drug may lead to worsening of the underlying condition.

Exceeding the dose An occasional unintentional extra dose is unlikely to cause problems. Large overdoses may cause a marked lowering of blood pressure. Tell your doctor immediately.

POSSIBLE ADVERSE EFFECTS

Amlodipine can cause a variety of minor adverse effects, including mild to moderate leg and ankle swelling, headache, dizziness (especially when rising from sitting or lying down, when it may be the result of an excessive reduction in blood pressure), fatigue, and flushing. If any of these become severe, discuss with your doctor. You should also consult your doctor if you have palpitations, nausea, abdominal pain, a rash, or breathing difficulties; if you have a rash or breathing difficulties, you should also stop taking the drug. The most serious adverse effect is the rare possibility of angina becoming worse after starting amlodipine treatment. If this occurs, you should stop taking the drug and consult your doctor immediately.

INTERACTIONS

Ketoconazole, itraconazole, and ritonavir These drugs may increase blood levels and adverse effects of amlodipine.

St John's wort This reduces the blood level of amlodipine.

Grapefruit juice This may increase the effects of amlodipine.

Alpha blockers, beta blockers, ACE inhibitors, and diuretics Amlodipine may increase the effects of these drugs and vice versa.

Antimalarials Taken with amlopidine, some antimalarials may cause an abnormally slow heart beat.

SPECIAL PRECAUTIONS

Be sure to tell your doctor if:

- You have long-term liver problems.
- You have heart failure or aortic stenosis.
- You have diabetes.
- You are taking other medicines.

Pregnancy Safety in pregnancy not established. Discuss with your doctor.

Breast-feeding It is not known if the drug passes into breast milk. Discuss with your doctor.

Infants and children Not recommended.

Over 60 No special problems.

Driving and hazardous work Avoid such activities until you have learned how amlodipine affects you because the drug can cause dizziness owing to lowered blood pressure.

Alcohol Avoid. Alcohol may further reduce blood pressure, causing dizziness or other symptoms.

Surgery and general anaesthetics Amlodipine may interact with some general anaesthetics, causing a fall in blood pressure. Discuss this with your doctor or dentist before any surgery.

PROLONGED USE

No problems expected.

AMOXICILLIN/ CO-AMOXICLAV

Brand name Amoxil

Used in the following combined preparations Augmentin, Co-amoxiclav

QUICK REFERENCE

Drug group Penicillin antibiotic (p.60)

Overdose danger rating Low

Dependence rating Low

Prescription needed Yes

Available as generic Yes

GENERAL INFORMATION

Amoxicillin is a penicillin antibiotic. It is prescribed to treat a variety of infections, but is particularly useful for treating ear, nose, and throat infections, respiratory tract infections, cystitis, uncomplicated gonorrhoea, and certain skin and soft tissue infections. The drug is sometimes combined with clavulanic acid (as co-amoxiclav) to prevent bacteria from breaking down the amoxicillin; this makes it effective against a wider range of bacteria than amoxicillin alone. Doses of co-amoxiclav are given as two numbers (e.g. 500/125 is 500mg amoxicillin plus 125mg clavulanic acid).

Amoxicillin/co-amoxiclav can cause minor stomach upsets and a rash. It can also provoke a severe allergic reaction with fever, swelling of the mouth and tongue, itching, and breathing difficulties.

INFORMATION FOR USERS

Your drug prescription is tailored for you. Do not alter dosage without checking with your doctor.

How taken/used Tablets, capsules, liquid, powder (dissolved in water), injection.

Frequency and timing of doses Normally 3 x daily.

Dosage range *Adults* 750mg–1.5g (of amoxicillin) daily. In some cases a short course of up to 6g (of amoxicillin) daily is given. A single dose of 3g (of amoxicillin) may be given as a preventative. However, dosage range depends on preparation and condition being treated. *Children* Reduced dose according to age and weight.

Onset of effect 1–2 hours.

Duration of action Up to 8 hours.

Diet advice Make sure you keep well hydrated.

Storage Keep in original container at room temperature out of the reach of children.

Missed dose Take as soon as you remember. Take your next dose at the scheduled time.

Stopping the drug Take the full course. Even if you feel better, the original infection may still be present if treatment is stopped too soon.

Exceeding the dose An occasional unintentional extra dose is unlikely to be a cause for concern. But if you notice any unusual symptoms, or if a large overdose has been taken, tell your doctor.

POSSIBLE ADVERSE EFFECTS

The most common adverse effects are diarrhoea and nausea. Talk to your doctor if these are severe or if you experience abdominal pain, unexplained bruising, or a sore throat or fever. If you develop a rash, itching, wheezing or breathing difficulties, or joint swelling, this may indicate an allergy to the drug. You should stop taking it and call your doctor immediately. Rarely, jaundice may occur, in some cases weeks or even months after finishing treatment. If you do develop jaundice, call your doctor immediately and stop taking the drug if you have not already done so.

INTERACTIONS

Anticoagulant drugs Amoxicillin and co-amoxiclav may alter the drugs' anticoagulant effect.

Allopurinol Amoxicillin may increase the likelihood of allergic skin reactions.

Oral typhoid vaccine Amoxicillin and co-amoxiclav inactivate this vaccine. Avoid taking them for 3 days before and after having the vaccine.

SPECIAL PRECAUTIONS

Be sure to tell your doctor if:

- ◆ You are allergic to penicillin antibiotics or cephalosporin antibiotics.
- ◆ You have glandular fever (infectious mononucleosis).
- ◆ You have a history of allergy.
- ◆ You have liver problems, or have had previous liver problems, with amoxicillin/co-amoxiclav.
- ◆ You have a kidney problem.
- ◆ You are taking other medicines.

Pregnancy No evidence of risk.

Breast-feeding No evidence of risk.

Infants and children Reduced dose necessary.

Over 60 No known problems.

Driving and hazardous work No known problems.

Alcohol No known problems.

PROLONGED USE

Amoxicillin and co-amoxiclav are usually given only for short courses of treatment.

AMPHOTERICIN (B)

Brand names Abelcet, AmBisome, Fungizone

Used in the following combined preparations None

QUICK REFERENCE

Drug group Antifungal drug (p.74)

Overdose danger rating Low

Dependence rating Low

Prescription needed Yes

Available as generic No

GENERAL INFORMATION

Amphotericin is a highly effective and powerful antifungal drug. Although previously given by mouth to treat candida (thrush) infections of the mouth or intestines, it is now only given by intravenous infusion to treat serious systemic fungal infections. All of the oral formulations have been discontinued in the UK. Administration is carefully supervised, usually in hospital, because of potentially serious adverse effects. A test dose for allergy may be given before treatment is started. The newer formulations of amphotericin appear to be less toxic than the original ones.

INFORMATION FOR USERS

Your drug prescription is tailored for you. Do not alter dosage without checking with your doctor.

How taken/used Intravenous infusion.

Frequency and timing of doses Once daily.

Dosage range Determined individually.

Onset of effect Improvement may be noticed after 2–4 days.

Duration of action Up to several days.

Diet advice The drug may reduce the levels of potassium and magnesium in the blood. To correct this, mineral supplements may be recommended by your doctor.

Storage Not applicable. The drug is not normally kept in the home.

Missed dose If you miss your scheduled dose, contact your doctor as soon as possible.

Stopping the drug Discuss with your doctor. Stopping the drug prematurely may lead to worsening of the underlying condition.

Exceeding the dose Unlikely, since treatment is carefully monitored and supervised.

POSSIBLE ADVERSE EFFECTS

The drug is given only by infusion under close medical supervision. Any adverse effects that develop are thus monitored closely and treated promptly. Common effects include nausea, vomiting, headache, fever, and rash. Rarer effects include unusual bleeding, muscle and joint pain, palpitations, or difficulty in breathing. Tell your doctor immediately if you have palpitations or breathing difficulties; in these cases the drug should be stopped.

INTERACTIONS

Digitalis drugs Amphotericin may increase the toxicity of digoxin.

Diuretics Amphotericin increases the risk of low potassium levels with diuretics.

Aminoglycoside antibiotics Taken with amphotericin, these increase the risk of kidney damage.

Corticosteroids may increase loss of potassium from the body caused by amphotericin.

Ciclosporin and tacrolimus increase the likelihood of kidney damage.

SPECIAL PRECAUTIONS

Be sure to tell your doctor if:

◆ You have long-term liver or kidney problems.

◆ You have previously had an allergic reaction to amphotericin.

◆ You are taking other medicines.

Pregnancy The drug is given only when the infection is very serious.

Breast-feeding It is not known whether the drug passes into the breast milk. Discuss with your doctor.

Infants and children Reduced dose may be necessary.

Over 60 No special problems.

Driving and hazardous work No known problems.

Alcohol No known problems.

PROLONGED USE

The drug may cause a reduction in blood levels of potassium and magnesium. It may also damage the kidneys and cause blood disorders.

Monitoring Regular blood tests to monitor liver and kidney function, blood cell counts, and potassium and magnesium levels are advised during treatment.

ANASTROZOLE

Brand name Arimidex

Used in the following combined preparations None

QUICK REFERENCE

Drug group Anticancer drug (p.94)

Overdose danger rating Low

Dependence rating Low

Prescription needed Yes

Available as generic Yes

GENERAL INFORMATION

Anastrozole is a potent non-steroidal inhibitor of the enzyme that makes oestradiol (natural oestrogen) in the body. It can reduce production of oestradiol by more than 80 per cent. It works by blocking oestradiol production in peripheral body tissues such as fat, rather than in the ovary itself, so it is generally not suitable for use in pre-menopausal women where the ovaries are still producing oestrogen. The drug is used in post-menopausal women to treat types of breast cancer in which the tumour cells have oestrogen receptors (oestrogen-receptor-positive breast cancer).

Anastrozole is generally well tolerated; adverse effects are mainly gastrointestinal or gynaecological, and are generally similar to menopausal symptoms. If there is any doubt about whether a woman to be treated is post-menopausal, a blood test may be performed.

INFORMATION FOR USERS

Your drug prescription is tailored for you. Do not alter dosage without checking with your doctor.

How taken/used Tablets.

Frequency and timing of doses Once daily.

Adult dosage range 1mg.

Onset of effect A few hours.

Duration of action More than 24 hours.

Diet advice None.

Storage Keep in original container at room temperature out of the reach of children.

Missed dose Take as soon as you remember. If your next dose is due within 2 hours, take a single dose now and skip the next.

Stopping the drug Do not stop the drug without consulting your doctor. Stopping may lead to worsening of the underlying condition.

Exceeding the dose An occasional unintentional extra dose is unlikely to be a cause for concern. But if you notice any unusual symptoms, or if a large overdose has been taken, tell your doctor.

POSSIBLE ADVERSE EFFECTS

Anastrozole is usually well tolerated and any side effects tend to be relatively minor, except for the increased risk of osteoporosis and bone fracture. Common effects include hot flushes, headache, fatigue, dizziness, joint pain or stiffness, muscle pain, vaginal dryness or bleeding, thinning hair, nausea, diarrhoea, and vomiting. Notify your doctor if mood disturbances occur. If you develop a rash, stop taking the drug and consult your doctor immediately.

INTERACTIONS

Tamoxifen and oestrogens oppose the effects of anastrozole and should be avoided.

SPECIAL PRECAUTIONS

Be sure to tell your doctor if:

- You are pre-menopausal.
- You have osteoporosis.
- You have kidney or liver problems.
- You are allergic to anastrozole.
- You are taking other medicines.

Pregnancy Not prescribed in pregnancy.

Breast-feeding Not prescribed.

Infants and children Not recommended.

Over 60 No special problems.

Driving and hazardous work Do not drive until you know how the drug affects you. It can cause drowsiness.

Alcohol No known problems.

PROLONGED USE

No known problems.

Monitoring Women with osteoporosis or at risk of osteoporosis will have their bone mineral density assessed at the start of treatment and at regular intervals. Cholesterol levels may also be monitored.

ASPIRIN

Brand names Aspro, Danamep, Disprin, Nu-Seals Aspirin, and others

Used in the following combined preparations Anadin, Beechams Powders, Codis, Migramax, and others

QUICK REFERENCE

Drug group Non-opioid analgesic (p.8), antiplatelet drug (p.37), and antipyretic

Overdose danger rating High

Dependence rating Low

Prescription needed No

Available as generic Yes

GENERAL INFORMATION

In use for over a century, aspirin relieves pain, reduces fever, and alleviates the symptoms of arthritis. In low doses, it helps to prevent blood clots, particularly in atherosclerosis or angina due to coronary artery disease, and it reduces the risk of heart attacks and strokes. It is present in many medicines for colds, flu, headaches, menstrual period pains, and joint or muscular aches.

Aspirin may irritate the stomach and even cause peptic ulcers or bleeding. Another drawback is that it can provoke asthma attacks. In children aspirin can cause Reye's syndrome, a rare but serious brain and liver disorder. For this reason, it should not be given to children under age 16 except on the advice of a doctor.

INFORMATION FOR USERS

Follow instructions on the label. Call your doctor if symptoms worsen.

How taken/used Tablets, slow release (SR) capsules, suppositories.

Frequency and timing of doses *Relief of pain or fever* Every 4–6 hours, as necessary, with or after food or milk. *Prevention of blood clots* Once daily.

Adult dosage range *Relief of pain or fever* 300–900mg per dose. *Prevention of blood clots* 75–300mg daily.

Onset of effect 30–60 minutes (regular aspirin); $1\frac{1}{2}$–8 hours (coated tablets or SR capsules).
Duration of action Up to 12 hours; persists for 7–10 days when used to prevent blood clotting.
Diet advice Take with or immediately after food.
Storage Keep in original container at room temperature out of the reach of children.
Missed dose Take as soon as you remember. If your next dose is due within 2 hours, take a single dose now and skip the next.
Stopping the drug If you have been prescribed aspirin by your doctor for a long-term condition, seek medical advice before stopping the drug. Otherwise it can be safely stopped.

OVERDOSE ACTION

Seek immediate advice in all cases. Take emergency action if there is restlessness, sweating, ringing noises in the ears, blurred vision, or vomiting.

POSSIBLE ADVERSE EFFECTS

Adverse effects are more likely to occur with high doses of aspirin but may be reduced by taking it with food or in buffered or enteric-coated forms. If it causes nausea, vomiting, or severe indigestion, consult your doctor. If you develop a rash, breathlessness, or wheezing, vomit blood, have black faeces, or experience ringing in the ears or dizziness, stop taking the drug and contact your doctor immediately.

INTERACTIONS

Anticoagulants Aspirin may add to the anticoagulant effect of these drugs, leading to an increased risk of abnormal bleeding.
Drugs for gout Aspirin may reduce their effect.
Non-steroidal anti-inflammatory drugs (NSAIDs) may increase the likelihood of stomach irritation with aspirin.
Methotrexate Aspirin may increase the toxicity of this drug.
Sulfonylurea antidiabetic drugs Aspirin may increase the effect of these drugs.
Corticosteroids and some SSRI antidepressants These may increase the risk of gastrointestinal bleeding with aspirin.

SPECIAL PRECAUTIONS

Be sure to consult your doctor or pharmacist before taking this drug if:
◆ You have long-term liver or kidney problems.
◆ You have asthma.
◆ You are allergic to aspirin or any NSAID.
◆ You have a blood clotting disorder.
◆ You have a history of peptic ulcer.
◆ You have glucose-6-phosphate dehydrogenase (G6PD) deficiency.
◆ You are taking other medicines.

Pregnancy Not usually recommended but may be prescribed to prevent pre-eclampsia if high risk. Discuss with your doctor.
Breast-feeding Avoid. Aspirin passes into breast milk and can cause Reye's syndrome in babies.
Infants and children Do not give to children under 16 years, except on a doctor's advice.
Over 60 Adverse effects more likely.
Driving and hazardous work No special problems.
Alcohol Avoid. Alcohol increases the likelihood of stomach irritation with this drug.
Surgery and general anaesthetics Regular treatment with aspirin may need to be stopped about 1 week before surgery. Discuss with your doctor or dentist before any operation.

PROLONGED USE

Aspirin should not be taken in high doses for prolonged periods. When taken long term, all doses increase the risk of peptic ulcers and gastrointestinal bleeding, so regular use should be avoided. Exceptions include long-term use of low-dose aspirin to prevent blood clots in people at high risk of cardiovascular disease, as this benefit outweighs the risk of bleeding.

ATENOLOL

Brand name Tenormin
Used in the following combined preparations Beta-Adalat, Co-tenidone, Kalten, Tenif, Tenoret, Tenoretic

QUICK REFERENCE

Drug group Beta blocker (p.28)
Overdose danger rating High
Dependence rating Low
Prescription needed Yes
Available as generic Yes

GENERAL INFORMATION

Atenolol is a cardioselective beta blocker (see p.28). It prevents the heart from beating too quickly and is used mainly to treat irregular heart rhythms (arrhythmias) and chest pain (angina). It may be given following a heart attack to protect the heart from further damage. Atenolol is also used to treat hypertension (high blood pressure) but is not usually used to initiate treatment. It is less likely than non-cardioselective beta blockers to cause breathing difficulties; nevertheless, it is not usually given to patients with asthma. It may slow the body's response to low blood sugar in people with diabetes who take insulin.

INFORMATION FOR USERS

Your drug prescription is tailored for you. Do not alter dosage without checking with your doctor.
How taken/used Tablets, liquid, injection.
Frequency and timing of doses 1–2 x daily.
Adult dosage range 25–100mg daily.
Onset of effect 2–4 hours.
Duration of action 20–30 hours.
Diet advice None.
Storage Keep in original container in a cool, dry place out of the reach of children. Protect from light.
Missed dose Take as soon as you remember. If your next dose is due within 6 hours, omit the missed dose but take the next scheduled dose.
Stopping the drug Do not stop without consulting your doctor; sudden withdrawal may lead to dangerous worsening of the underlying condition. It should be withdrawn gradually.

OVERDOSE ACTION

Seek immediate medical advice. Take emergency action if breathing difficulties, collapse, or loss of consciousness occur.

POSSIBLE ADVERSE EFFECTS

The adverse effects are common to most beta blockers and tend to diminish with long-term use. Lethargy, fatigue, and cold hands and feet are common. Other, rarer, adverse effects include nausea, vomiting, nightmares or vivid dreams, rash, dry eyes, and visual disturbances; these effects should be reported to your doctor. If you experience fainting, palpitations, breathlessness, or wheezing, stop taking the drug and consult your doctor immediately.

INTERACTIONS

Antihypertensive drugs Atenolol may enhance the blood-pressure-lowering effect.
Calcium channel blockers may cause low blood pressure, a slow heartbeat, and heart failure if used with atenolol.
Non-steroidal anti-inflammatory drugs (NSAIDs) may reduce antihypertensive effect of atenolol.
Cardiac glycosides (e.g. digoxin) may increase the heart-slowing effect of atenolol.
Antidiabetic drugs used with atenolol may increase the risk of low blood sugar or mask its symptoms.
Decongestants used with atenolol may increase blood pressure and heart rate.

SPECIAL PRECAUTIONS

Be sure to tell your doctor if:
- You have heart problems.
- You have a long-term kidney problem.
- You have diabetes.
- You have a lung disorder such as asthma or bronchitis.
- You have psoriasis.
- You are taking other medicines.

Pregnancy Safety in pregnancy not established. Discuss with your doctor.
Breast-feeding The drug passes into the breast milk. Discuss with your doctor.
Infants and children Not recommended.
Over 60 No special problems. Reduced dose may be needed if kidney function is impaired.
Driving and hazardous work Avoid until you have learned how atenolol affects you because the drug can cause dizziness.
Alcohol Avoid excessive intake. Alcohol may increase the blood-pressure-lowering effects of atenolol.
Surgery and general anaesthetics Occasionally, atenolol may need to be stopped before you have a general anaesthetic, but only do this after discussion with your doctor or dentist.

PROLONGED USE

No special problems expected.

ATORVASTATIN

Brand name Lipitor
Used in the following combined preparations None

QUICK REFERENCE

Drug group Lipid-lowering drug (p.35)
Overdose danger rating Medium
Dependence rating Low
Prescription needed Yes
Available as generic Yes

GENERAL INFORMATION

Atorvastatin is a member of the statin group of lipid-lowering drugs. It is used to treat hypercholesterolaemia (high blood cholesterol levels) in patients who have not responded to other treatments, such as a special diet or lifestyle changes, and who have, or are at risk of developing, heart disease. The drug is also used in patients with diabetes who are at high risk of heart attack or stroke. It blocks the action in the liver of an enzyme needed for the manufacture of cholesterol. As a result, blood levels of cholesterol are lowered, which can help to prevent coronary heart disease.

Rarely, atorvastatin can cause muscle pain, inflammation, and muscle damage.

INFORMATION FOR USERS

Your drug prescription is tailored for you. Do not alter dosage without checking with your doctor.

How taken/used Tablets, chewable tablets.

Frequency and timing of doses Once daily.

Adult dosage range 10–80mg.

Onset of effect Within 2 weeks. Full beneficial effects are usually seen within 4 weeks.

Duration of action 20–30 hours.

Diet advice A low-fat diet is usually recommended. Do not drink more than 2 small glasses of grapefruit juice per day.

Storage Keep in original container at room temperature out of the reach of children.

Missed dose Take as soon as you remember. If your next dose is due within 8 hours, do not take the missed dose, but take the next one on schedule.

Stopping the drug Do not stop without consulting your doctor. Stopping the drug may lead to a recurrence of the original condition.

Exceeding the dose An occasional unintentional extra dose is unlikely to cause problems, but large overdoses may cause liver problems. Notify your doctor.

POSSIBLE ADVERSE EFFECTS

The more common adverse effects include nausea, constipation or diarrhoea, headache, dizziness, tiredness, insomnia, back pain, and joint pain. They are usually mild and transient but should be discussed with your doctor if they are severe. Other, rarer effects include jaundice, rash, and muscle pain or weakness. Jaundice or a rash should always be reported to your doctor. If you have a rash, you should also stop taking the drug. Muscle damage is another rare possible adverse effect; if you develop muscle pain or weakness, notify your doctor immediately and stop taking the drug.

INTERACTIONS

Warfarin Atorvastatin may reduce the anticoagulant effect of warfarin. The dose of warfarin may need adjustment.

Macrolide antibiotics (e.g. erythromycin, clarithromycin), fusidic acid, and antifungals Taken with atorvastatin, these drugs may increase the risk of muscle damage.

Other lipid-lowering drugs Taken with atorvastatin, these drugs may increase the risk of muscle damage.

Ciclosporin and other immunosuppressant drugs Atorvastatin is not usually prescribed with these drugs because of the increased risk of muscle damage.

Oral contraceptives Atorvastatin increases blood levels of ethinylestradiol and norethisterone. The dose of these drugs may need adjustment.

Digoxin Atorvastatin increases blood levels of digoxin.

SPECIAL PRECAUTIONS

Be sure to tell your doctor if:

- You have had liver problems.
- You have kidney problems.
- You are a heavy drinker.
- You have an underactive thyroid.
- You or a family member have a muscle disorder.
- You have had muscle problems or other reactions with other lipid-lowering drugs.
- You are taking other medicines.

Pregnancy Not recommended. May affect fetal development. Discuss with your doctor if you are pregnant or intend to become pregnant.

Breast-feeding Safety not established. Discuss with your doctor.

Infants and children Not recommended.

Over 60 No special problems.

Driving and hazardous work No special problems.

Alcohol Avoid excessive amounts. Alcohol may increase the risk of developing liver problems with atorvastatin.

PROLONGED USE

Long-term use of atorvastatin may affect liver function.

Monitoring Regular blood tests to check liver function are needed. Tests of muscle function may be carried out if problems are suspected.

ATROPINE

Brand name Minims Atropine

Used in the following combined preparations Co-phenotrope, Lomotil, Minims Atropine

QUICK REFERENCE

Drug group Anti-arrhythmic (p.32), drug for irritable bowel syndrome (p.43), mydriatic drug (p.114)

Overdose danger rating High

Dependence rating Low

Prescription needed Yes

Available as generic Yes

GENERAL INFORMATION

Atropine is an anticholinergic drug. Because of its antispasmodic action, which relaxes the muscle wall of the gut, the drug has been used to relieve abdominal cramps in irritable bowel syndrome. It may be prescribed in combination with diphenoxylate, an antidiarrhoeal drug; however, the benefit may be outweighed by atropine-related side effects. This combination can be dangerous in overdose, particularly in young children.

Atropine eye drops are used to enlarge the pupil during eye examinations and to treat inflammatory eye disorders such as uveitis. Atropine may be used as part of premedication before a general anaesthetic, injected to restore normal heart beat in heart block (p.32), or given with pralidoxime to treat poisoning with organophosphates.

Atropine must be used with caution in children and older adults due to their sensitivity to the drug's effects.

INFORMATION FOR USERS

Your drug prescription is tailored for you. Do not alter dosage without checking with your doctor.

How taken/used Tablets, injection, eye ointment, eye drops.

Frequency and timing of doses Once only, or up to 4 times daily according to condition (eye drops); as directed (other forms).

Adult dosage range 1–2 drops as directed (eye drops); as directed (other forms).

Onset of effect Varies according to method of administration. 30 minutes (eye drops).

Duration of action 7 days or longer (eye drops); several hours (other forms).

Diet advice None.

Storage Keep in original container at room temperature out of the reach of children. Protect from light.

Missed dose Take as soon as you remember. If your next dose is due within 2 hours, take a single dose now and skip the next.

Stopping the drug Do not stop the drug without consulting your doctor.

OVERDOSE ACTION

Seek immediate medical advice in all cases. Take emergency action if palpitations, tremor, delirium, seizures, or loss of consciousness occur.

POSSIBLE ADVERSE EFFECTS

The use of atropine is limited by the frequency of anticholinergic effects. These commonly include blurred vision, dry mouth, and constipation; the drug may also cause nausea, vomiting, and dizziness. You should discuss with your doctor if any of these symptoms becomes severe or if you have difficulty in passing urine. If palpitations or confusion occur, you should stop taking the drug and contact your doctor immediately. The eye drops may cause stinging. If they also cause pain and irritation or if a rash develops on contact, stop using them and contact your doctor without delay.

INTERACTIONS

General note Atropine delays stomach emptying and may therefore alter the absorption of other drugs.

Anticholinergic drugs Atropine increases the risk of side effects from drugs that also have anticholinergic effects.

Ketoconazole Atropine reduces the absorption of this drug from the digestive tract. Increased dose may be necessary.

SPECIAL PRECAUTIONS

Be sure to tell your doctor if:

- ◆ You have long-term liver or kidney problems.
- ◆ You have prostate problems.
- ◆ You have gastro-oesophageal reflux.
- ◆ You have glaucoma.
- ◆ You have urinary difficulties.
- ◆ You have ulcerative colitis.
- ◆ You wear contact lenses (eye drops).
- ◆ You have heart problems.
- ◆ You are taking other medicines.

Pregnancy Safety in pregnancy not established. Discuss with your doctor.

Breast-feeding The drug may pass into the breast milk and affect the baby. Discuss with your doctor.

Infants and children Combination with diphenoxylate not recommended under 4 years; reduced dose necessary in older children.

Over 60 Increased likelihood of adverse effects.

Driving and hazardous work Avoid such activities until you have learned how atropine affects you because the drug can cause blurred vision and may impair concentration.

Alcohol Avoid. Alcohol increases the likelihood of confusion and affects your concentration when taken with atropine.

PROLONGED USE

No problems expected.

AZATHIOPRINE

Brand name Azapress, Imuran

Used in the following combined preparations None

QUICK REFERENCE

Drug group Disease-modifying antirheumatic drug (p.49) and immunosuppressant drug (p.97)

Overdose danger rating Medium

Dependence rating Low

Prescription needed Yes

Available as generic Yes

GENERAL INFORMATION

Azathioprine is an immunosuppressant drug used to prevent immune-system rejection of transplanted organs. It is also used to modify, halt, or slow the underlying disease process in severe rheumatoid arthritis (see Antirheumatic drugs, p.49) that has failed to respond to conventional drug therapy.

Autoimmune and collagen diseases (including polymyositis, systemic lupus erythematosus, myasthenia gravis, and dermatomyositis) may be treated with azathioprine, usually in combination with corticosteroids. Azathioprine is also occasionally used for other skin disorders, such as severe atopic eczema.

The drug is administered only under close supervision due to the risk of serious adverse effects, including reduced production of blood cells. For this reason, blood counts may be carried out before and during treatment.

INFORMATION FOR USERS

Your drug prescription is tailored for you. Do not alter dosage without checking with your doctor.

How taken/used Tablets, injection.

Frequency and timing of doses Usually once daily. Tablets taken 1 hour before or 3 hours after food.

Dosage range Initially according to body weight and disorder, then adjusted according to response.

Onset of effect 2–4 weeks. Antirheumatic effect may not be felt for 8 weeks or more.

Duration of action Immunosuppressant effects may last several weeks after drug is stopped.

Diet advice None.

Storage Keep in original container at room temperature out of the reach of children. Protect from light.

Missed dose Take as soon as you remember, then return to your normal schedule. If more than 2 doses are missed, consult your doctor

Stopping the drug Do not stop without consulting your doctor. If taken to prevent graft transplant rejection, stopping treatment could provoke the rejection of the transplant.

Exceeding the dose An occasional unintentional extra dose is unlikely to cause problems. Large overdoses may cause nausea, vomiting, abdominal pains, and diarrhoea. Tell your doctor.

POSSIBLE ADVERSE EFFECTS

The most common adverse effects are nausea, vomiting, loss of appetite, hair loss, and weakness. The drug may also cause unusual bleeding or bruising (which may be a sign of reduced levels of platelets in the blood), jaundice, rash, and fever or chills; if any of these symptoms develop, contact your doctor immediately. If jaundice, rash, fever, or chills occur, the drug should be stopped.

INTERACTIONS

Allopurinol This drug increases the effects and toxicity of azathioprine.

Warfarin Azathioprine may reduce the effect of this drug.

Live vaccines increase the risk of generalized infection when given with azathioprine.

Co-trimoxazole, trimethoprim, mesalazine, olsalazine, ribavirin, sulfasalazine may increase risk of blood problems if taken with azathioprine.

Corticosteroids may increase the risk of infections and bowel problems.

SPECIAL PRECAUTIONS

Be sure to tell your doctor if:

◆ You have long-term liver or kidney problems.

◆ You have had a previous allergic reaction to azathioprine or 6-mercaptopurine.

◆ You have hepatitis B infection or have recently had shingles or chickenpox.

◆ You have an infection.

◆ You have a blood disorder.

◆ You are taking other medicines.

Pregnancy Azathioprine has been taken in pregnancy without problems but safety is not certain. Discuss with your doctor.

Breast-feeding Not recommended.

Infants and children No special problems.

Over 60 Increased likelihood of adverse effects. Reduced dose necessary.

Driving and hazardous work Avoid until you have learned how azathioprine affects you because the drug can cause dizziness.

Alcohol No known problems.

PROLONGED USE

Prolonged use may reduce bone marrow activity, leading to a reduction of all types of blood cells. Some people have a genetic susceptibility to this effect. There is also a small increase in the risk of cancers affecting the immune system. Avoiding excessive exposure to sunlight may help to prevent adverse skin effects.

Monitoring Regular checks on blood chemistry and blood cell counts are carried out.

BACLOFEN

Brand names Lioresal, Lyflex

Used in the following combined preparations None

QUICK REFERENCE

Drug group Muscle relaxant drug (p.53)

Overdose danger rating Medium

Dependence rating Low

Prescription needed Yes

Available as generic Yes

GENERAL INFORMATION

Baclofen is a muscle relaxant that acts on the central nervous system, including the spinal cord. The drug relieves the spasms, cramping, and muscle rigidity (spasticity) caused by various disorders, including multiple sclerosis, spinal cord injury, brain injury, cerebral palsy, or stroke. Although it does not cure any of these disorders, it increases mobility, allowing other treatment, such as physiotherapy, to be carried out. It may also be used to treat hiccups due to distension of the stomach.

Baclofen is less likely to cause muscle weakness than similar drugs, and its side effects, such as dizziness or drowsiness, are usually temporary. Older people are more susceptible to side effects, especially during the early stages of treatment.

INFORMATION FOR USERS

Your drug prescription is tailored for you. Do not alter dosage without checking with your doctor.

How taken/used Tablets, liquid, injection (specialist use).

Frequency and timing of doses 3 x daily with food or milk.

Adult dosage range 15mg daily (starting dose). Daily dose may be increased by 15mg every 3 days as needed. Maximum daily dose: 100mg.

Onset of effect Some benefits may appear after 1–3 hours, but full beneficial effects may not be felt for several weeks. A dose 1 hour before a specific task will improve mobility.

Duration of action Up to 8 hours.

Diet advice None.

Storage Keep in original container at room temperature out of the reach of children. Protect liquid preparations from light.

Missed dose Take as soon as you remember. If your next dose is due within 2 hours, take a single dose now and skip the next.

Stopping the drug Do not stop the drug without consulting your doctor, who will supervise a gradual reduction in dosage. Abrupt cessation may cause hallucinations, confusion, anxiety, seizures, and worsening spasticity.

Exceeding the dose An occasional unintentional extra dose is unlikely to cause problems. Large overdoses may cause weakness, vomiting, and severe drowsiness. Notify your doctor.

POSSIBLE ADVERSE EFFECTS

The common adverse effects of baclofen, such as dizziness and drowsiness, are related to the sedative effects of the drug. Such effects may be minimized by starting with a low dose and gradually increasing it. Nausea and muscle fatigue or weakness may also occur. Rarer adverse effects include constipation or diarrhoea, headache, and difficulty in passing urine. If any of the adverse effects are severe, or if blurred vision, depression or euphoria, or confusion occur, you should consult your doctor immediately.

INTERACTIONS

Antihypertensive and diuretic drugs Baclofen may increase the blood-pressure-lowering effect of these drugs.

Drugs for parkinsonism Some drugs used for parkinsonism may cause confusion and hallucinations if taken with baclofen.

Sedatives All drugs with a sedative effect on the central nervous system may increase the sedative properties of baclofen.

Tricyclic antidepressants may increase the effects of baclofen, leading to muscle weakness.

SPECIAL PRECAUTIONS

Be sure to tell your doctor if:

- You have long-term liver or kidney problems.
- You have difficulty in passing urine.
- You have had a peptic ulcer.
- You have had epileptic seizures or a stroke.
- You have diabetes.
- You are being treated for hypertension.
- You have porphyria.
- You have Parkinson's disease.
- You have a history of psychiaatric illness.
- You have breathing problems.
- You are taking other medicines.

Pregnancy Safety in pregnancy not established. Discuss with your doctor.

Breast-feeding The drug passes into the breast milk, but at normal doses adverse effects are unlikely. Discuss with your doctor.

Infants and children Reduced dose necessary.

Over 60 Increased likelihood of adverse effects at start of treatment. Reduced initial dose may therefore be necessary.

Driving and hazardous work Avoid such activities until you have learned how baclofen affects you because the drug can cause drowsiness, decreased alertness, and blurred vision.

Alcohol Avoid. Alcohol may increase the sedative effects of this drug.

Surgery and general anaesthetics Be sure to tell the doctor or dentist that you are taking baclofen before you have a general anaesthetic.

PROLONGED USE

No problems expected.

BECLOMETASONE

Brand names Asmabec, Beclazone, Becodisks, Beconase, Clenil Modulite, Clipper, Pulvinal, Qvar, and others

Used in the following combined preparation Fostair

QUICK REFERENCE

Drug group Corticosteroid (p.78) and topical corticosteroid (p.118)

Overdose danger rating Low

Dependence rating Low

Prescription needed Yes (some preparations)

Available as generic Yes

GENERAL INFORMATION

Beclometasone is a corticosteroid drug that is prescribed to relieve the symptoms of allergic rhinitis (as a nasal spray) and to control asthma (as an inhalant). It controls nasal symptoms by reducing inflammation and mucus production in the nose. It also helps to reduce chest symptoms, such as wheezing and coughing. People with asthma may take it regularly to reduce the severity and frequency of attacks. However, once an attack has started, the drug does not relieve symptoms.

Beclometasone is given primarily to people whose asthma has not responded to bronchodilators alone (p.21). The drug is also given orally to help treat acute ulcerative colitis if there is an inadequate response to aminosalicylates such as mesalazine.

There are few serious adverse effects associated with beclometasone given by nasal spray or inhaler, although fungal infections of the mouth and throat (thrush) are a possible side effect of inhaling beclometasone. These infections can be mitigated by using a spacer device and by rinsing the mouth and gargling with water after use.

INFORMATION FOR USERS

Your drug prescription is tailored for you. Do not alter dosage without checking with your doctor.

How taken/used Inhaler, nasal spray, tablets.

Frequency and timing of doses 2–4 x daily.

Dosage range *Adults* 1–2 puffs 2–4 x daily according to preparation used (asthma); 1–2 sprays in each nostril 2–4 x daily (allergic rhinitis); 5mg daily orally for a maximum of 4 weeks. *Children* Reduced dose according to age and weight. Tablets not recommended.

Onset of effect Within 1 week (asthma); 1–3 days (allergic rhinitis). Full benefit may not be felt for up to 4 weeks (all conditions).
Duration of action Several days after stopping the drug.
Diet advice None.
Storage Keep in original container at room temperature out of the reach of children. Protect from light.
Missed dose Take as soon as you remember. If your next dose is due within 2 hours, take a single dose now and skip the next.
Stopping the drug Do not stop without consulting your doctor; symptoms may recur. Sometimes a gradual reduction in dosage is advised.
Exceeding the dose An occasional unintentional extra dose is unlikely to cause problems. But if you notice any unusual symptoms, or if a large overdose has been taken, notify your doctor. Adverse effects may occur if the recommended dose is regularly exceeded over a long period.

POSSIBLE ADVERSE EFFECTS

The occurrence and severity of adverse effects depend on the dose and duration of use. The main side effects are thrush of the throat and mouth with the inhaler, and irritation of the nose and throat with the nasal spray. Other possible effects of the inhaler or spray include cough, sore throat, hoarseness, and nosebleeds; contact your doctor if throat problems or nosebleeds occur.

INTERACTIONS

None.

SPECIAL PRECAUTIONS

Be sure to tell your doctor if:
- ◆ You have had tuberculosis or another nasal or respiratory infection.
- ◆ You have a skin infection (cream/ointment).
- ◆ You have had recent nasal ulcers or nasal surgery.

Pregnancy No evidence of risk.
Breast-feeding No evidence of risk.
Infants and children Reduced dose necessary.
Over 60 No known problems.
Driving and hazardous work No known problems.
Alcohol No known problems.

PROLONGED USE

Long-term use can lead to peptic ulcers, glaucoma, muscle weakness, osteoporosis, growth retardation in children, and, rarely, adrenal gland suppression. However, courses of oral beclometasone lasting more than 4 weeks are not generally recommended, which minimizes the risk of these side effects. Patients on long-term treatment should carry a steroid card or wear a MedicAlert bracelet.
Monitoring Periodic checks on adrenal gland function may be required if large doses are being taken. Children should have their height monitored.

BENDROFLUMETHIAZIDE (BENDROFLUAZIDE)

Brand name Aprinox
Used in the following combined preparation Prestim

QUICK REFERENCE

Drug group Thiazide diuretic (p.31)
Overdose danger rating Low
Dependence rating Low
Prescription needed Yes
Available as generic Yes

GENERAL INFORMATION

Bendroflumethiazide belongs to the thiazide diuretic group of drugs, which increase the amount of salt and water that the kidneys remove from the body. It is used predominantly for treating high blood pressure (see Antihypertensive drugs, p.34). The drug may also be used to reduce oedema (water retention) caused by heart, kidney, or liver conditions, and to treat premenstrual oedema. As with all thiazides, this drug increases the loss of potassium in the urine, which can cause various symptoms (see p.31), and increases the likelihood of irregular heart rhythms, particularly if taken with digoxin for heart failure. Although this effect is rare with low doses, potassium supplements may be given with bendroflumethiazide as a precaution.

INFORMATION FOR USERS

Your drug prescription is tailored for you. Do not alter dosage without checking with your doctor.
How taken/used Tablets.
Frequency and timing of doses Once daily, early in the day. (Sometimes 1–3 x per week.)
Adult dosage range 2.5–10g daily.

Onset of effect Within 2 hours but takes weeks to reach maximum effect on blood pressure.
Duration of action 6–18 hours.
Diet advice This drug may reduce potassium in the body, so you should eat plenty of fresh fruit and vegetables. Discuss with your doctor the advisability of reducing your salt intake as a further precaution for hypertension.
Storage Keep in original container at room temperature out of the reach of children.
Missed dose No cause for concern, but take as soon as you remember. However, if it is late in the day do not take the missed dose, or you may need to get up during the night to pass urine. Take the next scheduled dose as usual.
Stopping the drug Do not stop without consulting your doctor; symptoms may recur.
Exceeding the dose An occasional unintentional extra dose is unlikely to be a cause for concern. But if you notice any unusual symptoms, or if a large overdose has been taken, notify your doctor.

POSSIBLE ADVERSE EFFECTS

Some adverse effects, such as dizziness, nausea, fatigue, and leg cramps, are due to excessive potassium loss but can usually be corrected by taking potassium supplements. Bendroflumethiazide may precipitate gout in susceptible people, and diabetes may be more difficult to control. The blood cholesterol level may also rise slightly, and diarrhoea, constipation, or erectile dysfunction (impotence) may occur. Rarely, a rash may develop; if so, stop taking the drug and contact your doctor.

INTERACTIONS

Non-steroidal anti-inflammatory drugs (NSAIDs) may reduce the diuretic and antihypertensive effect of bendroflumethiazide, and bendroflumethiazide may increase the kidney toxicity of NSAIDs.
Digoxin The effects of digoxin may be increased if excessive potassium is lost.
Anti-arrhythmic drugs Low potassium levels may increase the toxicity of these drugs.
Lithium Bendroflumethiazide may increase lithium levels in the blood.
Corticosteroids These drugs further increase potassium loss if taken with bendroflumethiazide; potassium supplements may be needed to correct this. Corticosteroids may also reduce the diuretic effect of bendroflumethiazide.

SPECIAL PRECAUTIONS

Be sure to tell your doctor if:

- You have long-term liver or kidney problems.
- You have or have had gout.
- You have diabetes.
- You have Addison's disease.
- You have hyperparathyroidism.
- You have lactose intolerance.
- You have systemic lupus erythematosus.
- You are taking other medicines.

Pregnancy Not usually prescribed. Safety in pregnancy not established. Discuss with your doctor.
Breast-feeding The drug passes into breast milk but the level is usually too low to harm the baby. Discuss with your doctor.
Infants and children Not usually prescribed. Reduced dose necessary.
Over 60 Reduced dose may be necessary.
Driving and hazardous work No special problems.
Alcohol No problems expected if consumption is kept low.

PROLONGED USE

Prolonged use of bendroflumethiazide can lead to excessive loss of potassium and imbalances of other salts.
Monitoring Blood tests may be performed periodically to check kidney function and levels of potassium and other salts.

BENZOYL PEROXIDE

Brand names Acnecide, Brevoxyl, Oxy 10, Oxy On-the-Spot, PanOxyl
Used in the following combined preparations Duac Once Daily, Epiduo, Quinoderm

QUICK REFERENCE

Drug group Drug for acne (p.121)
Overdose danger rating Low
Dependence rating Low
Prescription needed No (most preparations)
Available as generic Yes

GENERAL INFORMATION

Benzoyl peroxide is used in a variety of topical preparations for treating acne. Available over the counter, it comes in concentrations of varying strengths for mild to moderate acne.

Benzoyl peroxide works by softening and shedding the top layer of skin and unblocking the sebaceous glands. It can also reduce inflammation of blocked hair follicles by killing the bacteria that infect them.

The drug may cause irritation due to its drying effect on the skin, but this generally diminishes with time. It should be applied to the affected areas as directed on the label. Washing the area prior to application greatly enhances the drug's beneficial effects.

Adverse effects are less likely if treatment is started with a preparation containing a low concentration of the drug and changed to a stronger preparation gradually and only if necessary. Marked dryness and peeling of the skin may occur, but can usually be controlled by reducing the frequency of application. Care should be taken to avoid contact of the drug with the eyes, mouth, and mucous membranes. It is also advisable to avoid excessive exposure to sunlight. Benzoyl peroxide preparations can bleach clothing and hair.

INFORMATION FOR USERS

Follow instructions on the label. Call your doctor if symptoms worsen.

How taken/used Cream, body wash, gel, lotion.

Frequency and timing of doses 1–2 x daily (after washing with soap and water).

Dosage range Start with lowest-strength preparation (2.5 per cent); if necessary, increase gradually to highest strength (10 per cent).

Onset of effect Reduces skin oiliness immediately. Acne usually improves within 4–6 weeks.

Duration of action 24–48 hours.

Diet advice None.

Storage Keep in original container at room temperature out of the reach of children.

Missed dose Apply as soon as you remember.

Stopping the drug Can be safely stopped as soon as you no longer need it.

Exceeding the dose A single extra application is unlikely to cause problems. Regular overuse may result in extensive irritation, peeling, redness, and swelling of the skin.

POSSIBLE ADVERSE EFFECTS

Application of benzoyl peroxide may cause temporary burning or stinging of the skin. Redness, peeling, and swelling may result from excessive drying of the skin and usually clears up if the treatment is stopped or used less frequently. If severe burning, blistering, or crusting occur, stop using benzoyl peroxide and consult your doctor.

INTERACTIONS

Skin-drying preparations Medicated cosmetics, soaps, toiletries, and other anti-acne preparations increase the likelihood of dryness and irritation of the skin with benzoyl peroxide.

SPECIAL PRECAUTIONS

Be sure to tell your doctor or pharmacist before using this drug if:

- You have eczema.
- You have sunburn.
- You have had a previous allergic reaction to benzoyl peroxide.
- You are taking other medicines.

Pregnancy No evidence of risk.

Breast-feeding No evidence of risk.

Infants and children Not usually recommended for children under 12 years except under medical supervision.

Over 60 Not usually required.

Driving and hazardous work No known problems.

Alcohol No known problems.

PROLONGED USE

Benzoyl peroxide usually takes 4–6 weeks to produce an effect. If the acne has not improved after 6 weeks, consult your doctor.

BETAHISTINE

Brand name Serc

Used in the following combined preparations None

QUICK REFERENCE

Drug group Drug for Ménière's disease (p.20)

Overdose danger rating High

Dependence rating Low

Prescription needed Yes

Available as generic Yes

GENERAL INFORMATION

Betahistine, a drug that resembles the natural substance histamine in some of its effects, was introduced in the 1970s as a treatment for Ménière's disease, which is caused by the pressure of excess fluid in the inner ear.

Taken regularly, betahistine reduces the frequency and severity of the nausea and vertigo attacks that characterize this condition. It may also be used to treat tinnitus (ringing in the ears) and hearing loss due to Ménière's disease. It is thought to work by reducing pressure in the inner ear, possibly by improving blood flow in the small blood vessels in that area. Drug treatment is not successful in all cases, however, and surgery may be needed.

INFORMATION FOR USERS

Your drug prescription is tailored for you. Do not alter dosage without checking with your doctor.

How taken/used Tablets.

Frequency and timing of doses 3 x daily with or after food.

Adult dosage range 24–48mg daily.

Onset of effect Usually within 1 hour, but full effect may not be reached for some time.

Duration of action 6–12 hours.

Diet advice None.

Storage Keep in original container at room temperature out of the reach of children.

Missed dose Take as soon as you remember. If your next dose is due within 2 hours, take a single dose now and skip the next.

Stopping the drug Do not stop the drug without consulting your doctor; symptoms may recur.

OVERDOSE ACTION

Seek immediate medical advice in all cases. Large overdoses may cause collapse and seizures requiring emergency action.

POSSIBLE ADVERSE EFFECTS

Adverse effects from betahistine are minor and rarely cause problems. Nausea, indigestion, headache, and itching may occur. Rarely, a rash may develop; if so, consult your doctor.

INTERACTIONS

Antihistamines Although unproven, there is a possibility that betahistine may reduce the effects of these drugs, and antihistamines may reduce the effects of betahistine.

SPECIAL PRECAUTIONS

Be sure to tell your doctor if:

- You have asthma.
- You have a history of peptic ulcers.
- You have lactose intolerance.
- You have phaeochromocytoma.
- You are taking other medicines.

Pregnancy Safety in pregnancy not established. Discuss with your doctor.

Breast-feeding The drug may pass into the breast milk, and effects on the baby areunknown. However, at normal doses, adverse effects are unlikely. Discuss with your doctor.

Infants and children Not recommended.

Over 60 No special problems.

Driving and hazardous work Avoid until you have learned how the drug affects you because rarely it may cause drowsiness.

Alcohol No special problems.

PROLONGED USE

No special problems.

BETAMETHASONE

Brand names Betacap, Betesil, Betnelan, Betnesol, Betnovate, Bettamousse, Diprosone, Vistamethasone

Used in the following combined preparations Betnesol-N, Betnovate-C, Diprosalic, Dovobet, Enstilar, Fucibet, Lotriderm

QUICK REFERENCE

Drug group Corticosteroid (p.78)

Overdose danger rating Low

Dependence rating Low

Prescription needed Yes

Available as generic Yes

GENERAL INFORMATION

Betamethasone is a corticosteroid drug used to treat a variety of conditions. Injected into joints, it relieves joint inflammation and the pain and stiffness of rheumatoid arthritis. It is given by mouth or injection to treat certain endocrine conditions affecting the pituitary and adrenal glands, and some blood disorders. It is also used topically (p.118) for skin disorders such as eczema and psoriasis.

When taken for short periods, low or moderate doses rarely cause serious side effects; however, high dosages or prolonged use can lead to many adverse effects (see below).

INFORMATION FOR USERS

Your drug prescription is tailored for you. Do not alter dosage without checking with your doctor.

How taken/used Tablets, injection, cream, ointment, rectal ointment, lotion, scalp solution, eye ointment, eye/ear/nose drops.

Frequency and timing of doses Usually once daily in the morning (systemic). Otherwise varies according to disorder being treated.

Dosage range Varies; follow your doctor's instructions.

Onset of effect Within 30 minutes (injection); within 48 hours (other forms).

Duration of action Up to 24 hours.

Diet advice A low-sodium and high-potassium diet may be recommended when the oral form of the drug is prescribed for extended periods. Follow the advice of your doctor.

Storage Keep in original container at room temperature out of the reach of children. Protect from light.

Missed dose Take as soon as you remember. If your next dose is due within 2 hours, take a single dose now and skip the next.

Stopping the drug Do not stop tablets without consulting your doctor, who may supervise a gradual reduction in dosage. Abrupt cessation after long-term treatment may cause problems with the pituitary and adrenal gland system.

Exceeding the dose An occasional unintentional extra dose is unlikely to cause problems. But if you notice any unusual symptoms, or if a large overdose has been taken, notify your doctor.

POSSIBLE ADVERSE EFFECTS

Topical preparations are unlikely to cause adverse effects unless overused. The possible effects of oral preparations include indigestion, weight gain, acne, muscle weakness, and mood changes. If any of these occur, discuss with your doctor. The drug may also cause bloody or tarry faeces; if so, stop taking it and call your doctor immediately. High oral doses taken for a long period may also cause more serious adverse effects (see Prolonged use).

INTERACTIONS

Insulin, antidiabetic drugs, and oral anticoagulants Betamethasone may alter insulin requirements and the effects of these drugs.

Antifungal drugs (e.g. itraconazole) may increase the effects of betamethasone.

Antihypertensive drugs and drugs used in myasthenia gravis Betamethasone may reduce the effects of these drugs.

Anticonvulsants and barbiturates These drugs may reduce the effects of betamethasone.

Vaccines Betamethasone can interact with some vaccines. Discuss with your doctor before having any vaccinations.

SPECIAL PRECAUTIONS

Be sure to tell your doctor if:

- You have a psychiatric disorder.
- You have a heart condition.
- You have glaucoma.
- You have high blood pressure.
- You have a history of epilepsy.
- You have had a peptic ulcer.
- You have had tuberculosis.
- You have any infection.
- You have diabetes.
- You have liver or kidney problems.
- You are taking other medicines.

Pregnancy No evidence of risk with topical preparations. Taken as tablets in low doses, harm to the baby is unlikely. Discuss with your doctor.

Breast-feeding No risk with topical preparations. Normal doses of tablets are unlikely to harm the baby. Discuss with your doctor.

Infants and children Reduced dose necessary.

Over 60 Reduced dose may be necessary.

Driving and hazardous work No known problems.

Alcohol Keep consumption low. Betamethasone tablets increase the risk of peptic ulcers.

Infection Avoid exposure to chickenpox, measles, or shingles with betamethasone tablets.

PROLONGED USE

Prolonged use by mouth can lead to peptic ulcers, glaucoma, osteoporosis, muscle weakness, and growth retardation in children. Prolonged use of topical treatment may also lead to skin thinning. People taking betamethasone tablets regularly should carry a steroid treatment card or wear a MedicAlert bracelet.

BEVACIZUMAB

Brand name Avastin, Zirabev
Used in the following combined preparations None

QUICK REFERENCE

Drug group Anticancer drug (p.94)
Overdose danger rating Medium
Dependence rating Low
Prescription needed Yes
Available as generic Not currently (available from 2022)

GENERAL INFORMATION

Bevacizumab is a monoclonal antibody (p.95) used in combination with other anticancer drugs to treat advanced cancer of the bowel, breast, lung, ovary, or kidney. It blocks vascular endothelial growth factor (VEGF), a protein produced by cancer metastases that promotes the growth of new blood vessels (angiogenesis). Blocking VEGF inhibits blood vessel growth and deprives metasases of nutrients and oxygen. However, bevacizumab does not destroy tumours and the cancer will eventually progress. On average, the drug improves survival for a few months.

A portion of the bevacizumab molecule is marketed separately under the generic name ranibizumab. This drug has the same anti-angiogenesis properties as bevacizumab and, given by injection into the eye, is used to treat wet age-related macular degeneration.

INFORMATION FOR USERS

This drug is given only under medical supervision and is not for self-administration.

How taken/used Intravenous infusion.

Frequency and timing of doses Once every 2–3 weeks.

Adult dosage range Dosage is determined individually according to the type of cancer and the patient's body weight.

Onset of effect 4–6 hours.

Duration of action 18–20 days.

Diet advice Bevacizumab can cause nausea and vomiting so it is advisable not to eat or drink for a few hours before treatment.

Storage Not applicable. This drug is not normally kept in the home.

Missed dose If you miss your scheduled dose, contact your doctor as soon as possible.

Stopping the drug Discuss with your doctor. Stopping the drug prematurely may lead to a worsening of the underlying condition.

Exceeding the dose Unlikely, as treatment is carefully monitored and supervised.

POSSIBLE ADVERSE EFFECTS

Bevacizumab is given only under medical supervision. Adverse effects are closely monitored. It frequently causes fatigue and gastrointestinal symptoms such as diarrhoea, nausea, and vomiting; increased blood pressure is also common. More serious, rare effects include internal bleeding from the cancer (which may cause coughing up of blood or blood in the faeces); abdominal or chest pain; breathlessness; loss of vision; seizures; heart attack; and stroke. Wound healing is also impaired, and there is a risk of jaw-bone problems, causing pain and swelling. If diarrhoea, nausea, or vomiting are severe, tell your doctor. Report any other side effects to the doctor immediately as it may be necessary to stop the drug.

INTERACTIONS

Bisphosphonates Those who have previously been treated with intravenous bisphosphonates or who are currently being treated with bisphosphonates are at increased risk of jaw-bone problems if also having bevacizumab.

Live vaccines (e.g. influenza; measles, mumps, rubella (MMR)) These are predicted to increase the risk of generalized infection if given with bevacizumab.

Anticoagulants (e.g. rivaroxaban, apixaban) are predicted to increase the risk of bleeding when given with bevacizumab.

SPECIAL PRECAUTIONS

Be sure to tell your doctor if:

- You have a history of colitis or have previously had a bowel perforation or fistula.
- You have recently had major surgery.
- You have high blood pressure, heart failure, or a history of thromboembolism, stroke or heart attacks.
- You have liver or kidney problems.
- You have a blood clotting disorder.
- You are pregnant, planning a pregnancy, or breast-feeding.
- You are taking other medicines, especially anticoagulants.

Pregnancy Must not be used during pregnancy. Women of childbearing age must use contraception during treatment and for up to 6 months afterwards.

Breast-feeding Women must not breast-feed during treatment and for at least 6 months afterwards.

Infants and children Unlikely to be necessary as the conditions for which the drug is used occur almost exclusively in adults.

Over 60 Increased risk of adverse effects.

Driving and hazardous work No known problems.

Alcohol No known problems.

PROLONGED USE

Prolonged treatment increases the risks of severe hypertension (high blood pressure), bleeding or clotting problems, and perforation of the bowel. The risks increase with the dose and duration of treatment.

Monitoring You will have blood tests to check your blood cell count and clotting, and regular checks of your blood pressure. Your urine will be tested for protein. You may need to have a dental check-up before starting treatment.

BEZAFIBRATE

Brand names Bezalip, Bezalip-Mono, Caberzol XL, Fibrazate (bezatard) XL

Used in the following combined preparations None

QUICK REFERENCE

Drug group Lipid-lowering drug (p.35)

Overdose danger rating Low

Dependence rating Low

Prescription needed Yes

Available as generic Yes

GENERAL INFORMATION

Bezafibrate belongs to a group of drugs called fibrates, which lower lipid (fat) levels in the blood. Fibrates are particularly effective in decreasing levels of triglycerides. They also reduce blood levels of cholesterol. Raised levels of lipids are associated with atherosclerosis (deposition of fat in blood vessel walls). This can lead to coronary heart disease (such as angina and heart attacks) and cerebrovascular disease (such as stroke). When bezafibrate is taken with a diet low in saturated fats, there is modest evidence that the risk of coronary heart disease is reduced. Bezafibrate should not be used with statins (another group of lipid-lowering drugs) due to the increased risk of muscle damage.

INFORMATION FOR USERS

Your drug prescription is tailored for you. Do not alter dosage without checking with your doctor.

How taken/used Tablets.

Frequency and timing of doses 1–3 x daily with a little liquid after a meal.

Adult dosage range 400–600mg daily.

Onset of effect It may take weeks for blood fat levels to be reduced, and it takes months or years for fat deposits in the arteries to be reduced. Treatment should be stopped if there is no adequate response within 3–4 months.

Duration of action About 6–24 hours. This may vary according to the individual.

Diet advice A low-fat and low-carbohydrate diet will have been recommended. Follow the advice of your doctor.

Storage Keep in original container at room temperature out of the reach of children.

Missed dose Take as soon as you remember. If your next dose is due within 4 hours (and you take it once daily), take a single dose now and skip the next. If you take the drug 2–3 times daily, take the next dose as normal.

Stopping the drug Do not stop the drug without consulting your doctor.

Exceeding the dose An occasional unintentional extra dose is unlikely to be a cause for concern. But if you notice unusual symptoms, notify your doctor.

POSSIBLE ADVERSE EFFECTS

The most common adverse effects involve the gastrointestinal tract, such as loss of appetite and nausea. These effects normally diminish as treatment continues. Less commonly, diarrhoea, dizziness or fatigue may occur; discuss with your doctor if these are severe. Rarely, there may be a rash, headache, muscle pain, cramp, or weakness, or abdominal pain; if any of these occur, discuss with your doctor.

INTERACTIONS

Anticoagulants Bezafibrate may increase the effect of anticoagulants such as warfarin. Your anticoagulant dose will be reduced when starting bezafibrate.

Monoamine oxidase inhibitors (MAOIs) There is a risk of liver damage when bezafibrate is taken with an MAOI.

Antidiabetic drugs These may interact with bezafibrate to lower blood sugar.

Simvastatin and other lipid-lowering statin drugs There is an increased risk of muscle damage if bezafibrate is taken with these drugs.

Ciclosporin This may interact with bezafibrate to impair kidney function. Bezafibrate may also raise blood levels of ciclosporin.

SPECIAL PRECAUTIONS

Be sure to tell your doctor if:

- You have long-term liver or kidney problems.
- You have a history of gallbladder disease.
- You are taking other medicines.

Pregnancy Safety in pregnancy not established. Discuss with your doctor.

Breast-feeding The drug may pass into the breast milk and may affect the baby. Discuss with your doctor.

Infants and children Not usually prescribed.

Over 60 No special problems expected.

Driving and hazardous work Avoid until you have learned how bezafibrate affects you because the drug can cause dizziness.

Alcohol No special problems.

PROLONGED USE
No problems expected, but patients with kidney disease will need special care as there is a high risk of muscle problems developing.

Monitoring Blood tests will be performed occasionally to monitor the drug's effect on lipids.

BISOPROLOL

Brand names Cardicor

Used in the following combined preparations None

QUICK REFERENCE
Drug group Beta blocker (p.28)

Overdose danger rating High

Dependence rating Low

Prescription needed Yes

Available as generic Yes

GENERAL INFORMATION
Bisoprolol is a cardioselective beta blocker (see p.28). It is used to treat angina and, usually in combination with an ACE inhibitor (see Vasodilators, p.30) and a diuretic (p.30), for treating heart failure. It is also used to treat high blood pressure, but is not usually used to initiate treatment. Bisoprolol is less likely than non-cardioselective beta blockers to provoke breathing difficulties; nevertheless, it is not usually given to people with asthma. It may slow the body's response to low blood sugar if you have diabetes and you are taking insulin.

INFORMATION FOR USERS
Your drug prescription is tailored for you. Do not alter dosage without checking with your doctor.

How taken/used Tablets.

Frequency and timing of doses Once daily.

Adult dosage range *Heart failure* 1.25mg per day (initial dose), increasing to 10mg. *Hypertension and angina* 5–20mg.

Onset of effect 2 hours. Full antihypertensive effect seen after 2 weeks.

Duration of action 24 hours.

Diet advice None.

Storage Keep in original container in a cool, dry place, out of the reach of children.

Missed dose If your next dose is due within 12 hours, take a single dose now. If more than 12 hours have passed, skip the missed dose and take the next dose at the scheduled time.

Stopping the drug Do not stop without consulting your doctor; abrupt cessation may lead to worsening of the underlying condition. The drug should be withdrawn gradually.

OVERDOSE ACTION
Seek immediate medical advice in all cases. Take emergency action if breathing difficulties, collapse, or loss of consciousness occur.

POSSIBLE ADVERSE EFFECTS
The adverse effects are common to most beta blockers; they are usually temporary and tend to diminish with long-term use. Dizziness, lethargy, fatigue, and cold hands and feet are common. If dizziness is severe or you experience any of these other adverse effects, you should report them to your doctor. Nausea and vomiting are also common but should be reported to your doctor. Rarely, bisoprolol may cause nightmares, vivid dreams, a rash, or dry eyes. If any of these occur, stop taking the drug and consult your doctor. If you experience fainting, palpitations, breathlessness, or wheezing, stop taking the drug and seek immediate medical attention.

INTERACTIONS
Other antihypertensive drugs may enhance the blood-pressure-lowering effect of bisoprolol and some may worsen heart failure.

Non-steroidal anti-inflammatory drugs (NSAIDs) may reduce the blood-pressure-lowering effect of bisoprolol.

Insulin and oral antidiabetics Bisoprolol may increase the blood-sugar-lowering effect of these drugs and may also mask symptoms of low blood sugar.

Calcium channel blockers These may cause low blood pressure, a slow heartbeat, and heart failure if taken with bisoprolol.

Cardiac glycosides (e.g. digoxin) These may increase the heart-slowing effect of bisoprolol.

SPECIAL PRECAUTIONS
Be sure to tell your doctor if:
- You have, or have had, asthma.
- You have heart problems.
- You have liver or kidney problems.
- You have diabetes.
- You have psoriasis.
- You have phaeochromocytoma.
- You are taking other medicines.

Pregnancy Not normally prescribed. May affect the developing baby. Discuss with your doctor.

Breast-feeding The drug passes into breast milk but the small amount present is unlikely to affect your baby. Discuss with your doctor.
Infants and children Not recommended.
Over 60 No special problems.
Driving and hazardous work Avoid until you have learned how bisoprolol affects you because it can cause fatigue and dizziness.
Alcohol Avoid excessive intake. Alcohol may increase the blood-pressure-lowering effect of bisoprolol.
Surgery and general anaesthetics Occasionally, bisoprolol may need to be stopped before you have a general anaesthetic, but only do this after discussion with your doctor or dentist.

PROLONGED USE

No special problems.

BOTULINUM TOXIN

Brand names Azzalure, Bocouture, Botox, Dysport, NeuroBloc, Xeomin
Used in the following combined preparations None

QUICK REFERENCE

Drug group Muscle relaxant (p.53)
Overdose danger rating High
Dependence rating Low
Prescription needed Yes
Available as generic No

GENERAL INFORMATION

Botulinum toxin is a neurotoxin (nerve poison) produced naturally by the bacterium *Clostridium botulinum*. It causes botulism, a rare but serious form of food poisoning.

Research has found several slightly different components in the toxin. Two are used medically: botulinum A toxin and botulinum B toxin. They are given to treat conditions in which there are painful muscle spasms, such as spastic foot deformity, blepharospasm (spasm of the eyelids, causing them almost to close), hemifacial spasm, and spasmodic torticollis (spasms of the neck muscles, causing the head to jerk). Toxin A is also used for very resistant, distressing hyperhidrosis (excessive sweating). The toxins' effects may last for 2–3 months, until new nerve endings have formed.

Botulinum toxin is used cosmetically to remove facial wrinkles by paralysing the muscles under the skin.

INFORMATION FOR USERS

This drug is given only under medical supervision and is not for self-administration.
How taken/used Injection.
Frequency and timing of doses Every 2–3 months, depending on response.
Adult dosage range Dose depends on the particular condition being treated. Individual injections may range from 1.25 units to 100 units. The number of injection sites depends on the size and number of the muscles to be paralysed. Specialist judgement is necessary.
Onset of effect Within 3 days to 2 weeks.
Duration of action 2–3 months.
Diet advice None.
Storage Not applicable as the drug is not normally kept in the home.
Missed dose Attend for treatment at the next possible time.
Stopping the drug If having botulinum toxin for medical reasons, discuss with your doctor whether you should stop receiving it. Cosmetic use can be stopped safely at any time.
Exceeding the dose When used for medical reasons, overdose is unlikely since treatment is carefully monitored. If the drug was injected into your face for cosmetic reasons, the effects of an overdose will develop gradually over several days. You should be especially alert for any weakness in your neck or any swallowing difficulty; if these occur, you should contact your doctor immediately.

POSSIBLE ADVERSE EFFECTS

Some of the adverse effects depend on the site of injection. Common ones include reduced blinking and dry eyes, headache, painful swallowing, and pain or weakness at the injection site. Misplaced injections may paralyse unintended muscle groups. All paralyses are likely to be long lasting. Rarely, the toxin may cause glaucoma or painful eyes, neck weakness, head tremor, or hypersensitivity reactions. Consult your doctor if any of these effects occur. Occasionally, it may cause difficulty swallowing (rather than just pain on swallowing); if so, call your doctor immediately.

INTERACTIONS

Aminoglycoside antibiotics and other drugs affecting neuromuscular transmission (e.g. curare-like muscle relaxant drugs) can intensify the effect of botulinum toxin.

SPECIAL PRECAUTIONS

Be sure to tell your doctor if:

- You have any difficulty in swallowing.
- You are taking an anticoagulant drug or have a bleeding disorder.
- You are allergic to botulinum toxin.
- You are taking other medicines.

Pregnancy Not prescribed.
Breast-feeding Not prescribed.
Infants and children Reduced dose necessary.
Over 60 No special problems.
Driving and hazardous work Do not drive until you know how botulinum toxin affects you; the drug may impair ability.
Alcohol No known problems.

PROLONGED USE

To maintain the desired effects, the drug may have to be administered at regular intervals.

BRIMONIDINE

Brand names Alphagan, Mirvaso
Used in the following combined preparations Combigan (with timolol), Simbrinza (with brinzolamide)

QUICK REFERENCE

Drug group Drug for glaucoma (p.112)
Overdose danger rating Medium
Dependence rating Low
Prescription needed Yes
Available as generic Yes

GENERAL INFORMATION

Brimonidine is a sympathomimetic drug (see p.7) available in the form of eye drops or gel.

As eye drops, brimonidine is used to reduce intra-ocular (inside the eye) pressure in the treatment of glaucoma, when patients cannot tolerate topical beta blockers (such as timolol). It may also be used in conjunction with other topical agents, when lower intra-ocular pressure is not achieved by a single agent. It works by reducing the production and increasing the outflow of the fluid inside the eye.

As a gel, it is used to treat facial redness caused by rosacea in adult patients. Side effects are usually limited to the area where the drug is applied; however, systemic side effects such as slowing of the heart rate, low blood pressure, and dizziness may occur. Care should be taken to minimize application just to irritated or damaged skin when using gel.

INFORMATION FOR USERS

Your drug prescription is tailored for you. Do not alter dosage without checking with your doctor.

How taken/used Eye drops, gel.
Frequency and timing of doses Twice daily (eye drops); once daily (gel on skin). If more than one type of eye drops is to be used, the different drugs should be instilled at least 5 minutes apart. The gel should be applied only to the face; any other products can be applied after the gel has dried. Wash your hands thoroughly after application.
Adult dosage range *Eye drops* 1 drop per eye, twice daily. *Gel* Once daily, max 1 g (pea-size drop) per application. Treatment should start with a smaller amount of gel for at least 1 week; it can then be gradually increased.
Onset of effect 0.5–2 hours.
Duration of action 12 hours.
Diet advice None.
Storage Keep the eye drops in the outer cardboard package to protect them from light. Store at room temperature, out of the reach of children. Discard any unused solution 4 weeks after opening.
Missed dose Apply the next dose as normal.
Stopping the drug Do not stop taking the drug without consulting your doctor; symptoms may recur.
Exceeding the dose An occasional unintentional extra application is unlikely to cause problems. Excessive use may irritate the eye and produce adverse effects in other parts of your body, notably low blood pressure, lethargy, and slow heart rate.

POSSIBLE ADVERSE EFFECTS

The most common side effects are redness, dryness, discharge, burning, or stinging of the eye; dry mouth; headache; and drowsiness or fatigue. These are usually transient and not severe enough to require stopping treatment. However, call your doctor if you develop a rash or itching. A rare adverse effect is swelling of the eye or face; if this develops, stop the drug immediately and call the doctor.

INTERACTIONS

Monoamine oxidase inhibitors (MAOIs) When used with brimonidine, these drugs may cause an increased systemic side effect such as hypotension (low blood pressure).

Tricyclic antidepressants (e.g. amitriptyline, imipramine) and mianserin When used with brimonidine, these drugs may cause an increased systemic side effect such as hypotension (low blood pressure).

SPECIAL PRECAUTIONS

Be sure to tell your doctor if:

- You wear contact lenses or have dry eyes.
- You are allergic to brimonidine or any of the ingredients in the formulation.
- You have heart or blood vessel problems (such as Raynaud's phenomenon).
- You are taking any other medicines, notably monoamine oxidase inhibitor (MAOI) therapy or other antidepressants.

Pregnancy Safety in pregnancy not established. Discuss with your doctor.

Breast-feeding Safety in breast-feeding not established. Discuss with your doctor.

Infants and children Not recommended for children under age 12 (eye drops) or 18 (gel).

Over 60 No dose adjustment required.

Driving and hazardous work Eye drops may cause fatigue, drowsiness, and blurred vision. Wait until the symptoms have cleared before such activities.

Alcohol Avoid. Alcohol may increase the sedative effect of the drug.

PROLONGED USE

There is no evidence that prolonged use of brimonidine causes any specific problems.

Monitoring Your doctor will continue to monitor the control of the glaucoma.

BRINZOLAMIDE

Brand name Azopt

Used in the following combined preparations Azarga (with timolol), Simbrinza (with brimonidine)

QUICK REFERENCE

Drug group Drug for glaucoma (p.112)

Overdose danger rating Low

Dependence rating Low

Prescription needed Yes

Available as generic Yes

GENERAL INFORMATION

Brinzolamide is a carbonic anhydrase inhibitor (a type of diuretic; see p.30) that is used in the form of eye drops to treat glaucoma and/or ocular hypertension (high pressure inside the eye). The drug inhibits the action of the enzyme carbonic anhydrase inside the eye; this decreases the amount of fluid that is produced inside the eye, thereby lowering the intra-ocular pressure.

Brinzolamide is used on its own in cases where beta blockers (see p.28) such as timolol are contraindicated, or as combined therapy with beta blockers or prostaglandin analogues when a beta blocker alone does not lower the pressure sufficiently. Most side effects are local to the eye, but systemic effects may occur occasionally if enough of the drug is absorbed into the bloodstream.

INFORMATION FOR USERS

Your drug prescription is tailored for you. Do not alter dosage without checking with your doctor.

How taken/used Eye drops.

Frequency and timing of doses 2–3 x daily.

Adult dosage range One drop in the affected eye(s) or as directed. If using additional eye drops, allow 5 minutes between using brinzolamide and applying the different drops into each eye.

Onset of effect 0.5–2 hours.

Duration of action 6–9 hours.

Diet advice None.

Storage Keep in original container at room temperature out of the reach of children. Protect from light. Discard eye drops 4 weeks after opening.

Missed dose Use the next dose as normal. Do not exceed one drop in the eye(s) three times daily.

Stopping the drug Do not stop without consulting your doctor; symptoms may recur.

Exceeding the dose An occasional unintentional extra dose is unlikely to cause problems. Overuse may irritate the eye and cause problems elsewhere in the body; consult your doctor.

POSSIBLE ADVERSE EFFECTS

The most common side effects are temporary blurred vision, stinging or burning eye(s), and a bitter or unusual taste in the mouth (possibly due to drops draining into the nose and throat). Pressing the inner corner of the eye or gently closing the eyelid after instillation may help to prevent it. Systemic side effects such as hair loss may also occur but are rare. If you faint or have palpitations, breathing difficulties, rash, or swollen lips or tongue, stop taking the drug and call your doctor immediately.

INTERACTIONS

Other carbonic anhydrase inhibitors taken orally Metabolic acid-base disturbance has been reported as there is a potential for additive effect (i.e. the drugs may enhance the effect of brinzolamide).

Antifungal drugs (ketoconazole, itraconazole, clotrimazole) and ritonavir may increase the level of brinzolamide.

SPECIAL PRECAUTIONS

Be sure to tell your doctor if:

- You wear contact lenses or have dry eyes.
- You are allergic to brinzolamide, sulfonamides (such as in co-trimoxazole), or any of the ingredients in the formulation including benzalkonium chloride.
- You have severe kidney problems.
- You are taking any other medicines.

Pregnancy Safety in pregnancy not established. Discuss with your doctor.

Breast-feeding Safety in breast-feeding not established. Discuss with your doctor.

Infants and children Safety has not been established, so not recommended for children and adolescents under the age of 17.

Over 60 No special problems.

Driving and hazardous work Avoid until you have learned how brinzolamide affects you because it can cause temporary blurred vision.

Alcohol No special problems.

PROLONGED USE

No particular problems associated with prolonged use.

Monitoring Your doctor will continue to monitor the control of the glaucoma.

BROMOCRIPTINE

Brand name Parlodel

Used in the following combined preparations None

QUICK REFERENCE

Drug group Drug for parkinsonism (p.16) and pituitary agent (p.83)

Overdose danger rating Low

Dependence rating Low

Prescription needed Yes

Available as generic Yes

GENERAL INFORMATION

Bromocriptine stimulates dopamine receptors in the brain, causing reduced secretion of the hormone prolactin from the pituitary gland. Hence it is used in treating conditions associated with excessive prolactin production, such as some types of female infertility and, occasionally, male infertility. It is also used to reduce the size of prolactin-secreting tumours in the brain, and may be used to suppress lactation in women who do not wish to breast-feed.

Bromocriptine may also be used to treat Parkinson's disease, especially when the disease is not controlled by levodopa. In addition, bromocriptine reduces the release of growth hormone and can therefore be used to treat acromegaly (see p.84).

INFORMATION FOR USERS

Your drug prescription is tailored for you. Do not alter dosage without checking with your doctor.

How taken/used Tablets, capsules.

Frequency and timing of doses 1–4 x daily with food.

Adult dosage range The dose given depends on the condition being treated and your response. In most cases treatment starts with a daily dose of 1–1.25mg. This is gradually increased until a satisfactory response is achieved.

Onset of effect Variable depending on the condition.

Duration of action 8–12 hours.

Diet advice None.

Storage Keep in original container at room temperature out of the reach of children. Protect from light.

Missed dose Take as soon as you remember. If your next dose is due within 2 hours, take a single dose now and skip the next.

Stopping the drug Do not stop the drug without consulting your doctor; symptoms may recur.

Exceeding the dose An occasional unintentional extra dose is unlikely to be a cause for concern. If you notice any unusual symptoms, or if a large overdose has been taken, tell your doctor.

POSSIBLE ADVERSE EFFECTS

Adverse effects such as nausea, vomiting, and constipation are usually dose-related. When it is used to treat Parkinson's disease, bromocriptine may cause abnormal movements. If you experience this problem or develop confusion, dizziness, headache, sudden drowsiness, palpitations, breathlessness, back pain, or swollen legs or feet, discuss with your doctor. Rarely, bromocriptine may cause hypersexuality and behavioural problems, such as compulsive gambling; if so, discuss with your doctor. When the drug is used for long periods, there is a small risk of fibrosis (see Prolonged use).

INTERACTIONS

Antipsychotic drugs oppose the action of bromocriptine and increase the risk of parkinsonism.

Phenylpropanolamine, ephedrine, and pseudoephedrine These drugs are found in some over-the-counter cough and cold remedies. Use of these with bromocriptine may lead to severe adverse effects.

Erythromycin and other macrolide antibiotics These drugs may lead to increased levels of bromocriptine and the risk of adverse effects.

Domperidone and metoclopramide These may reduce some of the effects of bromocriptine.

SPECIAL PRECAUTIONS

Be sure to tell your doctor if:

- You have a history of peptic ulcers.
- You have a history of psychiatric disorders.
- You have high blood pressure.
- You have porphyria.
- You have heart disease.
- You have liver disease.
- You are taking other medicines.

Pregnancy Safety in pregnancy not established. Discuss with your doctor.

Breast-feeding The drug suppresses milk production, and prevents it completely if given within 12 hours of delivery. If you wish to breast-feed, consult your doctor.

Infants and children Not usually prescribed under 15 years.

Over 60 Reduced dose may be necessary.

Driving and hazardous work Avoid until you know how bromocriptine affects you because it may cause dizziness and drowsiness.

Alcohol Avoid. Alcohol increases the likelihood of confusion and reduces tolerance to bromocriptine.

PROLONGED USE

Rarely, long-term use is associated with fibrosis (thickening of connective tissue) of the heart valves, lungs, and lining of the chest and abdominal cavities.

Monitoring Periodic blood tests may be performed to check hormone levels. To check for fibrosis, echocardiography may be carried out when starting treatment and at intervals during the treatment. Other tests, such as lung function tests, kidney function tests, or kidney scans, may also be carried out.

BUDESONIDE

Brand names Benacort, Budelin Novolizer, Budenofalk, Cortiment, Entocort, Jorveza, Pulmicort, Rhinocort Aqua

Used in the following combined preparations DuoResp Spiromax, Fobumix, Symbicort

QUICK REFERENCE

Drug group Corticosteroid drug (p.78)

Overdose danger rating Low

Dependence rating Low

Prescription needed Yes

Available as generic Yes

GENERAL INFORMATION

Budesonide is a corticosteroid given as slow-release (SR) capsules to relieve the symptoms of Crohn's disease, as an enema to treat ulcerative colitis, and via an inhaler as a maintenance treatment for asthma (see p.22). The inhaled corticosteroid is administered either on its own or in combination with a bronchodilator. Budesonide is also given in a nasal spray to relieve the symptoms of allergic rhinitis and for nasal polyps. Side effects are fewer and less serious with the inhaler or nasal spray because less of the drug is absorbed than with oral forms. Mouth and throat irritation can occur with the inhaler, but these effects can be minimized by thoroughly rinsing the mouth and gargling with water after each inhalation.

INFORMATION FOR USERS

Your drug prescription is tailored for you. Do not alter dosage without checking with your doctor.

How taken/used SR capsules, enema, inhaler, powder for inhalation, nasal spray.

Frequency and timing of doses 1–3 x daily (capsules); once daily at bedtime (enema); twice daily (inhaler); once or twice daily (nasal spray).

Dosage range 3–9mg (capsules); 2mg (enema); 200–1,600mcg (inhaler); 100–200mcg (nasal spray).

Onset of effect *Asthma* Within 1 week. *Other conditions* 1–3 days.

Duration of action 12–24 hours.
Diet advice None.
Storage Keep in original container at room temperature out of the reach of children.
Missed dose Take as soon as you remember. If your next dose is due within 2 hours, take a single dose now and skip the next.
Stopping the drug Do not stop taking the drug without consulting your doctor; symptoms may recur. The SR capsules used in Crohn's disease should be withdrawn gradually.
Exceeding the dose An occasional extra dose is unlikely to be a cause for concern. But if you notice any unusual symptoms, or if a large overdose has been taken, notify your doctor.

POSSIBLE ADVERSE EFFECTS
The main side effects of inhalers and nasal sprays are largely confined to the upper airway and mouth. They include cough, nasal irritation, bruising, sore throat, hoarseness, and, rarely, nosebleeds. Capsules and enemas may cause gastrointestinal disturbances, such as diarrhoea or constipation, and sometimes a rash and/or itching. High doses of budesonide by any route can cause weight gain and, if used for prolonged periods, other long-term side effects associated with corticosteroids (see Prolonged use). Contact your doctor if nosebleeds, sore throat, hoarseness, rash, itching, or weight gain occur, or if any of the other side effects are severe.

INTERACTIONS
Itraconazole, ritonavir, and telaprevir may increase the blood level of budesonide and the risk of adrenal gland suppression.

SPECIAL PRECAUTIONS
Be sure to tell your doctor if:
◆ You have had tuberculosis or another respiratory infection.
◆ You are taking other medicines.
Pregnancy Discuss with your doctor, especially if used for Crohn's disease.
Breast-feeding Discuss with your doctor, especially if used for Crohn's disease.
Infants and children Reduced dose necessary.
Over 60 No special problems.
Driving and hazardous work No special problems.
Alcohol No special problems.
Infection Avoid exposure to chickenpox.

PROLONGED USE
Prolonged use of budesonide may be required for asthma prevention. High doses inhaled over a long period can lead to peptic ulcers, osteoporosis, glaucoma, muscle weakness, and growth retardation in children. People taking the drug long term are advised to carry a steroid card or wear a MedicAlert bracelet.
Monitoring If budesonide is being taken in large doses, periodic checks may be needed to make sure that the adrenal glands are working properly. Children using inhalers should have their growth (height) monitored regularly.

BUMETANIDE

Brand name Burinex
Used in the following combined preparations None

QUICK REFERENCE
Drug group Loop diuretic (p.31)
Overdose danger rating Low
Dependence rating Low
Prescription needed Yes
Available as generic Yes

GENERAL INFORMATION
Bumetanide is a powerful, short-acting loop diuretic used to treat oedema (accumulation of fluid in tissue spaces) resulting from heart failure, nephrotic syndrome, and cirrhosis of the liver. The drug is particularly useful in treating people with impaired kidney function who do not respond well to thiazide diuretics.

Bumetanide increases potassium loss in the urine, which can result in a wide variety of symptoms (see p.31). For this reason, potassium supplements or a potassium-sparing diuretic may be given with the drug.

INFORMATION FOR USERS
Your drug prescription is tailored for you. Do not alter dosage without checking with your doctor.
How taken/used Tablets, liquid.
Frequency and timing of doses Usually once daily in the morning. In some cases, twice daily.
Dosage range 1–5mg daily. Dose may be increased if kidney function is impaired.
Onset of effect Within 30 minutes.
Duration of action 2–4 hours.
Diet advice Use of this drug may reduce potassium in the body. Eat plenty of fresh fruit and vegetables, such as bananas and tomatoes.

Storage Keep in original container at room temperature out of the reach of children. Protect from light.

Missed dose No cause for concern, but take as soon as you remember. However, if it is late in the day do not take the missed dose, or you may need to get up during the night to pass urine. Take the next scheduled dose as usual.

Stopping the drug Do not stop the drug without consulting your doctor; symptoms may recur.

Exceeding the dose An occasional unintentional extra dose is unlikely to be a cause for concern. But if you notice any unusual symptoms, or if a large overdose has been taken, tell your doctor.

POSSIBLE ADVERSE EFFECTS

Adverse effects are caused mainly by the rapid fluid loss produced by bumetanide, which can lead to dizziness and fainting. These usually diminish as the body adjusts to the drug. Bumetanide may precipitate gout in susceptible people and can affect the control of diabetes. The drug may also cause lethargy, fatigue, and muscle cramps; notify your doctor if these are severe. In all cases, you should contact your doctor if you experience a rash, photosensitivity, nausea, or vomiting.

INTERACTIONS

Anti-arrhythmic drugs Low potassium levels may increase these drugs' toxicity.

Antibacterials Very high doses of bumetanide can increase the ear damage that is caused by some antibiotics.

Digoxin Excessive potassium loss may increase the adverse effects of digoxin.

Non-steroidal anti-inflammatory drugs (NSAIDs) These drugs may reduce the diuretic effect of bumetanide.

Lithium Bumetanide may increase the blood levels of lithium, leading to an increased risk of lithium toxicity.

Amisulpride, sertindole, and pimozide Low potassium levels increase the risk of abnormal heart rhythms with these antipsychotic drugs.

Thiazides Extremely large amounts of urine may be produced when these drugs are taken with bumetanide.

SPECIAL PRECAUTIONS

Be sure to tell your doctor if:

- You have a long-term liver or kidney problem.
- You have prostate problems.
- You have gout.
- You have diabetes.
- You have low blood pressure.
- You are taking other medicines.

Pregnancy Not usually prescribed. May cause a reduction in blood supply to the developing baby. Discuss with your doctor.

Breast-feeding This drug may reduce your milk supply. Discuss with your doctor.

Infants and children Not usually prescribed. Reduced dose necessary.

Over 60 Dosage is often reduced.

Driving and hazardous work Avoid such activities until you have learned how bumetanide affects you because the drug may cause dizziness and faintness.

Alcohol Keep intake low. The drug increases the likelihood of dehydration and hangovers after drinking alcohol.

PROLONGED USE

Serious problems are unlikely, but the levels of certain salts in the body may occasionally become abnormal during prolonged use.

Monitoring Regular blood tests may be performed to check on kidney function and levels of body salts.

BUPROPION

Brand name Zyban
Used in the following combined preparations None

QUICK REFERENCE

Drug group Smoking cessation aid
Overdose danger rating High
Dependence rating Low
Prescription needed Yes
Available as generic No

GENERAL INFORMATION

Bupropion (also known as amfebutamone) is an antidepressant, although it is chemically unrelated to other classes of antidepressant. The drug has been used to treat depression but is generally used as an aid to giving up tobacco smoking.

The person who is being treated must commit in advance to a date for stopping smoking. Treatment is started while the patient is still smoking, and the "target stop date" is decided on within the first 2 weeks of treatment. Bupropion will be stopped after 7 weeks if the smoker has not given up tobacco smoking completely by then.

Bupropion should not be prescribed for people with a history of seizures or eating disorders, or those who are withdrawing from benzodiazepine or alcohol. In addition, it should not be used by people with bipolar disorder (manic depressive disorder) or psychosis because there is a risk of mania developing.

INFORMATION FOR USERS

Your drug prescription is tailored for you. Do not alter dosage without checking with your doctor.

How taken/used Slow-release (SR) tablets.

Frequency and timing of doses 1–2 x daily. Tablets should be swallowed whole.

Adult dosage range 150–300mg.

Onset of effect Up to 4 weeks for full effect.

Duration of action 12 hours.

Diet advice None.

Storage Keep in the original container at room temperature. Ensure the container is out of the reach of children.

Missed dose Take as soon as you remember. If your next dose is due within 2 hours, take a single dose now and skip the next.

Stopping the drug Do not stop the drug without consulting your doctor. The doctor may want to reduce the dose gradually.

OVERDOSE ACTION

Seek immediate medical advice in all cases. Take emergency action if consciousness is lost.

POSSIBLE ADVERSE EFFECTS

Common adverse effects associated with bupropion include insomnia, poor concentration, headache, dizziness, sweating, tremor, nausea, vomiting, and constipation; discuss with your doctor if these are severe. Rash, itching, fever, and depression are also common but should be discussed with your doctor in all cases. Some adverse effects, such as agitation, tremor, sweating, and insomnia, may be due to the withdrawal of nicotine rather than to the effects of bupropion itself.

Rarely, jaundice, confusion, or anxiety may occur with bupropion; if so, you should consult your doctor. If palpitations, fainting, chest pain, or seizures occur, you should stop taking the drug and consult your doctor at once.

INTERACTIONS

General note A wide range of drugs increases the likelihood of seizures when taken with bupropion. Check with your doctor if you are on other medications.

Ritonavir, amantadine, levodopa, and monoamine oxidase inhibitors increase the risk of adverse effects with bupropion.

Anticonvulsants Phenytoin and carbamazepine may reduce the blood levels and effects of bupropion. Valproate may increase its blood levels and effects.

Tamoxifen Bupropion may reduce blood levels and effects of tamoxifen.

SPECIAL PRECAUTIONS

Be sure to tell your doctor if:

- ◆ You have had a head injury or have a history of seizures or epilepsy.
- ◆ You have an eating disorder.
- ◆ You have cancer of the nervous system.
- ◆ You have diabetes.
- ◆ You have high blood pressure.
- ◆ You have bipolar disorder (manic depressive disorder) or a psychosis.
- ◆ You have kidney or liver problems.
- ◆ You are withdrawing from alcohol or benzodiazepine dependence.
- ◆ You are taking other medicines.

Pregnancy Safety not established. Try to give up smoking without using drugs.

Breast-feeding Safety not established. The drug passes into the breast milk and may affect the baby. Discuss with your doctor.

Infants and children Not recommended.

Over 60 Increased sensitivity to the effects of bupropion. Reduced dose may therefore be necessary.

Driving and hazardous work Avoid such activities until you have learned how bupropion affects you. The drug may cause impaired concentration and dizziness.

Alcohol Avoid. Alcohol will increase any sedative effects.

PROLONGED USE

Bupropion is used for up to 9 weeks for cessation of smoking.

Monitoring Progress will be reviewed after about 3–4 weeks, and the drug will be continued only if it is having some effect. Bupropion may increase blood pressure, so this should be monitored.

CALCIPOTRIOL

Brand name Dovonex
Used in the following combined preparations Dovobet, Enstilar, Xamiol

QUICK REFERENCE

Drug group Drug for psoriasis (p.122)
Overdose danger rating Low
Dependence rating Low
Prescription needed Yes
Available as generic Yes

GENERAL INFORMATION

Calcipotriol is a synthetic derivative of vitamin D used in the treatment of plaque psoriasis affecting the skin and scalp. Although similar to vitamin D, outside the skin calcipotriol is weak compared to vitamin D. In the skin, it is thought to work by reducing production of the skin cells that cause thickening and scaling, which are the most common symptoms of psoriasis. Because this drug is related to vitamin D, excessive use can lead to a rise of calcium levels in the body, although this is very uncommon; otherwise calcipotriol is unlikely to cause any serious adverse effects.

Calcipotriol is applied to the affected areas in the form of cream, ointment, foam, or scalp solution. The drug should not be used on the face, and it is important to wash the hands following application to the treatment area to avoid accidental transfer of the drug to unaffected areas. Local irritation may occur during the early stages of treatment. Excessive exposure to sunlight should be avoided while using calcipotriol.

INFORMATION FOR USERS

Your drug prescription is tailored for you. Do not alter dosage without checking with your doctor.
How taken/used Cream, ointment, scalp solution, foam.
Frequency and timing of doses 1–2 x daily.
Adult dosage range Maximum 100g each week (cream, ointment); maximum 60ml each week (scalp solution): maximum 15g each day (foam); less if more than one preparation is used at the same time.
Onset of effect Improvement is seen within 2 weeks.
Duration of action One application of cream, ointment, or scalp solution lasts up to 12 hours; one application of foam lasts for up to 24 hours. Beneficial effects are longer lasting.
Diet advice None.
Storage Store in original container at room temperature out of the reach of children.
Missed dose Apply the next dose at the scheduled time.
Stopping the drug Do not stop the drug without consulting your doctor; symptoms may recur.
Exceeding the dose Excessive prolonged use may lead to an increase in blood calcium levels, which can cause nausea, constipation, thirst, abdominal pain, weakness, tiredness, and frequent urination. Notify your doctor.

POSSIBLE ADVERSE EFFECTS

Temporary local irritation and itching may occur when treatment is started, and the skin may become dry. Other, less common adverse effects are usually due to heavy or prolonged use leading to high blood levels of calcium. They include a rash (which may be light-sensitive), thirst, frequent urination, nausea, and constipation. If you develop abdominal pain, weakness, tiredness, confusion, or worsening psoriasis, stop the drug and call your doctor.

INTERACTIONS

None known.

SPECIAL PRECAUTIONS

Be sure to tell your doctor if:
- You have a metabolic disorder.
- You have previously had a hypersensitivity reaction to the drug.
- You have long-term liver or kidney problems.
- You are taking other medicines.

Pregnancy Safety in pregnancy not established. Discuss with your doctor.
Breast-feeding Not known if excreted into breast milk. Discuss with your doctor.
Infants and children Not recommended.
Over 60 No problems expected.
Driving and hazardous work No problems expected.
Alcohol No problems expected.

PROLONGED USE

No problems expected from use of calcipotriol in low doses. If the effects of the skin preparation decline after several weeks, they may be regained by suspending use for a few weeks and then recommencing treatment.

Monitoring Regular checks on calcium levels in the blood or urine are required only during prolonged or heavy use.

CANDESARTAN

Brand name Amias, Atacand
Used in the following combined preparations None

QUICK REFERENCE

Drug group Vasodilator (p.30) and antihypertensive drug (p.34)
Overdose danger rating Low
Dependence rating Low
Prescription needed Yes
Available as generic No

GENERAL INFORMATION

Candesartan belongs to a group of vasodilator drugs called angiotensin II blockers. It is used to treat hypertension (high blood pressure) and heart failure (inability of the heart muscle to cope with its workload). The drug works by blocking the action of angiotensin II (a hormone that constricts blood vessels). This relaxes the blood vessels, so lowering blood pressure and easing the heart's workload.

Unlike ACE inhibitors, candesartan does not cause a persistent dry cough or angio-edema (tissue swelling) of the larynx or throat, and may be a useful alternative for people who have to discontinue treatment with an ACE inhibitor for those reasons.

INFORMATION FOR USERS

Your drug prescription is tailored for you. Do not alter dosage without checking with your doctor.
How taken/used Tablets.
Frequency and timing of doses Once daily.
Adult dosage range 4mg initially, increased to maximum of 32mg.
Onset of effect 2 hours.
Duration of action 24 hours.
Diet advice None.
Storage Keep in original container at room temperature out of the reach of children.
Missed dose Take as soon as you remember. If your next dose is due within 8 hours, take a single dose now and skip the next.
Stopping the drug Do not stop taking candesartan without consulting your doctor. Stopping the drug may lead to worsening of the underlying condition.
Exceeding the dose An occasional unintentional extra dose is unlikely to cause problems. Large overdoses may cause dizziness and fainting. Notify your doctor.

POSSIBLE ADVERSE EFFECTS

Adverse effects are usually mild and transient. Common effects include dizziness, headache, flushing, and nausea. More rarely, there may be muscle or joint pain. If you develop jaundice or swelling of the face or lips, stop taking the drug and consult your doctor immediately.

INTERACTIONS

ACE inhibitors (e.g. enalapril, captopril, lisinopril, or ramipril) may increase potassium levels when taken with candesartan. However, the combination of an ACE inhibitor with candesartan is not generally recommended.
Diuretics There is a risk of a sudden fall in blood pressure if these drugs are taken when candesartan is started. They may also affect sodium and potassium levels in the blood.
NSAIDs (e.g. diclofenac or ibuprofen) may reduce the effectiveness of candesartan.
Lithium Levels may be increased if lithium is combined with candesartan, leading to toxicity.
Ciclosporin may increase potassium levels when combined with candesartan.
Potassium salts may increase risk of high potassium levels with candesartan.

SPECIAL PRECAUTIONS

Be sure to tell your doctor if:
◆ You have heart problems, including heart failure.
◆ You have kidney problems or stenosis of the kidney's arteries.
◆ You have liver problems.
◆ You have lactose/galactose intolerance or glucose/galactose malabsorption.
◆ You are taking other medicines.
Pregnancy Not prescribed. If you become pregnant during treatment, consult your doctor without delay.
Breast-feeding Safety not established. Discuss with your doctor.
Infants and children Not prescribed.
Over 60 Increased risk of adverse effects. Reduced dose may therefore be necessary.
Driving and hazardous work Avoid until you know how candesartan affects you because the drug can cause dizziness and fatigue.

Alcohol Regular intake of excessive alcohol may raise blood pressure and reduce the effectiveness of candesartan.

PROLONGED USE

No special problems.

Monitoring Periodic checks on blood potassium levels and kidney function may be done.

CANNABIDIOL

Brand names Epidyolex, Sativex

Used in the following combined preparations None

QUICK REFERENCE

Drug group Anticonvulsants (p.14)

Overdose danger rating Medium

Dependence rating Low

Prescription needed Yes

Available as generic No

GENERAL INFORMATION

Cannabinoids are natural chemicals produced by the cannabis plant (*Cannabis sativa*) that affect signalling processes in the brain and nervous system.

In the UK two products are licensed: Epidyolex and Sativex. Epidyolex is an oral solution containing cannabidiol but lacking tetrahydrocannabinol (THC), the psychoactive chemical from the cannabis plant. It is used to treat rare forms of epilepsy, usually in combination with another anticonvulsant (clobazam). In contrast, Sativex contains both THC and cannabidiol. It is used to treat moderate to severe muscle spasms and stiffness in people with multiple sclerosis who have not derived benefit from other antispasmodic drugs.

INFORMATION FOR USERS

Your drug prescription is tailored for you. Do not alter dosage without checking with your doctor.

How taken/used Oral solution (Epidyolex); oral spray (Sativex).

Frequency and timing of doses Epidyolex: twice daily via measuring syringe. Sativex: 1–12 sprays a day inside cheeks or under tongue; dose is titrated for maximum relief with least side effects. Separate each spray by at least 15 minutes.

Adult dosage range Epidyolex: 2.5mg/kg to 10mg/kg twice daily. Sativex: two or more doses in a day.

Onset of effect Sativex: within 30 minutes, but may take weeks to stabilize.

Duration of action Both drugs have a duration of up to a week once the effect is stabilized.

Diet advice Epidyolex: take consistently with or without food.

Storage Epidyolex: no special conditions. Sativex: if unopened, store upright in a refrigerator. If opened, discard after 42 days. For both, ask pharmacist to dispose of unused drug.

Missed dose Epidyolex: take the next dose at the correct time. Sativex: use as soon as you remember or if you need it.

Stopping the drug Epidyolex should be discontinued gradually.

Exceeding the dose Epidyolex may cause diarrhoea and sleepiness; Sativex may cause dizziness, hallucinations, paranoia, altered heart rate, and low blood pressure. Seek medical attention in all cases.

POSSIBLE ADVERSE EFFECTS

Both drugs affect mood and thinking, but many effects settle over time. Common effects include impaired concentration or memory, insomnia, fatigue, altered appetite or taste, dry, blistered, or sore mouth, nausea, constipation or diarrhoea, rise in heart rate or blood pressure, fever, cough, sore throat, or feeling dizzy, agitated, or drunk. Epidyolex can cause liver injury, fever, rash, and respiratory symptoms. If you have more frequent seizures or a change in the colour of your mouth or teeth, tell your doctor. If you have suicidal or paranoid thoughts, hallucinations, fainting, or signs of liver damage (jaundice, itching, dark urine), stop the drug and call your doctor immediately.

INTERACTIONS

Many drugs, including antibiotics, sedatives, hormonal contraceptives, anticonvulsants, and antidepressants, may increase or reduce the effects of cannibidiol. Discuss with your doctor or pharmacist before taking other medications.

SPECIAL PRECAUTIONS

Be sure to tell your doctor if:

- You have a history of psychiatric disorders.
- You are allergic to cannabis, or (with Epidyolex) to alcohol or sesame oil.
- You have heart disease including fainting or an abnormal ECG.

◆ You have epilepsy.
◆ You have kidney or liver problems.
◆ You are taking any other medicines.
◆ You have previously misused any drug or other substance.
◆ You cannot take alcohol (Sativex).

Pregnancy Avoid. Use reliable barrier contraception with Sativex.

Breast-feeding Avoid. The drug may pass into breast milk and harm the baby.

Infants and children Sativex not recommended. Epidyolex can be used in children over 2 years.

Over 60 Increased risk of adverse effects involving the central nervous system.

Driving and hazardous work Cannabidiol may affect your ability to drive or work. Do not drive until you are on a stable dose and know how the medicine affects you.

Alcohol Avoid. The drug can impair reactions, concentration, and coordination.

Legal and safety information Taking cannabinoids is illegal in many countries.

Both men and women should take reliable contraception until 3 months after stopping therapy. Patients who are taking Sativex and who use hormonal contraceptives should add a barrier method.

PROLONGED USE

The value of continued treatment should be re-evaluated periodically.

Monitoring Liver function tests are monitored periodically for those on Epidyolex.

CAPTOPRIL

Brand names Noyada

Used in the following combined preparations None

QUICK REFERENCE

Drug group ACE inhibitor (p.30) and antihypertensive drug (p.34)

Overdose danger rating Medium

Dependence rating Low

Prescription needed Yes

Available as generic Yes

GENERAL INFORMATION

Captopril belongs to the class of drugs called ACE inhibitors, used to treat high blood pressure and heart failure. It acts by relaxing the muscles around blood vessels, allowing them to dilate and thereby easing blood flow.

Captopril lowers blood pressure rapidly but may require several weeks to achieve its full effect. People with heart failure may be given captopril in addition to diuretics. The drug can achieve dramatic results, relaxing muscle in blood vessel walls and reducing the workload of the heart.

The first dose is usually very small and taken while lying down as there is a risk of a sudden fall in blood pressure. Various minor side effects may occur. Some people experience loss of taste, while others get a persistent dry cough. The cough may be severe enough to necessitate switching to an angiotensin-blocking drug, such as losartan.

INFORMATION FOR USERS

Your drug prescription is tailored for you. Do not alter dosage without checking with your doctor.

How taken/used Tablets, oral solution.

Frequency and timing of doses 2–3 x daily.

Adult dosage range 6.25–25mg daily initially, gradually increased to 37.5–150mg daily.

Onset of effect 30–60 minutes; full beneficial effect may take several weeks.

Duration of action 6–8 hours.

Diet advice Your doctor may advise you to reduce your salt intake to help control your blood pressure.

Storage Keep in original container at room temperature out of the reach of children.

Missed dose Take as soon as you remember. If your next dose is due within 2 hours, take a single dose now and skip the next.

Stopping the drug Do not stop the drug without consulting your doctor; the underlying condition may worsen.

Exceeding the dose An occasional unintentional extra dose is not likely to cause problems. Large overdoses may cause dizziness or fainting. Notify your doctor.

POSSIBLE ADVERSE EFFECTS

Captopril causes a variety of minor adverse effects such as loss of taste, and gastrointestinal symptoms. These usually disappear soon after treatment has started. However, if you have a rash, persistent dry cough, sore or ulcerated mouth, dizziness, sore throat, or fever, discuss with your doctor. If you develop swelling of the mouth or lips, or breathing difficulties, stop taking the drug and call your doctor immediately.

INTERACTIONS

Non-steroidal anti-inflammatory drugs (NSAIDs) may reduce the effectiveness of captopril. There is also a risk of kidney damage when they are taken with captopril.
Vasodilators, diuretics, and other antihypertensives These drugs may increase the blood-pressure-lowering effect of captopril.
Potassium supplements and potassium-sparing diuretics These drugs increase the risk of high potassium levels in the blood when they are taken with captopril.
Ciclosporin This drug increases the risk of high potassium levels in the blood when it is taken with captopril.
Lithium Blood levels of lithium may be raised by captopril.

SPECIAL PRECAUTIONS

Be sure to tell your doctor if:
- ◆ You have long-term kidney or liver problems.
- ◆ You have heart problems.
- ◆ You have had angioedema or a previous allergic reaction to ACE inhibitors.
- ◆ You are pregnant or intend to become pregnant.
- ◆ You are taking other medicines.

Pregnancy Not prescribed in pregnancy. There is evidence of harm to fetus in second and third trimesters.
Breast-feeding Safety not established. Discuss with your doctor.
Infants and children Not recommended.
Over 60 Reduced dose may be necessary.
Driving and hazardous work Avoid such activities until you have learned how captopril affects you because the drug can cause dizziness and fainting.
Alcohol Avoid. Alcohol may increase the blood-pressure-lowering and adverse effects of the drug.
Surgery and general anaesthetics Captopril may need to be stopped before you have a general anaesthetic. Discuss with your doctor or dentist before any operation.

PROLONGED USE

No problems expected.
Monitoring Periodic checks on potassium levels, white blood cell count, kidney function, and urine are usually performed.

CARBAMAZEPINE

Brand names Carbagen SR, Curatil, Epimaz, Tegretol, Tegretol Retard
Used in the following combined preparations None

QUICK REFERENCE

Drug group Anticonvulsant drug (p.14)
Overdose danger rating Medium
Dependence rating Low
Prescription needed Yes
Available as generic Yes

GENERAL INFORMATION

Carbamazepine is used to treat several forms of epilepsy as it reduces the likelihood of seizures caused by abnormal nerve signals in the brain. The drug is also prescribed to relieve the intermittent severe pain caused by irritation of the cranial nerves in trigeminal neuralgia. It is prescribed to stabilize mood in bipolar disorder (manic depressive disorder), to reduce urine output in diabetes insipidus, and to relieve pain in diabetic neuropathy. Rarely, it may be used in the management of acute alcohol withdrawal.

In order to avoid side effects, carbamazepine therapy is usually commenced at a low dose and is gradually increased. It is recommended that patients stick to the same brand of carbamazepine prescribed.

INFORMATION FOR USERS

Your drug prescription is tailored for you. Do not alter dosage without checking with your doctor.
How taken/used Tablets, chewable tablets, liquid, suppositories.
Frequency and timing of doses 1–2 x daily.
Adult dosage range *Epilepsy* 100–2,000mg daily (low starting dose that is slowly increased every 2 weeks). *Pain relief* 100–1,600mg daily. *Psychiatric disorders* 400–1,600mg daily.
Onset of effect Within 4 hours.
Duration of action 12–24 hours.
Diet advice None.
Storage Keep in original container at room temperature out of the reach of children.
Missed dose Take as soon as you remember. If your next dose is due within 2 hours, take a single dose now and skip the next.
Stopping the drug Do not stop the drug without consulting your doctor; symptoms may recur.

Exceeding the dose An occasional unintentional extra dose is unlikely to cause problems. Large overdoses may cause tremor, seizures, and coma. Notify your doctor.

POSSIBLE ADVERSE EFFECTS

Most people have very few adverse effects with carbamazepine, although when blood levels get too high, adverse effects are common and the dose may need to be reduced. Dizziness, unsteadiness, drowsiness, nausea, and loss of appetite are common; discuss with your doctor if severe. Blurred vision is also common; it should be reported to your doctor in all cases. Rarer side effects include jaundice and swelling of the ankles, which should also be reported to your doctor. If you develop a sore throat, hoarseness, rash, fever, or abnormal bruising, stop taking the drug and contact your doctor immediately.

INTERACTIONS

General note Many drugs may increase or reduce the effects of carbamazepine. In addition, carbamazepine itself may reduce the blood levels and effectiveness of other drugs. Discuss with your doctor or pharmacist before taking other medications.

Other anticonvulsant drugs Complex and variable interactions can occur between these drugs and carbamazepine.

Contraceptive pill Carbamazepine may reduce the effectiveness of the contraceptive pill. Discuss this with your doctor.

SPECIAL PRECAUTIONS

Be sure to tell your doctor if:

- You have long-term liver or kidney problems.
- You have heart problems.
- You have had blood problems with other drugs.
- You are taking other medicines.

Pregnancy Avoid if possible. Associated with abnormalities in the fetus. Folic acid supplements should be taken before and during pregnancy. Discuss with your doctor.

Breast-feeding The drug passes into the breast milk and can affect the baby. Discuss with your doctor.

Infants and children Reduced dose necessary.

Over 60 May cause confused or agitated behaviour. Reduced dose may be necessary.

Driving and hazardous work Discuss with your doctor. Your underlying condition, as well as the possibility of reduced alertness while taking carbamazepine, may make such activities inadvisable.

Alcohol Avoid. Alcohol may increase the sedative effects of this drug.

PROLONGED USE

There is a slight risk of changes in liver function or of skin or blood abnormalities occurring during prolonged use.

Monitoring Periodic blood tests are usually performed to monitor levels of the drug, blood cell counts, and liver and kidney function.

CARBIMAZOLE

Brand names None

Used in the following combined preparations None

QUICK REFERENCE

Drug group Antithyroid drug (p.82)

Overdose danger rating Medium

Dependence rating Low

Prescription needed Yes

Available as generic Yes

GENERAL INFORMATION

Carbimazole is an antithyroid drug that suppresses the formation of thyroid hormones and is used to manage overactivity of the thyroid gland (hyperthyroidism). In Graves' disease, which is the most common cause of hyperthyroidism, a course of carbimazole alone or combined with thyroxine (so-called "block and replace" therapy) – usually given for 6–18 months – may cure the disorder. In other conditions, carbimazole is given until other treatments, such as surgery or radio-iodine, take effect. If other treatments are not possible or are declined by the patient, carbimazole can be given long term. The full effect of the drug may take several weeks to develop, and beta blockers may be given during this period to control symptoms.

The most important adverse effect is a reduction in white blood cells (agranulocytosis), increasing the risk of infection. Although this is rare, if you develop a sore throat, mouth ulcers, or a fever, you should see your doctor immediately to have your white blood cell count checked.

INFORMATION FOR USERS

Your drug prescription is tailored for you. Do not alter dosage without checking with your doctor.

How taken/used Tablets.

Frequency and timing of doses 1–3 x daily.

Adult dosage range 15–40mg daily (occasionally a larger dose may be needed). Once control is achieved, dose is reduced gradually to a maintenance dose of 5–15mg for about 18 months.

Onset of effect Some improvement is usually felt within 1–3 weeks. Full beneficial effects usually take 4–8 weeks.

Duration of action 12–24 hours.

Diet advice Your doctor may advise you to avoid foods that are high in iodine, such as cod and mackerel.

Storage Keep in original container at room temperature out of the reach of children.

Missed dose Take as soon as you remember. If next dose is due, take both doses together.

Stopping the drug Do not stop the drug without consulting your doctor; symptoms may recur.

Exceeding the dose An occasional unintentional extra dose is unlikely to cause problems. Large overdoses may cause nausea, vomiting, and headache. Notify your doctor.

POSSIBLE ADVERSE EFFECTS

The most serious adverse effect is a rare, life-threatening reduction in white blood cells (agranulocytosis), which may be indicated by sore throat, fever, or mouth ulcers. If these symptoms occur, stop the drug and notify your doctor immediately. If jaundice or unusual bleeding or bruising occur, you should also inform your doctor without delay. Other possible side effects include headache, dizziness, joint pain, nausea, and loss of sense of taste; discuss with your doctor if these are severe. You should also inform your doctor if you experience rash, itching, or hair loss.

INTERACTIONS

Theophylline Blood levels of this drug may increase when taken with carbimazole.

Erythromycin and prednisolone Blood levels may decrease if these are taken with carbimazole.

SPECIAL PRECAUTIONS

Be sure to tell your doctor if:

- You have a long-term liver problem.
- You are pregnant.
- You are taking other medicines.

Pregnancy May be associated with defects in the baby. Discuss with your doctor.

Breast-feeding The drug passes into the breast milk, but mothers may breast-feed as long as the lowest effective dose is used and the baby is monitored. Discuss with your doctor.

Infants and children Reduced dose necessary.

Over 60 No special problems.

Driving and hazardous work Avoid all such activities until you have learned how carbimazole affects you because the drug may cause dizziness.

Alcohol No known problems.

PROLONGED USE

Carbimazole may rarely cause a reduction in the number of white blood cells.

Monitoring Periodic tests of thyroid function are usually required. If you have a sore throat, fever, or mouth ulcers, your white blood cell count must be checked.

CEFALEXIN

Brand names Keflex

Used in the following combined preparations None

QUICK REFERENCE

Drug group Cephalosporin antibiotic (p.60)

Overdose danger rating Low

Dependence rating Low

Prescription needed Yes

Available as generic Yes

GENERAL INFORMATION

Cefalexin is a cephalosporin antibiotic used for a variety of mild to moderate infections. It does not have as wide a range of uses as some other antibiotics, but it is helpful for respiratory tract infections, cystitis, ear infections, and certain skin and soft tissue infections. In some cases it is prescribed as follow-up treatment for severe infections after a more powerful cephalosporin has been given by injection.

Diarrhoea is the most common adverse effect. Although this tends to be less severe than with other cephalosporins, the risk of the more dangerous *Clostridium difficile* diarrhoea is much higher for older adults taking cefalexin (or any other cephalosporin) than other classes of antibiotic. Some people may also find that they are allergic to cefalexin, especially if they are sensitive to penicillin.

INFORMATION FOR USERS

Your drug prescription is tailored for you. Do not alter dosage without checking with your doctor.

How taken/used Tablets, capsules, granules, liquid.

Frequency and timing of doses 2–4 x daily.

Dosage range *Adults* 1–4g daily. *Children* Reduced dose according to age and weight.

Onset of effect Within 1 hour.

Duration of action 6–12 hours.

Diet advice None.

Storage Keep tablets, capsules, and granules in their original container at room temperature; refrigerate liquid, but do not freeze, and keep for no longer than 10 days. Keep out of the reach of children and protect from light.

Missed dose Take the dose as soon as you remember. If your next dose is due at this time, take both doses now.

Stopping the drug Take the full course. Even if you feel better, the original infection may still be present and may recur if treatment is stopped too soon.

Exceeding the dose An occasional unintentional extra dose is unlikely to be a cause for concern. But if you notice any unusual symptoms, or if a large overdose has been taken, notify your doctor.

POSSIBLE ADVERSE EFFECTS

Most people do not experience serious adverse effects while taking cefalexin. Diarrhoea is common but tends not to be severe. Nausea and vomiting are less common but are also usually not severe. Abdominal pain may also be an adverse effect; if this occurs, report it to your doctor.

The rarer adverse effects, such as rash, itching, swelling, and wheezing, are usually due to an allergic reaction and may necessitate stopping the drug. If you experience any of these effects, consult your doctor at once and stop taking the drug.

INTERACTIONS

Probenecid This drug increases the level of cefalexin in the blood. If taken with cefalexin, the dosage of cefalexin may need to be adjusted accordingly.

Oral contraceptives Cefalexin may reduce the contraceptive effect of these drugs. Discuss with your doctor.

SPECIAL PRECAUTIONS

Be sure to tell your doctor if:

- You have a long-term kidney problem.
- You have had a previous allergic reaction to a penicillin or cephalosporin antibiotic.
- You have a history of blood disorders.
- You are taking other medicines.

Pregnancy No evidence of risk to fetus.

Breast-feeding The drug passes into breast milk but at normal doses adverse effects on the baby are unlikely. Discuss with your doctor.

Infants and children Reduced dose necessary.

Over 60 Avoid. Increased risk of *Clostridium difficile* diarrhoea.

Driving and hazardous work No known problems.

Alcohol No known problems.

PROLONGED USE

Cefalexin is usually given only for short courses of treatment.

CELECOXIB

Brand name Celebrex

Used in the following combined preparations None

QUICK REFERENCE

Drug group Analgesic (p.7) and non-steroidal anti-inflammatory drug (p.48)

Overdose danger rating Medium

Dependence rating Low

Prescription needed Yes

Available as generic Yes

GENERAL INFORMATION

Celecoxib is a type of NSAID called a cyclo-oxygenase-2 (COX-2) inhibitor. These drugs were originally thought to have a lower risk of irritating the upper gastrointestinal tract than other NSAIDs, but this is now disputed.

Celecoxib reduces the pain, stiffness, and inflammation that is caused by rheumatoid arthritis, osteoarthritis, or ankylosing spondylitis. Older patients may be more sensitive to the drug's effects, and for this reason they are usually prescribed a low dose to begin with.

The drug is not prescribed to anyone who has had a heart attack or stroke, because it slightly increases the risk of recurrence, nor is it prescribed to people with peripheral artery disease (poor circulation). Celecoxib is prescribed with caution to anyone at risk of any of these conditions.

INFORMATION FOR USERS

Your drug prescription is tailored for you. Do not alter dosage without checking with your doctor.

How taken/used Capsules.

Frequency and timing of doses 1–2 x daily.

Adult dosage range 200–400mg daily.

Onset of effect 1 hour.

Duration of action 8 hours.

Diet advice None.

Storage Keep in original container at room temperature out of the reach of children.

Missed dose Take as soon as you remember. If your next dose is due within 4 hours, take a single dose now and skip the next.

Stopping the drug If being used short-term, the drug can safely be stopped as soon as you no longer need it. If prescribed for long-term use, you should not stop taking the drug without consulting your doctor.

Exceeding the dose An occasional unintentional extra dose is unlikely to cause problems. Large overdoses may cause stomach and intestinal pain and damage. Notify your doctor.

POSSIBLE ADVERSE EFFECTS

Gastrointestinal, nervous, and respiratory symptoms are the most likely adverse effects. If you have severe indigestion, abdominal pain, diarrhoea, flatulence, nausea, dizziness, or insomnia, consult your doctor. In all cases, consult your doctor if a rash or swollen ankles develop, and call your doctor immediately if palpitations occur. If you experience wheezing, breathlessness, pain in the chest, groin, or leg, black or bloody vomit or faeces, or loss of consciousness, stop taking the drug and contact your doctor immediately.

INTERACTIONS

General note Celecoxib interacts with a wide range of drugs, including ACE inhibitors, SSRIs, antihypertensives, diuretics, and drugs that increase the risk of bleeding and/or peptic ulcers (e.g. aspirin and other NSAIDs).

Lithium Levels and effects of this drug are increased when taken with celecoxib.

Carbamazepine, fluconazole, rifampicin, and barbiturates reduce the effects of celecoxib.

SPECIAL PRECAUTIONS

Be sure to tell your doctor if:

- ◆ You have liver or kidney problems.
- ◆ You have epilepsy.
- ◆ You have asthma.
- ◆ You are allergic to aspirin or any other NSAIDs.
- ◆ You are allergic to sulfonamides.
- ◆ You have a history of peptic ulcers.
- ◆ You have high blood pressure.
- ◆ You have ankle swelling.
- ◆ You have heart problems.
- ◆ You have had a heart attack or stroke.
- ◆ You have inflammatory bowel disease.
- ◆ You are taking other medicines.

Pregnancy Not prescribed.

Breast-feeding Not prescribed.

Infants and children Not recommended.

Over 60 Older people may be more sensitive to the drug's effects. Lower doses may be needed.

Driving and hazardous work Avoid until you know how the drug affects you. It can cause dizziness, vertigo, and sleepiness.

Alcohol Avoid. Alcohol may increase drowsiness and the risk of stomach irritation.

PROLONGED USE

Long-term use increases the risk of a stroke or heart attack, so the lowest effective dose is given for the shortest duration.

Monitoring Periodic tests of kidney function may be performed.

CETIRIZINE/ LEVOCETIRIZINE

Brand names [cetirizine] Benadryl, Boots Hayfever and Allergy Relief, Piriteze, Pollenshield Hayfever, Zirtek; [levocetirizine] Xyzal

Used in the following combined preparations None

QUICK REFERENCE

Drug group Antihistamine (p.56)

Overdose danger rating Medium

Dependence rating Low

Prescription needed Yes (levocetirizine); No (cetirizine)

Available as generic Yes

GENERAL INFORMATION

Cetirizine and levocetirizine are long-acting antihistamines. Their main use is in treating allergic rhinitis, particularly hay fever. Both drugs are also used to treat a number of allergic skin conditions, such as urticaria (hives).

The principal difference between these medicines and traditional antihistamines such as chlorphenamine (chlorpheniramine) is that they have less of a sedative effect on the central nervous system and may therefore be suitable for people when they need to avoid sleepiness (for example, when driving or at work). However, because these drugs can cause drowsiness in some people, you should learn how cetirizine and levocetirizine affect you before you undertake any activities that require concentration.

INFORMATION FOR USERS

Your drug prescription is tailored for you. Do not alter dosage without checking with your doctor.

How taken/used Tablets, liquid.

Frequency and timing of doses 1–2 x daily.

Dosage range *Cetirizine* 10mg daily (adults and children over 12 years); 5mg twice daily (children 6–12 years); 2.5mg twice daily (children 2–6 years). *Levocetirizine* 5mg daily.

Onset of effect 1–3 hours. Some effects may not be felt for 1–2 days.

Duration of action Up to 24 hours.

Diet advice None.

Storage Keep in original container at room temperature out of the reach of children.

Missed dose No cause for concern, but take as soon as you remember. If your next dose is due within 8 hours, take a single dose now and skip the next.

Stopping the drug Can be safely stopped as soon as you no longer need it.

Exceeding the dose An occasional unintentional extra dose is unlikely to cause problems. Large overdoses may cause nausea or drowsiness and have adverse effects on the heart. Notify your doctor.

POSSIBLE ADVERSE EFFECTS

The most common side effects are drowsiness, dry mouth, and fatigue. Headache and diarrhoea may also occur. The side effects of cetirizine may be reduced if the dose is taken as 5mg twice a day (adults and children over 6 years). If the adverse effects are severe, discuss with your doctor.

INTERACTIONS

Anticholinergic drugs Anticholinergic effects of cetirizine and levocetirizine may be increased by all drugs with anticholinergic effects (p.7), including antipsychotics, tricyclic antidepressants, and some drugs for parkinsonism.

Sedatives Cetirizine and levocetirizine may increase the sedative effects of anti-anxiety drugs, sleeping drugs, antidepressants, and antipsychotic drugs.

Allergy tests Antihistamines should be discontinued about 3 days before allergy skin testing. Discuss details in advance with your allergy clinic; timings of discontinuation vary from clinic to clinic.

SPECIAL PRECAUTIONS

Be sure to consult your doctor if:

- You have long-term liver or kidney problems.
- You have glaucoma.
- You are taking other medicines.

Pregnancy Safety in pregnancy not established. Discuss with your doctor.

Breast-feeding The drug passes into the breast milk. Discuss with your doctor.

Infants and children Not recommended under 2 years (cetirizine). Not recommended under 6 years (levocetirizine).

Over 60 No problems expected.

Driving and hazardous work Avoid such activities until you have learned how cetirizine and levocetirizine affect you because the drugs can cause drowsiness in some people.

Alcohol Keep consumption low.

PROLONGED USE

No problems expected.

CHLORAMPHENICOL

Brand names Boots Antibiotic Eye Drops, Brochlor, Chloromycetin, Kemicetine, Minims Chloramphenicol, Optrex Infected Eyes

Used in the following combined preparation Actinac

QUICK REFERENCE

Drug group Antibiotic (p.60)

Overdose danger rating Low

Dependence rating Low

Prescription needed Yes (except some eye drops)

Available as generic Yes

GENERAL INFORMATION

Chloramphenicol is an antibiotic used topically to treat eye and ear infections. Eye drops are available over the counter. Given by mouth or injection, the drug is used to treat meningitis and brain abscesses. It is also effective in acute infections such as typhoid, pneumonia, epiglottitis, or meningitis caused by bacteria resistant to other antibiotics. Although most users experience few adverse effects, it occasionally causes serious or even fatal blood disorders. For this reason, chloramphenicol by mouth or injection is normally only given (usually in hospital) to treat life-threatening infections that do not respond to safer drugs.

INFORMATION FOR USERS

Your drug prescription is tailored for you. Do not alter dosage without checking with your doctor.

How taken/used Capsules, injection, lotion, eye ointment, eye and ear drops.

Frequency and timing of doses Every 6 hours (by mouth or injection); every 2–6 hours (eye preparations); 2–3 x daily (ear drops).

Adult dosage range Varies according to preparation and condition. Follow your doctor's instructions.

Onset of effect 1–3 days, depending on the condition and the preparation.

Duration of action 6–8 hours.

Diet advice None.

Storage Keep in original container at room temperature out of the reach of children.

Missed dose For skin, eye, and ear preparations, apply as soon as you remember. Other preparations are usually given in hospital.

Stopping the drug Take the full course. Even if you feel better the infection may still be present and may recur if treatment is stopped too soon.

Exceeding the dose An occasional unintentional extra dose is unlikely to be a cause for concern. But if you notice any unusual symptoms or a large overdose has been taken, tell your doctor.

POSSIBLE ADVERSE EFFECTS

Transient irritation may occur with eye or ear drops. Other forms of the drug may cause nausea, vomiting, diarrhoea, numbness or tingling in the hands or feet, or a rash or itching; discuss with your doctor if the gastrointestinal symptoms are severe or if you develop numbness, tingling, or rash. If you have impaired vision or a painful mouth or tongue, stop taking the drug and call your doctor immediately. Sore throat, fever, easy bruising, and unusual tiredness or weakness with any form of the drug may be signs of blood abnormalities and should be reported to your doctor without delay, even if treatment has stopped. If these effects occur during treatment, stop taking the drug and contact your doctor immediately.

INTERACTIONS (ORAL AND INJECTION ONLY)

General note Chloramphenicol may increase the effect of certain other drugs, including phenytoin, oral anticoagulant drugs, and oral antidiabetics; phenobarbital or rifampicin may reduce the effect of chloramphenicol.

Antidiabetic drugs The effect of sulfonylurea drugs may be increased by chloramphenicol.

Ciclosporin, tacrolimus, and sirolimus Chloramphenicol capsules, liquid, or injection may raise blood levels of these drugs.

Clozapine and other bone marrow suppressive drugs may increase the risk of bone marrow suppression (neutropenia) if they are used with chloramphenicol.

SPECIAL PRECAUTIONS

Be sure to tell your doctor if:

- You have long-term liver or kidney problems.
- You have porphyria.
- You have a blood disorder.
- You are taking other medicines.

Pregnancy No evidence of risk with eye or ear preparations. Safety in pregnancy of other methods of administration not established. Discuss with your doctor.

Breast-feeding No evidence of risk with eye or ear preparations. Taken by mouth, the drug passes into the breast milk and may increase the risk of blood disorders in the baby. Avoid unless essential.

Infants and children Over-the-counter preparations should not be used in infants under 2 years. Other preparations are rarely used in infants and children, and then only under medical supervision.

Over 60 No problems expected.

Driving and hazardous work Avoid such activities until you have learned how chloramphenicol eye drops affect your vision; the drug can cause transient stinging or blurred vision after application.

Alcohol No known problems.

PROLONGED USE

Rarely, prolonged or repeated use may increase the risk of serious blood disorders. Prolonged or repeated use of eye drops may make chloramphenicol less effective at treating eye infections.

Monitoring Patients given the drug by mouth or injection may have periodic blood cell counts and eye tests. In the rare cases when chloramphenicol is given to infants by mouth or injection, blood levels of the drug are usually monitored.

CHLOROQUINE

Brand names Avloclor, Malarivon
Used in the following combined preparations chloroquine with proguanil, Paludrine/Avloclor

QUICK REFERENCE

Drug group Antimalarial drug (p.73) and disease-modifying antirheumatic drug (p.49)
Overdose danger rating High
Dependence rating Low
Prescription needed No (malaria prevention); Yes (other uses)
Available as generic Yes

GENERAL INFORMATION

Chloroquine is used for the prevention and treatment of malaria. It usually clears an attack in 3 days. Injections may be given for a severe attack. To prevent malaria, a low dose is given once weekly, starting 1 week before visiting a high-risk area and continuing for 4 weeks after leaving. Chloroquine is not suitable for use in all parts of the world as resistance to the drug has developed in some areas. The other main use is in the treatment of autoimmune diseases, such as rheumatoid arthritis and lupus erythematosus.

Common side effects include nausea, headache, diarrhoea, and abdominal cramps. Occasionally a rash develops. Chloroquine can damage the retina during prolonged treatment, causing blurred vision that may progress to blindness. Regular eye examinations are performed to detect early changes.

INFORMATION FOR USERS

Follow the instructions on the label. Call your doctor if symptoms worsen.
How taken/used Tablets, liquid, injection.
Frequency and timing of doses *By mouth* 1 x weekly (prevention of malaria); 1–2 x daily (treatment of malaria); 1 x daily (arthritis); 1–2 x daily (lupus erythematosus).
Adult dosage range *Prevention of malaria* 310mg (2 tablets) as a single dose on the same day each week. Start 1 week before entering endemic area, and continue for 4 weeks after leaving. *Treatment of malaria* Initial dose 620mg (4 tablets) and following doses 310mg. *Rheumatoid arthritis* 150mg (1 tablet) per day.
Onset of effect 2–3 days. In rheumatoid arthritis, full effect may take up to 6 months.
Duration of action Up to 1 week.
Diet advice None.
Storage Keep in original container at room temperature out of the reach of children.
Missed dose Take as soon as you remember but if next dose is due within 24 hours (1 x weekly schedule), or 6 hours (1–2 x daily schedule), take a single dose now and skip the next.
Stopping the drug Do not stop the drug without consulting your doctor.

OVERDOSE ACTION

Seek immediate medical advice in all cases. Take emergency action if breathing difficulties, seizures, or loss of consciousness occur.

POSSIBLE ADVERSE EFFECTS

Common adverse effects, such as nausea, diarrhoea, and abdominal pain, may be avoided by taking chloroquine with food. More rarely, the drug may cause dizziness, hearing problems, hair loss, or depigmentation of the skin; if so, consult your doctor. If you develop a rash or notice any changes in vision, stop taking the drug and call your doctor promptly.

INTERACTIONS

Ciclosporin and digoxin Chloroquine increases blood levels of these drugs.
Anticonvulsant drugs Chloroquine may reduce the effect of these drugs.
Amiodarone, bosutinib, droperidol, and moxifloxacin Chloroquine may increase risk of abnormal heart rhythms if taken with these drugs.
Mefloquine may increase the risk of seizures if taken with chloroquine.
Thyroxine For chloroquine with proguanil, thyroxine dose may need to be increased.

SPECIAL PRECAUTIONS

Be sure to consult your doctor or pharmacist before taking this drug if:

- You have liver or kidney problems.
- You have heart problems.
- You have glucose-6-phosphate dehydrogenase (G6PD) deficiency.

- ◆ You have eye or vision problems.
- ◆ You have psoriasis.
- ◆ You have a history of epilepsy.
- ◆ You have porphyria.
- ◆ You are taking other medicines.

Pregnancy No evidence of risk with low doses. High doses may affect the baby. Discuss the benefits versus the risks of malaria prevention with your doctor.
Breast-feeding The drug may pass into breast milk in small amounts. At normal doses, effects on the baby are unlikely. At high doses in the long term, discuss with your doctor.
Infants and children Reduced dose necessary.
Over 60 No special problems, but it may be difficult to tell between changes in eyesight due to ageing and those that are drug induced.
Driving and hazardous work Avoid such activities until you have learned how chloroquine affects you because the drug may cause dizziness and changes in vision.
Alcohol Keep consumption low.

PROLONGED USE

Prolonged use may cause eye damage and blood disorders.
Monitoring Periodic eye tests and blood counts must be carried out. People taking choloroquine with proguanil and thyroxine need their thyroid function monitored.

CHLORPHENAMINE (CHLORPHENIRAMINE)

Brand names Allercalm, Allerief, Boots Allergy Relief, Hayleve, Numark, Piriton, Pollenase
Used in the following combined preparations Galpseud Plus, Haymine

QUICK REFERENCE

Drug group Antihistamine (p.56)
Overdose danger rating Medium
Dependence rating Low
Prescription needed No (tablets and liquid); yes (injection)
Available as generic Yes

GENERAL INFORMATION

Chlorphenamine is used to treat allergies such as hay fever, allergic conjunctivitis, urticaria (hives), insect bites and stings, and angioedema (allergic swellings). It is included in several over-the-counter cold remedies (p.26). Like other antihistamines, it relieves allergic skin symptoms such as itching, swelling, and redness. It reduces sneezing and the runny nose and itching eyes of hay fever. The drug also has a mild anticholinergic action (see p.7), which suppresses mucus secretion.

Chlorphenamine may be used to prevent or treat allergic reactions to blood transfusions or X-ray contrast material, and can be given with epinephrine (adrenaline) injections for acute allergic shock (anaphylaxis).

INFORMATION FOR USERS

Follow instructions on the label. Call your doctor if symptoms worsen.
How taken/used Tablets, liquid, injection.
Frequency and timing of doses 4–6 x daily (tablets, liquid); single dose as needed (injection).
Dosage range *Adults* 12–24mg daily (by mouth); up to 40mg daily (injection). *Children* Reduced dose according to age and weight.
Onset of effect Within 60 minutes (by mouth); within 20 minutes (injection).
Duration of action 4–6 hours (tablets, liquid, injection).
Diet advice None.
Storage Keep in original container at room temperature out of the reach of children.
Missed dose Take as soon as you remember. If your next dose is due within 2 hours, take a single dose now and skip the next.
Stopping the drug Can be safely stopped as soon as you no longer need it.
Exceeding the dose An occasional unintentional extra dose is unlikely to cause problems. Large overdoses may cause drowsiness or agitation, seizures, or heart problems; in these cases, notify your doctor.

POSSIBLE ADVERSE EFFECTS

Drowsiness is the most common adverse effect of chlorphenamine; another common effect is headache. Other side effects, such as dry mouth, blurred vision, and difficulty in passing urine, are due to its anticholinergic effects. Gastrointestinal irritation may be reduced by taking tablets or liquid with food or drink. Notify your doctor if these symptoms become severe or you have severe headaches, severe drowsiness or dizziness, or blurred vision. If you develop a rash, or if a child taking the drug becomes unusually excitable, stop the drug and call your doctor.

INTERACTIONS

Anticholinergic drugs All drugs, including some drugs for parkinsonism, that have an anticholinergic effect are likely to increase the anticholinergic effect of chlorphenamine.

Phenytoin The effects of phenytoin may be enhanced by chlorphenamine.

Monoamine oxidase inhibitors (MAOIs) and tricyclic antidepressants These drugs may increase the side effects of chlorphenamine.

Sedatives All drugs with a sedative effect are likely to increase the sedative properties of chlorphenamine.

SPECIAL PRECAUTIONS

Be sure to tell your doctor or pharmacist before taking this drug if:

- You have a long-term liver problem.
- You have had epileptic seizures.
- You have glaucoma.
- You have urinary difficulties.
- You are taking other medicines.

Pregnancy Safety in pregnancy not established. Discuss with your doctor.

Breast-feeding The drug passes into the breast milk and may cause drowsiness and poor feeding in the baby. Discuss with your doctor.

Infants and children Reduced dose necessary.

Over 60 Reduced dose may be necessary. Increased likelihood of adverse effects.

Driving and hazardous work Avoid such activities until you have learned how chlorphenamine affects you because the drug can cause drowsiness, dizziness, and blurred vision.

Alcohol Avoid. Alcohol may increase the sedative effects of this drug.

PROLONGED USE

No problems expected.

CHLORPROMAZINE

Brand name Largactil

Used in the following combined preparations None

QUICK REFERENCE

Drug group Phenothiazine antipsychotic and anti-emetic drug (p.19)

Overdose danger rating Medium

Dependence rating Low

Prescription needed Yes

Available as generic Yes

GENERAL INFORMATION

Chlorpromazine was the first antipsychotic drug to be marketed and it is still used today. It has a calming and sedative effect that is useful in the short-term treatment of anxiety, agitation, and aggressive behaviour.

Chlorpromazine is prescribed for the treatment of schizophrenia, psychosis, and mania. Other uses of this drug include the treatment of nausea and vomiting, especially when caused by drug or radiation treatment, and treating severe, prolonged hiccoughs.

The drug can produce a number of adverse effects, some of which may be serious. After continuous use over several years, eye changes and skin discoloration may occur.

INFORMATION FOR USERS

Your drug prescription is tailored for you. Do not alter dosage without checking with your doctor.

How taken/used Tablets, liquid, injection, suppositories (specialist manufacturers only).

Frequency and timing of doses 1–6 x daily.

Adult dosage range *Mental illness* 75–300mg daily; dose is started low and gradually increased. Some patients may need up to 1g daily. *Nausea and vomiting* 40–150mg daily.

Onset of effect 30–60 minutes (by mouth); 15–20 minutes (injection); up to 30 minutes (suppository).

Duration of action 8–12 hours (by mouth or injection); 3–4 hours (suppository). Some effects may persist for up to 3 weeks when stopping the drug after regular use.

Diet advice None.

Storage Keep in original container at room temperature out of the reach of children. Protect from light. Healthcare professionals should avoid direct contact with the drug because of the risk of contact sensitization; tablets should not be crushed, and liquids should be handled carefully.

Missed dose Take as soon as you remember. If your next dose is due within 2 hours, do not take the missed dose. Take your next scheduled dose as usual.

Stopping the drug Do not stop without consulting your doctor; symptoms may recur.

Exceeding the dose An occasional unintentional extra dose is unlikely to cause problems. Larger overdoses may cause unusual drowsiness, fainting, abnormal heart rhythms, muscle rigidity, and agitation. Notify your doctor.

POSSIBLE ADVERSE EFFECTS

The drug commonly causes mild drowsiness and has an anticholinergic effect (p.7), which can produce symptoms such as a dry mouth. Other side effects include weight gain and tremor or abnormal movements. If any of these symptoms is severe, consult your doctor. You should also consult your doctor if you develop blurred vision, dizziness or fainting, or, in women, menstrual irregularities. If a light-sensitive rash or jaundice occur, stop taking the drug and consult your doctor.

INTERACTIONS

Drugs for parkinsonism Chlorpromazine may reduce the effect of these drugs.

Anticholinergic drugs These may intensify the anticholinergic properties of chlorpromazine.

Sedatives All drugs with a sedative effect on the central nervous system are likely to increase the sedative properties of chlorpromazine.

SPECIAL PRECAUTIONS

Be sure to tell your doctor if:

- ◆ You have long-term liver or kidney problems.
- ◆ You have had heart problems or blood clots.
- ◆ You have Parkinson's disease or have had epileptic seizures or a stroke.
- ◆ You have any blood disorders.
- ◆ You have glaucoma.
- ◆ You have an underactive thyroid gland.
- ◆ You have prostate or urethra problems.
- ◆ You are taking other medicines.

Pregnancy Occasionally prescribed by specialist centres. Taken near the time of delivery, it may cause drowsiness in the newborn baby. Discuss with your doctor.

Breast-feeding Passes into breast milk and may affect the baby. Discuss with your doctor.

Infants and children Not recommended for infants under 1 year. Reduced dose necessary for older children.

Over 60 Initial dosage is low; it may be increased if there are no adverse reactions.

Driving and hazardous work Avoid until you know how chlorpromazine affects you as it can cause drowsiness and slowed reactions.

Alcohol Avoid. Alcohol may increase the sedative effects of this drug.

Surgery and general anaesthetics Chlorpromazine may need to be stopped before you have a general anaesthetic. Discuss this with your doctor or dentist.

PROLONGED USE

If used for many years, chlorpromazine may cause tardive dyskinesia (involuntary movements of the face, jaw, and tongue), which may be irreversible. It may also cause blood abnormalities, so regular blood tests may be done.

CICLOSPORIN

Brand names Capimune, Deximune, Neoral, Sandimmun, Vorkazia

Used in the following combined preparations None

QUICK REFERENCE

Drug group Immunosuppressant drug (p.97)

Overdose danger rating Medium

Dependence rating Low

Prescription needed Yes

Available as generic No

GENERAL INFORMATION

Ciclosporin is an immunosuppressant, a drug that suppresses the body's natural defences against infection and foreign cells. This action is of particular use following organ transplants, when the recipient's immune system may reject the transplanted organ unless the immune system is controlled.

Ciclosporin is widely used after many types of transplant, such as heart, bone marrow, kidney, liver, and pancreas; its use has considerably reduced the risk of rejection. It is sometimes used to treat rheumatoid arthritis, some severe types of dermatitis, severe psoriasis, and, as eye drops, to treat a severe dry eye condition (Sjögren's syndrome).

Because it reduces the immune system's effectiveness, it can make you more prone to infections. It can also cause kidney damage.

Different brands of ciclosporin may reach different levels in your blood. It is important to know which brand you are taking. Do not try to make dose changes on your own.

INFORMATION FOR USERS

Your drug prescription is tailored for you. Do not alter dosage without checking with your doctor.

How taken/used Capsules, liquid, injection, eye drops.

Frequency and timing of doses *Liquid* 1–2 x daily. The liquid can be mixed with water, apple juice, or orange juice just before taking. Do not mix with grapefruit juice.

Dosage range Dosage is calculated on an individual basis according to age and weight.
Onset of effect Within 12 hours.
Duration of action Up to 3 days.
Diet advice Avoid high-potassium foods, such as bananas and tomatoes; potassium supplements; and grapefruit, pomelo, and purple grape juice.
Storage Capsules should be left in the blister pack until required. Keep in original container at room temperature out of the reach of children. Do not refrigerate.
Missed dose Take as soon as you remember. If your dose is more than 36 hours late, consult your doctor.
Stopping the drug Do not stop taking the drug without consulting your doctor; stopping the drug may lead to transplant rejection.
Exceeding the dose An occasional unintentional extra dose is unlikely to cause problems. Large overdoses may cause vomiting and diarrhoea and affect kidney function. Notify your doctor.

POSSIBLE ADVERSE EFFECTS

The most common adverse effects are gum swelling, excessive hair growth, nausea, vomiting, and tremor, especially at the start of treatment. Headache, muscle cramps, and fatigue may also occur. Eye pain and discharge are commonly reported with eye drops. Less common effects include diarrhoea, facial swelling, flushing, "pins and needles", rash, and itching. Consult your doctor if headache, cramps, fatigue, or increased hair growth are severe or if you have nausea, tremor, or swollen gums.

INTERACTIONS

General note Ciclosporin may interact with a large number of drugs. Check with your doctor or pharmacist before taking any new prescription or over-the-counter medications. Grapefruit juice can increase blood levels of ciclosporin. Avoid all grapefruit flesh and juice while taking ciclosporin (see also Diet advice, above). St John's wort can reduce ciclosporin levels and even precipitate rejection of a transplanted organ. Avoid St John's wort completely while taking ciclosporin.

SPECIAL PRECAUTIONS

Ciclosporin is prescribed only under close medical supervision, taking account of your condition and medical history.

Pregnancy Use in pregnancy depends on the condition under treatment. Discuss with your doctor.
Breast-feeding Not recommended. The drug passes into the breast milk and safety has not been established. Discuss with your doctor.
Infants and children Used only by specialist children's doctors.
Over 60 Reduced dose may be necessary.
Driving and hazardous work No known problems with tablets, but eye drops may cause blurred vision.
Alcohol No known problems.
Vaccination Avoid vaccination with live attenuated vaccines. Discuss with your doctor.
Sunlight and sunbeds Avoid prolonged, unprotected exposure; apply sunscreen or sunblock.

PROLONGED USE

Long-term use, especially in high doses, can affect kidney and/or liver function. It may reduce numbers of white blood cells, thus increasing susceptibility to infection. It may also cause an increase in blood pressure.
Monitoring Regular blood tests should be carried out as well as tests for liver and kidney function. Ciclosporin blood levels should also be checked regularly, and blood pressure should be monitored.

CIMETIDINE

Brand name Tagamet
Used in the following combined preparations None

QUICK REFERENCE

Drug group Anti-ulcer drug (p.41)
Overdose danger rating Low
Dependence rating Low
Prescription needed No (some preparations)
Available as generic Yes

GENERAL INFORMATION

Cimetidine reduces the secretion of gastric acid and pepsin (an enzyme that helps in the digestion of protein) and thereby promotes ulcer healing in the stomach and duodenum. It is also used for reflux oesophagitis, in which acid stomach contents may flow up the oesophagus. Treatment is usually given in 4- to 8-week courses, with further short courses if symptoms recur. Cimetidine also affects the actions of certain enzymes in the liver. It is therefore prescribed with caution to people taking other drugs, particularly drugs whose levels need to be carefully controlled. Since the drug promotes healing of the stomach lining, it may mask symptoms of stomach cancer and delay diagnosis. It is therefore prescribed with caution to patients whose symptoms change or persist, and to middle-aged and older people.

INFORMATION FOR USERS

Follow the instructions on the label. Call your doctor if symptoms worsen.

How taken/used Tablets, liquid.

Frequency and timing of doses 1–4 x daily (after meals and at bedtime).

Adult dosage range 800–1,600mg daily (occasionally increased to 2,400mg daily)

Onset of effect Within 90 minutes.

Duration of action 2–6 hours.

Diet advice None.

Storage Keep in original container at room temperature out of the reach of children. Protect from light.

Missed dose Do not take the missed dose. Take your next dose as usual.

Stopping the drug If prescribed by your doctor, do not stop taking the drug without consulting the doctor because symptoms may recur.

Exceeding the dose An occasional unintentional extra dose is unlikely to be a cause for concern. But if you notice any unusual symptoms, or if a large overdose has been taken, tell your doctor.

POSSIBLE ADVERSE EFFECTS

Adverse effects are uncommon with cimetidine. They are usually related to dosage level and almost always disappear when the drug is stopped. The adverse effects include diarrhoea, dizziness, tiredness, headache, muscle or joint pain, and, in men, breast enlargement and erectile dysfunction (impotence). If any of these symptoms occur, seek medical advice. If the drug causes confusion or hallucinations, stop taking it and consult your doctor.

INTERACTIONS

Anticoagulant drugs Cimetidine may increase the effect of anticoagulants and their dose may need to be reduced.

Anticonvulsants, beta blockers, anti-arrhythmic drugs, and theophylline/aminophylline Cimetidine may increase the blood levels of these drugs, and their dose may need to be reduced.

Benzodiazepines Cimetidine may increase the blood levels of some of these drugs, increasing the risk of adverse effects.

Ciclosporin and tacrolimus Cimetidine may increase the blood levels of these drugs.

Itraconazole and posaconazole Cimetidine may reduce the absorption of these drugs.

Sildenafil Cimetidine may increase the blood level of this drug.

SPECIAL PRECAUTIONS

Be sure to consult your doctor or pharmacist before taking this drug if:

- You have long-term liver or kidney problems.
- You are taking other medicines.

Pregnancy Safety in pregnancy not established. Discuss with your doctor.

Breast-feeding The drug passes into breast milk but at normal doses adverse effects on the baby are unlikely. Discuss with your doctor.

Infants and children Reduced dose necessary.

Over 60 Risk of stomach cancer is higher in older people and this disorder must be excluded before cimetidine is prescribed. The drug is also more likely to cause confusion and depression in older people.

Driving and hazardous work Avoid such activities until you have learned how cimetidine affects you because the drug may cause dizziness and confusion.

Alcohol Avoid. Alcohol may aggravate the underlying condition and counter the beneficial effects of cimetidine.

PROLONGED USE

Courses of longer than 8 weeks are not usually necessary. If you have bought a preparation of cimetidine over the counter for indigestion, heartburn, or acid reflux and your symptoms persist for more than 2 weeks, you should consult your doctor.

CINNARIZINE

Brand names Cinarin, Cinaziere, Stugeron

Used in the following combined preparation Arlevert

QUICK REFERENCE

Drug group Antihistamine anti-emetic drug (p.19)

Overdose danger rating Medium

Dependence rating Low

Prescription needed No

Available as generic Yes

GENERAL INFORMATION
Cinnarizine is an antihistamine used mainly to control nausea and vomiting, especially motion (travel) sickness. The drug is also used to control the symptoms (nausea and vertigo) of inner ear disorders such as labyrinthitis and Ménière's disease. Taken in high doses, cinnarizine has a vasodilator effect.

The adverse effects are similar to those of most other antihistamines. Drowsiness is the most common problem, but it is usually less severe than with other antihistamines.

INFORMATION FOR USERS
Follow the instructions on the label. Call your doctor if symptoms worsen.

How taken/used Tablets, capsules.

Frequency and timing of doses 2–3 x daily. For the prevention of motion sickness, the first dose should be taken 2 hours before travel.

Dosage range *Adults* 90mg daily (nausea/vomiting); 30mg 2 hours before travel, then 15mg every 8 hours as needed (motion sickness). *Children aged 5–12* 15mg 2 hours before travel, then 7.5mg every 8 hours as needed (motion sickness).

Onset of effect Within 2 hours.

Duration of action Up to 8 hours.

Diet advice None.

Storage Keep in original container at room temperature out of the reach of children.

Missed dose Take as soon as you remember. If your next dose is due within 2 hours, take a single dose now and skip the next.

Stopping the drug If you are taking cinnarizine for an inner ear disorder, do not stop the drug without consulting your doctor; symptoms may recur. However, when taken for motion sickness, the drug can be safely stopped as soon as you no longer need it.

Exceeding the dose An occasional unintentional extra dose is unlikely to cause problems. Large overdoses may cause drowsiness or agitation. Notify your doctor.

POSSIBLE ADVERSE EFFECTS
Drowsiness is the main adverse effect. Anticholinergic effects (p.7), such as blurred vision and dry mouth, may also occur occasionally. Rarely, the drug may cause gastrointestinal problems. If these side effects become severe, notify your doctor. If you develop a rash, stop taking the drug and consult your doctor.

INTERACTIONS
General note All drugs with a sedative effect on the central nervous system may increase the sedative properties of cinnarizine. Such drugs include sleeping drugs, antidepressants, anti-anxiety drugs, and opioid analgesics.

SPECIAL PRECAUTIONS
Be sure to tell your doctor if:
- You have low blood pressure.
- You have Parkinson's disease.
- You have glaucoma.
- You have porphyria.
- You have an enlarged prostate.
- You are taking other medicines.

Pregnancy Safety in pregnancy not established. Discuss with your doctor.

Breast-feeding Safety not established. Discuss with your doctor.

Infants and children Reduced dose necessary.

Over 60 No special problems.

Driving and hazardous work Avoid such activities until you have learned how cinnarizine affects you because it can cause drowsiness.

Alcohol Avoid. Alcohol may increase the sedative effects of this drug.

PROLONGED USE
Development or aggravation of extrapyramidal symptoms (abnormal movements) may occur rarely in older people after prolonged use of cinnarizine. If such symptoms develop, treatment should be discontinued.

CIPROFLOXACIN

Brand names Cetraxal, Ciloxan, Ciproxin

Used in the following combined preparations None

QUICK REFERENCE
Drug group Antibacterial drug (p.64)

Overdose danger rating Medium

Dependence rating Low

Prescription needed Yes

Available as generic Yes

GENERAL INFORMATION
Ciprofloxacin, a quinolone antibacterial drug, is used to treat bacteria resistant to other commonly used antibiotics. It is especially useful for chest, intestine, urinary tract, and eye infections. When taken by mouth, ciprofloxacin works quickly and effectively. In more

severe systemic bacterial infections, however, it may be necessary to administer the drug by injection. Eye infections are usually treated with topical preparations.

The most common side effect of oral or injected ciprofloxacin is bowel disturbance. Occasionally it may cause tendon inflammation and damage (see advice for levofloxacin, p.295). Topical eye preparations may sometimes cause eye discomfort or blurred vision.

INFORMATION FOR USERS

Your drug prescription is tailored for you. Do not alter dosage without checking with your doctor.

How taken/used Tablets, liquid, injection, eye drops, eye ointment.

Frequency and timing of doses 2 x daily with plenty of fluids; variable with topical eye preparations.

Adult dosage range 500mg–1.5g daily (tablets); 400mg–1.2g daily (injection); variable with topical eye preparations.

Onset of effect Within a few hours, although full benefit may not be felt for several days.

Duration of action About 12 hours.

Diet advice Do not become dehydrated. Avoid dairy products; they may reduce the drug's absorption. No specal dietary precautions needed for topical eye preparations.

Storage Keep in original container at room temperature out of the reach of children. The injection must be protected from light.

Missed dose Take as soon as you remember, and take your next dose as usual.

Stopping the drug Take the full course. Even if you feel better the original infection may still be present, and symptoms may recur if treatment is stopped too soon.

Exceeding the dose An occasional unintentional extra dose is unlikely to cause problems. Large overdoses of oral or injected preparations may cause kidney problems, mental disturbance and seizures. Notify your doctor.

POSSIBLE ADVERSE EFFECTS

Blurred vision or eye discomfort may occur with topical ciprofloxacin. With oral or injected forms side effects are rare, except when very high doses are given. Nausea, vomiting, abdominal pain, diarrhoea, rash, and itching are the most common adverse effects. Others include dizziness, headache, disturbed sleep, sensitivity to light, jaundice, and confusion. Consult your doctor if you develop a rash or itching, sensitivity to light, jaundice, or confusion, or if any of the other symptoms are severe. If you have seizures or develop painful joints or tendons, stop taking the drug and contact your doctor immediately. With joint or tendon pain, you should also rest the affected limbs until the symptoms subside.

INTERACTIONS

General note A large number of drugs interact with ciprofloxacin. Do not take any over-the-counter or prescription medications without consulting your doctor or pharmacist.

Oral iron preparations and antacids Products containing magnesium or aluminium hydroxide interfere with absorption of ciprofloxacin. Do not take antacids within 2 hours of taking ciprofloxacin tablets.

SPECIAL PRECAUTIONS

Be sure to tell your doctor if:

- You have long-term liver or kidney problems.
- You have heart rhythm problems.
- You have had epileptic seizures.
- You have glucose-6-phosphate dehydrogenase (G6PD) deficiency.
- You have myasthenia gravis.
- You are taking other medicines.

Pregnancy Safety in pregnancy not established. Discuss with your doctor.

Breast-feeding The drug passes into the breast milk and may affect the baby adversely. Discuss with your doctor.

Infants and children Not usually recommended (oral and injected forms); reduced dose may be necessary (topical eye preparations).

Over 60 Reduced dose may be necessary.

Driving and hazardous work Avoid such activities until you have learned how ciprofloxacin affects you because the drug can cause dizziness and confusion. Topical eye preparations may cause blurred vision.

Alcohol Avoid if using oral or injected preparations as alcohol may increase the sedative effects of this drug.

Sunlight and sunbeds Avoid direct exposure to sunlight or sunlamps due to increased risk of a photosensitivity reaction.

PROLONGED USE

Ciprofloxacin is not usually prescribed for long-term use.

CISPLATIN

Brand name None
Used in the following combined preparations None

QUICK REFERENCE

Drug group Anticancer drug (p.94)
Overdose danger rating High
Dependence rating Low
Prescription needed Yes
Available as generic Yes

GENERAL INFORMATION

Cisplatin is an effective treatment for a wide variety of cancers including cancer of the ovaries, testes, head, neck, lung, bladder, and cervix, blood cancers, and certain children's cancers. It is usually given with other anticancer drugs and can be used with radiotherapy.

The most common and serious adverse effect of cisplatin is impaired kidney function. To reduce the risk of permanent kidney damage, the drug is usually given only once every 3 weeks, and plenty of fluid must be taken to minimize the effect on the kidneys. Cisplatin also frequently causes severe nausea and vomiting, usually starting within an hour and lasting for up to 24 hours, although in some cases persisting for up to a week. To prevent or control these symptoms, anti-emetic drugs are usually given. Damage to hearing is uncommon; it may be more severe in children and become more apparent at the end of treatment. Cisplatin may also increase the risk of anaemia, blood clotting disorders, and infection during treatment. It is likely to reduce fertility, especially in men, so approaches to preserve sperm may be offered.

INFORMATION FOR USERS

This drug is given only under medical supervision and is not for self-administration.
How taken/used Injection.
Frequency and timing of doses Every 3 weeks for up to 5 days; it may be given alone or in combination with other anticancer drugs.
Adult dosage range Dosage is determined individually by body height, weight, and response.
Onset of effect Some adverse effects, such as nausea and vomiting, may appear within 1 hour of starting treatment.
Duration of action Some adverse effects may last for up to 1 week after treatment has stopped.
Diet advice It is important that the body is well hydrated before treatment; 1–2 litres of fluid are usually given by infusion over 8–12 hours.
Storage Not applicable. The drug is not normally kept in the home.
Missed dose Not applicable. The drug is given only in hospital under medical supervision.
Stopping the drug Not applicable. The drug will be stopped under medical supervision.
Exceeding the dose Unlikely since treatment is carefully monitored, and the drug is given intravenously only under close supervision.

POSSIBLE ADVERSE EFFECTS

The most common adverse effects include loss of appetite or taste, nausea, and vomiting. More rarely, there may be ringing in the ears or hearing loss, wheezing or breathing difficulty, abnormal sensations, rash, or facial swelling. Most adverse effects appear within a few hours of injection and are carefully monitored in hospital after each dose. Some wear off within about 24 hours, although nausea and vomiting may last for up to a week. The most common serious adverse effect of cisplatin is impaired kidney function, which may cause reduced urine output. If this occurs, inform medical staff immediately.

INTERACTIONS

General note A number of drugs (e.g. antibacterials such as gentamicin) increase the adverse effects of cisplatin. Because cisplatin is given only under close medical supervision, these interactions are carefully monitored and the dosage is adjusted accordingly.

SPECIAL PRECAUTIONS

Cisplatin is prescribed only under close medical supervision, taking account of your present condition and your medical history. However, be sure to tell your doctor if:
- You have impaired kidney function.
- You are planning to have children.
- You are taking other medicines.

Pregnancy Not usually prescribed. Cisplatin may cause birth defects or premature birth. Discuss with your doctor.
Breast-feeding Not advised. The drug passes into the breast milk and may affect the baby adversely. Discuss with your doctor.
Infants and children The risk of hearing loss is increased. Reduced dose used.

Over 60 Reduced dose may be necessary. Increased likelihood of adverse effects.
Driving and hazardous work No known problems.
Alcohol No known problems.

PROLONGED USE

There is an increased risk of long-term damage to the kidneys, nerves, and bone marrow, and to hearing. The drug may also increase the risk of further cancers later in life.
Monitoring Hearing tests and blood checks to monitor kidney function and bone marrow activity are carried out regularly.

CITALOPRAM/ ESCITALOPRAM

Brand name [escitalopram] Cipralex; [citalopram] Cipramil
Used in the following combined preparations None

QUICK REFERENCE

Drug group Antidepressant drug (p.12)
Overdose danger rating Medium
Dependence rating Low
Prescription needed Yes
Available as generic Yes (both drugs)

GENERAL INFORMATION

Citalopram and escitalopram are selective serotonin re-uptake inhibitor (SSRI) antidepressants used for depressive illness and panic disorder; escitalopram is also used for social and generalized anxiety disorders. They gradually improve mood, increase physical activity, and restore interest in everyday pursuits. Both are generally well tolerated. Any gastrointestinal adverse effects, such as nausea, vomiting, or diarrhoea, are dose related and usually diminish with continued use. Like other SSRIs, these drugs cause fewer anticholinergic side effects (p.7) and are less sedating than tricyclic antidepressants. They are also less likely to be harmful in overdose, but can cause drowsiness and impair performance of tasks such as driving.

INFORMATION FOR USERS

Your drug prescription is tailored for you. Do not alter dosage without checking with your doctor.
How taken/used Tablets, oral drops.
Frequency and timing of doses Once daily in the morning or evening.
Adult dosage range *Depressive illness* 20–40mg (citalopram); 10–20mg (escitalopram). *Panic attacks* 10–40mg (citalopram); 5–20mg (escitalopram). *Social anxiety disorder* 5–20mg (escitalopram). *Generalized anxiety disorder* 10–20mg (escitalopram).
Onset of effect Some benefit may appear within 7 days, but full benefits may take 2–6 weeks (panic attacks may take longer to resolve).
Duration of action Antidepressant effect may persist for some weeks following prolonged treatment.
Diet advice None.
Storage Keep in original container at room temperature out of the reach of children.
Missed dose Take as soon as you remember. If your next dose is due within 8 hours, take a single dose now and skip the next.
Stopping the drug Do not stop the drug without consulting your doctor. Stopping abruptly can cause withdrawal symptoms.
Exceeding the dose An occasional unintentional extra dose is unlikely to be a cause for concern. If you notice any unusual symptoms, or if a large overdose has been taken, tell your doctor.

POSSIBLE ADVERSE EFFECTS

Common effects include nausea, vomiting, indigestion, diarrhoea or constipation, sexual dysfunction, anxiety, insomnia, headache, tremor, dizziness, drowsiness, dry mouth, and sweating. They usually diminish with reduced dose; contact your doctor if they are severe. If seizures, rash, or heart rate or rhythm problems occur, consult your doctor immediately. If you have suicidal thoughts or attempts, stop the drug and seek urgent medical help.

INTERACTIONS

Sumatriptan, other 5HT1 agonists, and lithium There is an increased risk of adverse effects when citalopram and escitalopram are taken with these drugs.
St. John's wort may increase the adverse effects of citalopram and escitalopram.
Monoamine oxidase inhibitors (MAOIs) may cause a severe reaction if taken with citalopram and escitalopram; avoid if MAOIs have been taken in the last 14 days.
Anticoagulants The effects of these drugs may be increased by citalopram and escitalopram. Bruising may occur if citalopram/escitalopram and anticoagulants are used together.

SPECIAL PRECAUTIONS

Be sure to tell your doctor if:

◆ You have epilepsy.
◆ You have diabetes.
◆ You have liver or kidney problems.
◆ You have had bipolar (manic-depressive) disorder and/or suicidal thoughts.
◆ You have or have had heart problems, particularly heart rhythm disturbances.
◆ You have been taking monoamine oxidase inhibitors (MAOIs) or other antidepressants.
◆ You are taking other medicines.

Pregnancy Safety in pregnancy not established. Discuss with your doctor.
Breast-feeding Drug may pass into breast milk and affect the baby. Discuss with your doctor.
Infants and children Not generally recommended under 18 years.
Over 60 Reduced dose may be necessary.
Driving and hazardous work Avoid such activities until you have learned how the drugs affect you because they can cause drowsiness.
Alcohol No special problems.

PROLONGED USE

No problems expected in healthy adults. However, high doses are linked with an increased risk of heart problems, especially in those over 65. There is a small risk of suicidal thoughts and self-harm in children and adolescents, although the drugs are rarely used for them.
Monitoring Any person experiencing drowsiness, confusion, muscle cramps, or seizures should be monitored for low sodium levels in the blood. Under-18s should be monitored for suicidal thoughts and self-harm.

CLARITHROMYCIN

Brand names Clarosip, Febzin XL, Klaricid, Klaricid XL, Mycifor XL
Used in the following combined preparations None

QUICK REFERENCE

Drug group Antibiotic (p.60)
Overdose danger rating Low
Dependence rating Low
Prescription needed Yes
Available as generic No

GENERAL INFORMATION

Clarithromycin is a macrolide antibiotic drug similar to erythromycin (p.236), from which it is derived. It has similar actions and uses to erythromycin, but is slightly more active. Clarithromycin is used for ear, nose, and throat infections, such as middle ear infections, sinusitis, and pharyngitis, and for respiratory tract infections, including whooping cough, bronchitis, and pneumonia, as well as for skin and soft tissue infections. Given with anti-ulcer drugs (p.41) and other antibiotics, it is used to eradicate *Helicobacter pylori*, the bacterium that causes many peptic ulcers. Prolonged use is not usually necessary.

INFORMATION FOR USERS

Your drug prescription is tailored for you. Do not alter dosage without checking with your doctor.
How taken/used Tablets, liquid, granules, injection.
Frequency and timing of doses 2 x daily, up to 14 days; 1 x daily (extra-long release (XL) forms).
Adult dosage range 500mg–1g daily.
Onset of effect 1–4 hours.
Duration of action 1–12 hours; 24 hours (XL preparations).
Diet advice None.
Storage Keep in original container at room temperature out of the reach of children. Protect from light.
Missed dose Take as soon as you remember. If your next dose is due within 2 hours, take a single dose now and skip the next.
Stopping the drug Take the full course. Even if you feel better, the infection may still be present and symptoms may recur if treatment is stopped too soon.
Exceeding the dose An occasional unintentional extra dose is unlikely to be a cause for concern. But if you notice any unusual symptoms, or if a large overdose has been taken, tell your doctor.

POSSIBLE ADVERSE EFFECTS

Clarithromycin is generally well tolerated. Gastrointestinal disturbances such as nausea, vomiting, diarrhoea, and indigestion, headache, and joint and muscle pain are the most common side effects. Hearing loss is a rare risk but usually reverses on stopping the drug. If digestive problems, headaches, or joint or muscle pain are severe, discuss with your doctor. Tell your doctor if you have altered sense of taste or smell, anxiety, insomnia, confusion, or hallucinations. If a rash or jaundice develop, stop the drug and consult your doctor.

INTERACTIONS

Warfarin, midazolam, disopyramide, lovastatin, repaglinide, rifabutin, ranolazine, ticagrelor, ciclosporin, tacrolimus, sildenafil, ergotamine, and valproate Blood levels and effects of all these drugs are increased by clarithromycin.

Carbamazepine, phenytoin, theophylline, digoxin, and colchicine Blood levels and toxicity of these drugs are increased by clarithromycin.

Amiodarone, citalopram, domperidone, ondansetron, quinine, and ranolazine Avoid taking these drugs with clarithromycin as they may cause cardiac arrhythmias.

Lipid-lowering statin drugs Risk of rhabdomyolysis (muscle damage) with clarithromycin.

Zidovudine Blood levels of zidovudine are reduced if this drug is taken at the same time as clarithromycin.

SPECIAL PRECAUTIONS

Be sure to tell your doctor if:

- You have liver or kidney problems.
- You have had an allergic reaction to erythromycin or clarithromycin.
- You have a heart problem.
- You have porphyria.
- You are taking other medicines.

Pregnancy Safety has not been established. Discuss with your doctor.

Breast-feeding Clarithromycin passes into the breast milk and may affect the baby. Discuss with your doctor.

Infants and children Reduced dose necessary.

Over 60 No special problems.

Driving and hazardous work No known problems.

Alcohol No known problems.

PROLONGED USE

In courses of over 14 days, there is a risk of developing antibiotic-resistant infections.

CLINDAMYCIN

Brand names Dalacin, Dalacin C, Dalacin T, Zindaclin

Used in the following combined preparations Duac Once Daily, Treclin

QUICK REFERENCE

Drug group Antibiotic (p.60)

Overdose danger rating Low

Dependence rating Low

Prescription needed Yes

Available as generic Yes

GENERAL INFORMATION

Clindamycin is an antibiotic that is effective against a broad range of bacteria. This action, combined with the fact that it reaches good concentrations in the bones and skin, makes it especially useful for treating diseases such as the bone infection osteomyelitis and the skin infections erysipelas and cellulitis.

The drug is also effective against protozoa, such as those causing toxoplasmosis and falciparum malaria. However, it may cause proliferation of other bacteria such as *Clostridium difficile*, especially in the intestines when used in oral or intravenous forms. Clindamycin-induced *Clostridium difficile* diarrhoea is a serious, sometimes life-threatening side effect, which limits the use of this antibiotic. For this reason the drug should be used under specialist supervision and avoided in older people.

Clindamycin may also be used topically for acne as well as vulval and vaginal infections.

INFORMATION FOR USERS

Your drug prescription is tailored for you. Do not alter dosage without checking with your doctor.

How taken/used Capsules, injection, topical solution, vaginal cream.

Frequency and timing of doses 4 x daily with plenty of water (capsules); 2–4 x daily (injection); 1–2 x daily (topical solution or vaginal cream).

Adult dosage range 600mg–1.8g daily (capsules); 0.6–4.8g daily in divided doses (injection); 5g daily (vaginal cream): 1 pre-prepared applicator daily (topical solution).

Onset of effect 1 hour.

Duration of action 6 hours.

Diet advice None.

Storage Keep in original container at room temperature out of the reach of children.

Missed dose Take as soon as you remember, and take your next dose as usual.

Stopping the drug Take the full course. Even if you feel better the original infection may still be present, and symptoms may recur if treatment is stopped too soon.

Exceeding the dose An occasional unintended extra dose is unlikely to cause problems. Large overdoses may cause nausea or, in rare cases, seizures. Notify your doctor immediately.

POSSIBLE ADVERSE EFFECTS

Most side effects are rare. Rash and/or itching are the only likely adverse reactions to the topical solution or vaginal cream; if these occur, discuss with your doctor. You should also consult your doctor if you are taking the oral or injected form and it causes severe nausea or a hypersensitivity reaction (which may produce a range of allergylike symptoms). Rarely, clindamycin may cause jaundice; if so, stop taking the drug and consult your doctor.

The most serious adverse effect of clindamycin is *Clostridium difficile* diarrhoea, which may be life-threatening. You should therefore report any diarrhoea to your doctor immediately and stop taking the drug.

INTERACTIONS

General note Interactions are unlikely with the topical solution and vaginal cream.

Warfarin Clindamycin may alter the effectiveness of warfarin.

Muscle relaxants Clindamycin may enhance the action of neuromuscular blocking drugs.

Pyridostigmine and neostigmine Clindamycin reduces the effectiveness of these drugs.

Oral typhoid vaccine Clindamycin may make this vaccine less effective if taken at the time of vaccination.

SPECIAL PRECAUTIONS

Be sure to tell your doctor if:

◆ You have a history of antibiotic-associated or *Clostridium difficile* diarrhoea.

◆ You have gastrointestinal disease.

◆ You have kidney or liver problems.

Pregnancy Use in pregnancy only if clearly needed. Discuss with your doctor.

Breast-feeding The drug passes into the breast milk, but if taken at normal doses adverse effects on the baby are unlikely. Discuss with your doctor.

Infants and children Reduced dose necessary.

Over 60 Not recommended.

Driving and hazardous work No special problems with this drug.

Alcohol No special problems.

PROLONGED USE

No major problems with the topical solution or vaginal cream. Oral and injected forms of the drug carry an ongoing risk of *Clostridium difficile* diarrhoea.

Monitoring Liver and kidney function will need to be monitored if oral or injected treatment exceeds 10 days.

CLOBETASOL

Brand names Clarelux, Clobaderm, Dermovate, Etrivex

Used in the following combined preparation
Dermovate-NN

QUICK REFERENCE

Drug group Topical cortisosteroid (p.118)

Overdose danger rating Low

Dependence rating Low

Prescription needed Yes

Available as generic Yes

GENERAL INFORMATION

Clobetasol is a very potent corticosteroid drug (p.78) used for the short-term treatment of inflammatory skin conditions that have not responded to treatment with a less potent corticosteroid. It is used for conditions such as resistant eczema, discoid lupus erythematosus, lichen planus, and lichen simplex.

Because clobetasol is one of the strongest topical corticosteroids, it should be applied sparingly only to affected areas, and for the shortest possible duration. This is to prevent skin damage and to avoid rare systemic side effects, which can result from absorption of the drug through the skin. Such side effects include pituitary or adrenal gland suppression and Cushing's syndrome. In addition, the drug should not be used on untreated bacterial, fungal, or viral skin infections.

Treatment of psoriasis with clobetasol must only be carried out under specialist care and supervision.

INFORMATION FOR USERS

Your drug prescription is tailored for you. Do not alter dosage without checking with your doctor.

How taken/used Cream, ointment, scalp application.

Frequency and timing of doses 1–2 x daily. If treating the face (only under specialist advice), use for no more than 5 days.

Dosage range Usually limited to 50g weekly, but prescribed dose depends on the condition and its extent.

Onset of effect 12 hours. Full beneficial effect after 48 hours.

Duration of action Up to 24 hours.

Diet advice None.

Storage Keep in original container at room temperature out of the reach of children.

Missed dose Use as soon as you remember. If your next application is due within 8 hours, apply the usual amount now and skip the next application.
Stopping the drug Do not stop using the drug without consulting your doctor, who may advise a gradual reduction in dosage to reduce the likelihood of a flare-up of symptoms.
Exceeding the dose An occasional unintentional extra application is unlikely to cause problems. But if you notice any unusual symptoms, notify your doctor.

POSSIBLE ADVERSE EFFECTS

Most people who use clobetasol as directed do not have problems. Adverse effects mainly affect the skin. They include thinning of the skin, stretch marks, thread veins, enlargement of blood capillaries in the skin, acne, and dermatitis. Rarely, there may be growth of unwanted hair and loss of skin pigmentation. Some of these effects may not be reversible. You should talk to your doctor if loss of pigmentation or unwanted hair growth are severe or if any other side effects occur.

INTERACTIONS

None.

SPECIAL PRECAUTIONS

Be sure to tell your doctor if:
- You have a cold sore or chickenpox.
- You have any other infection.
- You have psoriasis.
- You have acne or rosacea.
- You are taking other medicines.

Pregnancy Safety in pregnancy not established. Discuss with your doctor.
Breast-feeding The drug passes into the breast milk and may affect the baby. Discuss with your doctor.
Infants and children Not recommended for infants under 1 year. Used only with great caution for short periods in older children as over-use increases the risk of side effects.
Over 60 No special problems.
Driving and hazardous work No special problems.
Alcohol No special problems.

PROLONGED USE

Clobetasol is not normally used for more than 4 weeks. If the condition has not improved in 2 to 4 weeks, you should notify your doctor.

CLOMIFENE

Brand name Clomid
Used in the following combined preparations None

QUICK REFERENCE

Drug group Drug for infertility (p.107)
Overdose danger rating Low
Dependence rating Low
Prescription needed Yes
Available as generic Yes

GENERAL INFORMATION

Clomifene is used to treat female infertility due to failure of ovulation, by increasing production of hormones by the hypothalamus and pituitary gland. Tablets are taken within about 5 days of the onset of each menstrual cycle. If ovulation has not occurred after several months, other drugs may be prescribed.

Multiple pregnancies (usually twins) occur more commonly in women taking clomifene. Adverse effects include an increased risk of ovarian cysts and ectopic pregnancy. Ovarian hyperstimulation syndrome (over-stimulation of the ovaries) has also been reported; symptoms include pain and swelling of the abdomen, swelling of the hands and legs, shortness of breath, weight gain, nausea, and vomiting. You should consult your doctor immediately if any of these symptoms develop.

INFORMATION FOR USERS

Your drug prescription is tailored for you. Do not alter dosage without checking with your doctor.
How taken/used Tablets.
Frequency and timing of doses Once daily for 5 days in each menstrual cycle.
Dosage range 50mg daily initially; dose may be increased up to 100mg daily.
Onset of effect Ovulation occurs 11–12 days after the last dose in any cycle. However, ovulation may not occur for several months.
Duration of action 5 days.
Diet advice None.
Storage Keep in original container at room temperature out of the reach of children. Protect from light.
Missed dose Take as soon as you remember. If next dose is due at this time, take the missed dose and the next scheduled dose together.
Stopping the drug Take as directed by doctor. Stopping will reduce the chance of conception.

Exceeding the dose An occasional unintentional extra dose is unlikely to be a cause for concern. If you notice any unusual symptoms, or if a large overdose has been taken, tell your doctor.

POSSIBLE ADVERSE EFFECTS

Most adverse effects are related to the dose. Common side effects include hot flushes and breakthrough vaginal bleeding, which should be reported to your doctor if severe; and nausea, vomiting, and abdominal discomfort or bloating, which should be reported in all cases. More rarely, there may be headaches, breast tenderness, dry skin, hair loss, rash, or dizziness; if headaches are severe or if any of these other side effects occur, notify your doctor. Ovarian enlargement and cyst formation may also sometimes occur but usually resolve within a few weeks of stopping the drug. If blurred or disturbed vision, seizures, limb swelling, shortness of breath, or severe pain in the chest or abdomen occur, stop taking the drug and consult your doctor immediately.

INTERACTIONS

None.

SPECIAL PRECAUTIONS

Be sure to tell your doctor if:

- You have a long-term liver problem.
- You are pregnant.
- You have uterine fibroids, ovarian cysts, or abnormal vaginal bleeding.
- You are taking other medicines.

Pregnancy Not prescribed. The drug is stopped as soon as pregnancy occurs.
Breast-feeding Not prescribed.
Infants and children Not prescribed.
Over 60 Not prescribed.
Driving and hazardous work Avoid until you have learned how clomifene affects you because the drug can cause blurred vision.
Alcohol Keep consumption low.

PROLONGED USE

Prolonged use of clomifene may cause visual impairment. Also, no more than 6 courses of treatment are recommended since this may lead to an increased risk of ovarian cancer.
Monitoring Eye tests may be recommended if symptoms of visual impairment are noticed. Monitoring of body temperature and blood or urine hormone levels, or ultrasound scans of the ovaries, are performed to detect signs of ovulation and pregnancy.

CLOMIPRAMINE

Brand names Anafranil
Used in the following combined preparations None

QUICK REFERENCE

Drug group Tricyclic antidepressant drug (p.12)
Overdose danger rating High
Dependence rating Low
Prescription needed Yes
Available as generic Yes

GENERAL INFORMATION

Clomipramine belongs to the tricyclic class of antidepressant drugs. It is used mainly in the long-term treatment of depression.

The drug is particularly useful in treating obsessive and phobic disorders. In these cases, it has to be taken for many months to achieve its full effect. It is also used to treat cataplexy (sudden loss of muscle tone) and narcolepsy (attacks of sleepiness).

Clomipramine has similar adverse effects to other tricyclics, such as drowsiness, dizziness, dry mouth, and constipation. In overdose, the drug may cause coma and dangerously abnormal heart rhythms.

INFORMATION FOR USERS

Your drug prescription is tailored for you. Do not alter dosage without checking with your doctor.
How taken/used Tablets, capsules.
Frequency and timing of doses 1–3 x daily.
Adult dosage range 10–250mg daily but 30–50mg is often effective.
Onset of effect Some effects, a few days; full antidepressant effect, up to 6 weeks; phobic and obsessional disorders, full effect up to 12 weeks.
Duration of action During prolonged treatment antidepressant effect may last up to 2 weeks.
Diet advice Avoid grapefruit and cranberry juice because they may interact with clomipramine and increase the drug's effects.
Storage Keep in original container at room temperature out of the reach of children.
Missed dose Take as soon as you remember. If your next dose is due within 3 hours, take a single dose now and skip the next.
Stopping the drug Stopping abruptly can cause withdrawal symptoms and a recurrence of the

original disorder. Consult your doctor, who will supervise a gradual reduction in dosage.

OVERDOSE ACTION

Seek immediate medical advice in all cases. Take emergency action if palpitations are noted or consciousness is lost.

POSSIBLE ADVERSE EFFECTS

The adverse effects of clomipramine are mainly the result of its anticholinergic action (p.7); they include drowsiness, dizziness, dry mouth, sweating, flushing, blurred vision, and constipation. Weight gain may also occur. Discuss with your doctor if any of these are severe. If you experience difficulty in passing urine, stop taking the drug and talk to your doctor. If you have palpitations, stop taking the drug and consult your doctor urgently.

INTERACTIONS

Sedatives All drugs that have a sedative effect may intensify those of clomipramine.
Anticonvulsants Clomipramine may reduce the effects of these drugs and vice versa.
Antihypertensives Clomipramine may enhance the effect of some of these drugs.
Monoamine oxidase inhibitors (MAOIs) A serious reaction may occur if these drugs are given with clomipramine.
Grapefruit and cranberry juice These may increase the effects of clomipramine.
Cigarette smoking and St. John's wort may decrease the effects of clomipramine.

SPECIAL PRECAUTIONS

Be sure to tell your doctor if:
- You have heart problems.
- You have had epileptic seizures.
- You have long-term liver or kidney problems.
- You have had glaucoma.
- You have had prostate problems.
- You have had mania or a psychotic illness.
- You are taking other medicines.

Pregnancy Safety in pregnancy not established. Discuss with your doctor.
Breast-feeding The drug passes into the breast milk and may affect the baby. Discuss with your doctor.
Infants and children Not recommended.
Over 60 Increased likelihood of adverse effects. Reduced dose may therefore be necessary.
Driving and hazardous work Avoid until you know how the drug affects you as it may cause blurred vision, drowsiness, and dizziness.
Alcohol Avoid. Alcohol may increase the sedative effects of this drug.
Surgery and general anaesthetics Clomipramine treatment may need to be stopped before you have a general anaesthetic. Discuss with your doctor or dentist before any operation.

PROLONGED USE

No problems expected.
Monitoring Regular checks on heart and liver function are recommended.

CLONAZEPAM

Brand names None
Used in the following combined preparations None

QUICK REFERENCE

Drug group Benzodiazepine anticonvulsant drug (p.14)
Overdose danger rating Medium
Dependence rating Medium
Prescription needed Yes
Available as generic Yes

GENERAL INFORMATION

Clonazepam belongs to the benzodiazepine group of drugs, which are mainly used in the treatment of anxiety and insomnia (see Anti-anxiety drugs, p.11). However, it is usually used as an anticonvulsant to prevent and treat epileptic seizures. It is particularly useful for preventing brief muscle spasms (myoclonus) and absence seizures (petit mal) in children, but other forms of epilepsy, such as sudden flaccidity or seizures induced by flashing lights, also respond to this treatment. Being a benzodiazepine, it also has sedative effects.

Clonazepam is used either alone or together with other anticonvulsant drugs. Its anticonvulsant effect may begin to wear off after some months, which often limits its long-term use.

INFORMATION FOR USERS

Your drug prescription is tailored for you. Do not alter dosage without checking with your doctor.
How taken/used Tablets, liquid.
Frequency and timing of doses 1–4 x daily.
Dosage range *Adults* 1mg daily at night (starting dose), increased gradually to 4–8mg daily (maintenance dose). *Children* Reduced dose according to age and weight.

Onset of effect 1–4 hours.
Duration of action 24–48 hours.
Diet advice None.
Storage Keep in original container at room temperature out of the reach of children.
Missed dose No cause for concern, but take as soon as you remember. Take next dose when due.
Stopping the drug Do not stop without consulting your doctor because symptoms may recur, and withdrawal symptoms may occur.
Exceeding the dose An occasional unintentional extra dose is unlikely to cause problems. Larger overdoses may cause excessive drowsiness and confusion. Notify your doctor.

POSSIBLE ADVERSE EFFECTS

The main adverse effects are related to the drug's sedative and tranquillizing action. They include daytime drowsiness, dizziness, unsteadiness, altered behaviour, and, less commonly, forgetfulness, confusion, and muscle weakness. Consult your doctor if drowsiness or dizziness are severe or for any of these other effects. Side effects normally lessen after the first few days of treatment and can often be reduced by medically supervised adjustment of the dose.

INTERACTIONS

Sedatives All drugs with a sedative effect on the central nervous system are likely to increase the sedative properties of clonazepam. Such drugs include anti-anxiety and sleeping drugs, antihistamines, opioid analgesics, antidepressants, and antipsychotics.
Other anticonvulsants Clonazepam may alter the effects of other anticonvulsants you are taking, or they may alter its effect. Adjustment of dosage or change of drug may be necessary.

SPECIAL PRECAUTIONS

Be sure to tell your doctor if:
- You have severe respiratory disease, including sleep apnoea.
- You have long-term liver or kidney problems.
- You have porphyria.
- You have myasthenia gravis.
- You have misused drugs or alcohol.
- You have mental health problems.
- You are taking other medicines.

Pregnancy May adversely affect baby if used in late pregnancy or labour. Discuss with doctor.
Breast-feeding Passes into breast milk and may adversely affect baby. Discuss with doctor.
Infants and children Reduced dose necessary.
Over 60 Reduced dose may be necessary.
Driving and hazardous work Your underlying condition, and the risk of drowsiness while taking clonazepam, may make such activities inadvisable. Discuss with your doctor.
Alcohol Avoid. Alcohol may increase the sedative effects of this drug.

PROLONGED USE

Both beneficial and adverse effects of clonazepam may become less marked during prolonged treatment as the body adapts to it. Prolonged use may also result in dependence and difficulty in withdrawing.

CLOPIDOGREL

Brand names Grepid, Plavix
Used in the following combined preparations None

QUICK REFERENCE

Drug group Antiplatelet drug (p.37)
Overdose danger rating Medium
Dependence rating Low
Prescription needed Yes
Available as generic Yes

GENERAL INFORMATION

Clopidogrel is an antiplatelet drug used to prevent blood clots from forming. It is prescribed to patients with a tendency to form clots in the fast-flowing blood of the arteries and heart, or those who have had a stroke or heart attack. It is also widely used to prevent clots forming in metal stents inserted into coronary arteries. It may be used alone or together with aspirin.

The drug reduces the tendency of platelets (clot-forming particles) to stick together, which can lead to abnormal bleeding. You should therefore report any unusual bleeding to your doctor at once, and, if you require dental treatment, tell your dentist that you are taking clopidogrel. Adverse effects are common and usually associated with bleeding.

INFORMATION FOR USERS

Your drug prescription is tailored for you. Do not alter dosage without checking with your doctor.
How taken/used Tablets.
Frequency and timing of doses Once daily.
Dosage range 75mg; up to 300mg as initial dose in hospital.

Onset of effect 1 hour.
Duration of action Antiplatelet effect may last up to 1 week.
Diet advice None.
Storage Keep in original container at room temperature out of the reach of children.
Missed dose Take as soon as you remember. If your next dose is due within 4 hours, take a single dose now and skip the next.
Stopping the drug Do not stop without consulting your doctor. Stopping the drug may lead to a recurrence of the original condition.
Exceeding the dose An occasional unintentional extra dose is unlikely to be a cause for concern. But if you notice any unusual symptoms, or if a large overdose has been taken, tell your doctor.

POSSIBLE ADVERSE EFFECTS

The most frequent adverse effects are bruising and bleeding, such as nosebleeds; diarrhoea; or abdominal pain. Rarer adverse effects include nausea, vomiting, headache, dizziness, and constipation; tell your doctor if these are severe. Report any unusual bleeding or bruising, blood in the urine or faeces, rash, itching, sore throat, or fever to your doctor at once.

INTERACTIONS

Aspirin and other non-steroidal anti-inflammatory drugs (NSAIDs) Clopidogrel increases the effect of aspirin on platelets. The risk of gastrointestinal bleeding is increased when clopidogrel is used with these drugs.
Anticoagulant drugs (e.g. warfarin) The risk of bleeding with these drugs is increased if they are taken with clopidogrel.
Proton pump inhibitors (especially omeprazole and esomeprazole) These may reduce the antiplatelet effect of clopidogrel and should be avoided.

SPECIAL PRECAUTIONS

Be sure to tell your doctor if:
- You have liver or kidney problems.
- You have a history of peptic ulcers.
- You have had a bleed into your gut or brain.
- You have a bleeding disorder.
- You are taking other medicines.

Pregnancy Safety in pregnancy not established. Discuss with your doctor.
Breast-feeding Drug passes into breast milk and may affect baby. Discuss with your doctor.
Infants and children Not recommended.
Over 60 No special problems.
Driving and hazardous work No special problems.
Alcohol Avoid. Stomach irritation from alcohol can increase the risk of bleeding.
Surgery and general anaesthetics Clopidogrel may need to be stopped a week before surgery. Discuss this with your doctor or dentist.

PROLONGED USE

Increased risk of bleeding from any trauma, even a minor head injury.

CLOTRIMAZOLE

Brand names Boots Thrush Cream, Canesten, Care Clotrimazole Cream
Used in the following combined preparations Canesten HC, Lotriderm

QUICK REFERENCE

Drug group Antifungal drug (p.74)
Overdose danger rating Low
Dependence rating Low
Prescription needed Yes (for combined preparations)
Available as generic Yes

GENERAL INFORMATION

Clotrimazole is an antifungal drug commonly used to treat fungal and yeast infections such as tinea (ringworm) infections of the skin, and candida (thrush) infections of the ear, mouth, vagina, or penis. It is applied as a cream, spray, topical solution, or dusting powder to the affected area and inserted as pessaries or cream for vaginal conditions such as candida.

Adverse effects are very rare, although some people may experience burning and irritation on the skin where the drug has been applied.

INFORMATION FOR USERS

Your drug prescription is tailored for you. Do not alter dosage without checking with your doctor.
How taken/used Pessaries, cream, topical solution, spray, dusting powder.
Frequency and timing of doses 2–3 x daily (skin cream, spray, solution); once daily at bedtime (pessaries, vaginal cream). Solutions for ear infections should be continued for at least 14 days after the infection has disappeared.
Dosage range *Vaginal infections* One applicatorful (5g) per dose (vaginal cream); 100–500mg per dose (pessaries). *Skin infections* (skin cream, spray, solution) as directed.
Onset of effect Within 2–3 days.

Duration of action Up to 12 hours.
Diet advice None.
Storage Keep in original container at room temperature out of the reach of children.
Missed dose No cause for concern, but make up the missed dose as soon as you remember.
Stopping the drug Apply the full course. Even if symptoms disappear, the original infection may still be present and symptoms may recur if treatment is stopped too soon.
Exceeding the dose An occasional unintentional extra dose is unlikely to cause problems. But if you notice unusual symptoms or if a large amount has been swallowed, tell your doctor.

POSSIBLE ADVERSE EFFECTS
The drug rarely causes adverse effects. Topical preparations may occasionally cause localized burning, stinging, or irritation. If you have a rash, stop using the drug and tell your doctor.

INTERACTIONS
Latex contraceptives The drug may damage the latex; additional precautions are needed during use of clotrimazole and for at least 5 days after the end of treatment.

SPECIAL PRECAUTIONS
Be sure to tell your doctor if:
- You are taking other medicines.

Pregnancy No evidence of risk to the fetus, but only use with the advice of your doctor.
Breast-feeding No evidence of risk.
Infants and children No special problems, but use of pessaries not recommended.
Over 60 No special problems.
Driving and hazardous work No known problems.
Alcohol No known problems.

PROLONGED USE
No problems expected.

CLOZAPINE

Brand names Clozaril, Denzapine, Zaponex
Used in the following combined preparations None

QUICK REFERENCE
Drug group Antipsychotic drug (p.13)
Overdose danger rating Medium
Dependence rating Low
Prescription needed Yes
Available as generic No

GENERAL INFORMATION
Clozapine is an atypical antipsychotic drug for schizophrenia and for psychosis in Parkinson's disease. It is given to patients who have not responded to other treatments or who have experienced intolerable side effects with other drugs. Clozapine helps to control severe resistant schizophrenia. The improvement is gradual, and relief of severe symptoms can take several weeks to months.

All treatment is supervised by a consultant psychiatrist. The patient and pharmacist must be registered with the drug manufacturer. Clozapine can cause a very serious side effect: agranulocytosis (a large decrease in white blood cells). Blood tests are done before and during treatment; the drug is supplied only if results are normal. The drug may also cause heart muscle problems; monitoring is necessary to avoid such problems.

INFORMATION FOR USERS
This drug is given only under strict medical supervision and continual monitoring.
How taken/used Tablets, liquid.
Frequency and timing of doses 1–2 x daily; a larger dose may be given at night.
Adult dosage range 12.5–900mg daily.
Onset of effect Gradual. Some effect may appear within 3–5 days, but the full beneficial effect may not be felt for some months.
Duration of action Up to 16 hours.
Diet advice None.
Storage Keep in original container at room temperature out of the reach of children.
Missed dose Take as soon as you remember. If next dose is due within 2 hours, take a single dose now and skip the next. If you miss more than 2 days of tablets, notify your doctor as you may need to re-start at a lower dose.
Stopping the drug Do not stop without consulting your doctor because symptoms may recur.
Exceeding the dose An occasional unintentional extra dose is unlikely to cause problems. Large overdoses may cause unusual drowsiness, seizures, and agitation. Notify your doctor.

POSSIBLE ADVERSE EFFECTS
Clozapine is less likely to cause parkinsonian side effects (tremor and stiffness) than other antipsychotics. The most serious side effect is a large decrease in white blood cells (agranulocytosis), and strict monitoring of the white

cell count is therefore necessary. Common adverse effects include drowsiness, tiredness, dry mouth or excessive salivation, and weight gain; tell your doctor if severe. Tell your doctor in any case of fast heartbeat, dizziness, fainting, constipation, or blurred vision. Rarely, clozapine may cause fever, sore throat, or seizures; if so, seek urgent medical advice.

INTERACTIONS

General note A number of drugs increase the risk of adverse effects on the blood. Do not take other medication without checking with your doctor or pharmacist. Smoking lowers clozapine levels, which may reduce its effect

Sedatives Drugs with a sedative effect on the central nervous system are likely to increase the sedative properties of clozapine.

Anticholinergic drugs There is a risk of severe constipation or even bowel obstruction when these drugs are used with clozapine.

SPECIAL PRECAUTIONS

Be sure to tell your doctor if:

- You have long-term liver or kidney problems.
- You have a history of blood disorders.
- You have had epileptic seizures.
- You have heart problems.
- You have colon problems or have had bowel surgery.
- You have diabetes.
- You have glaucoma.
- You have prostate problems.
- You are taking other medicines.

Pregnancy Not usually prescribed. Safety not established. Discuss with your doctor.

Breast-feeding The drug passes into the breast milk and may affect the baby adversely. Discuss with your doctor.

Infants and children Not prescribed.

Over 60 Adverse effects are more likely. Initial dose is low and is slowly increased.

Driving and hazardous work Avoid such activities until you know how clozapine affects you because the drug can cause blurred vision, drowsiness, and dizziness.

Alcohol Avoid. Alcohol may increase the sedative effects of this drug.

PROLONGED USE

Agranulocytosis and heart muscle problems may occur. Occasionally liver function may be upset. Significant weight gain may also occur.

Monitoring Blood tests are carried out weekly for 18 weeks, fortnightly until the end of the first year, and, if blood counts are stable, every 4 weeks thereafter. Liver function tests, weighing, and tests for diabetes are performed every 3–6 months. Heart function is also monitored.

CODEINE

Used in the following combined preparations Aspirin with codeine, Co-codamol, Codafen Continus, Cuprofen Plus, Galcodine, Migraleve, Nurofen Plus, Panadol Ultra, Paracodol, Pulmo Bailly, Solpadeine, Solpadol, Syndol, Veganin, and others

QUICK REFERENCE

Drug group Opioid analgesic (p.8), antidiarrhoeal drug (p.42), and cough suppressant (p.25)

Overdose danger rating High

Dependence rating High

Prescription needed Yes (some preparations)

Available as generic Yes

GENERAL INFORMATION

Codeine is a mild opioid analgesic similar to, but weaker than, morphine. It has been in common medical use since the early 19th century, although raw opium, of which codeine is a constituent, has been used for much longer.

Codeine is prescribed mainly to relieve mild to moderate pain, and is often combined with a non-opioid analgesic such as paracetamol. It is also an effective cough suppressant, so it is included in many non-prescription cough syrups and cold relief preparations.

Like other opioid drugs, codeine is constipating; this characteristic sometimes makes it useful in the short-term control of diarrhoea.

Although codeine is habit-forming, addiction seldom occurs if it is used for a limited time and the recommended dosage is followed.

INFORMATION FOR USERS

Your drug prescription is tailored for you. Do not alter dosage without checking with your doctor.

How taken/used Tablets, liquid, injection.

Frequency and timing of doses 4–6 x daily (pain); 3–4 x daily when necessary (cough); every 6–8 hours when necessary (diarrhoea).

Adult dosage range 120–240mg daily (pain); 45–120mg daily (cough); 30–120mg daily (diarrhoea).

Onset of effect 30–60 minutes.

Duration of action 4–6 hours.
Diet advice None.
Storage Keep in original container at room temperature out of the reach of children. Protect from light.
Missed dose Take as soon as you remember if needed for relief of symptoms. If not needed, do not take the missed dose, and return to your normal dose schedule when necessary.
Stopping the drug Can be safely stopped as soon as you no longer need it.

OVERDOSE ACTION
Seek immediate medical advice in all cases. Take emergency action if there are symptoms such as slow or irregular breathing, severe drowsiness, or loss of consciousness.

POSSIBLE ADVERSE EFFECTS
Serious adverse effects are rare with codeine. Constipation is common, especially with prolonged use, but other common effects (such as nausea, vomiting, drowsiness, and dizziness) are not usually troublesome at the recommended dose and usually disappear if the dose is reduced; discuss with your doctor if severe. If you have restlessness or agitation, stop taking the drug and tell your doctor. If you develop a rash, hives, wheezing, or breathlessness, stop the drug and seek urgent medical advice.

INTERACTIONS
Sedatives All drugs that have a sedative effect on the central nervous system are likely to increase sedation with codeine. Such drugs include sleeping drugs, antidepressant drugs, antihistamines, antipsychotics, and alcohol.

SPECIAL PRECAUTIONS
Be sure to consult your doctor or pharmacist before taking this drug if:
- You have long-term liver, kidney, or bowel problems.
- You have a lung disorder such as asthma or bronchitis.
- You are taking other medicines.

Pregnancy No evidence of risk, but regular use may cause withdrawal symptoms in the baby and if used during delivery can reduce the baby's breathing.
Breast-feeding Should not be used as it passes into the breast milk and may harm the baby.
Infants and children Not for use in children under 12 years, nor for children under 18 years having tonsillectomy or adenoidectomy for obstructive sleep apnoea. Not advised for any child with respiratory problems.
Over 60 Reduced dose may be necessary.
Driving and hazardous work Avoid until you have learned how codeine affects you because the drug may cause dizziness and drowsiness.
Alcohol Avoid. Alcohol may increase the sedative effects of this drug.

PROLONGED USE
Codeine is normally used only for short-term relief of symptoms. It can be habit-forming if taken for extended periods, especially if higher-than-average doses are taken.

COLCHICINE

Brand name None
Used in the following combined preparations None

QUICK REFERENCE
Drug group Drug for gout (p.51)
Overdose danger rating High
Dependence rating Low
Prescription needed Yes
Available as generic Yes

GENERAL INFORMATION
Colchicine, a drug originally extracted from the autumn crocus flower and later synthesized, has been used since the 18th century for gout. It has now, to an extent, been superseded by newer drugs but is still often used to relieve joint pain and inflammation in flare-ups. It is most effective when taken at the first sign of symptoms, and almost always produces an improvement. Its use is limited by side effects such as nausea, vomiting, and diarrhoea at high doses. It may also be given at a lower dose in the first few months of treatment with allopurinol or probenecid (other drugs for gout), as these may at first increase the frequency of gout attacks. Colchicine is occasionally prescribed to relieve symptoms of familial Mediterranean fever (a rare congenital condition).

INFORMATION FOR USERS
Your drug prescription is tailored for you. Do not alter dosage without checking with your doctor.
How taken/used Tablets.

Frequency and timing of doses *Prevention of gout attacks* Twice daily. *Relief of gout attacks* Every 4 hours.
Adult dosage range *Prevention of gout attacks* 0.5mg 2 x daily. *Relief of gout attacks* 0.5mg 2–4 x daily, until relief of pain, vomiting, or diarrhoea occurs, or until a total dose of 6mg is reached. This course must not be repeated within 3 days.
Onset of effect Relief of symptoms in an attack of gout may be felt in 6–24 hours. Full effect in gout prevention may take several days.
Duration of action Up to 2 hours. Some effects may last longer.
Diet advice Certain foods are known to make gout worse. Discuss with your doctor.
Storage Keep in original container at room temperature out of the reach of children. Protect from light.
Missed dose Take as soon as you remember. If your next dose is due within 30 minutes, take a single dose now and skip the next.
Stopping the drug When taking colchicine frequently during an acute attack of gout, stop if diarrhoea or abdominal pain develop. In other cases, do not stop without consulting your doctor.

OVERDOSE ACTION

Seek immediate medical advice in all cases. Some reactions can be fatal. Take emergency action if severe nausea, vomiting, bloody diarrhoea, severe abdominal pain, or loss of consciousness occur.

POSSIBLE ADVERSE EFFECTS

The appearance of any symptom that may be an adverse effect of colchicine is a sign that you should stop taking it until you have received medical advice. The more common adverse effects are nausea, vomiting, diarrhoea, and abdominal pain. More rarely, colchicine may cause numbness and tingling, unusual bleeding or bruising, and a rash.

INTERACTIONS

Ciclosporin, clarithromycin, erythromycin, itraconazole, ketoconazole, and verapamil These drugs may significantly increase the adverse effects of colchicine.
Statins Taking statins with colchicine may increase the risk of adverse effects involving the muscles.
Protease inhibitors may increase the risk of colchicine toxicity.

SPECIAL PRECAUTIONS

Be sure to tell your doctor if:
- You have long-term liver or kidney problems.
- You have heart problems.
- You have a blood disorder.
- You have stomach ulcers.
- You have chronic inflammation of the bowel.
- You are taking other medicines.

Pregnancy Not recommended. May cause defects in the fetus. Discuss with your doctor.
Breast-feeding The drug passes into the breast milk and may affect the baby. Discuss with your doctor.
Infants and children Not recommended.
Over 60 Increased likelihood of adverse effects.
Driving and hazardous work No special problems.
Alcohol Avoid. Alcohol may increase stomach irritation caused by colchicine.

PROLONGED USE

Prolonged use may lead to hair loss, rashes, tingling in the hands and feet, muscle pain and weakness, and blood disorders.
Monitoring Periodic blood checks are usually required.

COLESTYRAMINE

Brand names Questran, Questran Light
Used in the following combined preparations None

QUICK REFERENCE

Drug group Lipid-lowering drug (p.35)
Overdose danger rating Low
Dependence rating Low
Prescription needed Yes
Available as generic Yes

GENERAL INFORMATION

Colestyramine is a resin that binds bile acids in the intestine, preventing their reabsorption. Cholesterol in the body is normally converted to bile acids; therefore, colestyramine reduces cholesterol levels in the blood. The drug's action on the bile acids also adds bulk to faeces, giving an antidiarrhoeal effect (hence its use in diarrhoea associated with, for example, Crohn's disease, gallbladder removal, removal of part of the intestine, or radiotherapy). The drug is used to treat hyperlipidaemia (high levels of fat in the blood) in people who have not responded to dietary changes. In liver disorders such as primary biliary cirrhosis, bile salts sometimes accumulate in the bloodstream, and colestyramine may be prescribed to alleviate any accompanying itching.

Taken in large doses, colestyramine often causes bloating, mild nausea, and constipation. It may also impair the body's ability to absorb fat and certain fat-soluble vitamins, causing pale, bulky, foul-smelling faeces.

INFORMATION FOR USERS

Your drug prescription is tailored for you. Do not alter dosage without checking with your doctor.
How taken/used Powder mixed with water, juice, or soft food.
Frequency and timing of doses 1–6 x daily before meals and at bedtime.
Adult dosage range 4–36g daily.
Onset of effect May take several weeks to achieve full beneficial effects.
Duration of action 12–24 hours.
Diet advice A low-fat, low-calorie diet may be advised for patients who are overweight. Use of this drug may deplete levels of certain vitamins. Supplements may be advised.
Storage Keep in original container at room temperature out of the reach of children.
Missed dose Take as soon as you remember.
Stopping the drug Do not stop taking the drug without consulting your doctor.
Exceeding the dose An occasional unintentional extra dose is unlikely to cause problems. But if you notice any unusual symptoms, or if a large overdose has been taken, notify your doctor.

POSSIBLE ADVERSE EFFECTS

Adverse effects are more likely in people over 60 who take large doses. Minor effects, such as indigestion, abdominal discomfort, constipation, nausea, and vomiting, are rarely a cause for concern; notify your doctor only if they are severe. High doses may cause diarrhoea; other serious adverse effects, such as bruising or increased bleeding, are usually due to vitamin deficiency. If these occur, consult your doctor.

INTERACTIONS

General note Colestyramine reduces the body's ability to absorb other drugs. If you are taking other medicines, tell your doctor or pharmacist so that they can discuss with you the best way to take all your drugs. To avoid any problems, take other drugs at least 1 hour before, or 4–6 hours after, colestyramine. The dosage of other drugs may need to be adjusted.

SPECIAL PRECAUTIONS

Be sure to tell your doctor if:
- You have jaundice.
- You have a peptic ulcer.
- You have diabetes.
- You have haemorrhoids.
- You are taking other medicines.

Pregnancy Safety in pregnancy not established. Discuss with your doctor.
Breast-feeding Safety not established. The drug binds fat-soluble vitamins long term and may cause vitamin deficiency in the baby. Discuss with your doctor.
Infants and children Not recommended under 6 years. Reduced dose needed in older children.
Over 60 Increased likelihood of adverse effects.
Driving and hazardous work No special problems.
Alcohol Although this drug does not interact with alcohol, your underlying condition may make it inadvisable to take alcohol.

PROLONGED USE

As this drug reduces vitamin absorption, supplements of vitamins A, D, and K and folic acid may be advised.
Monitoring Periodic blood checks are usually required to monitor the level of cholesterol in the blood.

CONJUGATED OESTROGENS

Brand name Premarin
Used in the following combined preparations Duavive, Premique

QUICK REFERENCE

Drug group Female sex hormone (p.86) and drug for bone disorders (p.54)
Overdose danger rating Low
Dependence rating Low
Prescription needed Yes
Available as generic Yes

GENERAL INFORMATION

Conjugated oestrogens are preparations of naturally occurring oestrogens. Taken by mouth, they are used to relieve menopausal symptoms such as hot flushes and sweating, but are usually only advised for short-term use around the menopause and are not normally recommended for long-term use or for the treatment of osteoporosis.

As replacement therapy, the drugs are usually taken on a cyclic dosing schedule, in conjunction with a progestogen, to simulate the hormonal changes of a normal menstrual cycle. On their own, they are not recommended for women with an intact uterus.

Conjugated oestrogens do not provide contraception. Pregnancy is still possible for 2 years after a woman's last period (if she is under 50 years) or 1 year after the end of menstruation (if she is over 50).

INFORMATION FOR USERS

Your drug prescription is tailored for you. Do not alter dosage without checking with your doctor.

How taken/used Tablets.

Frequency and timing of doses Once daily.

Adult dosage range *Replacement therapy* 0.625–1.25mg daily. *Osteoporosis prevention* 0.625–1.25mg daily.

Onset of effect 5–20 days.

Duration of action 1–2 days.

Diet advice None.

Storage Keep in original container at room temperature out of the reach of children.

Missed dose Take as soon as you remember.

Stopping the drug Do not stop the drug without consulting your doctor; symptoms may recur.

Exceeding the dose An occasional unintentional extra dose is unlikely to be a cause for concern. But if you notice any unusual symptoms, or if a large overdose has been taken, notify your doctor.

POSSIBLE ADVERSE EFFECTS

The most common adverse effects are similar to symptoms of early pregnancy, such as nausea, vomiting, breast swelling or tenderness, weight changes, and abdominal bloating or pain. These generally diminish or disappear after 2–3 months of treatment. Women on a cyclic schedule will have a menstrual bleed each month. The drugs may also reduce sex drive. If headaches, migraines, depression, or unusual vaginal bleeding occur, tell your doctor. If you develop jaundice, stop taking the drug and contact your doctor promptly. Sudden sharp pain in the chest, groin, or legs may indicate a blood clot that requires urgent medical attention; call your doctor immediately.

INTERACTIONS

General note A number of medications can alter oestrogen levels, including some antibiotics, anticonvulsants, antifungals, anti-HIV drugs, and St John's wort. Check with your doctor or pharmacist before taking any other medicines.

Tobacco smoking increases the risk of serious adverse effects on the heart and circulation with conjugated oestrogens.

Oral anticoagulants Their anticoagulant effect is reduced by conjugated oestrogens.

SPECIAL PRECAUTIONS

Be sure to tell your doctor if:

- ◆ You have heart disease, high blood pressure, or thrombophilia (abnormal clotting) or have had blood clots or a stroke.
- ◆ You have porphyria or diabetes.
- ◆ You have a history of breast disease or breast cancer.
- ◆ You have had uterine fibroids, abnormal vaginal bleeding, or endometrial cancer.
- ◆ You have migraine or epilepsy.
- ◆ You have long-term liver or kidney problems.
- ◆ You are taking other medicines.

Pregnancy Not prescribed. May affect the baby adversely. Discuss with your doctor.

Breast-feeding Not prescribed. The drug passes into the breast milk and may inhibit its flow. Discuss with your doctor.

Infants and children Not prescribed.

Over 60 No special problems.

Driving and hazardous work No known problems.

Alcohol No known problems.

Surgery and general anaesthetics Conjugated oestrogens may need to be stopped several weeks before surgery. Discuss with your doctor.

PROLONGED USE

Conjugated oestrogens are normally only advised for use around the menopause. Long-term use may increase the risk of breast, endometrial, or ovarian cancer, venous thrombosis, heart attack, and stroke.

Monitoring Regular physical examinations (e.g. mammograms) and blood pressure checks are advised.

CO-PHENOTROPE

Brand name Lomotil
Used in the following combined preparations None

QUICK REFERENCE

Drug group Opioid antidiarrhoeal (p.42)
Overdose danger rating Medium
Dependence rating Medium
Prescription needed Yes
Available as generic Yes

GENERAL INFORMATION

Co-phenotrope is an antidiarrhoeal drug containing diphenoxylate and atropine. It reduces bowel contractions and the fluidity and frequency of bowel movements. It is used to relieve sudden or recurrent bouts of diarrhoea. It may also be used to control the consistency of faeces after colostomy or ileostomy.

Co-phenotrope is not suitable for treating diarrhoea caused by infections, poisons, or antibiotics as it may delay recovery by slowing expulsion of harmful substances from the bowel. The drug can cause toxic megacolon, which is a dangerous dilation of the bowel that shuts off the blood supply to the wall of the bowel and increases the risk of perforation.

At recommended doses, serious adverse effects are rare. However, if taken in excessive amounts, the atropine will cause highly unpleasant anticholinergic effects (p.7). This drug is especially dangerous for young children and should be stored out of their reach.

INFORMATION FOR USERS

Your drug prescription is tailored for you. Do not alter dosage without checking with your doctor.

How taken/used Tablets.

Frequency and timing of doses 3–4 x daily.

Dosage range *Adults* 4 tablets (equivalent to 10mg diphenoxylate) initially, then 2 tablets (5mg) every 6 hours until diarrhoea controlled. *Children* Reduced dose necessary according to age (not recommended under 4 years).

Onset of effect Within 1 hour. Control of diarrhoea may take some hours.

Duration of action 3–4 hours (single dose).

Diet advice Always drink plenty of water during an attack of diarrhoea.

Storage Keep in original container at room temperature out of the reach of children. Protect from light.

Missed dose Take as soon as you remember. If your next dose is due within 3 hours, take a single dose now and skip the next.

Stopping the drug Can be safely stopped as soon as you no longer need it.

Exceeding the dose An occasional unintentional extra dose is unlikely to cause problems. Large overdoses may cause unusual drowsiness, dry mouth and skin, restlessness, and in extreme cases, loss of consciousness. Symptoms of overdose may be delayed. Notify your doctor urgently if you have taken a large overdose.

POSSIBLE ADVERSE EFFECTS

Drowsiness is the most common adverse effect of co-phenotrope. Other adverse effects, such as restlessness, headache, rash, and itching, are infrequent; call your doctor only if these are severe. If dizziness occurs or it becomes difficult to pass urine, stop taking the drug and consult your doctor. If nausea, vomiting, or abdominal pain or distension occur, stop the drug and call your doctor promptly.

INTERACTIONS

Sedatives All drugs that have a sedative effect on the central nervous system may increase co-phenotrope's sedative effect. They include anti-anxiety and sleeping drugs, antihistamines, opioid analgesics, antidepressants, and antipsychotics.

Monoamine oxidase inhibitors (MAOIs) There is a risk of a dangerous rise in blood pressure if MAOIs are taken with co-phenotrope.

SPECIAL PRECAUTIONS

Be sure to tell your doctor if:

- You have long-term liver or kidney problems.
- You have severe abdominal pain.
- You have bloodstained diarrhoea.
- You have recently taken antibiotics.
- You have ulcerative colitis.
- You have prostate problems.
- You have recently travelled abroad.
- You are taking other medicines.

Pregnancy Safety in pregnancy not established. Discuss with your doctor.

Breast-feeding The drug passes into the breast milk and may cause drowsiness in the baby. Discuss with your doctor.

Infants and children Not recommended under 4 years. Reduced dose needed for older children.

Over 60 Reduced dose may be necessary.

Driving and hazardous work Avoid such activities until you have learned how co-phenotrope affects you because the drug may cause drowsiness and dizziness.
Alcohol Avoid. Alcohol may increase the sedative effects of this drug.

PROLONGED USE
Not usually recommended.

CO-TRIMOXAZOLE

Brand name None
Used in the following combined preparation
(Co-trimoxazole is a combination of two drugs)

QUICK REFERENCE
Drug group Antibacterial drug (p.64)
Overdose danger rating Medium
Dependence rating Low
Prescription needed Yes
Available as generic Yes

GENERAL INFORMATION
Co-trimoxazole is a mixture of two antibacterial drugs: trimethoprim and sulfamethoxazole. It is prescribed for serious respiratory and urinary tract infections only when they cannot be treated with other drugs. Co-trimoxazole is also used to treat pneumocystis pneumonia, toxoplasmosis, and the bacterial infection nocardiasis. The drug may also be used for otitis media in children if no safer drug is suitable. Although co-trimoxazole was widely prescribed in the past, its use has greatly declined in recent years with the introduction of new, more effective, and safer drugs.

The drug may cause rare but serious adverse effects including skin rashes, blood disorders, and liver or kidney damage.

INFORMATION FOR USERS
Your drug prescription is tailored for you. Do not alter dosage without checking with your doctor.
How taken/used Tablets, liquid, injection.
Frequency and timing of doses Normally 2 x daily, preferably with food.
Adult dosage range Usually 4 tablets daily (each standard tablet is 480mg). Higher doses may be used for the treatment of pneumocystis pneumonia, toxoplasmosis, and nocardiasis.
Onset of effect 1–4 hours.
Duration of action 24 hours.
Diet advice Drink plenty of fluids, particularly in warm weather.
Storage Keep in original container at room temperature out of the reach of children. Protect from light.
Missed dose Take as soon as you remember. If your normal dose is 480mg, double this; if it is more than 480mg, take one dose only.
Stopping the drug Take the full course. Even if you feel better, the original infection may still be present and symptoms may recur if treatment is stopped too soon.
Exceeding the dose An occasional unintentional extra dose is unlikely to be a cause for concern. Large overdoses may cause nausea, vomiting, dizziness, and confusion. Notify your doctor.

POSSIBLE ADVERSE EFFECTS
The most common adverse effects are nausea, rash, and itching. If either of the last two occur, you should stop taking the drug and consult your doctor without delay. Diarrhoea and headache are also relatively common; consult your doctor if they are severe. More rarely, mouth ulcers, sore tongue, or jaundice may occur; in these cases, stop taking the drug and consult your doctor promptly.

INTERACTIONS
Warfarin Co-trimoxazole may increase the anticoagulant effect of warfarin; the warfarin dose may have to be reduced. Blood-clotting status may have to be checked.
Ciclosporin Taking ciclosporin together with co-trimoxazole can impair kidney function.
Phenytoin Co-trimoxazole may cause a build-up of phenytoin in the body; the dose of phenytoin may have to be reduced.
Amiodarone Co-trimoxazole may increase the risk of irregular heart beats when given with amiodarone.
Methotrexate Co-trimoxazole may increase the blood level of methotrexate, and regular blood tests may be necessary.

SPECIAL PRECAUTIONS
Be sure to tell your doctor if:
- You have long-term liver or kidney problems.
- You have a blood disorder.
- You have asthma.
- You have glucose-6-phosphate dehydrogenase (G6PD) deficiency.
- You are allergic to sulfonamide drugs.

◆ You have porphyria.
◆ You are taking other medicines.

Pregnancy Not prescribed. May cause defects in the baby.

Breast-feeding The drug passes into the breast milk, but normal levels are unlikely to affect the baby adversely. Discuss with your doctor.

Infants and children Not recommended for infants under 6 weeks old. Reduced dose necessary in older children.

Over 60 Side effects are more likely. Used only when necessary.

Driving and hazardous work No known problems.

Alcohol No known problems.

PROLONGED USE

Long-term use of this drug may lead to folic acid deficiency, which can cause anaemia. Folic acid supplements may be needed.

Monitoring Regular blood tests are recommended.

CYCLOPHOSPHAMIDE

Brand name None
Used in the following combined preparations None

QUICK REFERENCE

Drug group Anticancer drug (p.94)
Overdose danger rating Medium
Dependence rating Low
Prescription needed Yes
Available as generic Yes

GENERAL INFORMATION

Cyclophosphamide belongs to a group of anticancer drugs known as alkylating agents. It is used in treating a wide range of cancers, including lymphomas (lymph gland cancers), leukaemias, and solid tumours. It is commonly given together with radiotherapy or other drugs. Cyclophosphamide has also been used for autoimmune diseases, such as rheumatoid arthritis and systemic lupus erythematosus when it involves the kidneys.

The drug causes nausea, vomiting, and hair loss, and can affect the heart, lungs, and liver. It can cause bladder damage in susceptible people because it produces a toxic substance called acrolein. To reduce toxicity, people considered to be at risk may be given a drug called mesna before and after each dose of cyclophosphamide. In addition, because the drug often reduces production of blood cells, it may lead to abnormal bleeding and increased risk of infection. It may also reduce fertility in both men and women; approaches to preserve sperm are likely to be offered with treatment.

INFORMATION FOR USERS

Your drug prescription is tailored for you. Do not alter dosage without checking with your doctor.

How taken/used Tablets, injection.

Frequency and timing of doses Varies from once daily to every 3 weeks, depending on the condition being treated.

Dosage range Dosage is determined individually according to the nature of the condition, body weight, and response.

Onset of effect Some effects may appear within hours of starting treatment. Full beneficial effects may not be felt for many weeks.

Duration of action Several weeks.

Diet advice High fluid intake with frequent bladder emptying is recommended. This will usually prevent the drug irritating the bladder.

Storage Keep in original container at room temperature out of the reach of children. Protect from light.

Missed dose Injections are given only in hospital. If you are taking tablets, take the missed dose as soon as you remember. If your next dose is due within 6 hours, take a single dose now and skip the next. Tell your doctor that you missed a dose.

Stopping the drug The drug will be stopped under medical supervision (injection). Do not stop taking the drug without consulting your doctor (tablets); stopping the drug may lead to worsening of the underlying condition.

Exceeding the dose An occasional unintentional extra dose is unlikely to cause problems. Large overdoses may cause nausea, vomiting, and bladder damage. Notify your doctor.

POSSIBLE ADVERSE EFFECTS

Cyclophosphamide often causes nausea and vomiting, which usually lessen as your body adjusts to the drug; hair loss is also common. Discuss with your doctor if severe. Women often have irregular menstrual periods; if affected, discuss with your doctor. More rarely, fever, breathlessness, and mouth ulcers may occur; if so, you should discuss with your doctor. Blood in the urine may be a sign of bladder damage and needs prompt medical attention. Those thought to be at risk of bladder damage may be given mesna before and after doses of cyclophosphamide.

INTERACTIONS

General note A number of drugs reduce the effects of cyclophosphamide and increase the risk of side effects. They include allopurinol, chloramphenicol, chloroquine, imipramine, and phenothiazines (e.g. chlorpromazine).

SPECIAL PRECAUTIONS

Cyclophosphamide is given only under close medical supervision, taking account of your present condition and medical history. However, be sure to tell your doctor if:

- You have liver or kidney problems.
- You have porphyria.
- You plan to have children in the future.

Pregnancy Not usually prescribed. Cyclophosphamide may cause birth defects. Pregnancy should be avoided during, and for 3 months after, treatment. Discuss with your doctor.
Breast-feeding Not advised. The drug passes into the breast milk and may affect the baby adversely. Discuss with your doctor.
Infants and children Reduced dose necessary.
Over 60 No special problems.
Driving and hazardous work No known problems.
Alcohol Cyclophosphamide may increase nausea and vomiting.

PROLONGED USE

Prolonged use of this drug may reduce the production of blood cells in the bone marrow. It may also cause pigmentation of the nails, palms, and soles of the feet.
Monitoring Periodic checks on blood composition and blood chemistry are usually required.

CYPROTERONE

Brand names Androcur, Cyprostat
Used in the following combined preparations Co-Cyprindiol (Dianette)

QUICK REFERENCE

Drug group Male sex hormone (p.85)
Overdose danger rating Low
Dependence rating Low
Prescription needed Yes
Available as generic Yes

GENERAL INFORMATION

Cyproterone reduces the action and production of androgens (male sex hormones) in the body. It is used in males to treat conditions that are due to the action of androgens, such as prostate cancer, hypersexuality, sexual deviation, and precocious puberty in boys. It is used in women to treat certain conditions due to abnormally high androgen levels, such as hirsutism, male-pattern baldness, and severe acne. For women taking cyproterone combined with an oestrogen for acne or hirsutism, the drug also provides contraception.

Cyproterone alone is also used to facilitate hormonal male-to-female gender reassignment. Common side effects in men include reduced libido, erectile dysfunction (impotence), and infertility, which is usually reversible. Occasionally, the drug may disrupt liver function, and it significantly increases the risk of thrombosis.

INFORMATION FOR USERS

Your drug prescription is tailored for you. Do not alter dosage without checking with your doctor.
How taken/used Tablets.
Frequency and timing of doses 1–3 x daily, with liquid after meals. *Oral contraceptives* Once daily on certain days of the menstrual cycle.
Adult dosage range 50–300mg daily, usually in divided doses. *Oral contraceptives* 2mg daily.
Onset of effect Up to a week; longer for acne, possibly several months.
Duration of action Several days.
Diet advice None.
Storage Keep at room temperature, away from heat, moisture, and direct light and out of the reach of children.
Missed dose Take as soon as you remember and take the next dose when it is due.
Stopping the drug Do not stop taking the drug without consulting your doctor; stopping may lead to recurrence or worsening of your symptoms. If you have diabetes, stopping may upset control of your blood sugar levels.

POSSIBLE ADVERSE EFFECTS

Cyproterone may cause a wide range of adverse effects, although serious ones are rare. In men, common adverse effects include decreased libido, erectile dysfunction (impotence), and infertility. In both sexes, the drug may cause fluid retention, weight changes, restlessness, low mood, breast swelling or tenderness, hot flushes, sweating, dry skin and hair loss; consult your doctor if severe. If you develop persistent abdominal pain, abnormal itching, jaundice, breathlessness, chest pain, or swollen or painful calves, stop taking the drug and contact your doctor immediately.

INTERACTIONS

Thiazolidinedione antidiabetic drugs (e.g. pioglitazone) The dose may need to be reduced when taken with cyproterone.
Rifampicin, phenytoin, and St John's wort may reduce the level of cyproterone.
Ketoconazole, itraconazole, and clotrimazole may increase the level of cyproterone.
Statins may increase the risk of muscle side effects when taken with cyproterone.

SPECIAL PRECAUTIONS

Be sure to tell your doctor if:
◆ You have liver problems.
◆ You have diabetes.
◆ You have sickle cell anaemia.
◆ You have a history of depression.
◆ You have a family history of venous thrombosis or have had blood clots, stroke, or a heart attack.
◆ You have or have had a meningioma.
◆ You are taking other medicines.

Pregnancy Not prescribed. Cyproterone can feminize a male fetus.
Breast-feeding Not prescribed.
Infants and children Reduced dose necessary.
Over 60 No special problems.
Driving and hazardous work Avoid such activities until you have learned how cyproterone affects you because the drug may cause tiredness and weakness.
Alcohol Avoid. Alcohol can reduce the effect of cyproterone.

PROLONGED USE

Long-term use of high doses of cyproterone has been associated with certain tumours and alteration of liver and adrenal gland function. The development of meningiomas (a type of brain tumour), abnormal liver function, suppression of adrenal gland function, and very rarely, liver tumours have been reported with prolonged use of cyproterone at high doses. Meningiomas are not a risk with co-cyprindiol (Dianette).

Monitoring Your blood count and liver function will be checked regularly, and your adrenal function may be monitored. If you have diabetes, blood sugar control will be monitored. Men may have their sperm count checked.

DABIGATRAN

Brand name Pradaxa
Used in the following combined preparations None

QUICK REFERENCE

Drug group Anticoagulant drug (p.37)
Overdose danger rating High
Dependence rating Low
Prescription needed Yes
Available as generic No

GENERAL INFORMATION

Dabigatran is an oral anticoagulant drug with a rapid onset of action. It is used to treat or prevent deep-vein thrombosis (blood clots that form in veins, such as the leg veins) and pulmonary embolism (blockage of blood vessels in the lungs by clots from elsewhere in the body). It is also used to prevent strokes and blood clots in the arteries in patients with the heart rhythm problem atrial fibrillation.

The most serious side effect is an increased risk of bleeding. The drug should not be used in people with damaged or artificial heart valves, for whom warfarin is usually more suitable. In emergencies Praxbind (idarucizumab) may be used to reverse the effects of dabigatran.

INFORMATION FOR USERS

Your drug prescription is tailored for you. Do not alter dosage without checking with your doctor.
How taken/used Capsules.
Frequency and timing of doses 1–2 x daily.
Dosage range 75–300mg daily.
Onset of effect 1 hour.
Duration of action 12–24 hours.
Diet advice None.
Storage Keep in original container at room temperature out of the reach of children.
Missed dose Take as soon as you remember. If next dose is due within 6 hours, take a single dose now and skip the next dose. Do not take a double dose to make up for missed doses.
Stopping the drug Do not stop taking the drug without consulting your doctor; stopping may lead to worsening of the underlying condition.

OVERDOSE ACTION
Seek immediate medical advice in all cases. Take emergency action if bleeding, severe headache, or loss of consciousness occur.

POSSIBLE ADVERSE EFFECTS
Bleeding is the most common adverse effect of dabigatran. If you notice excessive bruising or bleeding from a minor wound, vomit blood, or pass bloody or black stools, consult your doctor immediately. You should also call your doctor at once if you develop jaundice. Other adverse effects include abdominal pain, diarrhoea, nausea, vomiting, rash, and itching. If these occur, notify your doctor.

INTERACTIONS
Other anticoagulants, antiplatelet drugs, non-steroidal anti-inflammatory drugs, and SSRI antidepressants There is an increased risk of bleeding if these are used with dabigatran.
Anticonvulsant drugs, rifampicin, and St John's wort may lower the blood concentration of dabigatran and reduce its effectiveness.
Antibacterial drugs, antifungal drugs, amiodarone, verapamil, ciclosporin, and tacrolimus may increase the blood concentration of dabigatran and increase the risk of bleeding.
Itraconazole, dronedarone, and the fixed-dose combination glecaprevir/pibrentasvir significantly increase the risk of bleeding.

SPECIAL PRECAUTIONS
Be sure to tell your doctor if:
- You have had a stroke or a brain haemorrhage.
- You have liver or kidney problems.
- You have high blood pressure.
- You have a bleeding disorder.
- You have peptic ulcers.
- You have had recent surgery.
- You have had a metal heart valve fitted.
- You are taking other medicines.

Pregnancy Safety not established. Discuss with your doctor.
Breast-feeding Safety not established. Discuss with your doctor.
Infants and children Safety not established. Discuss with your doctor.
Over 60 Reduced dose recommended if over 75.
Driving and hazardous work Use caution. Even minor injuries may cause severe bruising and excessive bleeding.
Alcohol Avoid excessive intake.
Surgery and general anaesthetics Dabigatran may need to be stopped before surgery. Discuss with your doctor or dentist.

PROLONGED USE
No special problems known, but the need for continued treatment should be reviewed.
Monitoring Kidney function should be monitored at least annually.

DAPAGLIFLOZIN

Brand name Forxiga
Used in the following combined preparations Qtern (with saxagliptin), Xigduo (with metformin)

QUICK REFERENCE
Drug group Drug for diabetes (p.80)
Overdose danger rating Low
Dependence rating Low
Prescription needed Yes
Available as generic No

GENERAL INFORMATION
Dapagliflozin is an oral antidiabetic drug used to treat type 2 diabetes in adults if the diabetes cannot be controlled with other medicines, diet, and exercise. It reduces blood glucose levels by increasing the amount of glucose removed from the blood by the kidneys and excreted in the urine. It can be used alone or in combination with other glucose-lowering medications, including insulin. Common side effects of dapagliflozin include urinary and genital yeast infections, dehydration, low blood pressure, and, if taken with certain other diabetes medications, low blood sugar.

INFORMATION FOR USERS
Your drug prescription is tailored for you. Do not alter dosage without checking with your doctor.
How taken/used Tablets.
Frequency and timing of doses Once daily with half a glass of water; can be taken with or without food.
Dosage range 5 or 10mg daily.
Onset of effect Within hours, but may take a week to develop full effect.
Duration of action 24 hours.
Diet advice Your doctor will advise an individualized diet for you to ensure good control of your diabetes.

Storage Keep in original container at room temperature out of the reach of children.

Missed dose If it is less than 12 hours until next dose, skip missed dose and take next dose at the usual time. If it is more than 12 hours to next dose, take as soon as you remember.

Stopping the drug Do not stop taking the drug without consulting your doctor; stopping may lead to worsening of your diabetes control.

Exceeding the dose An occasional unintentional extra dose is unlikely to be a cause for concern. If symptoms of low blood sugar develop, such as sweating, hunger, trembling, confusion, headache, or feeling faint, eat or drink something sugary. If a large overdose has been taken, seek immediate medical attention.

POSSIBLE ADVERSE EFFECTS

Common side effects are urinary or genital infections (causing genital itching, discharge, cloudy or smelly urine, or rash) and faintness or light-headedness. Low blood sugar (causing dizziness, confusion, sweating, and shaking) may occur when dapagliflozin is taken with insulin or sulfonylureas. If you feel faint or dizzy or have signs of low blood sugar, stop taking the drug and consult your doctor. A rare but potentially serious effect is diabetic ketoacidosis: a build-up of ketones in the body, producing nausea, vomiting, stomach pains, excessive thirst, breathing problems, unusual tiredness, or confusion. Another serious effect is Fournier's gangrene: severe swelling, pain and redness of the perineal area (between the genitals and anus), with fever or malaise. Stop taking the drug and seek immediate medical attention if any of these symptoms develops.

INTERACTIONS

Diuretics When these drugs are taken with dapagliflozin, there is a risk of dehydration and low blood pressure.

SPECIAL PRECAUTIONS

Be sure to tell your doctor if:

- You have liver or kidney problems.
- You have or have had bladder cancer.
- You get frequent urinary tract infections.
- You have a history of heart disease or stroke.
- You have low blood pressure.
- You are taking other medicines.

Pregnancy Not prescribed in pregnancy. Discuss with your doctor.

Breast-feeding May pass into breast milk and affect the baby. Discuss with your doctor.

Infants and children Not recommended.

Over 60 Increased risk of adverse effects. Reduced dose may therefore be necessary.

Driving and hazardous work Avoid if you have warning signs of low blood sugar.

Alcohol Avoid excessive intake as alcohol may upset blood sugar control.

Surgery and general anaesthetics Dapagliflozin should be stopped before any major surgical procedure or during severe illness due to increased risk of ketoacidosis.

PROLONGED USE

No problems expected.

Monitoring Regular checks of blood sugar control and kidney function are necessary. Urine will test positive for glucose while on dapagliflozin but this is no cause for concern unless there are other indications of poor blood sugar control. Blood cholesterol levels should be monitored as dapagliflozin may cause an increase in blood cholesterol.

DESMOPRESSIN

Brand names DDAVP, DDAVP Melt, DesmoMelt, Desmospray, Desmotabs, Noqdirna, Octim

Used in the following combined preparations None

QUICK REFERENCE

Drug group Drug for diabetes insipidus (p.84)

Overdose danger rating Medium

Dependence rating Low

Prescription needed Yes

Available as generic Yes

GENERAL INFORMATION

Desmopressin is a synthetic form of the hormone vasopressin. Low levels of vasopressin in the body can lead to diabetes insipidus, which causes excess urine production and continual thirst; desmopressin can be used to correct this deficiency. It is also used to test for diabetes insipidus, to check kidney function, and to treat nocturnal enuresis (bedwetting) in both children and adults. When given by injection, it helps to boost clotting factors in haemophilia and von Willebrand's disease.

Side effects include low blood sodium and fluid retention (which sometimes requires monitoring of body weight and blood pressure to check the body's water balance). Desmopressin should not be taken during an episode of vomiting and diarrhoea because the body's fluid balance may be upset.

INFORMATION FOR USERS

Your drug prescription is tailored for you. Do not alter dosage without checking with your doctor.

How taken/used Tablets, sublingual tablets, injection, nasal solution, nasal spray.

Frequency and timing of doses *Diabetes insipidus* 3 x daily (tablets/sublingual tablets); 1–2 x daily (nasal spray/solution). *Nocturnal enuresis* At bedtime (tablets/sublingual tablets, nasal spray/solution). Avoid fluids from 1 hour before bedtime to 8 hours afterwards.

Dosage range *Diabetes insipidus: Adults* 300–600mcg daily (tablets/sublingual tablets); 1–4 puffs (nasal spray); 10–40mcg daily (nasal solution). *Diabetes insipidus: Children* 300–600mcg daily (tablets/sublingual tablets); up to 2 puffs (nasal spray); 20mcg (nasal solution). *Nocturnal enuresis* 200–400mcg for adults and children over 5 years only (tablets/sublingual tablets); 20–40mcg (nasal solution); 2–4 puffs (nasal spray).

Onset of effect A few minutes. Full effects: a few hours (injection, nasal solution/spray); 30–90 minutes (tablets/sublingual tablets).

Duration of action Tablets/sublingual tablets 6–12 hours; injection, nasal solutions, and nasal spray 5–21 hours.

Diet advice Your doctor may advise you to avoid excessive fluid intake.

Storage Keep in original container at room temperature (tablets/sublingual tablets) or in a refrigerator, without freezing (nasal solution and nasal spray), out of the reach of children. Protect from light.

Missed dose Take as soon as you remember. If your next dose is due within 2 hours, take a single dose now and skip the next.

Stopping the drug Do not stop without consulting your doctor, because symptoms may recur.

Exceeding the dose An occasional unintentional extra dose is unlikely to cause problems. Large overdoses may cause seizures. Notify your doctor without delay.

POSSIBLE ADVERSE EFFECTS

Adverse effects with desmopressin are uncommon. However, it may cause fluid retention (which may cause weight gain) and low blood sodium, especially if fluid intake is too high. In serious cases, this can lead to seizures; if so, stop taking the drug and contact your doctor immediately. Headache, nausea, vomiting, nasal congestion, and nosebleeds may also occur; if these symptoms are severe, discuss with your doctor. You should also consult your doctor if you experience stomach pain with the drug.

INTERACTIONS

Antidepressants, chlorpropamide, chlorpromazine, fludrocortisone, and carbamazepine These drugs may increase the effects of desmopressin.

Non-steroidal anti-inflammatory drugs (NSAIDs) These may increase the body's response to desmopressin.

Loperamide This drug may significantly increase blood levels of desmopressin.

SPECIAL PRECAUTIONS

Be sure to tell your doctor if:

- You have heart problems.
- You have high blood pressure.
- You have kidney problems.
- You have cystic fibrosis.
- You have asthma or allergic rhinitis.
- You have epilepsy.
- You are taking other medicines.

Pregnancy Safety in pregnancy not established. Discuss with your doctor.

Breast-feeding The drug passes into breast milk, in small amounts, but adverse effects on the baby are unlikely.

Infants and children No special problems in children; infants may need monitoring to ensure that fluid balance is correct.

Over 60 May need monitoring to ensure that fluid balance is correct.

Driving and hazardous work No known problems.

Alcohol Your doctor may advise on fluid intake.

PROLONGED USE

Diabetes insipidus: no problems expected. Nocturnal enuresis: the drug will be withdrawn for at least a week after 3 months for assessment of the need to continue treatment.

Monitoring The levels of electrolytes (such as sodium) in the blood should be monitored periodically, as well as blood pressure and the levels of electrolytes in the urine.

DESOGESTREL

Brand name Aizea, Cerazette, Cerelle, Desomono, Desorex, Feanolla, Zelleta, and others

Used in the following combined preparations Alenvona, Bimizza, Cimizt, Gedarel, Marvelon, Mercilon, Munalea, and others

QUICK REFERENCE

Drug group Female sex hormone (p.86) and oral contraceptive (p.103)

Overdose danger rating Low

Dependence rating Low

Prescription needed Yes

Available as generic Yes

GENERAL INFORMATION

Desogestrel is a synthetic hormone similar to the natural female sex hormone progesterone. It is used alone as a progestogen-only pill, or POP (p.104), and is especially helpful as contraception in women who do not tolerate oestrogens or those who are breast-feeding. The drug works by thickening the mucus at the neck of the cervix, making it difficult for sperm to enter. Unlike other POPs, it also acts by preventing ovulation (release of an egg from an ovary). In addition, it changes the quality of the endometrium (lining of the uterus), preventing implantation of a fertilized egg.

Desogestrel is also used in combination with the oestrogen drug ethinylestradiol (see p.242) as an oral contraceptive.

When the drug is taken without an oestrogen, irregular vaginal bleeding may occur in the form of slight spotting, heavier bleeding, or no bleeding at all. Desogestrel, either alone or in a combined oral contraceptive, also carries a significant risk of venous thrombosis.

INFORMATION FOR USERS

Your drug prescription is tailored for you. Do not alter dosage without checking with your doctor.

How taken/used Tablets.

Frequency and timing of doses One tablet at the same time each day.

Adult dosage range 75mcg daily.

Onset of effect Within a few hours.

Duration of action 24 hours.

Diet advice None.

Storage Keep in original container at room temperature out of the reach of children. Protect from light.

Missed dose If a tablet is delayed by 12 hours or more, regard it as a missed pill. See What to do if you miss a pill (p.107).

Stopping the drug The drug can be safely stopped as soon as contraceptive protection is no longer required. If used for treatment of menstrual symptoms, consult your doctor before stopping the drug.

Exceeding the dose An occasional unintentional dose is unlikely to be a cause for concern. But if you notice any unusual symptoms, or if a large overdose has been taken, call your doctor.

POSSIBLE ADVERSE EFFECTS

Irregular vaginal bleeding is the most common side effect of desogestrel taken alone. If you have heavy or prolonged bleeding, consult your doctor. Other common side effects include nausea, vomiting, headache, breast discomfort or tenderness, weight changes, acne, mood changes, and reduced libido. More rarely, the drug may cause changes in skin pigmentation. Discuss with your doctor if you have any changes in mood or libido, or if any of these other symptoms becomes severe.

If you vomit within 3–4 hours of taking a tablet, absorption of the drug may be reduced and you should use additional contraceptive measures for the next 7 days.

INTERACTIONS

General note The beneficial effects of many drugs, including oral anticoagulants, anticonvulsants, antihypertensives, and antidiabetic drugs, may be affected by desogestrel. Many drugs may also reduce the contraceptive effect of desogestrel. These include anticonvulsants, antituberculous drugs, antidepressants, and the herbal remedy St John's wort.

SPECIAL PRECAUTIONS

Be sure to tell your doctor if:

- You have jaundice or a liver problem.
- You have diabetes.
- You have a history of breast cancer.
- You have had an ectopic pregnancy.
- You have unexplained abnormal vaginal bleeding.
- You have had epileptic seizures.
- You have had venous thrombosis or a stroke.
- You are taking other medicines.

Pregnancy Not prescribed. May cause defects in the fetus. Discuss with your doctor.

Breast-feeding The drug passes into the breast milk, but normal doses are unlikely to affect the baby adversely. Discuss with your doctor.
Infants and children Not prescribed.
Over 60 Not prescribed.
Driving and hazardous work No known problems.
Alcohol No known problems.

PROLONGED USE

There is a small increase in the risk of breast cancer in women who have used a progestogen-only pill. However, the risk is related to the age at which the pill is stopped rather than duration of use. The increased risk reduces to zero over 10 years after stopping use.
Monitoring Regular blood pressure checks may be carried out.

DEXAMETHASONE

Brand names Dexsol, Dropodex, Eythalm, Glensoludex, Martapan, Maxidex, Neofordex, Ozurdex
Used in the following combined preparations Maxitrol, Otomize, Sofradex, Tobradex, and others

QUICK REFERENCE

Drug group Corticosteroid (p.78)
Overdose danger rating Low
Dependence rating Low
Prescription needed Yes
Available as generic Yes

GENERAL INFORMATION

Dexamethasone is a long-acting, potent corticosteroid used to suppress inflammatory and allergic disorders, shock, and brain swelling (due to injury or tumour), and to relieve the lung complications of COVID-19 coronavirus infection. It is also used with other drugs to alleviate nausea and vomiting associated with chemotherapy. It is available in different forms, including tablets, oral solution, injection, and eye and ear drops. Low doses taken for short periods rarely cause serious side effects. However, as with other corticosteroids, long-term treatment, especially with high doses, can cause significant adverse effects.

INFORMATION FOR USERS

Your drug prescription is tailored for you. Do not alter dosage without checking with your doctor.
How taken/used Tablets, liquid, injection, eye ointment, eye/ear drops, ear/nasal spray.
Frequency and timing of doses 1–4 x daily with food (by mouth); 1–6 hourly (eye drops); 1–4 x daily (ear drops/spray, eye ointment); 2–6 x daily (nasal spray).
Dosage range Usually 0.5–10mg daily (by mouth).
Onset of effect 1–4 days.
Duration of action Some effects may last for several days.
Diet advice None.
Storage Keep in original container at room temperature out of the reach of children. Protect from light.
Missed dose Take as soon as you remember. If your next dose is due within 2 hours, take a single dose now and skip the next.
Stopping the drug Do not stop taking the drug without consulting your doctor. It may be necessary to withdraw the drug gradually.
Exceeding the dose An occasional unintentional extra dose is unlikely to be a cause for concern. But if you notice any unusual symptoms, or if a large overdose has been taken, call your doctor.

POSSIBLE ADVERSE EFFECTS

Indigestion, acne and other skin changes, weight gain, fluid retention, or mood changes are common adverse effects; discuss with your doctor if any of these become severe. More serious adverse effects occur only with high doses taken for long periods (see Prolonged use); these are carefully monitored during long-term treatment. Rarely, severe mental effects, such as depression or suicidal thoughts or behaviour, may occur. If this happens, consult your doctor without delay.

INTERACTIONS

Antidiabetic drugs Dexamethasone reduces the action of these drugs. Dosage may need to be adjusted accordingly to prevent abnormally high blood sugar.
Barbiturates, phenytoin, rifampicin, and carbamazepine These drugs may reduce the effectiveness of dexamethasone. The dosage may need to be adjusted accordingly.
Oral anticoagulant drugs Dexamethasone may increase the effects of these drugs.
Non-steroidal anti-inflammatory drugs These drugs may increase the likelihood of indigestion from dexamethasone.
Antacids Take at least 2 hours apart from dexamethasone as they may reduce its effect.

Vaccines Dexamethasone can interact with some vaccines. Discuss with your doctor before having any vaccinations.

SPECIAL PRECAUTIONS

Be sure to tell your doctor if:

- You have had a peptic ulcer.
- You have glaucoma.
- You have high blood pressure.
- You have congestive heart failure.
- You have diabetes.
- You have epilepsy.
- You have had tuberculosis.
- You have had depression or mental illness.
- You are taking other medicines.

Pregnancy Safety in pregnancy not established. Discuss with your doctor.

Breast-feeding Safety not established. The drug passes into breast milk. Consult your doctor.

Infants and children Reduced dose necessary.

Over 60 No known problems.

Driving and hazardous work No known problems, although eye drops or ointment may cause temporary visual disturbances.

Alcohol Avoid. Alcohol may increase the risks of indigestion and peptic ulcer with this drug.

Surgery and general anaesthetics Tell doctor or anaesthetist that you take dexamethasone; close monitoring is required during surgery.

Infection Avoid exposure to chickenpox, shingles, and measles if you are on systemic dexamethasone treatment.

PROLONGED USE

Prolonged use by mouth can lead to peptic ulcers, glaucoma, fragile bones, muscle weakness, and growth retardation in children. People receiving long-term treatment are advised to carry a steroid treatment card.

DIAZEPAM/LORAZEPAM

Brand names [diazepam] Diazemuls, Diazepam Rectubes, Stesolid, Valclair; [lorazepam] Ativan

Used in the following combined preparations None

QUICK REFERENCE

Drug group Benzodiazepine anti-anxiety drug (p.11), muscle relaxant (p.53), and anticonvulsant (p.14)

Overdose danger rating High

Dependence rating High

Prescription needed Yes

Available as generic Yes

GENERAL INFORMATION

Introduced in the early 1960s, diazepam is the best known and most widely used benzodiazepine, and lorazepam is closely related to it. Benzodiazepines help to relieve tension and nervousness, relax muscles, and encourage sleep. Their actions and adverse effects are described more fully on p.11.

Diazepam and lorazepam have a wide range of uses. Besides being commonly used to treat anxiety and anxiety-related insomnia, they are used to treat alcohol withdrawal and to relieve epileptic seizures. Diazepam is also used as a muscle relaxant. Given intravenously, they are used to sedate people undergoing certain uncomfortable medical procedures.

Diazepam and lorazepam can be habit-forming if taken regularly over a long period. Their effects may also diminish with time. For these reasons, courses of treatment are limited to 2 weeks whenever possible.

INFORMATION FOR USERS

Your drug prescription is tailored for you. Do not alter dosage without checking with your doctor.

How taken/used Tablets, liquid, injection, suppositories, rectal solution.

Frequency and timing of doses 1–4 x daily.

Dosage range Anxiety 2–30mg daily (diazepam); 1–4mg daily (lorazepam).

Onset of effect Immediate effect (injection); 30 minutes–2 hours (other methods of administration).

Duration of action Up to 24 hours; some effect: up to 4 days.

Diet advice None.

Storage Keep in original container at room temperature out of the reach of children.

Missed dose Take as soon as you remember. If your next dose is due within 2 hours, take a single dose now and skip the next.

Stopping the drug If you have been taking the drug for less than 2 weeks, it can be stopped as soon as no longer needed. If taking it for longer, consult your doctor, who will supervise a gradual reduction in dosage. Stopping abruptly may lead to withdrawal symptoms (see p.11).

OVERDOSE ACTION

Seek immediate medical advice. Large overdoses may cause excessive drowsiness and possibly even deep coma, requiring emergency action.

POSSIBLE ADVERSE EFFECTS

The principal adverse effects of diazepam and lorazepam are due to their sedative properties. They include daytime drowsiness, dizziness, unsteadiness, forgetfulness, and confusion. More rarely, the drugs may also cause headache and blurred vision. Drowsiness and headache normally diminish after a few days and may be reduced by adjusting the dosage; consult your doctor if severe. However, if you experience dizziness, forgetfulness, confusion, or blurred vision, call your doctor promptly.

INTERACTIONS

Sedatives All drugs that have a sedative effect on the central nervous system can increase the sedative properties of diazepam and lorazepam. If combined with opiates, both diazepam and lorazepam carry a risk of potentially fatal respiratory depression.

Omeprazole (diazepam), cimetidine, isoniazid, fosamprenavir, and ritonavir These drugs may increase blood levels of diazepam and lorazepam and the risk of adverse effects.

Rifampicin may reduce the effects of diazepam.

SPECIAL PRECAUTIONS

Be sure to tell your doctor if:

- You have severe respiratory disease.
- You have long-term liver or kidney problems.
- You have had problems with alcohol or drug misuse.
- You have myasthenia gravis or muscle weakness.
- You have sleep apnoea.
- You have a marked personality disorder.
- You have porphyria.
- You are taking other medicines.

Pregnancy Not usually recommended; may cause adverse effects on newborn baby at the time of delivery. Discuss with your doctor.

Breast-feeding The drugs pass into breast milk and affect the baby. Discuss with your doctor.

Infants and children Reduced dose necessary.

Over 60 Increased likelihood of adverse effects. Reduced dose may therefore be necessary.

Driving and hazardous work Avoid such activities until you have learned how diazepam or lorazepam affect you because the drugs can cause reduced alertness, slowed reactions, and increased aggression.

Alcohol Avoid. Alcohol may increase the sedative effects of these drugs.

PROLONGED USE

Regular use of these drugs over several weeks can lead to a reduction in their effect as the body adapts. They may also be habit-forming when taken for extended periods, and severe withdrawal reactions can occur if they are stopped abruptly.

DICLOFENAC

Brand names Dicloflex, Diclomax SR, Dyloject, Fenactol, Motifene, Voltarol, and many others

Used in the following combined preparation Arthrotec (with misoprostol)

QUICK REFERENCE

Drug group Non-steroidal anti-inflammatory drug (p.48), analgesic (p.7), and drug for gout (p.51)

Overdose danger rating Medium

Dependence rating Low

Prescription needed Yes (except for some gel formulations)

Available as generic Yes

GENERAL INFORMATION

Taken as a single dose, diclofenac has analgesic properties similar to those of paracetamol. It is taken to relieve mild to moderate headache, menstrual pain, and pain following minor surgery. When taken regularly over a long period, it has an anti-inflammatory effect and is used to relieve pain and stiffness associated with rheumatoid arthritis and advanced osteoarthritis. It may also be prescribed to treat acute gout attacks, and may be given as eye drops to relieve eye inflammation.

The combined preparation Arthrotec contains diclofenac and misoprostol (see p.328). Misoprostol helps prevent gastroduodenal ulceration, which is sometimes caused by diclofenac, and may be particularly useful in patients at risk of developing this problem.

INFORMATION FOR USERS

Your drug prescription is tailored for you. Do not alter dosage without checking with your doctor.

How taken/used Tablets, slow-release (SR) tablets, dispersible tablets, capsules, SR capsules, injection, suppositories, gel, eye drops.

Frequency and timing of doses 1–3 x daily with food.

Adult dosage range 75–150mg daily.

Onset of effect Around 1 hour (pain relief); full anti-inflammatory effect may take 2 weeks.

Duration of action Up to 12 hours; up to 24 hours (SR preparations).
Diet advice None.
Storage Keep in original container at room temperature out of the reach of children.
Missed dose Take as soon as you remember. If your next dose is due within 2 hours, take a single dose now and skip the next.
Stopping the drug If used for short-term pain relief, you can stop as soon as you no longer need it. If prescribed for long-term treatment, speak to your doctor before stopping.
Exceeding the dose An occasional unintentional extra dose is unlikely to be a cause for concern. But if you notice any unusual symptoms or if a large overdose has been taken, tell your doctor.

POSSIBLE ADVERSE EFFECTS

The most common adverse effects are gastro-intestinal disturbances, such as heartburn, indigestion, nausea, and vomiting. More rarely, headache, dizziness, drowsiness, swelling of the feet or legs, or weight gain may occur. If any of these symptoms are severe, discuss with your doctor. If the drug causes a rash, itching, wheezing, breathlessness, or black or blood-stained vomit or faeces, stop taking it and consult your doctor without delay.

INTERACTIONS

General note Diclofenac interacts with other NSAIDs, oral anticoagulants, corticosteroids, and SSRI antidepressants to increase the risk of bleeding and/or peptic ulceration.
Ciclosporin and tacrolimus Diclofenac may increase the risk of kidney problems.
Antihypertensive drugs and diuretics Benefits of these drugs may be reduced with diclofenac.
Lithium, digoxin, and methotrexate Diclofenac may increase the blood levels of these drugs to an undesirable extent.

SPECIAL PRECAUTIONS

Be sure to tell your doctor if:
- You have long-term liver or kidney problems.
- You have a bleeding disorder.
- You have had a peptic ulcer or you have indigestion.
- You have porphyria.
- You are allergic to aspirin or other NSAIDs.
- You have asthma, heart problems, or high blood pressure.
- You are taking other medicines.

Pregnancy The drug may increase the risks of adverse effects on the baby's heart and may prolong labour if taken in the third trimester. Discuss with your doctor.
Breast-feeding Small amounts of the drug pass into the breast milk, but adverse effects on the baby are unlikely. Discuss with your doctor.
Infants and children Reduced dose necessary.
Over 60 Increased risk of adverse effects. Reduced dose may be necessary.
Driving and hazardous work Avoid such activities until you have learned how diclofenac affects you; the drug can cause dizziness, drowsiness and vertigo.
Alcohol Avoid. Alcohol may increase the risk of stomach irritation.
Surgery and general anaesthetics Discuss with your doctor or dentist before any surgery.

PROLONGED USE

There is an increased risk of ulceration, perforation, or bleeding from the bowel wall with prolonged use of diclofenac. There is also a small risk of a heart attack or stroke. To minimize these risks, the lowest effective dose is given for the shortest duration.

DICYCLOVERINE (DICYCLOMINE)

Brand name None
Used in the following combined preparation Kolanticon

QUICK REFERENCE

Drug group Drug for irritable bowel syndrome (p.43)
Overdose danger rating Medium
Dependence rating Low
Prescription needed No (doses of 10mg or less); Yes (doses of more than 10mg)
Available as generic Yes

GENERAL INFORMATION

Dicycloverine is a mild anticholinergic drug that relieves painful abdominal cramps caused by spasms of the smooth muscle in the wall of the gastrointestinal tract. It can be used for irritable bowel syndrome, and colicky conditions in babies (only those over 6 months).

Because the drug has anticholinergic properties (p.7), it is also included in some combined preparations used to treat flatulence, indigestion, and diarrhoea. Dicycloverine relieves the symptoms but does not cure the underlying condition. Additional treatment with other drugs and self-help measures, such as dietary changes, may be recommended by your doctor.

Side effects with dicycloverine are rare, but they include headaches, constipation, urinary difficulties, and palpitations.

INFORMATION FOR USERS

Follow instructions on the label. Call your doctor if symptoms worsen.

How taken/used Tablets, liquid.

Frequency and timing of doses 3–4 x daily before or after meals.

Dosage range *Adults* 30–60mg daily. *Children* Reduced dose according to age and weight.

Onset of effect Within 1–2 hours.

Duration of action 4–6 hours.

Diet advice None.

Storage Keep in original container at room temperature out of the reach of children. Protect from light.

Missed dose Take as soon as you remember. If your next dose is due within 2 hours, take a single dose now and skip the next.

Stopping the drug The drug can be stopped without causing problems as soon as it is no longer needed.

Exceeding the dose An occasional unintentional extra dose is unlikely to cause problems. However, large overdoses may cause drowsiness, dizziness, and difficulty in swallowing. Notify your doctor.

POSSIBLE ADVERSE EFFECTS

Most people do not notice any adverse effects from dicycloverine. Those that do occur are related to its anticholinergic effect and include drowsiness, dry mouth, constipation, headache, and blurred vision. These symptoms may be reduced by adjusting the dose, or may disappear after a few days as your body adjusts to the drug; consult your doctor if severe. If you develop palpitations or difficulty in passing urine, discuss with your doctor.

INTERACTIONS

Sedatives All drugs that have a sedative effect on the central nervous system may increase the sedative properties of dicycloverine.

Anticholinergic drugs These drugs may increase the adverse effects of dicycloverine.

SPECIAL PRECAUTIONS

Be sure to tell your doctor if:

- You have glaucoma.
- You have urinary problems and/or an enlarged prostate gland.
- You have a hiatus hernia or you have heartburn or acid reflux.
- You have any heart condition.
- You have myasthenia gravis.
- You are taking other medicines.

Pregnancy No evidence of risk.

Breast-feeding The drug passes into the breast milk, but normal doses are unlikely to affect the baby adversely. Discuss with your doctor.

Infants and children Reduced dose necessary. Not recommended in infants under 6 months.

Over 60 Reduced dose may be necessary. Older people are more susceptible to anticholinergic side effects.

Driving and hazardous work Avoid until you know how dicycloverine affects you; the drug can cause drowsiness and blurred vision.

Alcohol Caution. Alcohol may increase the sedative effects of this drug.

PROLONGED USE

No problems expected.

DIGOXIN

Brand name Lanoxin

Used in the following combined preparations None

QUICK REFERENCE

Drug group Digitalis drug (p.27)

Overdose danger rating High

Dependence rating Low

Prescription needed Yes

Available as generic Yes

GENERAL INFORMATION

Digoxin is the most widely used extract of digitalis, a compound originally obtained from the leaves of the foxglove plant. The drug is given in the treatment of irregular heart rhythms such as atrial fibrillation or atrial flutter; it may also sometimes be used to treat congestive heart failure.

Digoxin increases the force of the heart beat, making it more effective in pumping blood around the body. This in turn helps to control breathlessness, fluid retention, and tiredness in people with heart failure.

The effective dose of digoxin can be close to the toxic dose, so treatment needs careful monitoring to prevent toxic doses being reached. Adverse effects may indicate that the toxic level is close and should be reported to your doctor.

INFORMATION FOR USERS

Your drug prescription is tailored for you. Do not alter dosage without checking with your doctor.

How taken/used Tablets, liquid, injection.

Frequency and timing of doses Up to 3 x daily (starting dose); once daily, or divided to reduce nausea (maintenance dose).

Adult dosage range Usually 0.0625–0.25mg daily (by mouth), but doses of up to 0.5mg are occasionally used.

Onset of effect Within a few minutes (injection); within 1–2 hours (by mouth).

Duration of action Up to 4 days.

Diet advice Drug may be more toxic if potassium levels are low. Include potassium-rich fruit and vegetables, such as bananas and tomatoes, in your diet.

Storage Keep in original container at room temperature out of the reach of children. Protect from light.

Missed dose Take as soon as you remember. If your next dose is due within 8 hours, take a dose now and skip the next.

Stopping the drug Do not stop the drug without consulting your doctor; stopping may lead to worsening of the underlying condition.

OVERDOSE ACTION

Seek immediate medical advice in all cases. Take emergency action if palpitations, severe weakness, chest pain, or loss of consciousness occur.

POSSIBLE ADVERSE EFFECTS

Adverse effects are usually due to high blood levels of the drug. Common effects include tiredness, nausea, and loss of appetite. More rarely, confusion, visual disturbance, and palpitations may occur. Any symptoms should be reported to your doctor without delay. If you experience palpitations and/or visual disturbances, stop taking the drug.

INTERACTIONS

General note Many drugs interact with digoxin. Do not take any medication without consulting your doctor or pharmacist.

Diuretics may increase the risk of adverse effects from digoxin if they lower potassium levels.

Ciclosporin and tacrolimus may increase blood levels of digoxin.

Calcium channel blockers and anti-arrhythmic drugs (e.g. amiodarone and quinidine) may increase blood levels of digoxin.

Antacids may reduce the effects of digoxin. The effect of digoxin may increase when antacids are stopped.

SPECIAL PRECAUTIONS

Be sure to tell your doctor if:

- ◆ You have had previous problems with your heart rhythm.
- ◆ You have kidney problems.
- ◆ You have a thyroid disorder.
- ◆ You are taking other medicines.

Pregnancy No evidence of risk, but adjustment in dose may be necessary.

Breast-feeding The drug passes into breast milk, but normal doses are unlikely to affect the baby adversely. Discuss with your doctor.

Infants and children Reduced dose necessary.

Over 60 Increased likelihood of adverse effects. Reduced dose may therefore be necessary.

Driving and hazardous work Special problems are unlikely, but do not undertake these activities until you know how digoxin affects you as it can cause tiredness and visual disturbances.

Alcohol No special problems.

PROLONGED USE

No problems expected.

Monitoring Periodic checks on blood levels of digoxin and body salts may be advised.

DIHYDROCODEINE

Brand names DF118 Forte, DHC Continus

Used in the following combined preparations Co-dydramol, Paramol

QUICK REFERENCE

Drug group Opioid analgesic (p.8)

Overdose danger rating High

Dependence rating Medium

Prescription needed Yes (most preparations)

Available as generic Yes

GENERAL INFORMATION

Dihydrocodeine is an opioid analgesic related to codeine and of similar potency if taken by mouth. It is used mainly to relieve moderately severe pain but has also been used as a cough suppressant. As with codeine, side effects limit the dose that can be taken; the drug causes constipation, nausea, and vomiting.

Dihydrocodeine is also used in combination with paracetamol; in this way, a lower dose of the opioid can be used to give pain relief with fewer side effects. A preparation containing dihydrocodeine and paracetamol is available under the generic name of co-dydramol.

INFORMATION FOR USERS

Your drug prescription is tailored for you. Do not alter dosage without checking with your doctor.

How taken/used Tablets, slow release (SR) tablets, liquid, injection.

Frequency and timing of doses 2–6 x daily.

Adult dosage range 120–240mg daily.

Onset of effect 30–60 minutes (tablets, liquid); 3–4 hours (SR tablets).

Duration of action 4–6 hours (tablets, liquid); 12 hours (SR tablets).

Diet advice None.

Storage Keep in original container at room temperature out of the reach of children.

Missed dose Take as soon as you remember if needed for relief of symptoms. If not needed, do not take the missed dose, and return to your normal dosage schedule when necessary.

Stopping the drug Can usually be safely stopped as soon as you no longer need it. However, if you have been taking it for a long time or at high doses, you may experience withdrawal effects. Discuss with your doctor.

OVERDOSE ACTION

Seek immediate medical advice in all cases. Take emergency action if slow or irregular breathing, severe drowsiness, or loss of consciousness occur.

POSSIBLE ADVERSE EFFECTS

The most common effects are constipation, nausea, vomiting, drowsiness, dizziness, headache, and vertigo. More rarely, the drug may cause abdominal pain. If these symptoms are severe, discuss with your doctor. If rash, itching, confusion, hallucinations, or breathing difficulties occur, seek medical advice promptly; you should also stop taking the drug if you have breathing difficulties. Tolerance and dependence may occur with long-term use.

INTERACTIONS

Sedatives All drugs with a sedative effect on the central nervous system increase the sedative properties of dihydrocodeine. These include other opioid analgesics, sleeping drugs, antihistamines, antipsychotics, and antidepressants.

Monoamine oxidase inhibitors (MAOIs) may cause a dangerous rise in blood pressure. Avoid using dihydrocodeine together with MAOIs and for 14 days after stopping MAOIs.

SPECIAL PRECAUTIONS

Be sure to tell your doctor if:

- You have liver or kidney problems.
- You have a phaeochromocytoma.
- You have a lung disorder such as asthma or bronchitis.
- You have a problem with alcohol misuse.
- You have an enlarged prostate.
- You have low blood pressure.
- You have an underactive thyroid.
- You are taking other medicines.

Pregnancy Safety in pregnancy not established, although drug has been used for many years without obvious effect (except near delivery).

Breast-feeding Safety not established. Discuss with your doctor.

Infants and children Not recommended under 4 years. Over 4 years a reduced dose is necessary.

Over 60 Reduced dose necessary.

Driving and hazardous work Avoid until you know how the drug affects you as it may cause drowsiness, dizziness, and confusion.

Alcohol Avoid. Alcohol may increase the sedative effects of the drug.

PROLONGED USE

The drug is generally only used short term as it can be habit forming if used long term.

DILTIAZEM

Brand names Adizem-SR, Dilzem SR, Dilzem XL, Slozem, Tildiem, and others

Used in the following combined preparations None

QUICK REFERENCE

Drug group Calcium channel blocker (p.33) and antihypertensive drug (p.34)

Overdose danger rating Medium

Dependence rating Low

Prescription needed Yes

Available as generic Yes

GENERAL INFORMATION

Diltiazem is a calcium channel blocker (p.33). This group of drugs interrupts the conduction of nerve signals in the muscles of the heart and blood vessels.

The drug is used to treat angina, and longer-acting formulations are used for high blood pressure. Taken regularly, it reduces the frequency of angina attacks, but it does not work fast enough to reduce the pain of an angina attack that is already in progress. Topical diltiazem is used to treat chronic anal fissure.

Diltiazem does not adversely affect breathing, so the drug is valuable for people with asthma, for whom other anti-angina drugs may not be suitable.

Different brands of sustained-release (SR) diltiazem may not be equivalent, so you should always take the same brand.

INFORMATION FOR USERS

Your drug prescription is tailored for you. Do not alter dosage without checking with your doctor.

How taken/used Tablets, SR tablets, capsules, SR capsules, cream.

Frequency and timing of doses 3 x daily (tablets/capsules); 1–2 x daily (SR tablets/SR capsules); 2 x daily (cream).

Adult dosage range *Angina/high blood pressure* 180–480mg daily. *Anal fissure* 1 inch of cream applied to anal area twice daily for 2 months.

Onset of effect 2–3 hours.

Duration of action 6–8 hours.

Diet advice None.

Storage Keep in original container at room temperature out of the reach of children.

Missed dose Take as soon as you remember. If your next dose is due within 2 hours, take a single dose now and skip the next.

Stopping the drug Do not stop without consulting your doctor; symptoms may recur. Stopping suddenly may worsen angina.

Exceeding the dose An occasional unintentional extra dose is unlikely to cause problems. Large overdoses may cause dizziness or collapse. Notify your doctor urgently.

POSSIBLE ADVERSE EFFECTS

Diltiazem can cause various minor side effects that are also common to other calcium channel blockers. These include headache, nausea, vomiting, dry mouth, and ankle swelling. If any of these symptoms are severe, discuss with your doctor. More rarely, the drug may cause breast and/or gum enlargement, a rash, and, more seriously, a slowed heartbeat, which may cause dizziness or tiredness. If you develop any of these symptoms, contact your doctor. It is sometimes possible to control the adverse effects by adjusting the dosage.

INTERACTIONS

Antihypertensive drugs Diltiazem increases the effects of these drugs, leading to a further reduction in blood pressure.

Anticonvulsant drugs Levels of these drugs may be altered by diltiazem.

Anti-arrhythmic drugs There is a risk of side effects on the heart if these are taken with diltiazem.

Beta blockers increase the risk of the heart slowing.

Digoxin Blood levels and adverse effects of this drug may be increased if it is taken with diltiazem. The dosage of digoxin may need to be reduced.

Simvastatin Diltiazem may increase blood levels and adverse effects of this drug. The dosage of simvastatin may need to be reduced.

Theophylline/aminophylline Diltiazem may increase the levels of this drug.

SPECIAL PRECAUTIONS

Be sure to tell your doctor if:

- You have long-term liver or kidney problems.
- You have heart failure, heart block, or heart valve problems.
- You have acute porphyria.
- You are taking other medicines.

Pregnancy Not usually prescribed. Discuss with your doctor.

Breast-feeding The drug passes into the breast milk and may affect the baby. Discuss with your doctor.

Infants and children Not recommended.

Over 60 Increased likelihood of adverse effects. Reduced dose may therefore be necessary.

Driving and hazardous work Avoid such activities until you have learned how diltiazem affects you because the drug can cause dizziness due to lowered blood pressure.

Alcohol Avoid excessive amounts. Alcohol may lower blood pressure, causing dizziness.

PROLONGED USE

No problems expected.

DIPYRIDAMOLE

Brand names Attia, Ofcram PR, Trolactin
Used in the following combined preparation Molita (dipyridamole with aspirin)

QUICK REFERENCE

Drug group Antiplatelet drug (p.37)
Overdose danger rating Medium
Dependence rating Low
Prescription needed Yes
Available as generic Yes

GENERAL INFORMATION

Dipyridamole was introduced to improve the capability for exercise in people with angina. More effective drugs are now available, but dipyridamole is still used as an antiplatelet drug. It acts by reducing the ability of platelets to stick to each other and to blood vessel walls, which reduces the likelihood of clots forming. This is especially important in people who have had a stroke or transient ischaemic attack (TIA) or after heart valve replacement surgery. It is usually given with other drugs such as warfarin or aspirin. It can also be given by injection in certain diagnostic tests on the heart.

Side effects may occur, especially during the early days of treatment. If they persist, your doctor may advise a reduction in dosage.

INFORMATION FOR USERS

Your drug prescription is tailored for you. Do not alter dosage without checking with your doctor.
How taken/used Tablets, capsules, modified release (MR) capsules, liquid, injection (for diagnostic tests only).
Frequency and timing of doses 3–4 x daily, 1 hour before meals (tablets, capsules, liquid). 2 x daily with food (MR capsules).
Adult dosage range 300–600mg daily (tablets, capsules, liquid); 400mg daily (MR capsules).
Onset of effect Within 1 hour. Full therapeutic effect may not be reached for 2–3 weeks.
Duration of action Up to 8 hours. Up to 12 hours (MR capsules).
Diet advice None.
Storage Keep in original container at room temperature out of the reach of children. Protect from light.
Missed dose Take as soon as you remember. If your next dose is due within 2 hours, take a single dose now and skip the next.
Stopping the drug Do not stop without consulting your doctor; withdrawal of the drug could lead to abnormal blood clotting.
Exceeding the dose An occasional unintentional extra dose is unlikely to be a cause for concern. Large overdoses may cause dizziness or vomiting. Notify your doctor.

POSSIBLE ADVERSE EFFECTS

Adverse effects are rare. Possible symptoms include nausea, stomach upsets, diarrhoea, headache, and flushing. Discuss with your doctor if these are severe or if the drug causes dizziness and fainting. If a rash, breathing difficulties, or swollen lips occur, stop taking the drug and consult your doctor promptly. In rare cases, dipyridamole may aggravate angina.

INTERACTIONS

Anticoagulant drugs The effect of these drugs may be increased by dipyridamole, thereby increasing the risk of uncontrolled bleeding. The dosage of the anticoagulant may need to be adjusted accordingly.
Adenosine should not be given together with dipyridamole as the combination can cause a serious drop in blood pressure.
Antihypertensives Dipyridamole may increase the effect of these drugs.
Cholinesterase inhibitors Used to treat myasthenia gravis, the effect of these drugs may be reduced by dipyridamole.
Antacids may reduce the effectiveness of dipyridamole.

SPECIAL PRECAUTIONS

Be sure to tell your doctor if:
- You have low blood pressure.
- You have a blood clotting disorder.
- You have migraine.
- You have angina or heart valve problems.
- You have myasthenia gravis.
- You have had a recent heart attack.
- You are taking other medicines.

Pregnancy Safety in pregnancy not established. Discuss with your doctor.
Breast-feeding The drug passes into breast milk but at normal doses adverse effects on the baby are unlikely. Discuss with your doctor.
Infants and children Reduced dose necessary.
Over 60 No special problems.
Driving and hazardous work Avoid such activities until you have learned how dipyridamole

affects you because the drug may cause dizziness and faintness.

Alcohol Avoid until you have learned how dipyridamole affects you as it may cause dizziness and faintness when taken with alcohol.

PROLONGED USE

No known problems.

DISULFIRAM

Brand name Antabuse, Esperal

Used in the following combined preparations None

QUICK REFERENCE

Drug group Alcohol abuse deterrent

Overdose danger rating Medium

Dependence rating Low

Prescription needed Yes

Available as generic Yes

GENERAL INFORMATION

Disulfiram is used to help people who misuse alcohol to abstain from drinking. It does not cure alcoholism but provides a powerful deterrent to drinking.

If you are taking disulfiram and drink even a small amount of alcohol, highly unpleasant reactions follow (see Possible adverse effects, below). These are due to high levels of acetaldehyde in the body, because disulfiram prevents the breakdown of this substance.

It is important not to drink any alcohol for at least 24 hours before beginning treatment, and for at least a week after stopping. Foods, medicines, and even toiletries containing alcohol should also be avoided. Disulfiram treatment is usually only started by specialist services in conjunction with social support.

INFORMATION FOR USERS

Your drug prescription is tailored for you. Do not alter dosage without checking with your doctor.

How taken/used Tablets.

Frequency and timing of doses Once daily.

Adult dosage range 800mg initially, gradually reduced over 5 days to 100–200mg (maintenance dose).

Onset of effect Interaction with alcohol occurs within a few minutes of taking alcohol.

Duration of action Interaction with alcohol can occur for up to 6 days after the last dose of disulfiram.

Diet advice Avoid all alcoholic drinks, even in very small amounts. Food, fermented vinegar, medicines, mouthwashes, and lotions containing alcohol should also be avoided.

Storage Keep in original container at room temperature out of the reach of children. Protect from light.

Missed dose Take as soon as you remember. If your next dose is due within 2 hours, take a single dose now and skip the next.

Stopping the drug Do not stop taking the drug without consulting your doctor.

Exceeding the dose An occasional unintentional extra dose is unlikely to cause problems. Large overdoses may cause a temporary increase in adverse effects. Notify your doctor.

POSSIBLE ADVERSE EFFECTS

Adverse effects such as drowsiness, fatigue, nausea, vomiting, bad breath, and reduced libido may occur but usually disappear when you get used to the drug. If they persist or become severe, discuss with your doctor; the dosage may need to be adjusted.

The most potentially severe effects are due to interaction with alcohol (see above). Flushing, throbbing headache, nausea, breathlessness, thirst, palpitations, dizziness, and fainting may be experienced. Such reactions may last from 30 minutes to several hours, leaving you feeling drowsy and fatigued. The reactions can also include unconsciousness, so it is wise to carry a card stating the person to be notified in an emergency.

INTERACTIONS

General note A number of drugs can produce an adverse reaction when taken with disulfiram. You are advised to check with your doctor or pharmacist before taking any other medication.

Phenytoin Disulfiram increases the blood levels of this drug.

Anticoagulant drugs (e.g. warfarin) Disulfiram increases the effect of these drugs.

Metronidazole A severe reaction can occur if this drug is taken with disulfiram.

Theophylline Disulfiram may increase the toxic effects of this drug.

Diazepam/chlordiazepoxide Disulfiram increases the effect of these drugs.

Tricyclic antidepressants Disulfiram increases the blood levels of these drugs.

SPECIAL PRECAUTIONS

Be sure to tell your doctor if:

- ◆ You have long-term liver or kidney problems.
- ◆ You have heart problems, coronary artery disease, or high blood pressure, or have had a previous stroke.
- ◆ You have had epileptic seizures.
- ◆ You have diabetes.
- ◆ You have breathing problems.
- ◆ You have depression.
- ◆ You are taking other medicines.

Pregnancy Safety in pregnancy not established. Discuss with your doctor.

Breast-feeding Avoid. No information available on whether the drug passes into breast milk. Discuss with your doctor.

Infants and children Not recommended.

Over 60 Reduced dose may be necessary.

Driving and hazardous work Avoid until you know how disulfiram affects you because the drug can cause drowsiness and dizziness.

Alcohol Never drink alcohol while being treated with disulfiram, and avoid foods, medicines, and toiletries containing alcohol. This drug may interact dangerously with alcohol.

PROLONGED USE

Not usually prescribed for longer than 6 months without review. It is wise to carry a card indicating that you are taking disulfiram, with instructions as to who should be notified in an emergency.

DOMPERIDONE

Brand name Motilium

Used in the following combined preparations None

QUICK REFERENCE

Drug group Anti-emetic drug (p.19)

Overdose danger rating Medium

Dependence rating Low

Prescription needed Yes

Available as generic Yes

GENERAL INFORMATION

Domperidone, an anti-emetic drug, was first introduced in the early 1980s. It is particularly effective for treating nausea and vomiting caused by gastroenteritis, chemotherapy, or radiotherapy. It is not effective for motion sickness or nausea caused by inner ear disorders such as Ménière's disease.

The main advantage of domperidone over other anti-emetic drugs is that it does not usually cause drowsiness or other adverse effects such as abnormal movement. It is not suitable, however, for the long-term treatment of gastrointestinal disorders, for which an alternative drug treatment is often prescribed.

Domperidone is now restricted to use in the relief of nausea and vomiting. It is sometimes given in single doses to manage acute attacks of migraine by enhancing the absorption of other drugs for migraine, such as paracetamol.

INFORMATION FOR USERS

Follow instructions on the label. Call your doctor if symptoms worsen.

How taken/used Tablets, liquid.

Frequency and timing of doses 1–3 x daily.

Adult dosage range Up to a maximum of 30mg daily.

Onset of effect Within 1 hour. Effects may be delayed if taken after the onset of nausea.

Duration of action Approximately 6 hours.

Diet advice Avoid taking domperidone with grapefruit juice because it may increase the risk of heart rhythm problems.

Storage Keep in original container at room temperature out of the reach of children. Protect from light.

Missed dose If your next dose is due within 4 hours, take a single dose now and skip the next. Then return to normal dose schedule.

Stopping the drug Can be stopped when you no longer need it.

Exceeding the dose An occasional unintentional extra dose is unlikely to cause problems, but large overdoses may cause dizziness. Notify your doctor.

POSSIBLE ADVERSE EFFECTS

Adverse effects are rare but may include breast enlargement or milk secretion, muscle spasms, tremors, reduced libido, and a rash. Consult your doctor if any of these effects occur. Rarely, it may cause an irregular heartbeat or fainting; if either of these occur, stop taking the drug and seek immediate medical attention.

INTERACTIONS

Anticholinergic drugs These may reduce the beneficial effects of domperidone.

Opioid analgesics These may reduce the beneficial effects of domperidone.

Bromocriptine and cabergoline Domperidone may reduce these drugs' effects in some users.
Ketoconazole and erythromycin These drugs should not be taken while also taking domperidone as the combination increases the risk of heart rhythm problems.

SPECIAL PRECAUTIONS
Be sure to consult your doctor or pharmacist before taking this drug if:
- ◆ You have a long-term kidney problem or liver disease.
- ◆ You have thyroid disease.
- ◆ You have a pituitary tumour.
- ◆ You are taking other medicines.

Pregnancy Safety in pregnancy not established. Discuss with your doctor.
Breast-feeding The drug may pass into breast milk, but normal doses are unlikely to affect the baby adversely. Discuss with your doctor.
Infants and children Do not use in children under 16 years, except on a doctor's advice.
Over 60 Reduced dose may be necessary.
Driving and hazardous work No special problems.
Alcohol No special problems, but alcohol is best avoided in cases of nausea and vomiting.

PROLONGED USE
Treatment should be reviewed after 1 week and the need for continued treatment reassessed. In people with heart disease, there is a small increased risk of collapse or sudden death.

DONEPEZIL

Brand names Aricept, Aricept Evess
Used in the following combined preparations None

QUICK REFERENCE
Drug group Drug for dementia (p.17)
Overdose danger rating Medium
Dependence rating Low
Prescription needed Yes
Available as generic Yes

GENERAL INFORMATION
Donepezil is an inhibitor of the enzyme acetylcholinesterase. This enzyme breaks down the neurotransmitter acetylcholine (see p.7) to limit its effects. Blocking the enzyme raises levels of acetylcholine; in the brain, this increases awareness and memory. Donepezil has been found to improve the symptoms of dementia in mild to moderate Alzheimer's disease and is used to slow the deterioration. It is not currently recommended for dementia due to other causes. Treatment is initiated under specialist supervision. Those being treated are usually assessed at 6-monthly intervals to decide whether the drug is helping.

Side effects may include bladder outflow obstruction and psychiatric problems, such as agitation and aggression, that may be due to the disease itself.

INFORMATION FOR USERS
Your drug prescription is tailored for you. Do not alter dosage without checking with your doctor.
How taken/used Tablets, dispersible tablets, liquid.
Frequency and timing of doses Once daily at bedtime.
Adult dosage range 5–10mg.
Onset of effect 1 hour. Full effects may take up to 3 months.
Duration of action Usually 1–2 days.
Diet advice None.
Storage Keep in original container at room temperature out of the reach of children.
Missed dose Take as soon as you remember. A carer should ensure that the maximum dose taken in 24 hours does not exceed 10mg.
Stopping the drug Do not stop without consulting your doctor; symptoms may recur.
Exceeding the dose An occasional unintentional extra dose is unlikely to be a cause for concern. But if you notice any unusual symptoms, or if a large overdose has been taken, tell your doctor.

POSSIBLE ADVERSE EFFECTS
Adverse effects include such problems as accidents and falls, which are common in people with dementia, even those not being treated. Other side effects include nausea, vomiting, diarrhoea, fatigue, insomnia, muscle cramps, and headache. Consult your doctor if any of these are severe. You should also consult your doctor if you experience urinary incontinence or difficulty in passing urine, fainting, dizziness, or palpitations. If you have seizures, stop taking the drug and seek urgent medical help.

INTERACTIONS
Muscle relaxants used in surgery Donepezil may increase the effect of some muscle relaxants, but it may also block some others.

Fluoxetine, erythromycin, and ketoconazole can increase levels and adverse effects of donepezil.

SPECIAL PRECAUTIONS

Be sure to tell your doctor if:

- You have liver or kidney problems.
- You have a heart problem.
- You have asthma or respiratory problems.
- You have had a gastric or duodenal ulcer.
- You are taking a non-steroidal anti-inflammatory drug (NSAID) regularly.
- You are taking other medicines.

Pregnancy Not recommended. Safety in pregnancy not established.
Breast-feeding Not recommended.
Infants and children Not recommended.
Over 60 Treatment may have to be stopped if you develop low heart rate, heart block, or unexplained fainting.
Driving and hazardous work Your underlying condition may make such activities inadvisable. Discuss with your doctor.
Alcohol Avoid. Alcohol may reduce the effect of donepezil.
Surgery and general anaesthetics Treatment with donepezil may need to be stopped before you have a general anaesthetic. Discuss this with your doctor or dentist before any operation.

PROLONGED USE

May be continued for as long as there is benefit. Stopping the drug leads to a gradual loss of the improvements over several weeks.
Monitoring Periodic checks should be carried out at 6-monthly intervals to test whether the drug is still providing some benefit.

DORZOLAMIDE

Brand name Eydelto, Trusopt
Used in the following combined preparation Cosopt, Eylamdo, Tidomat

QUICK REFERENCE

Drug group Drug for glaucoma (p.112)
Overdose danger rating Low
Dependence rating Low
Prescription needed Yes
Available as generic Yes

GENERAL INFORMATION

Dorzolamide is a carbonic anhydrase inhibitor (a kind of diuretic) that is used, in the form of eye drops only, to treat glaucoma. It is also used for ocular hypertension (high pressure inside the eye). The drug relieves the pressure by reducing production of aqueous humour, the fluid in the front chamber of the eye.

The drug may be used either alone or combined with a beta blocker (p.28) by people who are resistant to the effects of beta blockers or for whom beta blockers are not suitable.

Most side effects are local to the eye, but systemic effects may occur if enough of the drug is absorbed by the body. Systemic absorption from eye drops may also result in an increase in the effects of other carbonic acid inhibitors taken orally (such as acetazolamide) if they are used concurrently.

INFORMATION FOR USERS

Your drug prescription is tailored for you. Do not alter dosage without checking with your doctor.
How taken/used Eye drops.
Frequency and timing of doses 3 x daily (on its own); 2 x daily (combined preparation).
Adult dosage range 1 drop in the affected eye(s) or as directed. If using additional eye drops, allow 5 minutes between applying the different types of drop.
Onset of effect 15–30 minutes.
Duration of action 4–8 hours.
Diet advice None.
Storage Keep in original container at room temperature out of the reach of children. Protect from light. Discard eye drops 4 weeks after opening.
Missed dose Use as soon as you remember. If next dose is due, skip the missed dose and then go back to your normal dosing schedule.
Stopping the drug Do not stop the drug without consulting your doctor; symptoms may recur.
Exceeding the dose An occasional unintentional extra application is unlikely to cause problems. Excessive use may provoke side effects as described below.

POSSIBLE ADVERSE EFFECTS

Local side effects include inflammation of the eye surface and the skin of the eyelids, which may lead to burning, stinging, or watery eyes, inflamed or sore eyes, or blurred vision. The drug may also cause a bitter taste in the mouth and headaches. Consult your doctor if any of these become severe. Systemic side effects may also occur but are rare. If you develop an itchy rash, swelling of the lips or tongue, or breathing difficulties, you should stop taking the drug and consult your doctor urgently.

INTERACTIONS

None.

SPECIAL PRECAUTIONS

Be sure to tell your doctor if:

- You have liver or kidney problems.
- You are allergic to sulfonamide drugs.
- You are allergic to benzalkonium chloride.
- You are taking other medicines.

Pregnancy Not prescribed. Discuss with your doctor.
Breast-feeding Not recommended. Discuss with your doctor.
Infants and children Not recommended.
Over 60 No special problems.
Driving and hazardous work Avoid until you have learned how dorzolamide affects you because the drug can affect your vision.
Alcohol No special problems.

PROLONGED USE

Rarely, prolonged use of this drug may lead to development of kidney stones.

DOSULEPIN (DOTHIEPIN)

Brand name Prothiaden
Used in the following combined preparations None

QUICK REFERENCE

Drug group Tricyclic antidepressant drug (p.12)
Overdose danger rating High
Dependence rating Low
Prescription needed Yes
Available as generic Yes

GENERAL INFORMATION

Dosulepin belongs to the tricyclic class of antidepressants and is used in the long-term treatment of depression. It is particularly useful for depression accompanied by anxiety and insomnia. The drug elevates mood, increases physical activity, improves appetite, and restores interest in everyday activities. Taken at night, it encourages sleep and helps eliminate the need for additional sleeping drugs.

Dosulepin takes several weeks to achieve its full antidepressant effect. It has adverse effects common to all of the tricyclics, including a risk of dangerous heart rhythms, seizures, and coma, if taken in overdose. The drug should not be taken by anyone who has a serious heart condition.

INFORMATION FOR USERS

Your drug prescription is tailored for you. Do not alter dosage without checking with your doctor.
How taken/used Tablets, capsules.
Frequency and timing of doses 2–3 x daily or once at night.
Adult dosage range 75–150mg daily (a maximum dose of up to 225mg may be given in some circumstances).
Onset of effect Full antidepressant effect may not be felt for 2–6 weeks, but adverse effects may be noticed within a day or two.
Duration of action Several days.
Diet advice None.
Storage Keep in original container at room temperature out of the reach of children.
Missed dose Take as soon as you remember. If your next dose is due within 2 hours, take a single dose now and skip the next.
Stopping the drug Do not stop taking the drug without consulting your doctor, who may supervise a gradual reduction in dosage. Abrupt cessation may cause withdrawal symptoms and a recurrence of the original problem.

OVERDOSE ACTION

Seek immediate medical advice in all cases. Take emergency action if palpitations or loss of consciousness occur.

POSSIBLE ADVERSE EFFECTS

The adverse effects of dosulepin, such as drowsiness, dry mouth, sweating, and blurred vision, are mainly the result of its anticholinergic action (p.7) and are more common early in treatment. The drug can also affect normal heart rhythm. If blurred vision, dizziness, or fainting occur, consult your doctor. If you have difficulty in passing urine or palpitations, stop the drug and call your doctor urgently.

INTERACTIONS

Antiarrhythmics Dosulepin should be avoided in patients on amiodarone, sotalol, and other medications that can affect heart rhythms.
Monoamine oxidase inhibitors (MAOIs) In the rare cases where these drugs are given with dosulepin, serious interactions may occur.

Sedatives All drugs that have a sedative effect on the central nervous system increase the sedative properties of dosulepin.
Anticonvulsant drugs Dosulepin may reduce the effectiveness of these drugs.

SPECIAL PRECAUTIONS

Be sure to tell your doctor if:

- You have heart problems.
- You have had epileptic seizures.
- You have long-term liver or kidney problems.
- You have glaucoma.
- You have had mania or a psychotic illness.
- You are taking other medicines.

Pregnancy Safety in pregnancy not established. Discuss with your doctor.
Breast-feeding The drug passes into the breast milk, but effects on the baby are unlikely. Discuss with your doctor.
Infants and children Not recommended.
Over 60 Greater risk of adverse effects. Reduced dose necessary.
Driving and hazardous work Avoid until you know how dosulepin affects you because the drug can reduce alertness and may cause blurred vision, dizziness, and drowsiness.
Alcohol Avoid. Alcohol may increase the sedative effects of this drug.
Surgery and general anaesthetics Treatment with dosulepin may need to be stopped before you have a general anaesthetic. Discuss this with your doctor or dentist before any operation.

PROLONGED USE

No problems expected.

DOXAZOSIN

Brand names Cardozin, Cardura, Cardura XL, Doxadura, Raporsin, Slocinx XL
Used in the following combined preparations None

QUICK REFERENCE

Drug group Vasodilator (p.30), antihypertensive drug (p.34), and drug for urinary disorders (p.110)
Overdose danger rating Medium
Dependence rating Low
Prescription needed Yes
Available as generic Yes

GENERAL INFORMATION

Doxazosin is an antihypertensive vasodilator drug that relieves hypertension (high blood pressure) by relaxing the muscles in the blood vessel walls. It may be administered together with other antihypertensive drugs, including beta blockers, because its effects on blood pressure are increased when it is combined with most other antihypertensives.

The drug can also be given to men with an enlarged prostate gland. It relaxes the muscles around the prostate gland and bladder exit, making bladder emptying easier. However, this effect may cause incontinence when it is used in women.

Doxazosin may cause dizziness and fainting. Typically, this occurs on standing and may improve with continued use but it may limit the drug's use, especially in older people. It may be better tolerated if it is taken at night.

INFORMATION FOR USERS

Your drug prescription is tailored for you. Do not alter dosage without checking with your doctor.
How taken/used Tablets, modified release (MR) tablets.
Frequency and timing of doses 1–2 x daily.
Adult dosage range *Hypertension* 1mg (starting dose for tablets), increased gradually as necessary up to 16mg; or 4mg (starting dose for MR tablets) increased as necessary to 8mg. *Enlarged prostate* 1mg (starting dose), increased gradually at 1–2-week intervals up to 8mg.
Onset of effect Within 2 hours.
Duration of action 24 hours.
Diet advice None.
Storage Keep in original container at room temperature out of the reach of children.
Missed dose If you forget to take a tablet, skip that dose completely but carry on as normal the following day.
Stopping the drug Do not stop taking the drug without consulting your doctor; stopping the drug may lead to a rise in blood pressure.
Exceeding the dose An occasional unintentional extra dose is unlikely to be a cause for concern. Larger overdoses may cause dizziness or fainting. Notify your doctor.

POSSIBLE ADVERSE EFFECTS

Nausea, weakness, drowsiness, and swollen ankles are common adverse effects of doxazosin, but the main problem is that it may cause dizziness or fainting when you stand up, especially when first using the drug. It may also cause a stuffy or runny nose, headache, sleepiness, and sleep disturbances. Consult your doctor if any of these symptoms are severe, if you develop a rash, or if you are a woman and the drug causes incontinence. Consult your doctor urgently if you experience palpitations or chest pain.

INTERACTIONS

General note Any other drugs that can reduce blood pressure are likely to increase the blood-pressure-lowering effect of doxazosin. These drugs include diuretics, beta blockers, ACE inhibitors, calcium channel blockers, nitrates, some antipsychotics and antidepressants, and drugs for erectile dysfunction (sildenafil and tadalafil).

SPECIAL PRECAUTIONS

Be sure to tell your doctor if:

- ◆ You have long-term liver problems.
- ◆ You have heart problems.
- ◆ You have problems with urinary incontinence.
- ◆ You have attacks of fainting, especially on standing up or while urinating.
- ◆ You have had an allergic reaction to doxazosin in the past.
- ◆ You are due to have cataract surgery or another operation.
- ◆ You are taking other medicines.

Pregnancy Safety in pregnancy not established. Discuss with your doctor.

Breast-feeding Safety not established. The drug passes into the breast milk. Discuss with your doctor.

Infants and children Not recommended.

Over 60 Reduced dose may be necessary. Take extra care when standing up until you have learned how the drug affects you.

Driving and hazardous work Avoid such activities until you have learned how doxazosin affects you because the drug can cause drowsiness, dizziness, and fainting.

Alcohol Avoid excessive amounts. Alcohol may increase some of the adverse effects of doxazosin, such as dizziness, drowsiness, and fainting.

Surgery and general anaesthetics A general anaesthetic may increase the low blood pressure effect of doxazosin.

PROLONGED USE

No known problems.

DOXORUBICIN

Brand names Caelyx, Myocet

Used in the following combined preparations None

QUICK REFERENCE

Drug group Cytotoxic anticancer drug (p.94)

Overdose danger rating Medium

Dependence rating Low

Prescription needed Yes

Available as generic Yes

GENERAL INFORMATION

Doxorubicin is one of the most effective anticancer drugs. It is prescribed to treat a wide variety of cancers, usually in conjunction with other anticancer drugs. It is used in cancer of the lymph nodes (Hodgkin's disease), lung, breast, bladder, stomach, thyroid, and reproductive organs. It is also used to treat Kaposi's sarcoma in AIDS patients.

Nausea and vomiting after injection are the most common side effects. Although unpleasant, they tend to become less severe as the body adjusts to treatment. The drug may stain the urine bright red, but this is not harmful. More seriously, because doxorubicin interferes with the production of blood cells, blood clotting disorders, anaemia, and infections may occur. Hair loss is also a common side effect. Heart rhythm disturbance and heart failure are possible, although less common, dose-dependent effects. The heart failure is usually irreversible and is worsened by trastuzumab (Herceptin). The brand-name drugs Caelyx and Myocet are formulations in which doxorubicin is enclosed in fatty spheres. This makes it more suitable for certain types of cancer, such as AIDS-related Kaposi's sarcoma.

INFORMATION FOR USERS

This drug is given only under medical supervision and is not for self-administration.

How taken/used Injection, bladder instillation.

Frequency and timing of doses Every 1–3 weeks (injection); once a month (bladder instillation).

Adult dosage range Dosage is determined individually according to body height, weight, and response.

Onset of effect Some adverse effects may appear within 1 hour of starting treatment, but full benefits may not be felt for up to 4 weeks.

Duration of action Adverse effects can persist for up to 2 weeks after stopping treatment.
Diet advice None.
Storage Not applicable. The drug is not normally kept in the home.
Missed dose The drug is administered in hospital under close medical supervision. If for some reason you miss your dose, contact your doctor as soon as you can.
Stopping the drug Discuss with your doctor. Stopping the drug prematurely may lead to a worsening of the underlying condition.
Exceeding the dose Unlikely, since treatment is carefully monitored and supervised.

POSSIBLE ADVERSE EFFECTS

Nausea and vomiting are common and generally occur within an hour of injection. Many people also have hair loss, loss of appetite, bruising, and fever. Other effects include diarrhoea, mouth ulcers, skin irritation or ulcers, breathlessness, and palpitations (which may indicate that the drug is adversely affecting the heart). Since doxorubicin is administered under close supervision in hospital, all adverse effects are monitored, but call your doctors promptly if you develop fever, palpitations, or breathlessness.

INTERACTIONS

General note A wide range of drugs can interact with doxorubicin. Consult your doctor or pharmacist before using any other medications.

SPECIAL PRECAUTIONS

Doxorubicin is prescribed only under close medical supervision, taking account of your present condition and medical history. Be sure to tell your doctor if:

- You have heart problems or have had a previous heart attack.
- You have kidney or liver problems.

Pregnancy Not usually prescribed. Doxorubicin may cause birth defects or premature birth. Discuss with your doctor.
Breast-feeding Not advised. The drug passes into the breast milk and may affect the baby adversely. Discuss with your doctor.
Infants and children Reduced dose necessary.
Over 60 Increased risk of adverse effects. Reduced dose may be necessary.
Driving and hazardous work No known problems.
Alcohol No known problems.

PROLONGED USE

Prolonged use of doxorubicin may suppress the activity of the bone marrow, leading to reduced production of all types of blood cell. It may also adversely affect the pumping capacity of the heart.
Monitoring Periodic checks on blood counts and liver function are required. Regular heart examinations are also carried out.

DOXYCYCLINE

Brand names Doxylar, Efracea, Periostat, Vibramycin, Vibramycin-D
Used in the following combined preparations None

QUICK REFERENCE

Drug group Tetracycline antibiotic (p.61)
Overdose danger rating Low
Dependence rating Low
Prescription needed Yes
Available as generic Yes

GENERAL INFORMATION

Doxycycline is a tetracycline antibiotic. It is used to treat infections of the urinary, respiratory, and gastrointestinal tracts. It is also prescribed for some oral and dental infections; sexually transmitted diseases; skin, eye, and prostate infections; acne; and malaria prevention (in some parts of the world, see p.73).

Doxycycline is less likely to cause diarrhoea than other tetracyclines, and milk and food do not significantly impair its absorption. It can therefore be taken with meals to reduce side effects such as nausea or indigestion. It is also safer than most other tetracyclines for people with impaired kidney function. However, like other tetracyclines, it can stain developing teeth and may affect development of bone; it is therefore usually avoided for children under 12 years old and for pregnant women.

INFORMATION FOR USERS

Your drug prescription is tailored for you. Do not alter dosage without checking with your doctor.
How taken/used Tablets, dispersible tablets, capsules.
Frequency and timing of doses 1–2 x daily with plenty of water, or with or after food, in a sitting or standing position, well before going to bed to avoid risk of throat irritation.
Dosage range 100–200mg daily.

Onset of effect 1–12 hours; several weeks (acne).
Duration of action Up to 24 hours; several weeks (acne).
Diet advice None.
Storage Keep in original container at room temperature out of the reach of children.
Missed dose Take as soon as you remember. If your next dose is due within 6 hours, take a single dose now and skip the next.
Stopping the drug Take the full course. Even if you feel better, the original infection may still be present and symptoms may recur if treatment is stopped too soon.
Exceeding the dose An occasional unintentional extra dose is unlikely to be a cause for concern. But if you notice any unusual symptoms, or if a large overdose has been taken, tell your doctor.

POSSIBLE ADVERSE EFFECTS

Adverse effects from doxycycline are rare, although it may cause nausea, vomiting, or diarrhoea. If a rash, itching, or abnormal sensitivity of the skin to light occur, stop taking the drug and talk to your doctor. If you experience headache or visual disturbances, stop the drug and consult your doctor urgently.

INTERACTIONS

Penicillin antibiotics Doxycycline interferes with the antibacterial action of these drugs.
Barbiturates, carbamazepine, and phenytoin All of these drugs reduce the effectiveness of doxycycline. Doxycycline dosage may need to be increased.
Oral contraceptives There is a slight risk of doxycycline reducing the effectiveness of oral contraceptives. Discuss with your doctor.
Oral anticoagulants Doxycycline may increase the anticoagulant action of these drugs.
Antacids and preparations containing iron, calcium, or magnesium may impair absorption of this drug. Do not take within 2–3 hours of doxycycline.
Ciclosporin and lithium Doxycycline may increase levels of these drugs in the blood.
Methotrexate Doxycycline may increase the risk of methotrexate toxicity.

SPECIAL PRECAUTIONS

Be sure to tell your doctor if:
- You have a long-term liver problem.
- You have previously had an allergic reaction to a tetracycline antibiotic.
- You have porphyria.
- You have systemic lupus erythematosus.
- You have myasthenia gravis.
- You have a history of angioedema.
- You are taking other medicines.

Pregnancy Not used in pregnancy. May discolour the teeth of the developing baby.
Breast-feeding The drug passes into the breast milk. It may lead to discoloration of the baby's teeth and may also have other adverse effects. Discuss with your doctor.
Infants and children Not recommended under 12 years. Reduced dose needed for older children.
Over 60 No special problems. Dispersible tablets should be used as they are less likely to cause oesophageal irritation or ulceration.
Driving and hazardous work Avoid if drug causes visual disturbances, such as blurred vision.
Alcohol Excessive amounts may decrease the effectiveness of doxycycline.
Surgery and general anaesthetics Notify your doctor or dentist beforehand that you are taking doxycycline.

PROLONGED USE

Not usually prescribed long term, except for acne and a few other skin conditions including the blistering disorder bullous pemphigoid.

DULAGLUTIDE

Brand names Trulicity
Used in the following combined preparations None

QUICK REFERENCE

Drug group Drug for diabetes (p.80)
Overdose danger rating High
Dependence rating Low
Prescription needed Yes
Available as generic No

GENERAL INFORMATION

Dulaglutide is a long-acting injectable antidiabetic drug used to treat Type 2 diabetes mellitus together with diet, exercise, and weight control. The drug is usually combined with other diabetes medications.

Dulaglutide mimics the action of a hormone called GLP-1, which is produced by the gut and parts of the brain and is involved in regulating blood sugar levels. The drug works by increasing the secretion of insulin in response to high blood sugar levels and lowering the secretion of the hormone glucagon, which leads to a decreased output of glucose from the liver. It also slows emptying of the stomach, so smoothing out the rise in blood sugar after meals. Nausea, vomiting, diarrhoea, and abdominal discomfort are common side effects but often subside within a few weeks.

INFORMATION FOR USERS

Your drug prescription is tailored for you. Do not alter dosage without checking with your doctor.
How taken/used Injection (subcutaneous) in stomach or thigh.
Frequency and timing of doses Once a week.
Dosage range 0.75–1.5mg weekly.
Onset of effect A few days to a few weeks.
Duration of action At least 1 week.
Diet advice An individualized diabetic diet must be followed for the drug to be fully effective.
Storage Store unused injection pens in a refrigerator. After first use a pen may be stored at room temperature for up to 14 days, away from heat and light and out of the reach of children.
Missed dose If 3 days or more until next dose, administer as soon as possible; if less than 3 days, skip missed dose.
Stopping the drug Do not stop the drug without consulting your doctor. Stopping may lead to worsening of the underlying condition.

OVERDOSE ACTION

Seek immediate medical advice. If you have nausea and vomiting and signs of low blood sugar (hunger, anxiety, slurred speech, tremor, cold sweats, blurred vision, headache), eat or drink something sugary. Take emergency action if seizures or unconsciousness occur.

POSSIBLE ADVERSE EFFECTS

Common adverse effects include nausea, vomiting, and diarrhoea; reduced appetite; weight loss; dizziness; headache; fatigue; and low blood sugar. Less commonly, a reaction at the injection site may occur. Consult your doctor if any of these are severe. If you have persistent abdominal pain, or allergic reactions such as wheezing, itchy rash, or swollen face and lips, seek immediate medical help.

INTERACTIONS

General note Many drugs, especially other antidiabetic drugs, may interact with dulaglutide to affect blood sugar levels. The dose of diabetes medication such as insulin and sulfonylureas may have to be reduced. Consult your doctor or pharmacist before taking other drugs.

SPECIAL PRECAUTIONS

Be sure to tell your doctor if:

- You have Type 1 diabetes mellitus.
- You have long-term kidney problems.
- You have stomach or bowel problems.
- You have a history of pancreatitis.
- You have a gallbladder disorder.
- You have a history or family history of medullary thyroid cancer or multiple endocrine neoplasia 2 (MEN 2).
- You are taking other medicines.

Pregnancy Not prescribed. May harm the baby.
Breast-feeding Unknown if the drug passes into breast milk. Not prescribed. May have to switch to insulin.
Infants and children Not usually prescribed.
Over 60 No special problems.
Driving and hazardous work Usually no problem, but be aware of warning signs of low blood sugar and avoid such activities if you have these signs.
Alcohol Avoid. Alcohol may upset diabetic control.

Diabetic ketoacidosis has occurred in patients who had their insulin doses reduced rapidly. This can present as excessive thirst, passing urine more often than normal, excessive tiredness, rapid breathing, nausea and vomiting, and "fruity" smelling breath.

PROLONGED USE

Monitoring Regular monitoring of your diabetes control is necessary. You may also have periodic assessment of your eyes, heart, and kidneys, and of the lipids in your blood.

DYDROGESTERONE

Brand name None
Used in the following combined preparations Femapak, Femoston 1/10 and 2/10, Femoston-conti

QUICK REFERENCE

Drug group Female sex hormone (p.86)
Overdose danger rating Low
Dependence rating Low
Prescription needed Yes
Available as generic No

GENERAL INFORMATION

Dydrogesterone is a synthetic version of the natural female sex hormone progesterone that has more specific hormonal effects and greater potency than progesterone itself. The drug is no longer used alone but is still available together with an oestrogen as part of hormone replacement therapy (HRT) following the menopause. Dydrogesterone is added either to each HRT tablet (continuous combined HRT) or only the tablets taken during the second half of each 28-day cycle (cyclical HRT). Only cyclical HRT produces regular shedding of the lining of the uterus, mimicking a menstrual period. However, both types prevent the risk of endometrial cancer in women on HRT who have an intact uterus. Dydrogesterone with estradiol may also be used to prevent osteoporosis in women with an intact uterus.

INFORMATION FOR USERS

Your drug prescription is tailored for you. Do not alter dosage without checking with your doctor.

How taken/used Tablets.

Frequency and timing of doses Once daily.

Adult dosage range 5–10mg daily in combined preparations.

Onset of effect Beneficial effects of this drug may not be felt for several months.

Duration of action 12–24 hours.

Diet advice None.

Storage Keep in original container at room temperature out of the reach of children. Protect from light.

Missed dose Take as soon as you remember. If your next dose is due within 2 hours, take a single dose now and skip the next.

Stopping the drug Take as soon as you remember. If more than 24 hours have elapsed, do not take the missed tablet and take the next tablet at the normal time. Missed doses may increase the risk of irregular menstrual bleeding or spotting.

Exceeding the dose An occasional unintentional extra dose is unlikely to be a cause for concern. But if you notice any unusual symptoms, or if a large overdose has been taken, notify your doctor.

POSSIBLE ADVERSE EFFECTS

Irregular periods and breakthrough bleeding are the most common adverse effects of this drug. Consult your doctor if these symptoms occur; they may be helped by adjusting the dosage of the drug. Other common adverse effects include swelling of the feet or ankles, rash, and weight gain. More rarely, the drug may cause nausea, vomiting, and breast tenderness. Talk to your doctor if any of these symptoms become severe or if the drug causes headache or dizziness.

INTERACTIONS

Anticonvulsants Some of these may reduce the effect of dydrogesterone, and dydrogesterone may reduce the effect of lamotrigine.

Ciclosporin Dydrogesterone increases the effects of this drug.

St. John's wort may reduce the effect of dydrogesterone.

SPECIAL PRECAUTIONS

Be sure to tell your doctor if:

- You have long-term liver or kidney problems.
- You have heart or circulatory problems, especially a history of venous or pulmonary thrombosis.
- You have diabetes.
- You have high blood pressure.
- You have porphyria.
- You or a family member have had breast cancer.
- You are taking other medicines.

Pregnancy Not used. If you become pregnant, stop taking the drug immediately and contact your doctor.

Breast-feeding Not used.

Infants and children Not prescribed.

Over 60 No special problems.

Driving and hazardous work Avoid until you have learned how dydrogesterone affects you because the drug may rarely cause dizziness.

Alcohol No special problems.

PROLONGED USE

As part of HRT, dydrogesterone is usually only advised for short-term use after the menopause. It is not normally recommended for long-term use or for treating osteoporosis. HRT increases the risk of both venous thrombosis and breast cancer. This risk diminishes after stopping the drug, disappearing entirely after 10 years.

Monitoring Blood-pressure checks and physical examinations, including regular mammograms, may be performed.

EFAVIRENZ

Brand name Sustiva
Used in the following combined preparation Atripla

QUICK REFERENCE

Drug group Drug for HIV and immune deficiency (p.98)
Overdose danger rating Medium
Dependence rating Low
Prescription needed Yes
Available as generic Yes

GENERAL INFORMATION

Efavirenz is a non-nucleoside reverse transcriptase inhibitor, which is a type of antiretroviral drug used to treat HIV infection; it is active against HIV type 1 but not against type 2 (which is rare in the UK). Efavirenz is never used alone but is combined with other antiretrovirals – for example, two nucleoside analogues – to reduce viral replication. The aim of this treatment is to minimize viral damage to the immune system and to make the emergence of drug resistance less likely. Combination antiretroviral therapy (ART) is not a cure for HIV, but if the drugs are taken regularly on a long-term basis, they can reduce the viral load and improve the outlook for the patient. However, the patient remains infectious and will experience a relapse if treatment is stopped.

INFORMATION FOR USERS

Your drug prescription is tailored for you. Do not alter dosage without checking with your doctor.
How taken/used Tablets, capsules, oral solution.
Frequency and timing of doses Once daily, usually at night to minimize adverse effects; best taken on an empty stomach.
Adult dosage range Up to 600mg, according to body weight (tablets/capsules); patients over 3 years: according to body weight (liquid).
Onset of effect 1 hour.
Duration of action 24 hours.
Diet advice None.
Storage Keep in the original container in a cool, dry place out of the reach of children.
Missed dose Take as soon as you remember. If your next dose is due within 2 hours, take a single dose now and skip the next. It is very important not to miss doses on a regular basis as this can lead to the development of drug-resistant HIV.
Stopping the drug Do not stop taking the drug without consulting your doctor. It may be necessary to withdraw all your drugs gradually, starting with efavirenz.
Exceeding the dose An occasional unintentional extra dose is unlikely to cause problems. But if you notice any unusual symptoms, or if a large overdose has been taken, notify your doctor.

POSSIBLE ADVERSE EFFECTS

Gastrointestinal upsets, including nausea, vomiting, and diarrhoea, and a rash are the most common adverse effects. Efavirenz can also cause vivid dreams and changes in sleep patterns, but these tend to wear off with time. If any of these symptoms are severe, or you have mood changes, discuss with your doctor. If a rash develops, call your doctor without delay.

INTERACTIONS

General note A wide range of drugs may interact with efavirenz, causing either an increase in adverse effects or a reduction in the effect of the antiretroviral drugs. Check with your doctor or pharmacist before taking any new drugs, including those from the dentist and supermarket, and herbal medicines.

SPECIAL PRECAUTIONS

Be sure to tell your doctor if:
- You have liver or kidney problems.
- You have lactose or galactose intolerance.
- You have an infection such as hepatitis B or C.
- You are pregnant or planning a pregnancy.
- You have a mental health disorder.
- You have porphyria.
- You have epilepsy.
- You are taking other medicines.

Pregnancy Should not be used in pregnancy except on strict medical advice. Pregnancy should be avoided; use barrier methods of contraception in addition to other methods.
Breast-feeding Safety not established. Breast-feeding is not recommended for HIV-positive mothers as the virus may pass to the baby.
Infants and children Not prescribed to children under 3 years. Reduced dose necessary in older children.
Over 60 Reduced dose may be necessary to minimize adverse effects.
Driving and hazardous work Avoid until you know how efavirenz affects you because the drug can cause dizziness.

Alcohol No known problems, although some people may find the effects of alcohol are more pronounced while taking efavirenz.

PROLONGED USE

No known problems.

Monitoring Your doctor will take regular blood samples to check the drug's effects on the viral load. Blood will also be checked for changes in lipid, cholesterol, and sugar levels.

EMTRICITABINE

Brand name Emtriva

Used in the following combined preparations Atripla, Descovy, Genova, Ictastan, Odefsey, Stribild, Truvada

QUICK REFERENCE

Drug group Drug for HIV and immune deficiency (p.98)

Overdose danger rating Medium

Dependence rating Low

Prescription needed Yes

Available as generic No

GENERAL INFORMATION

Emtricitabine is an antiviral drug used to treat (but not cure) HIV. It is a type of drug known as a nucleoside reverse transcriptase inhibitor, which blocks reverse transcriptase, an enzyme that HIV needs to multiply. Emtricitabine is usually used in combination with other anti-HIV drugs to reduce production of new viruses before the immune system is irreversibly damaged. This combined therapy (antiretroviral therapy, or ART) reduces the viral load in people with HIV but does not completely rid the body of the virus. HIV may still be transmitted to other people, so it is important to continue taking precautions to avoid infecting others.

INFORMATION FOR USERS

Your drug prescription is tailored for you. Do not alter dosage without checking with your doctor.

How taken/used Capsules, oral solution.

Frequency and timing of doses Once daily. Swallow capsules whole with water. If you vomit within 1 hour of a dose, take another one; if you vomit more than 1 hour after a dose, do not take another one.

Adult dosage range *People over 33kg* 200mg daily capsules, or 240ml daily liquid. (Reduced dose for children/people under 33kg. Less frequent doses for those with renal problems.)

Onset of effect May take from many weeks to a year before virus levels reduce significantly.

Duration of action Up to several days.

Diet advice None.

Storage Keep in original container at room temperature and out of the reach of children.

Missed dose Take the missed dose as soon as you remember unless your next dose is due within 12 hours, in which case omit the missed dose and take the next as scheduled.

Stopping the drug Do not stop without consulting your doctor; your condition may worsen.

Exceeding the dose An occasional unintentional extra dose is unlikely to cause problems. However, a large overdose may cause serious side effects; notify your doctor immediately.

POSSIBLE ADVERSE EFFECTS

The most common adverse effects are headache, diarrhoea, nausea, muscle aches, and dizziness; combination therapy may cause rash, darkening of the skin, and redistribution of body fat. Consult your doctor if any of these are severe or if you develop fever, sore throat, tiredness, lethargy, or joint stiffness or pain. If you have rapid breathing or drowsiness, contact your doctor promptly. Long-term use may affect blood sugar and lipid levels and cause bone problems (see Prolonged use).

INTERACTIONS

General note Various drugs that affect the kidneys may affect blood levels of emtricitabine. Discuss with your doctor before taking any other medications.

Lamivudine and zalcitabine should not be used with emtricitabine because all three drugs are chemically similar and there is therefore a risk of increased toxicity.

Orlistat may reduce the absorption of emtricitabine.

SPECIAL PRECAUTIONS

Be sure to tell your doctor if:

- You have kidney or liver disease.
- You have had hepatitis B or C.
- You have diabetes.
- You have a high blood cholesterol level.
- You are or intend to become pregnant.
- You are taking other medicines, especially corticosteroids.

Pregnancy Safety not established. Discuss with your doctor. If you receive nucleoside reverse transcriptase inhibitors in pregnancy, the baby should be monitored during and after birth.

Breast-feeding It is not known if this drug passes into breast milk. However, HIV can be passed to the baby in breast milk so breast-feeding is not recommended.

Infants and children Not recommended under 4 months.

Over 60 No known problems.

Driving and hazardous work Avoid such activities until you have learned how the drug affects you because it may cause dizziness.

Alcohol Avoid. Alcohol increases the risk of developing serious bone problems.

PROLONGED USE

Emtricitabine as part of ART may cause redistribution of body fat and abnormal blood sugar and lipid levels. Rarely, it may also cause bone destruction, especially in the hip.

Monitoring Liver function tests are routine. People being treated for HIV will also have regular checks of blood cell counts (including CD4 counts), viral load, blood sugar and cholesterol levels, and response to treatment.

ENALAPRIL

Brand name Innovace

Used in the following combined preparation Innozide

QUICK REFERENCE

Drug group ACE inhibitor (p.30) and antihypertensive drug (p.34)

Overdose danger rating Medium

Dependence rating Low

Prescription needed Yes

Available as generic Yes

GENERAL INFORMATION

Enalapril belongs to the ACE inhibitor group of vasodilator drugs, which are used to treat hypertension (high blood pressure) and heart failure (reduced ability of the heart to pump blood). It is also given to patients following a heart attack. Enalapril may be given with a diuretic to increase its effect.

The first dose may cause a sudden drop in blood pressure. For this reason, you should be resting at the time and be able to lie down for 2 to 3 hours afterwards. The more common adverse effects (see below) often lessen with long-term treatment or disappear when the drug is stopped. In some cases, they clear up on their own despite continued treatment.

INFORMATION FOR USERS

Your drug prescription is tailored for you. Do not alter dosage without checking with your doctor.

How taken/used Tablets.

Frequency and timing of doses 1–2 x daily.

Adult dosage range 2.5–5mg daily (starting dose), increased to 10–40mg daily (maintenance dose).

Onset of effect 30–60 minutes; full beneficial effect may take several weeks.

Duration of action 24 hours.

Diet advice Your doctor may advise you to reduce your salt intake to help control your blood pressure.

Storage Keep in original container below 25°C, out of the reach of children. Protect from light.

Missed dose Take as soon as you remember. If your next dose is due within 8 hours, take a single dose now and skip the next.

Stopping the drug Do not stop the drug without consulting your doctor; stopping may lead to worsening of the underlying condition.

Exceeding the dose An occasional unintentional extra dose is unlikely to be a cause for concern. Large overdoses may cause dizziness or fainting. Notify your doctor.

POSSIBLE ADVERSE EFFECTS

The more common adverse effects, such as a persistent dry cough, often diminish with long-term treatment. Less common effects, such as dizziness, mouth ulcers or a sore mouth, sore throat, or fever, may also reduce with time, although it may be necessary to adjust the drug dosage. Rashes may occur but usually disappear when the drug is stopped. If you experience any side effects, discuss with your doctor. If you develop swelling of the mouth or lips or breathing difficulty, stop the drug and contact your doctor immediately.

INTERACTIONS

Potassium supplements and potassium-sparing diuretics Enalapril may enhance the effect of these drugs, leading to raised levels of potassium in the blood.

Non-steroidal anti-inflammatory drugs (NSAIDs) Some of these drugs may reduce the effectiveness of enalapril. There is also risk of kidney damage when they are taken with enalapril.

Vasodilators, diuretics, and other antihypertensives These may increase the blood-pressure-lowering effect of enalapril.
Lithium Enalapril increases the levels of lithium in the blood, and serious adverse effects from lithium excess may occur.
Ciclosporin Taken with enalapril, this drug may increase blood levels of potassium.

SPECIAL PRECAUTIONS

Be sure to tell your doctor if:

- You have kidney or liver problems.
- You have heart problems.
- You have had angioedema or a previous allergic reaction to ACE inhibitors.
- You are taking other medicines.
- You are or intend to become pregnant.

Pregnancy Not prescribed. There is evidence of harm to the developing fetus.
Breast-feeding May be used, but there is a risk of low blood pressure in the baby, especially if baby was preterm. Discuss with your doctor.
Infants and children Not recommended.
Over 60 Reduced dose may be necessary.
Driving and hazardous work Avoid until you have learned how enalapril affects you because the drug can cause dizziness and fainting.
Alcohol Avoid. Alcohol may increase the blood-pressure-lowering and adverse effects of the drug.
Surgery and general anaesthetics Enalapril may have to be stopped before you have a general anaesthetic. Discuss with your doctor or dentist before any operation.

PROLONGED USE

No problems expected.
Monitoring Periodic checks on potassium levels, white blood cell count, kidney function, and urine are usually performed.

EPHEDRINE

Brand name None
Used in the following combined preparations None

QUICK REFERENCE

Drug group Bronchodilator (p.21) and decongestant (p.24)
Overdose danger rating Medium
Dependence rating Low
Prescription needed No
Available as generic Yes

GENERAL INFORMATION

Chemically related to amfetamines, ephedrine promotes the release of the neurotransmitter norepinephrine (noradrenaline). It was once widely prescribed to relax constricted muscles around the airways due to asthma, bronchitis, and emphysema but more effective drugs have now replaced it for these purposes. Its main use is as a nasal decongestant. In addition, ephedrine injections may be used to restore normal blood pressure after anaesthesia, especially spinal and epidural anaesthesia.

Adverse effects are unusual from nasal drops used in moderation. However, if the drug is taken by mouth or injection it may stimulate the heart and central nervous system, causing palpitations and anxiety. It is best avoided by people with high blood pressure.

Ephedrine was also widely used in dietary supplements and is present in the Chinese herbal medicine *ma huang*.

INFORMATION FOR USERS

Follow instructions on the label. Call your doctor if symptoms worsen.
How taken/used Tablets, injection, nasal drops.
Frequency and timing of doses *By mouth* 3 x daily. *Nasal drops* 3–4 x daily.
Dosage range *Adults* 45–180mg daily (by mouth); 1–2 drops into each nostril per dose (drops); 3–6mg every 3–4 minutes to a maximum of 30mg (injection). *Children* Reduced dose according to age and weight.
Onset of effect Within 15–60 minutes.
Duration of action 3–6 hours.
Diet advice None.
Storage Keep in original container at room temperature out of the reach of children. Protect from light.
Missed dose Do not take the missed dose. Take your next dose as usual.
Stopping the drug Can be safely stopped as soon as you no longer need it.
Exceeding the dose An occasional unintentional extra dose is unlikely to cause problems. Large overdoses may cause shortness of breath, high fever, seizures, or loss of consciousness. Notify your doctor immediately.

POSSIBLE ADVERSE EFFECTS

Adverse effects from ephedrine nasal drops are uncommon, although local irritation may occur. When taken by mouth, the drug may affect the central nervous system, causing anxiety, restlessness, and insomnia. Taking the last dose before 4pm may help to prevent insomnia. Other adverse effects include cold hands and feet, dry mouth, tremor, and urinary difficulties; discuss with your doctor in all cases of urinary difficulties or if these other symptoms are severe. Ephedrine may also affect the cardiovascular system, causing palpitations or chest pain; if these occur, stop taking the drug and seek urgent medical advice. Long-term use may cause other problems and is not advised (see Prolonged use).

INTERACTIONS

Monoamine oxidase inhibitors (MAOIs) Ephedrine may interact with these drugs to cause a dangerous rise in blood pressure.

Beta blockers may interact with ephedrine to cause a dangerous rise in blood pressure.

Antihypertensive drugs Ephedrine may counteract the effects of some antihypertensive drugs.

Theophylline taken with ephedrine can lower potassium levels in children. The two drugs should not be given together.

SPECIAL PRECAUTIONS

Be sure to tell your doctor or pharmacist before taking this drug if:

- You have a long-term kidney problem.
- You have heart disease.
- You have high blood pressure.
- You have diabetes.
- You have an overactive thyroid gland.
- You have had glaucoma.
- You have urinary difficulties.
- You are taking other medicines, especially an MAOI antidepressant (see p.12).

Pregnancy Safety in pregnancy not established. Discuss with your doctor.

Breast-feeding Passes into breast milk and may affect the baby. Discuss with your doctor.

Infants and children Not recommended under 6 years. Should only be used in children 6–12 years under medical supervision.

Over 60 Not usually prescribed.

Driving and hazardous work Avoid until you have learned how ephedrine affects you. No special problems with nasal drops.

Alcohol No special problems.

Surgery and general anaesthetics May need to be stopped before you have a general anaesthetic. Discuss with doctor or dentist before surgery.

PROLONGED USE

Prolonged use is not recommended. Excessive use in nasal drops leads to reduced decongestant effects and rebound congestion when the drug is stopped. Long-term use of ephedrine-containing herbal preparations is associated with stroke.

EPINEPHRINE (ADRENALINE)

Brand names Emerade, EpiPen, Jext

Used in the following combined preparation Several local anaesthetics (e.g. bupivacaine and xylocaine)

QUICK REFERENCE

Drug group Drug for cardiac resuscitation and anaphylaxis

Overdose danger rating High

Dependence rating Low

Prescription needed Yes

Available as generic Yes

GENERAL INFORMATION

Epinephrine is a neurotransmitter (p.7) that is produced in the centre (medulla) of the adrenal glands – hence its original name, adrenaline. Synthetic epinephrine is given in an emergency to stimulate heart activity and raise low blood pressure. It also narrows blood vessels in the skin and intestine.

Epinephrine is injected to counteract cardiac arrest, or to relieve severe allergic reactions (anaphylaxis) to drugs, food, or insect stings. For patients who are at risk of anaphylactic shock, it is provided as a pre-filled syringe for immediate self-injection into a muscle at the start of an attack.

Because it constricts blood vessels, epinephrine is used in preparations of local anaesthetics to slow dispersal of the drug through the body and thereby prolong its effect.

INFORMATION FOR USERS

Your drug prescription is tailored for you. Do not alter dosage without checking with your doctor.

How taken/used *Self-administration* Injection into thigh muscle. *Cardiac arrest* Injection into vein.

Frequency and timing of doses *Self-administration* As directed, in emergency.

Dosage range *Pre-filled syringe (e.g. EpiPen)* Usually 300 mcg. *Hospital* 500mcg ampoules.

Onset of effect Within 5 minutes.
Duration of action Up to 4 hours.
Diet advice None.
Storage Keep in original container at room temperature out of the reach of children. Protect from light.
Missed dose Not applicable. By itself, the drug is used for one-off emergencies.
Stopping the drug Not applicable. By itself, the drug is used for one-off emergencies.

OVERDOSE ACTION

Seek immediate medical advice in all cases. Take emergency action if palpitations, breathing difficulties, or loss of consciousness occur.

POSSIBLE ADVERSE EFFECTS

The principal adverse effects of epinephrine are related to its stimulant action on the heart and central nervous system. Dry mouth, nervousness, restlessness, nausea, vomiting, cold hands and feet, palpitations, headache, and blurred vision are common. As epinephrine by itself is used in emergencies, medical help should always be sought after its use.

INTERACTIONS

General note Epinephrine may interact with a wide variety of drugs, including monoamine oxidase inhibitors (MAOIs; see p.12); tricyclic antidepressants such as amitriptyline; some beta blockers, such as propranolol; and antidiabetic drugs. However, because epinephrine is usually used only to treat life-threatening medical emergencies, possible drug interactions are usually of secondary importance.

SPECIAL PRECAUTIONS

Be sure to tell your doctor if:
- You have a heart problem.
- You have an overactive thyroid gland.
- You have high blood pressure.
- You are taking other medications, especially a beta blocker.

Pregnancy Discuss with your doctor. Although it may cause defects in the fetus and prolong labour, epinephrine by itself is used only for medical emergencies and may be life-saving.
Breast-feeding Adverse effects on the baby are unlikely. Discuss with your doctor.
Infants and children Reduced dose necessary.
Over 60 Increased likelihood of adverse effects. Reduced dose may therefore be necessary.
Driving and hazardous work Not applicable. By itself, the drug is used for one-off emergencies.
Alcohol No known problems.
Surgery and general anaesthetics Epinephrine may interact with some general anaesthetics. If you have used or been treated with epinephrine within the past 24 hours, discuss this with your doctor or dentist before surgery.

PROLONGED USE

Epinephrine is not normally used long term.

ERGOTAMINE

Brand names None
Used in the following combined preparations
Cafergot, Migril

QUICK REFERENCE

Drug group Drug for migraine (p.18)
Overdose danger rating Medium
Dependence rating Medium
Prescription needed Yes
Available as generic Yes

GENERAL INFORMATION

Ergotamine is used to treat migraine attacks, but it has largely been superseded by newer agents with fewer adverse effects. It may also be used to prevent or treat cluster headaches. For migraine, its use should be restricted to occasions when other treatments are ineffective, and it should be taken only at the first sign of migraine (the "aura"); later use may be ineffective and cause stomach upset. Ergotamine causes temporary narrowing of blood vessels, so it should not be used by people with poor circulation. If taken too often, it can dangerously reduce circulation to the hands and feet (ergotism); it should never be taken regularly. Frequent migraine attacks may indicate the need for a drug to prevent migraine.

INFORMATION FOR USERS

Your drug prescription is tailored for you. Do not alter dosage without checking with your doctor.
How taken/used Tablets, suppositories.
Frequency and timing of doses Once at the onset, repeated if needed after 30 minutes (tablets) up to the maximum dose (see below).
Adult dosage range Varies according to product. Generally, 1–2mg per dose. Take no more than 4mg in 24 hours or 8mg in 1 week. Treatment

should not be repeated within 4 days or more than twice a month.

Onset of effect 15–30 minutes.

Duration of action Up to 24 hours.

Diet advice Changes in diet are unlikely to affect the action of this drug, but certain foods may provoke migraine attacks in some people.

Storage Keep in original container at room temperature out of the reach of children. Protect from light.

Missed dose Regular doses of this drug are not necessary and may be dangerous. Take only when you have symptoms of migraine.

Stopping the drug Can be safely stopped as soon as you no longer need it.

Exceeding the dose An occasional unintentional extra dose is unlikely to cause problems. Large overdoses may cause vomiting, thirst, diarrhoea, dizziness, seizures, or coma. Notify your doctor immediately.

POSSIBLE ADVERSE EFFECTS

Digestive disturbances, abdominal pain, muscle cramps, and nausea and vomiting (for which an anti-emetic may be given) are common with ergotamine. Consult your doctor if any of these symptoms are severe or if you experience dizziness, muscle pain or stiffness, or severe diarrhoea. Cold or numb fingers and toes are rare but serious side effects that may result from arterial spasm. If these symptoms occur or if you experience chest pain, leg pain, or groin pain, stop taking the drug and seek immediate medical advice.

INTERACTIONS

Beta blockers These drugs may increase circulatory problems with ergotamine.

Sumatriptan and related drugs Increased risk of adverse effects on the blood circulation if ergotamine is used with these drugs.

Erythromycin and related antibiotics and antivirals taken with ergotamine increase the likelihood of adverse effects.

Oral contraceptives There is an increased risk of blood clotting in women taking these drugs with ergotamine.

SPECIAL PRECAUTIONS

Be sure to tell your doctor if:

- You have long-term liver or kidney problems.
- You have heart problems.
- You have poor circulation.
- You have high blood pressure.
- You have had a recent stroke.
- You have an overactive thyroid gland.
- You have anaemia.
- You are taking other medicines.

Pregnancy Not prescribed. Ergotamine can cause contractions of the uterus.

Breast-feeding Not recommended. The drug passes into the breast milk and may have adverse effects on the baby. It may also reduce your milk supply.

Infants and children Not usually prescribed.

Over 60 Not recommended. May aggravate existing heart or circulatory problems.

Driving and hazardous work Avoid until you have learned how ergotamine affects you because the drug can cause dizziness.

Alcohol No special problems, but some spirits may provoke migraine in some people.

Surgery and general anaesthetics Notify your doctor if you have used ergotamine within 48 hours prior to surgery.

PROLONGED USE

Reduced circulation to the hands and feet may result if doses near to the maximum are taken for too long. Never exceed the recommended dosage and length of treatment. Rebound headache may occur if the drug is taken too frequently. Cardiovascular complications, such as heart rhythm problems or problems with the heart valves or coronary blood vessels, may also develop with prolonged use.

ERYTHROMYCIN

Brand names Erythrocin, Erythrolar, Erythroped

Used in the following combined preparations Aknemycin Plus, Isotrexin, Zineryt

QUICK REFERENCE

Drug group Antibiotic (p.60)

Overdose danger rating Low

Dependence rating Low

Prescription needed Yes

Available as generic Yes

GENERAL INFORMATION

One of the safest and most widely used antibiotics, erythromycin is effective against many bacteria. It is commonly used as an alternative in people who are allergic to penicillin and related antibiotics.

Erythromycin is used to treat throat, middle ear, and chest infections (including some rare types of pneumonia, such as Legionnaires' disease). It is also used for sexually transmitted diseases such as chlamydial infections, and in some forms of gastroenteritis. Erythromycin may be included as part of the treatment for diphtheria. It is sometimes given to treat pertussis (whooping cough) and reduce the likelihood of infecting others with this disease. Oral administration or topical application is sometimes helpful in treating acne.

When taken by mouth, erythromycin may sometimes cause nausea and vomiting or rash, and may pose a rare risk of liver disorders.

INFORMATION FOR USERS

Your drug prescription is tailored for you. Do not alter dosage without consulting your doctor.

How taken/used Tablets, capsules, gastro-resistant (GR) capsules, liquid, injection, topical solution.

Frequency and timing of doses Every 6–12 hours before or with meals.

Dosage range 1–4g daily.

Onset of effect 1–4 hours.

Duration of action 6–12 hours.

Diet advice None.

Storage Keep in original container at room temperature out of the reach of children.

Missed dose Take as soon as you remember. If your next dose is due within 2 hours, take a single dose now and skip the next.

Stopping the drug Take the full course. Even if you feel better, the original infection may still be present and symptoms may recur if treatment is stopped too soon.

Exceeding the dose An occasional unintentional extra dose is unlikely to be a cause for concern. But if you notice any unusual symptoms, or if a large overdose has been taken, tell your doctor.

POSSIBLE ADVERSE EFFECTS

Nausea and vomiting are common adverse effects and most likely with large doses taken by mouth. Diarrhoea is also common. Consult your doctor if these are severe. Deafness may rarely occur with high doses; if you develop impaired hearing, consult your doctor without delay. Symptoms such as rash, itching, skin blisters or ulcers, jaundice, or fever may also occur. If you develop any of these, stop taking the drug and consult your doctor immediately.

INTERACTIONS

General note Erythromycin interacts with a number of other drugs, particularly:

Mizolastine Erythromycin increases the risk of adverse effects on the heart with this drug.

Warfarin Erythromycin increases the risk of bleeding with warfarin.

Ergotamine Erythromycin increases the risk of side effects with this drug.

Carbamazepine, digoxin, and some immunosuppressants Erythromycin may increase blood levels of these drugs.

Theophylline/aminophylline Erythromycin increases the risk of adverse effects with these drugs.

Simvastatin and other statins Erythromycin should not be used with simvastatin; increased risk of muscle aches with other statins.

SPECIAL PRECAUTIONS

Be sure to tell your doctor if:

- You have a long-term liver problem.
- You have had a previous allergic reaction to erythromycin.
- You have porphyria.
- You have myasthenia gravis.
- You are taking other medicines.

Pregnancy No evidence of risk to the developing fetus. Discuss with your doctor.

Breast-feeding Passes into breast milk. Drug should be avoided in newborns under 2 weeks old, but at normal doses adverse effects on the baby are unlikely. Discuss with your doctor.

Infants and children Reduced dose necessary.

Over 60 No special problems.

Driving and hazardous work No known problems.

Alcohol No known problems.

PROLONGED USE

Oral courses of longer than 14 days may increase the risk of liver damage.

ERYTHROPOIETIN

Brand names Aranesp, Binocrit, Eprex, Mircera, NeoRecormon, Retacrit

Used in the following combined preparations None

QUICK REFERENCE

Drug group Kidney hormone (p.78)

Overdose danger rating Low

Dependence rating Low

Prescription needed Yes

Available as generic No

GENERAL INFORMATION

Erythropoietin is a naturally occurring hormone produced by the kidneys; it stimulates the body to produce red blood cells. In medicine, artificially produced erythropoietin is used to treat anaemia associated with chronic kidney disease, and with certain cancer treatments and certain dysfunctions of the bone marrow. It is also used to boost the level of red blood cells before surgery. In addition, it may be used as an alternative to blood transfusions in major orthopaedic (bone) surgery.

Erythropoietin has been used by athletes to enhance their performance. However, this is not a recognized use and the drug is banned by sport governing bodies.

The drug may worsen hypertension (high blood pressure), and blood pressure should therefore be monitored during treatment.

INFORMATION FOR USERS

Your drug prescription is tailored for you. Do not alter dosage without checking with your doctor.

How taken/used Injection.

Frequency and timing of doses 1–3 x weekly, depending on product and disorder.

Dosage range Dosage is calculated on an individual basis according to body weight. The dosage also varies depending on the product and the condition being treated.

Onset of effect Active in body within 4 hours, but effects may not be noted for 2–3 months.

Duration of action Some effects may persist for several days.

Diet advice None. However, if you have kidney failure, you may have to follow a special diet.

Storage Store at 2–8°C, out of the reach of children. Do not freeze or shake. Protect from light.

Missed dose Do not make up any missed doses.

Stopping the drug Discuss with your doctor.

Exceeding the dose A single excessive dose is unlikely to be a cause for concern, but too high a dose over a long period can increase the likelihood of adverse effects.

POSSIBLE ADVERSE EFFECTS

The most common effects are raised blood pressure and problems at the injection site. More rarely there may be flulike symptoms, bone pain, chest pain, swelling in one leg, seizures, rash, or a stabbing headache. Discuss all such symptoms with your doctor immediately, especially seizures or stabbing headache.

INTERACTIONS

Ciclosporin Erythropoietin may affect the blood level of ciclosporin; ciclosporin blood levels should therefore be monitored more often when erythropoietin treatment starts.

SPECIAL PRECAUTIONS

Be sure to tell your doctor if:

- You have high blood pressure.
- You have a long-term liver problem.
- You have previously had allergic reactions to any drugs.
- You have peripheral vascular disease.
- You have had epileptic fits.
- You are taking other medicines.

Pregnancy Not usually prescribed. Safety in pregnancy not established. Discuss with your doctor.

Breast-feeding Safety not established. Discuss with your doctor.

Infants and children Reduced dose necessary.

Over 60 No known problems.

Driving and hazardous work Not applicable.

Alcohol Follow your doctor's advice.

PROLONGED USE

If the level of anaemia is overcorrected, there is an increased risk of thrombosis. This is potentially fatal, hence the need for careful monitoring. Prolonged use of erythropoietin may also reduce the chance of survival in some patients with cancer.

Monitoring Regular blood tests to monitor blood composition, and blood pressure monitoring, are required.

ESTRADIOL

Brand names Climaval, Elleste, Estraderm, FemSeven, Oestrogel, Progynova, Zumenon, and others

Used in the following combined preparations Angeliq, Climesse, Trisequens, and others

QUICK REFERENCE

Drug group Female sex hormone (p.86)

Overdose danger rating Low

Dependence rating Low

Prescription needed Yes

Available as generic Yes

GENERAL INFORMATION

Estradiol is a natural oestrogen (female sex hormone). It is used mainly as hormone replacement therapy (HRT) for menopausal and post-menopausal symptoms (see p.87). The drug is often given with a progestogen, either separately or as a combined product. Estradiol alone is associated with an increased risk of cancer of the uterus, but combining it with a progestogen reduces the risk; it is usually used alone only in women who have had a hysterectomy. HRT is usually only advised for short-term use around the menopause or in women with premature failure of the ovaries.

Estradiol may help to prevent osteoporosis in women at high risk of fractures who are intolerant of other medication.

INFORMATION FOR USERS

Your drug prescription is tailored for you. Do not alter dosage without checking with your doctor.

How taken/used Tablets, implants, pessaries, vaginal rings, skin gel, patches.

Frequency and timing of doses Once daily (tablets, gel); every 1–7 days (skin patches); every 4–8 months (implants); every 1–7 days (pessaries); every 3 months (vaginal ring).

Adult dosage range 1–2mg daily (tablets); as per instructions (skin gel); 25–100mcg daily (skin patches); 25–100mg per dose (implants); 25mcg per dose (pessaries); 7.5mcg daily (vaginal ring).

Onset of effect 10–20 days.

Duration of action Up to 24 hours; some effects may be longer lasting.

Diet advice None.

Storage Keep in original container at room temperature out of the reach of children.

Missed dose Take as soon as you remember. If next daily treatment is due within 4 hours, take a single dose now and skip the next.

Stopping the drug Do not stop the drug without consulting your doctor; symptoms may recur.

Exceeding the dose An occasional unintentional extra dose is unlikely to be a cause for concern. But if you notice any unusual symptoms, or if a large overdose has been taken, tell your doctor.

POSSIBLE ADVERSE EFFECTS

The most common adverse effects are similar to symptoms of early pregnancy and generally lessen with time. They include nausea, vomiting, abdominal pain, tender or swollen breasts, weight gain or fluctuations, fluid retention, and swollen legs. Headaches, depression, or mood alterations may also occur. Discuss with your doctor if you experience breast symptoms, depression, or mood alterations or if any of the other symptoms are severe. Sudden, sharp pain in the chest, groin, or legs may indicate a blood clot; if this occurs, stop taking the drug and seek urgent medical help.

INTERACTIONS

Tobacco smoking increases the risk of heart and circulatory damage with estradiol.

Anticonvulsants The effects of estradiol are reduced by topiramate, carbamazepine, phenytoin, and phenobarbital; estradiol reduces the effects of lamotrigine.

Anticoagulants Effects are reduced by estradiol.

St John's wort and rifampicin may reduce the effects of estradiol.

Lenalidomide and tranexamic acid may increase the risk of blood clots with estradiol.

Thyroxine If taken with estradiol, the dose may need to be adjusted.

SPECIAL PRECAUTIONS

Be sure to tell your doctor if:

◆ You have a long-term liver problem, gallstones, or raised blood triglycerides.

◆ You have hypertension, or heart or circulation problems.

◆ You have a personal or family history of blood clots or stroke.

◆ You have diabetes, porphyria, or lupus erythematosus.

◆ You have breast cancer or abnormal vaginal bleeding.

◆ You are a smoker.

◆ You have migraine or epilepsy.

◆ You are taking other medicines.

Pregnancy Not prescribed.

Breast-feeding Not prescribed. The drug passes into breast milk. Discuss with your doctor.

Infants and children Not usually prescribed.

Over 60 No special problems.

Driving and hazardous work No problems expected.

Alcohol No known problems.

Surgery and general anaesthetics You may need to stop estradiol before having major surgery. Discuss this with your doctor.

PROLONGED USE

As part of HRT, estradiol is usually only advised for short-term use around the menopause and is not normally recommended for

long-term use or for treatment of osteoporosis. Long-term use increases the risk of breast, uterine, and ovarian cancer, venous thrombosis, heart attack, and stroke.
Monitoring Blood pressure checks and physical examinations, including regular mammograms, may be performed.

ETANERCEPT

Brand name Benepali, Enbrel, Erelzi
Used in the following combined preparations None

QUICK REFERENCE

Drug group Drug for psoriasis (p.122) and disease-modifying antirheumatic drug (p.49)
Overdose danger rating Low
Dependence rating Low
Prescription needed Yes
Available as generic No

GENERAL INFORMATION

Etanercept is a synthetic protein. One part acts like an antibody (see p.56) and the other part blocks a molecule called tumour necrosis factor (TNF); in this way it alters the functioning of the immune system. As a result, etanercept reduces inflammation and improves the course of diseases such as psoriasis and rheumatological conditions including rheumatoid arthritis and juvenile idiopathic arthritis. It is given by injection once or twice weekly. The injections are often given in hospital initially but can be self-administered after you have been trained how to use them yourself.

Like many drugs that alter the immune system, etanercept increases the risk of infections, from common colds and flu to more unusual ones like tuberculosis. In addition, there may be a slightly higher risk of immune system cancers and skin cancer, but these risks have to be balanced against the benefits from the treatments.

INFORMATION FOR USERS

This drug is usually given under medical supervision. If you need to administer it yourself at home, you will be taught how to do so.
How taken/used Subcutaneous injection.
Frequency and timing of doses 1–2 x weekly.
Adult dosage range 25–50mg weekly for up to 24 weeks.
Onset of effect 12–24 hours. Full beneficial effect may take several weeks.
Duration of action 2–8 weeks.
Diet advice None.
Storage Store in a refrigerator (2–8°C). Do not freeze. Keep the pre-filled pens in the outer carton to protect the drug from light. If you need to keep the drug at home, you will be instructed about its storage.
Missed dose If you are using the drug at home and forget a dose, inject it as soon as you remember, unless the next scheduled dose is the next day, in which case you should skip the missed dose, then take the next on the usual day(s). Do not take a double dose on the same day to make up for a missed dose. If you are having the drug in hospital and miss your dose, contact your doctor as soon as possible.
Stopping the drug Discuss with your doctor. Stopping the drug prematurely may lead to worsening of the underlying condition.
Exceeding the dose Overdosage is unlikely since treatment is closely monitored and supervised. If you think you have received an overdose, tell your doctor as soon as possible.

POSSIBLE ADVERSE EFFECTS

The main side effects at the start of treatment are injection site reactions, such as bruising, redness, and itching; discuss any severe reaction with your doctor. Contact your doctor if you have fever or headache. If you develop wheezing or tight chest, rash or itching, sore throat, spontaneous bleeding, or easy bruising, stop the drug and call your doctor immediately.

INTERACTIONS

Anakinra and abatacept should not be used together with etanercept because there is an increased risk of side effects.
Vaccines Effectiveness of some vaccines may be reduced by etanercept. Live vaccines must not be given during a course of etanercept.

SPECIAL PRECAUTIONS

Be sure to tell your doctor if:
- You have had or been exposed to chickenpox, shingles, hepatitis B or C, or tuberculosis.
- You have signs of infection (e.g. fever, shivering).
- You have liver or kidney problems.
- You have recently had, or are scheduled to have, a vaccination.
- You have a central nervous system disorder, such as multiple sclerosis.

◆ You have heart problems.
◆ You have diabetes.
◆ You are taking other medicines.

Pregnancy Not recommended. Women of childbearing age should avoid becoming pregnant. Discuss with your doctor.
Breast-feeding Not recommended. Discuss with your doctor.
Infants and children Reduced dose necessary.
Over 60 No special problems.
Driving and hazardous work Avoid until you have learned how etanercept affects you.
Alcohol No special problems.

PROLONGED USE

There is an increased risk of infections and of some cancers, particularly skin cancers, following etanercept treatment.
Monitoring Periodic blood tests will be carried out to monitor response to treatment. Body temperature, heart rate, and blood pressure may be monitored when you start the drug.

ETHAMBUTOL

Brand name Myambutol
Used in the following combined preparations Rimstar, Voractiv

QUICK REFERENCE

Drug group Antituberculous drug (p.65)
Overdose danger rating Medium
Dependence rating Low
Prescription needed Yes
Available as generic Yes

GENERAL INFORMATION

Ethambutol is an antibiotic used in treating tuberculosis. It is combined with other antituberculous drugs to enhance its effect and reduce the risk of the infection becoming drug resistant. It is not used in all cases of tuberculosis, but is more likely to be used in people with a history of tuberculosis; those with a low immune status; and those whose infection may be caused by a resistant organism.

Although ethambutol has few common adverse effects, it may occasionally cause optic neuritis, a type of eye damage leading to blurring and fading of vision. As a result, it is not usually prescribed for children under 6 years of age or for other patients who cannot communicate their symptoms adequately. Before starting treatment, a full ophthalmic examination is recommended.

INFORMATION FOR USERS

Your drug prescription is tailored for you. Do not alter dosage without checking with your doctor.
How taken/used Tablets.
Frequency and timing of doses Once daily.
Adult dosage range According to body weight.
Onset of effect It may take several days for symptoms to improve.
Duration of action Up to 24 hours.
Diet advice None.
Storage Keep in original container at room temperature out of the reach of children.
Missed dose Take as soon as you remember. If your next dose is due within 6 hours, take a single dose now and skip the next.
Stopping the drug Take the full course. Even if you feel better the original infection may still be present and may recur if treatment is stopped too soon.
Exceeding the dose An occasional unintentional extra dose is unlikely to cause problems. Large overdoses may cause headache and abdominal pain. Notify your doctor.

POSSIBLE ADVERSE EFFECTS

Side effects are uncommon but are more likely after prolonged treatment with high doses. They include nausea, vomiting, and dizziness; discuss with your doctor if these are severe, or if you develop numbness or tingling in the hands or feet. If a rash or itching develops, stop taking the drug and consult your doctor. If you develop blurred vision, eye pain, or loss of colour vision, stop taking the drug and seek prompt medical attention.

INTERACTIONS

Antacids Those containing aluminium salts may decrease levels of ethambutol and should be taken at least 2 hours before ethambutol or 4 hours afterwards.

SPECIAL PRECAUTIONS

Be sure to tell your doctor if:
◆ You have a kidney problem.
◆ You have cataracts or other eye problems.
◆ You have gout.
◆ You have had a previous allergic reaction to this drug.
◆ You are taking other medicines.

Pregnancy No evidence of risk. Discuss with your doctor.
Breast-feeding The drug passes into the breast milk, but normal doses are unlikely to affect the baby adversely. Discuss with your doctor.
Infants and children Not generally prescribed under 6 years unless the child can reliably report any vision changes.
Over 60 Increased risk of adverse effects. Reduced dose may therefore be necessary.
Driving and hazardous work Avoid until you have learned how ethambutol affects you because the drug may cause dizziness.
Alcohol No known problems.

PROLONGED USE

Prolonged use of this drug may increase the risk of eye damage.
Monitoring Regular eye tests are usually necessary if you are taking ethambutol.

ETHINYLESTRADIOL

Used in the following combined preparations
Co-cyprindiol, combined oral contraceptives (e.g. Akizza, Brevinor, Dianette, Elevin, Femodene, Katya, Loestrin, Marvelon, Mercilon, Microgynon 30, Norimin, Ovranette, Rigevidon, Yacella, Yasmin)

QUICK REFERENCE

Drug group Female sex hormone (p.86) and oral contraceptive (p.103)
Overdose danger rating Low
Dependence rating Low
Prescription needed Yes
Available as generic Yes

GENERAL INFORMATION

Ethinylestradiol is a synthetic oestrogen similar to estradiol, a natural female sex hormone. It is widely used in oral contraceptives in combination with a synthetic progestogen. These drugs can also be used to treat an irregular menstrual cycle; for conditions in women due to high levels of androgen (male sex hormones), such as polycystic ovary syndrome and hirsutism; or as HRT (p.87) for the short-term relief of menopausal symptoms. Ethinylestradiol may be used to treat hypogonadism (late or absent sexual development) in women. More rarely, it may be used for osteoporosis, prostate cancer and, in combination with cyproterone, acne in women.

Women taking an oral contraceptive containing ethinylestradiol have an increased risk of venous thrombosis. This risk is greater in overweight women and smokers.

INFORMATION FOR USERS

Your drug prescription is tailored for you. Do not alter dosage without checking with your doctor.
How taken/used Tablets.
Frequency and timing of doses Once daily. Often at certain times of the menstrual cycle.
Adult dosage range *Menopausal symptoms* 10–20mcg daily. *Hormone deficiency* 10–50mcg daily. *Combined contraceptive pills* 20–40mcg daily, depending on preparation. *Acne* 35mcg daily. *Prostate cancer* 0.15–1.5mg daily.
Onset of effect 10–20 days. Contraceptive protection is effective after 7 days in most cases.
Duration of action 1–2 days.
Diet advice None.
Storage Keep in original container at room temperature out of the reach of children.
Missed dose Take as soon as you remember. If your next dose is due within 4 hours, take a single dose now and skip the next. If you are taking the drug for contraceptive purposes, see What to do if you miss a pill (p.107).
Stopping the drug Do not stop the drug without consulting your doctor. Contraceptive protection is lost unless an alternative is used.
Exceeding the dose An occasional unintentional extra dose is unlikely to be a cause for concern. But if you notice any unusual symptoms, or if a large overdose has been taken, notify your doctor.

POSSIBLE ADVERSE EFFECTS

The most common adverse effects of ethinylestradiol include nausea, vomiting, breast swelling or tenderness, weight gain, fluid retention, and bleeding between menstrual periods. They generally diminish with time, but discuss with your doctor if they are severe or if you experience headaches or depression. Sudden, sharp pain in the chest, groin, or legs may indicate a blood clot. If you experience such pain or you develop sudden breathlessness, jaundice, or itching, stop taking the drug and seek urgent medical attention. Long-term use of ethinylestradiol is not advised because it carries an increased risk of various disorders (see Prolonged use).

INTERACTIONS

Tobacco smoking This increases the risk of serious adverse effects on the heart and circulation with ethinylestradiol.
Rifampicin and anticonvulsants These drugs significantly reduce the effectiveness of oral contraceptives containing ethinylestradiol.
Antihypertensive drugs, anticoagulants, and diuretics Ethinylestradiol may reduce the effectiveness of these drugs.
Antibiotics and St John's wort may reduce the effectiveness of oral contraceptives containing ethinylestradiol.

SPECIAL PRECAUTIONS

Be sure to tell your doctor if:
◆ You have heart failure, high blood pressure, or high blood triglyceride (lipid) levels.
◆ You have had venous thrombosis or a stroke.
◆ You have gallstones or a long-term liver or kidney problem.
◆ You have had breast or endometrial cancer.
◆ You have diabetes, porphyria, sickle cell anaemia, or lupus erythematosus.
◆ You are a smoker.
◆ You have migraine or epilepsy.
◆ You are taking other medicines.
Pregnancy Not prescribed. High doses may adversely affect the developing fetus. Discuss with your doctor.
Breast-feeding The drug passes into the breast milk; it may also inhibit milk flow. Discuss with your doctor.
Infants and children Not usually prescribed.
Over 60 No special problems.
Driving and hazardous work No known problems.
Alcohol No known problems.
Surgery and general anaesthetics The drug may need to be stopped before major surgery. Discuss with your doctor.

PROLONGED USE

When given as part of HRT, ethinylestradiol is usually only advised for short-term use around the menopause and is not normally recommended for long-term use or for treatment of osteoporosis. Long-term use increases the risk of breast cancer, venous thrombosis, heart attack, and stroke.
Monitoring Physical examinations and blood pressure checks may be performed.

EVOLOCUMAB

Brand names Repatha, Repatha SureClick
Used in the following combined preparations None

QUICK REFERENCE

Drug group Lipid-lowering drug (p.35)
Overdose danger rating Low
Dependence rating Low
Prescription needed Yes
Available as generic No

GENERAL INFORMATION

Evolocumab (and the related drug alirocumab) is a monoclonal antibody. It belongs to a new drug class called PCSK9 inhibitors and is used to lower blood cholesterol in patients who have not responded adequately to other therapies (e.g. statins) or patients who have a genetic predisposition to high cholesterol (e.g. homozygous familial hypercholesterolaemia). It works by reducing blood levels of a protein called PCSK9, which leads to increased uptake of harmful cholesterol (LDL-cholesterol) from the blood into the liver. PCSK9 inhibition is highly effective at lowering LDL-cholesterol and is generally better tolerated than statins.

The drugs are given as an injection under the skin. Injection site reactions and flulike symptoms are the most common side effects.

INFORMATION FOR USERS

Your drug prescription is tailored for you. Do not alter dosage without checking with your doctor.
How taken/used Injection under the skin; recommended sites include thigh, abdomen, or upper arm. Injections should not be given into areas where skin is red, bruised, tender, or hard.
Frequency and timing of doses Every 2–4 weeks.
Adult dosage range 140–420mg every 2 weeks.
Onset of effect It may take weeks for blood cholesterol to be reduced. Response to treatment should be reviewed at 12 weeks.
Duration of action Up to 4 weeks.
Diet advice Your doctor will recommend a low-fat diet.
Storage Store in a refrigerator (2–8°C).
Missed dose Take as soon as you remember. Delaying by a few days is expected to have negligible effect.
Stopping the drug Do not stop the drug without consulting your doctor; the underlying condition may worsen.

Exceeding the dose An unintentional extra dose is unlikely to be a cause for concern. But if you notice any unusual symptoms, tell your doctor.

POSSIBLE ADVERSE EFFECTS
Mild side effects are common and include a runny or stuffy nose, back pain, joint aches, and nausea; discuss with your doctor if severe. If you develop a reaction at the injection site, a rash, or signs of infection, notify your doctor. Serious side effects are rare.

INTERACTIONS
There are no known interactions.

SPECIAL PRECAUTIONS
Be sure to tell your doctor if:

◆ You have long-term liver or kidney problems.

Pregnancy Safety in pregnancy not established. Discuss with your doctor.

Breast-feeding Safety not established. Discuss with your doctor.

Infants and children The safety and effectiveness have not been established.

Over 60 No special problems.

Driving and hazardous work No special problems.

Alcohol No known problems.

PROLONGED USE
Prolonged use can be associated with injection site reactions such as bruising, bleeding, pain, and swelling. Rotation of the injection site, using different areas of skin, reduces this risk.

EXENATIDE

Brand names Bydureon, Byetta

Used in the following combined preparations None

QUICK REFERENCE
Drug group Drug for diabetes (p.80)

Overdose danger rating High

Dependence rating Low

Prescription needed Yes

Available as generic No

GENERAL INFORMATION
Exenatide is an injected antidiabetic drug used to treat Type 2 diabetes together with other antidiabetic drugs, as well as diet, exercise, and weight control. It is a synthetic protein that mimics the action of a natural hormone called GLP-1, which is involved in regulating blood sugar levels. The drug works by increasing insulin secretion in response to high blood sugar levels and lowering the secretion of the hormone glucagon, which leads to a decreased output of glucose from the liver. It also slows emptying of the stomach, so smoothing out the rise in blood sugar after meals.

INFORMATION FOR USERS
Your drug prescription is tailored for you. Do not alter dosage without checking with your doctor.

How taken/used Injection under the skin.

Frequency and timing of doses 2 x daily, doses at least 6 hours apart. Take within 1 hour before a meal (do not take after a meal). Bydureon is injected once weekly, same day each week, at any time of the day.

Adult dosage range 10–20mcg daily. Bydureon: 2mg per week.

Onset of effect Within 1 hour.

Duration of action 8–12 hours.

Diet advice An individualized diabetic diet must be maintained for the drug to be fully effective. Follow your doctor's advice.

Storage Store unused exenatide injection pens in the refrigerator, protected from light. After first use of a pen, it may be stored at room temperature, away from heat and bright light. Keep out of the reach of children.

Missed dose Take as soon as you remember, but only if you have not yet had a meal. If you have already eaten, wait until next scheduled dose.

Stopping the drug Do not stop without consulting your doctor. Stopping the drug may lead to worsening of the underlying condition.

OVERDOSE ACTION
Seek immediate medical help. If you have severe nausea and vomiting or warning signs of low blood sugar (e.g. faintness, dizziness, headache, confusion, sweating, or tremor), eat or drink something sugary. Take emergency action if seizures or unconsciousness occur.

POSSIBLE ADVERSE EFFECTS
Exenatide commonly causes gastrointestinal side effects, such as nausea, vomiting, diarrhoea, decreased appetite, and weight loss, but these generally improve with continued use. It may also cause symptoms of low blood sugar (see Overdose action, above). Discuss with your doctor if any of these symptoms are

severe. Very rarely, exenatide may cause severe inflammation of the pancreas. If you develop severe abdominal pain, wheezing, an itchy rash, swelling of the face or lips, you notice that you are bleeding or bruising easily, or you have a reaction at the injection site, you should stop taking the drug and contact your doctor without delay.

INTERACTIONS

General note Many drugs, especially other antidiabetic drugs, may interact with exenatide to affect blood sugar levels. Exenatide can affect the absorption of some drugs, so the timing of doses may need to be changed. Check with your doctor or pharmacist.

Anticoagulants (e.g. warfarin) Exenatide may increase their anticoagulant effect.

Oral contraceptives and antibiotics These should be taken at least 1 hour before exenatide to ensure adequate absorption.

SPECIAL PRECAUTIONS

Be sure to tell your doctor if:

- You have long-term kidney problems.
- You have stomach or bowel problems.
- You have a history of pancreatitis.
- You are taking other medicines.

Pregnancy Safety not established. Switching to insulin is safe. Discuss with your doctor.

Breast-feeding Safety not established. Switching to insulin is safe. Discuss with your doctor.

Infants and children Not prescribed.

Over 60 No special problems.

Driving and hazardous work Usually the drug causes no problems, but be aware of warning signs of low blood sugar and avoid such activities if you have these signs.

Alcohol Avoid. Alcohol may upset diabetic control.

Surgery and general anaesthetics Notify your doctor or dentist that you have diabetes. Surgery may affect diabetic control, and therefore your diabetes treatment may need to be adjusted or, in some cases, insulin may need to be substituted.

PROLONGED USE

No problems expected.

Monitoring Regular monitoring of your diabetes control is necessary. You may also have periodic assessment of your eyes, heart, and kidneys and of the lipids in your blood.

EZETIMIBE

Brand name Ezetrol

Used in the following combined preparation Inegy

QUICK REFERENCE

Drug group Lipid-lowering drug (p.35)

Overdose danger rating Low

Dependence rating Low

Prescription needed Yes

Available as generic Yes

GENERAL INFORMATION

Ezetimibe is a lipid-lowering drug that is used to treat hypercholesterolaemia (high blood levels of cholesterol) in people at risk of developing heart disease. It acts in the small intestine to reduce the absorption of cholesterol.

Ezetimibe is prescribed in conjunction with a low-fat diet and usually in combination with a statin (a drug that blocks the action, in the liver, of an enzyme needed for the manufacture of cholesterol). It is also prescribed alone to people in whom a statin is considered inappropriate or is not tolerated.

Common adverse effects include headache, abdominal pain, and diarrhoea. You need to notify your doctor if you are taking over-the-counter statins; when ezetimibe is combined with statins, it can, rarely, cause marked muscle pain, weakness, or tenderness, which should be reported to your doctor immediately. This is less likely to occur if ezetimibe is used alone.

INFORMATION FOR USERS

Your drug prescription is tailored for you. Do not alter dosage without checking with your doctor.

How taken/used Tablets.

Frequency and timing of doses Once daily.

Adult dosage range 10mg daily.

Onset of effect 2 weeks.

Duration of action 24 hours.

Diet advice A low-fat diet is usually recommended.

Storage Keep in original container at room temperature out of the reach of children.

Missed dose Take as soon as you remember. If your next dose is due within 12 hours, do not take the missed dose but take the next one on schedule.

Stopping the drug Do not stop taking the drug without consulting your doctor. Stopping may lead to a recurrence of the original condition.

Exceeding the dose An occasional unintentional extra dose is unlikely to cause problems. But if you notice any unusual symptoms or if a large overdose has been taken, notify your doctor.

POSSIBLE ADVERSE EFFECTS

The most common side effects include headache, fatigue, abdominal pain, and diarrhoea. More rarely, ezetimibe may cause nausea or joint pain. Discuss with your doctor if these symptoms are severe or if you have bleeding or bruising. If you develop a rash, swelling of the face or tongue, or muscle pain or weakness, stop the drug and call your doctor immediately.

INTERACTIONS

Fibrates (e.g. gemfibrozil, bezafibrate) These drugs, which also reduce cholesterol, may raise levels of ezetimibe.
Colestyramine may reduce the effects of ezetimibe. Ezetimibe should be taken either 2 hours before or 4 hours after colestyramine.
Ciclosporin The levels of both drugs may be increased when they are taken together.
Warfarin If ezetimibe is added to warfarin, the INR (International Normalized Rate, a standardized measure of blood clotting) should be closely monitored.

SPECIAL PRECAUTIONS

Be sure to tell your doctor if:

- You have liver problems.
- You are taking a statin.
- You have lactose intolerance or glucose-galactose malabsorption.
- You are taking other medicines.

Pregnancy Not usually prescribed. Safety not established. Discuss with your doctor.
Breast-feeding Not usually prescribed. It is not known whether the drug passes into the breast milk. Discuss with your doctor.
Infants and children Not recommended under 10 years.
Over 60 Increased likelihood of adverse effects.
Driving and hazardous work No special problems.
Alcohol No special problems.

PROLONGED USE

No known problems.
Monitoring Regular blood tests to check the drug's effectiveness in reducing cholesterol levels may be performed. Blood tests of liver and muscle function may also be carried out.

FELODIPINE

Brand names Cardioplen, Felotens, Folpik, Keloc, Neofel, Parmid, Plendil, Vascalpha
Used in the following combined preparation Triapin

QUICK REFERENCE

Drug group Anti-angina drug (p.33) and antihypertensive drug (p.34)
Overdose danger rating Medium
Dependence rating Low
Prescription needed Yes
Available as generic Yes

GENERAL INFORMATION

Felodipine belongs to a group of drugs known as calcium channel blockers. It is used either alone or with another antihypertensive, such as an ACE inhibitor or a diuretic, in treating hypertension (high blood pressure). It may be used alone or with a beta blocker for angina.

The drug works by relaxing the lining of the muscles in small blood vessels, thus dilating the vessels. This enables blood to be pumped more easily throughout the body, thereby lowering blood pressure and reducing the strain on the heart.

Felodipine is not usually prescribed to people with unstable angina or uncontrolled heart failure. It is prescribed with caution to people whose liver function is impaired.

As with other drugs of its class, felodipine may cause the blood pressure to fall too low at the start of treatment.

INFORMATION FOR USERS

Your drug prescription is tailored for you. Do not alter dosage without checking with your doctor.
How taken/used Tablets, modified release (MR) tablets.
Frequency and timing of doses Once daily, in the morning, swallowed whole with at least half a glass of water; do not chew or crush.
Adult dosage range *Hypertension* 5mg (2.5mg for older people) daily (initial dose), increased to 10mg daily (maintenance dose). *Angina* 5mg daily, increased to 10mg if needed.
Onset of effect 1–2 hours.
Duration of action 24 hours.
Diet advice Felodipine should not be taken with grapefruit juice.
Storage Keep in original container at room temperature out of the reach of children.

Missed dose Take as soon as you remember. Take the next dose as scheduled. Do not take an extra dose to make up.
Stopping the drug Do not stop without consulting your doctor. Stopping abruptly may worsen the underlying condition.
Exceeding the dose An occasional unintentional extra dose is unlikely to cause problems. Large overdoses may cause dizziness or collapse. Notify your doctor urgently.

POSSIBLE ADVERSE EFFECTS

Flushing, headache, and palpitations are common side effects of felodipine. These are usually transient and are most likely at the start of treatment or after an increase in dosage. Other common side effects include dizziness (which may be due to excessively lowered blood pressure) and ankle swelling; more rarely, you may have fatigue. Discuss with your doctor if any of these are severe. Felodipine may also rarely cause gingivitis or worsening of angina; if these occur, consult your doctor.

INTERACTIONS

Other antihypertensives may increase felodipine's blood-pressure-lowering effects.
Erythromycin, itraconazole, ketoconazole, atazanavir, and ritonavir may increase the effects of felodipine.
Anticonvulsant drugs may reduce the effectiveness of felodipine.
Ciclosporin, tacrolimus, and theophylline/aminophylline Toxicity of these drugs may be increased with felodipine.
Grapefruit juice may block the breakdown of felodipine, increasing its effects.

SPECIAL PRECAUTIONS

Be sure to tell your doctor if:
- You have liver problems.
- You have angina.
- You have heart problems (especially aortic stenosis).
- You have had a recent heart attack.
- You have lactose intolerance.
- You are taking other medicines.

Pregnancy Not prescribed. May cause defects in the unborn baby.
Breast-feeding Not recommended. Drug passes into breast milk and may adversely affect baby.
Infants and children Not recommended. Safety not established.
Over 60 Increased likelihood of adverse effects. Reduced dose may therefore be necessary.
Driving and hazardous work Avoid until you have learned how felodipine affects you because the drug can cause dizziness.
Alcohol Avoid. Alcohol may increase dizziness and the blood-pressure-lowering effect of felodipine, especially at the start of treatment.

PROLONGED USE

No problems expected.

FILGRASTIM

Brand names Accofil, Neupogen, Nivestim, Zarzio
Used in the following combined preparations None

QUICK REFERENCE

Drug group Blood stimulant
Overdose danger rating Medium
Dependence rating Low
Prescription needed Yes
Available as generic No

GENERAL INFORMATION

Filgrastim is a synthetic form of a naturally occurring protein called G-CSF (granulocyte-colony stimulating factor). This protein is responsible for the manufacture of white blood cells, which fight infection.

The drug acts by stimulating bone marrow to produce white blood cells. It also causes bone marrow cells to move into the bloodstream, where they can be collected for use in treating bone marrow disease, or to replace bone marrow lost during intensive cancer treatment. Filgrastim is used to treat patients with congenital neutropenia (deficiency of G-CSF from birth), some AIDS patients, and those who have recently received high doses of chemo- or radiotherapy during bone-marrow transplantation or cancer treatment. Such patients are prone to frequent and severe infections.

Bone pain is a common adverse effect, but it can be controlled using painkillers. There is an increased risk of leukaemia (cancer of white blood cells) if filgrastim is given to patients with certain rare blood disorders.

INFORMATION FOR USERS

Your drug prescription is tailored for you. Do not alter dosage without checking with your doctor.
How taken/used Injection.

Frequency and timing of doses Once daily.
Adult dosage range 0.1–1.2 million units/kg body weight, depending upon condition being treated and response to treatment.
Onset of effect 24 hours (increase in numbers of white blood cells); several weeks (recovery of normal numbers of white blood cells).
Duration of action 1–7 days.
Diet advice None.
Storage Store in a refrigerator out of the reach of children.
Missed dose Take as soon as you remember. If your next dose is due within 6 hours, do not take the missed dose. Take the next scheduled dose as usual.
Stopping the drug Do not stop without consulting your doctor; stopping the drug may lead to worsening of the underlying condition.
Exceeding the dose An occasional unintentional extra dose is unlikely to cause problems. But if you notice any unusual symptoms or if a large overdose has been taken, notify your doctor.

POSSIBLE ADVERSE EFFECTS

Adverse effects from short courses of filgrastim are unusual. The most common is bone pain, which is probably linked to the stimulant effect of the drug on bone marrow. Muscle pain is another common side effect. Discuss with your doctor if either of these is severe or if you have abdominal pain. More rarely, the drug may cause a rash, cough, or breathlessness. If you have any of these symptoms, consult your doctor. If you develop abdominal or more generalized swelling, consult your doctor without delay. Prolonged use of filgrastim may also cause various adverse effects (see below).

INTERACTIONS

Cytotoxic chemotherapy or radiotherapy should not be administered within 24 hours of taking filgrastim because of the risk of increasing the damage that these treatments inflict on the bone marrow.

SPECIAL PRECAUTIONS

Be sure to tell your doctor if:
- You have any blood disorders.
- You have sickle-cell disease.
- You have a history of lung problems or lung infections.
- You have osteoporosis.
- You are taking other medicines.

Pregnancy Safety in pregnancy not established. Discuss with your doctor.
Breast-feeding Safety in breast-feeding not established. Discuss with your doctor.
Infants and children No special problems.
Over 60 No special problems.
Driving and hazardous work No known problems.
Alcohol No known problems.

PROLONGED USE

Prolonged use may lead to a slightly increased risk of certain leukaemias. Cutaneous vasculitis (inflammation of blood vessels of the skin), osteoporosis (weakening of the bones), hair thinning, enlargement of the spleen and liver, and bleeding due to reduction in platelet numbers may also occur.
Monitoring Blood checks and regular physical examinations are performed, as well as bone scans to check for bone thinning.

FINASTERIDE

Brand names Aindeem, Propecia, Proscar
Used in the following combined preparations None

QUICK REFERENCE

Drug group Drug for urinary disorders (p.110)
Overdose danger rating Low
Dependence rating Low
Prescription needed Yes
Available as generic Yes

GENERAL INFORMATION

Finasteride is an anti-androgen drug (see Male sex hormones, p.85) that blocks the conversion of testosterone to the more potent dihydrotestosterone in the body. It is used to treat benign prostatic hyperplasia (BPH), in which the prostate gland enlarges, making urination difficult. The drug gradually shrinks the prostate, improving urine flow and other symptoms such as difficulty in starting urination.

Because it is excreted in semen and can feminize a male fetus, you should use a condom if your sexual partner may be, or is likely to become, pregnant. Women of childbearing age should not handle broken or crushed tablets because small quantities of the drug are absorbed through the skin.

The symptoms of BPH are similar to those of prostate cancer, so the drug is used only when the possibility of cancer has been ruled out.

Finasteride is also used, at a lower dose, to reverse male-pattern baldness by preventing the hair follicles from becoming inactive. Noticeable improvements may take about 3–6 months but will disappear within a year of treatment being stopped.

INFORMATION FOR USERS

Your drug prescription is tailored for you. Do not alter dosage without checking with your doctor.
How taken/used Tablets.
Frequency and timing of doses Once daily.
Adult dosage range *Prostate disease* 5mg. *Male-pattern baldness* 1mg.
Onset of effect The drug action takes effect within 1 hour, but effects on the prostate and scalp hair may take months to appear.
Duration of action 24 hours.
Diet advice None.
Storage Keep in original container at room temperature out of the reach of children. Protect from light.
Missed dose Do not take the missed dose, but take your next scheduled dose as usual.
Stopping the drug Do not stop without consulting your doctor; stopping the drug may lead to worsening of the underlying condition.
Exceeding the dose An occasional unintentional extra dose is unlikely to cause problems. But if you notice any unusual symptoms, or if a large overdose has been taken, notify your doctor.

POSSIBLE ADVERSE EFFECTS

Most people experience very few adverse effects when taking finasteride; the most common are erectile dysfunction (impotence), decreased libido, reduced semen volume, and breast swelling or tenderness. Report any sexual problems to your doctor. Any changes in the breast tissue, such as lumps, pain, enlargement, or nipple discharge, should be reported promptly to your doctor. More rarely, testicular pain, mood alterations, or depression may occur; discuss with your doctor if you have testicular pain or severe mood changes or depression. If a rash, swelling of the lips, or wheezing develop, stop taking the drug and seek urgent medical attention.

INTERACTIONS

No drug interactions, but finasteride does interfere with the prostate specific antigen (PSA) screening test for prostate cancer.

SPECIAL PRECAUTIONS

Be sure to tell your doctor if:
- You have liver problems.
- You are taking other medicines.

Pregnancy Not prescribed.
Breast-feeding Not applicable.
Infants and children Not prescribed.
Over 60 No special problems.
Driving and hazardous work No special problems.
Alcohol No special problems.

PROLONGED USE

Treatment for benign prostatic hyperplasia and male-pattern baldness is reviewed after about 6 months to see if it has been effective. Long-term use of finasteride carries a small increase in the risk of breast cancer in men.

FLUCLOXACILLIN

Brand names Floxapen, Fluclomix, Ladropen
Used in the following combined preparations Co-Fluampicil, Flu-Amp, Magnapen

QUICK REFERENCE

Drug group Penicillin antibiotic (p.60)
Overdose danger rating Low
Dependence rating Low
Prescription needed Yes
Available as generic Yes

GENERAL INFORMATION

Flucloxacillin is a penicillin antibiotic. It was developed to deal with staphylococci bacteria that are resistant to other antibiotics. Such bacteria make enzymes (penicillinases) that neutralize the antibiotics, but flucloxacillin is not inactivated by penicillinases and is therefore effective for treating penicillin-resistant staphylococcal infections. The drug is used to treat ear infections, pneumonia, impetigo, cellulitis, osteomyelitis, and endocarditis. Flucloxacillin is also available combined in equal parts with ampicillin; this drug is known as co-fluampicil. It is used to treat mixed infections of penicillinase-producing organisms.

Staphylococci have now evolved so that some strains are now resistant to flucloxacillin as well. These are the so-called methicillin-resistant *Staphylococcus aureus* infections (MRSA). Only a few antibiotics held in reserve can deal with them.

INFORMATION FOR USERS

Your drug prescription is tailored for you. Do not alter dosage without checking with your doctor.

How taken/used Capsules, liquid, injection.

Frequency and timing of doses 4 x daily at least 30 minutes before food.

Adult dosage range 1–2g daily (oral); 1–8g daily (injection); 8–12g daily (endocarditis).

Onset of effect 30 minutes.

Duration of action 4–6 hours.

Diet advice Make sure you keep well hydrated.

Storage Keep in original container at room temperature out of the reach of children.

Missed dose Take as soon as you remember. Take your next dose at the scheduled time.

Stopping the drug Take the full course. Even if you feel better, the original infection may still be present and symptoms may recur if treatment is stopped too soon.

Exceeding the dose An occasional unintentional extra dose is unlikely to be a cause for concern. But if you notice any unusual symptoms, or if a large overdose has been taken, notify your doctor.

POSSIBLE ADVERSE EFFECTS

The most common adverse effects of flucloxacillin are gastrointestinal: diarrhoea and nausea. Other adverse effects include abdominal pain, bruising, sore throat, and fever. Consult your doctor if you have any of these symptoms or if gastrointestinal symptoms are severe. If you develop a rash, itching, breathing difficulties, wheezing, or swollen joints (all signs of an allergic reaction), stop taking the drug and contact your doctor at once. If jaundice develops, even weeks or months after treatment, consult your doctor promptly and stop taking the drug if you have not already done so.

INTERACTIONS

Oral typhoid vaccine Flucloxacillin inactivates the vaccine. Avoid taking flucloxacillin for 3 days before and after having the vaccine.

Methotrexate Flucloxacillin reduces the excretion of methotrexate, thereby increasing the risk of toxicity.

SPECIAL PRECAUTIONS

Be sure to tell your doctor if:

- ◆ You are allergic to penicillin antibiotics or cephalosporin antibiotics.
- ◆ You have a history of allergy.
- ◆ You have liver problems, or you have had previous liver problems with flucloxacillin.
- ◆ You are taking other medicines.

Pregnancy No evidence of risk.

Breast-feeding No evidence of risk.

Infants and children Reduced dose necessary.

Over 60 No known problems.

Driving and hazardous work No known problems.

Alcohol No known problems.

PROLONGED USE

Although flucloxacillin is not normally necessary for long-term use, osteomyelitis and endocarditis may require longer than usual courses of treatment.

Monitoring Regular tests of liver and kidney function will be performed if a longer course of treatment is prescribed.

FLUCONAZOLE

Brand names Azocan, Azocan-P, Canestan Oral, Care Fluconazole, Diflucan

Used in the following combined preparations None

QUICK REFERENCE

Drug group Antifungal drug (p.74)

Overdose danger rating Medium

Dependence rating Low

Prescription needed Yes (except for oral treatments for vaginal infections)

Available as generic Yes

GENERAL INFORMATION

Fluconazole is an antifungal drug that is used to treat local candida infections (thrush) affecting the vagina, mouth, and skin as well as systemic or more widespread candida infections. The drug is also used to treat some more unusual fungal infections, including cryptococcal meningitis, and may be used to prevent fungal infections in patients with defective immunity. The dosage and length of course will depend on the condition being treated.

Fluconazole is generally well tolerated, although side effects such as nausea and vomiting, diarrhoea, and abdominal discomfort are common.

INFORMATION FOR USERS

Your drug prescription is tailored for you. Do not alter dosage without checking with your doctor.

How taken/used Capsules, liquid, injection.
Frequency and timing of doses Once daily.
Adult dosage range 50–400mg daily.
Onset of effect Within a few hours, but full beneficial effects may take several days.
Duration of action Up to 24 hours.
Diet advice None.
Storage Keep in original container at room temperature out of the reach of children. Store liquid in a refrigerator (do not freeze) for no longer than 14 days.
Missed dose Take as soon as you remember. If your next dose is due within 6 hours, take a single dose now and skip the next.
Stopping the drug Take the full course. Even if you feel better, the original infection may still be present and may recur if treatment is stopped too soon.
Exceeding the dose An occasional unintentional extra dose is unlikely to be a cause for concern. But if you notice any unusual symptoms, or if a large overdose has been taken, tell your doctor.

POSSIBLE ADVERSE EFFECTS
Fluconazole is generally well tolerated. Most side effects involve the gastrointestinal tract and include nausea, vomiting, abdominal discomfort, diarrhoea, and flatulence. Headache is also a common side effect. If any of these are severe, discuss with your doctor. Rarely, a rash may occur; if so, you should stop taking the drug and consult your doctor.

INTERACTIONS
General note Interactions with other drugs relate to multiple doses of fluconazole. The relevance of a single dose is not established, but is likely to be small. As well as the drugs listed below, fluconazole interacts with and can affect the breakdown of numerous other drugs. Consult your doctor or pharmacist before using any other drug with fluconazole.
Rifampicin may reduce the effect of fluconazole. Avoid using both drugs together.
Oral antidiabetics Fluconazole may increase the risk of hypoglycaemia with sulfonylureas and drugs such as nateglinide and repaglinide.
Anticoagulants Fluconazole may increase the effect of oral anticoagulants such as warfarin.
Theophylline/aminophylline, midazolam, ciclosporin, tacrolimus, zidovudine, phenytoin, and carbamazepine Fluconazole may increase the blood levels of these drugs.
Bosentan, eletriptan, ergotamine, erythromycin, ivabradine, methysergide, and pimozide These drugs should not be used with flucanazole because of potentially dangerous interactions that can affect the rhythm of your heart beat.

SPECIAL PRECAUTIONS
Be sure to tell your doctor if:
- You have long-term liver or kidney problems.
- You have a history of heart rhythm problems.
- You have previously had an allergic reaction to antifungal drugs.
- You have acute porphyria.
- You are taking other medicines.

Pregnancy May adversely affect the fetus if taken during pregnancy; should be avoided.
Breast-feeding The drug passes into the breast milk, although probably in amounts too small to be harmful. Discuss with your doctor.
Infants and children Reduced dose necessary.
Over 60 Normal dose used as long as kidney function is not impaired.
Driving and hazardous work No known problems.
Alcohol No known problems.

PROLONGED USE
Fluconazole is usually given for short courses of treatment, although long-term courses may be prescribed for those with recurrent candidiasis. To prevent relapse of cryptococcal meningitis in patients with defective immunity, it may be administered indefinitely.

FLUOROURACIL

Brand names Efudix 5% Cream
Used in the following combined preparations Actikerall

QUICK REFERENCE
Drug group Anticancer drug (p.94)
Overdose danger rating Low
Dependence rating Low
Prescription needed Yes
Available as generic Yes

GENERAL INFORMATION
Fluorouracil (5-FU) is a chemotherapy drug for cancers including colon and breast cancer. It may be used on its own or combined with other chemotherapy drugs. It is thought to act by stopping the production of DNA. The drug is usually given by injection or infusion. It can also be applied as a cream for pre-cancerous

areas of sun-damaged skin, and for skin cancers called superficial basal cell carcinomas.

Patients having fluorouracil injections or infusions should first be screened for deficiency of an enzyme called dihydropyramidine dehydrogenase (DPD), which could lead to severe or fatal toxicity with fluorouracil.

INFORMATION FOR USERS

Your drug prescription is tailored for you. Do not alter dosage without checking with your doctor.

How taken/used Injection/infusion; cream.

Frequency and timing of doses Regime decided by doctor (injection/infusion). 1–2 x daily for 3–4 weeks (cream).

Adult dosage range Injection/infusion dose determined by weight. For cream, maximum area of skin to be treated at one time is 500cm^2 (23cm x 23cm).

Onset of effect Benefits and adverse effects of cream usually develop within 1–2 weeks.

Duration of action Effects of cream should settle by 4–6 weeks.

Diet advice Drink plenty of liquid before, during, and after injections or infusions.

Storage The cream is flammable. Store at room temperature and out of the reach of children.

Missed dose If you miss a dose of cream, apply as soon as possible. If next dose is nearly due, skip the missed dose and continue as before.

Stopping the drug Try to complete courses of cream as prescribed. If the skin inflammation is intolerable, seek advice from your doctor.

Exceeding the dose Unlikely to occur; call doctor about any concerns or unusual symptoms.

POSSIBLE ADVERSE EFFECTS

Side effects are common with the injections. If loss of appetite, hair loss, weakness, or fatigue are severe, discuss with your doctor. Tell your doctor in all cases of nausea, vomiting, diarrhoea, nosebleed, or mouth or lip ulcers; call the doctor promptly for rash, chest pain, or palpitations. The cream may cause significant inflammatory skin reactions as well as abdominal pain and diarrhoea; if symptoms are severe, consult your doctor.

INTERACTIONS

Cimetidine and metronidazole increase the blood level and toxicity of systemic fluorouracil.

Phenytoin Systemic fluorouracil increases the concentration of phenytoin so blood levels of phenytoin should be monitored and dose adjusted if necessary.

Live vaccines e.g. influenza should be avoided with systemic fluorouracil due to risk of generalized/life-threatening infection.

Warfarin Systemic fluorouracil increases the anticoagulant effect of warfarin.

Methotrexate may increase the risk of a severe skin reaction to topical fluorouracil.

SPECIAL PRECAUTIONS

Fluorouracil injections or infusions are prescribed under close medical supervision, taking into account your present condition and medical history. However, tell your doctor if:

- ◆ You have impaired liver function.
- ◆ You have impaired kidney function.
- ◆ You have a known personal or family history of DPD enzyme deficiency.
- ◆ You are pregnant or planning a pregnancy.
- ◆ You are breast-feeding.
- ◆ You have a known allergy to fluorouracil.
- ◆ You take any other medications, including over-the-counter treatments.

Pregnancy Strictly contraindicated. Women having fluorouracil in any form should avoid pregnancy during and for 6 months after treatment. Men should avoid fathering a child during and for 6 months after treatment.

Breast-feeding Not advised. Discuss with doctor.

Infants and children Safety and efficacy have not been established.

Over 60 Dose reduction may be required.

Driving and hazardous work No known problems, but see how the drug affects you as it can cause nausea.

Alcohol Alcohol can be taken in moderation.

PROLONGED USE

No specific problems, but the length of the course will be decided by your doctor.

FLUOXETINE

Brand names Olena, Prozac, Prozep

Used in the following combined preparations None

QUICK REFERENCE

Drug group Antidepressant drug (p.12)

Overdose danger rating Low

Dependence rating Low

Prescription needed Yes

Available as generic Yes

GENERAL INFORMATION

Fluoxetine belongs to the group of antidepressant drugs called selective serotonin re-uptake inhibitors (SSRIs). These tend to cause less sedation, have different side effects, and are safer if taken in overdose than older antidepressants. Fluoxetine elevates mood, increases physical activity, and restores interest in everyday pursuits. The drug is broken down slowly and remains in the body for several weeks after treatment is stopped. It is used to treat depression, to reduce binge eating and purging activity (bulimia nervosa), and to treat obsessive-compulsive disorder.

INFORMATION FOR USERS

Your drug prescription is tailored for you. Do not alter dosage without checking with your doctor.

How taken/used Capsules, dispersible tablets, liquid.

Frequency and timing of doses Once daily in the morning.

Adult dosage range 20–60mg daily.

Onset of effect Some benefits may appear in 14 days, but full benefits may not be felt for 6 weeks or more. Obsessive-compulsive disorder and bulimia may take longer to respond.

Duration of action Beneficial effects may last for up to 6 weeks following prolonged treatment. Adverse effects may wear off within 1–2 weeks.

Diet advice None.

Storage Keep in original container at room temperature out of the reach of children.

Missed dose Take as soon as you remember. If your next dose is due within 8 hours, take a single dose now and skip the next.

Stopping the drug Do not stop the drug without consulting your doctor, who may supervise a gradual reduction in dosage.

Exceeding the dose An occasional unintentional extra dose is unlikely to cause problems, but large overdoses may cause adverse effects. Notify your doctor.

POSSIBLE ADVERSE EFFECTS

The most common adverse effects of fluoxetine are restlessness, anxiety, insomnia, nausea, diarrhoea, and headache. Rarely, it may cause sexual dysfunction. Discuss with your doctor if any of these symptoms are severe. If a rash develops or you have suicidal thoughts or attempts, the drug should be stopped and medical advice sought at once. Fluoxetine produces fewer anticholinergic side effects (p.7) than the tricyclic antidepressants.

INTERACTIONS

Sedatives All drugs having a sedative effect may increase the sedative effects of fluoxetine.

Monoamine oxidase inhibitors (MAOIs; p.12) Fluoxetine should not be started less than 14 days after stopping an MAOI (except moclobemide) as serious adverse effects can occur. An MAOI should not be started less than 5 weeks after stopping fluoxetine.

Tricyclic antidepressants Fluoxetine reduces the breakdown of tricyclics and may increase the toxicity of these drugs.

Antipsychotics The levels and effects of some of these drugs can be increased by fluoxetine.

SPECIAL PRECAUTIONS

Be sure to tell your doctor if:

- You have long-term liver or kidney problems.
- You have a history of mania.
- You have diabetes.
- You have had epileptic seizures.
- You have previously had an allergic reaction to fluoxetine or other SSRIs.
- You are taking other medicines.

Pregnancy Avoid if possible. Discuss with your doctor.

Breast-feeding The drug passes into the breast milk. Discuss with your doctor.

Infants and children Not generally recommended under 18 years.

Over 60 Reduced dose may be necessary.

Driving and hazardous work Avoid until you have learned how fluoxetine affects you because the drug can cause drowsiness and can affect your judgement and coordination.

Alcohol No special problems.

PROLONGED USE

No problems expected in adults. Side effects tend to decrease with time. There is a small risk of suicidal thoughts and self-harm in children and adolescents, although the drug is rarely used for this age group.

Monitoring Any person experiencing drowsiness, confusion, muscle cramps, or seizures should be monitored for low sodium levels in the blood. Under-18s should be monitored for suicidal thoughts and self-harm.

FLUPENTIXOL

Brand names Depixol, Fluanxol, Psytixol
Used in the following combined preparations None

QUICK REFERENCE

Drug group Antipsychotic drug (p.13)
Overdose danger rating Medium
Dependence rating Low
Prescription needed Yes
Available as generic No

GENERAL INFORMATION

Flupentixol is an antipsychotic drug that is prescribed to treat schizophrenia and similar illnesses. It is also occasionally used as an antidepressant for mild to moderate depression. The side effects from flupentixol are similar to those of phenothiazines, but flupentixol is less sedating.

The drug is not suitable for any patients who experience mania because it may worsen the symptoms. It has fewer anticholinergic effects (p.7) than the phenothiazines but, because it has antidopaminergic effects, it can cause side effects such as parkinsonism (p.16).

INFORMATION FOR USERS

Your drug prescription is tailored for you. Do not alter dosage without checking with your doctor.
How taken/used Tablets, injection.
Frequency and timing of doses 1–2 x daily no later than 4 pm (tablets); every 2–4 weeks (injection).
Adult dosage range *Schizophrenia and other psychoses* 6–18mg daily (tablets); from 20mg every 4 weeks to a maximum of 400mg weekly (injection). *Depression* 1–3mg daily (tablets).
Onset of effect 10 days (side effects may appear much sooner).
Duration of action Up to 12 hours (by mouth); 1–2 months (by depot injection).
Diet advice None.
Storage Store at room temperature out of the reach of children. Protect injections from light.
Missed dose Take as soon as you remember. If next dose is due within 2 hours, skip missed dose, but take next scheduled dose as usual.
Stopping the drug Do not stop without consulting your doctor, who will supervise a gradual reduction in dosage. Abrupt cessation of the drug may result in withdrawal symptoms and a recurrence of the original problem.
Exceeding the dose An occasional unintentional extra dose is unlikely to cause problems, but larger overdoses may cause severe drowsiness, seizures, low blood pressure, or shock. Notify your doctor.

POSSIBLE ADVERSE EFFECTS

The adverse effects of flupentixol are mainly due to its anticholinergic and antidopaminergic actions and its blocking action on the transmission of signals through the heart. Weight gain, nausea, drowsiness, sexual dysfunction, breast growth, and absent menstrual periods are common; discuss with your doctor if they are severe. Blurred vision, parkinsonism, tremor, palpitations, and jaundice may also occur. If you have any of these adverse effects, you should consult your doctor; you should also stop taking the drug if you develop jaundice. If you experience dizziness, fainting, or confusion with flupentixol, you should contact your doctor immediately.

INTERACTIONS

Anti-arrhythmic drugs and antibiotics (e.g. erythromycin and moxifloxacin) Taken with these drugs, flupentixol may increase the risk of arrhythmias.
Antihypertensive drugs Flupentixol may increase the effects of some antihypertensives.
Anticholinergic drugs Flupentixol may increase the effects of these drugs.
Antiparkinson drugs and anticonvulsants Flupentixol may reduce the effects of these drugs.
Sedatives Flupentixol enhances the effect of all sedative drugs.

SPECIAL PRECAUTIONS

Be sure to tell your doctor if:

- You have long-term liver or kidney problems.
- You have heart problems.
- You have had epileptic seizures.
- You have Parkinson's disease.
- You have glaucoma.
- You have porphyria.
- You have lactose intolerance.
- You are taking other medicines.

Pregnancy Not usually prescribed. May cause lethargy in the baby during labour. Discuss with your doctor.
Breast-feeding The drug passes into the breast milk and may affect the baby. Discuss with your doctor.

Infants and children Not recommended.
Over 60 Reduced dose necessary. Increased risk of late-appearing movement disorders or of confusion.
Driving and hazardous work Avoid such activities until you have learned how flupentixol affects you because the drug can cause drowsiness and slowed reactions.
Alcohol Avoid. Flupentixol enhances the sedative effect of alcohol.
Surgery and general anaesthetics Treatment may need to be stopped before you have any surgery. Discuss this with your doctor or dentist.

PROLONGED USE
The risk of late-appearing movement disorders increases as flupentixol treatment continues. Blood disorders, as well as jaundice and other liver disorders, are occasionally seen.

FLUTAMIDE

Brand names None
Used in the following combined preparations None

QUICK REFERENCE
Drug group Anticancer drug (p.94)
Overdose danger rating Medium
Dependence rating Low
Prescription needed Yes
Available as generic Yes

GENERAL INFORMATION
Flutamide is an anti-androgen drug (see Male sex hormones, p.85) used in the treatment of advanced prostate cancer, often in combination with drugs such as goserelin that control the production of the male sex hormones (androgens). Both drugs are effective because the cancer is dependent on androgens for its continued development.

Treatment with goserelin-type drugs causes an initial increase in release of the hormone testosterone, leading to a growth spurt of the cancer (a "tumour flare"), which flutamide is prescribed to stop. Flutamide is also used to treat prostate cancer when goserelin-type drugs are not prescribed.

Flutamide may discolour the urine amber or yellow-green, but this is harmless. However, you should notify your doctor straight away if your urine becomes dark-coloured, because this may be an indication of liver damage.

INFORMATION FOR USERS
Your drug prescription is tailored for you. Do not alter dosage without checking with your doctor.
How taken/used Tablets.
Frequency and timing of doses 3 x daily, starting 3 days before the goserelin-type drug and continuing for 3 weeks.
Adult dosage range 250mg.
Onset of effect 1 hour.
Duration of action 8 hours.
Diet advice None.
Storage Keep in original container at room temperature out of the reach of children.
Missed dose Take as soon as you remember. If your next dose is due within 2 hours, take a single dose now and skip the next.
Stopping the drug Do not stop taking the drug without consulting your doctor because the condition may worsen rapidly.
Exceeding the dose An occasional unintentional extra dose is unlikely to be a cause for concern. But if you notice any unusual symptoms, or if a large overdose has been taken, tell your doctor.

POSSIBLE ADVERSE EFFECTS
Nausea, vomiting, diarrhoea, insomnia, tiredness, headache, breast swelling or tenderness, decreased libido, hot flushes, and thirst are common adverse effects of flutamide; discuss with your doctor if they are severe. Breast swelling and tenderness may occur if the drug is given at an effective dose; these are usually reversible when it is stopped or reduced. More rarely, dizziness, blurred vision, fluid retention, and stomach or chest pain may occur; if you have stomach or chest pain, or severe dizziness or fluid retention, consult your doctor. If you develop a rash or jaundice or your urine becomes dark in colour, you should stop taking the drug and contact your doctor immediately.

INTERACTIONS
Warfarin Flutamide increases the anticoagulant effect of warfarin.
Theophylline Flutamide may increase blood levels of theophylline.
Idelalisib and ivacaftor severely increase flutamide levels in the body and should be avoided. Several antiretrovirals can also increase flutamide levels to a lesser degree.
Drugs that increase the risk of heart arrhythmias These drugs, which include amiodarone,

sotalol, moxifloxacin, and methadone, should be used with caution when taking flutamide. ECG monitoring is advised.

SPECIAL PRECAUTIONS

Be sure to tell your doctor if:

◆ You have heart problems.

◆ You have had a blood clot, such as a deep vein thrombosis.

◆ You have liver problems.

◆ You are taking other medicines.

Pregnancy Not prescribed to women. The drug causes fetal abnormalities in animals; for safety, barrier contraception must be used by men when on flutamide, and their female partners should also use effective contraception.
Breast-feeding Not prescribed.
Infants and children Not prescribed.
Over 60 No special problems.
Driving and hazardous work Avoid until you know how flutamide affects you because the drug can cause blurred vision and dizziness.
Alcohol No special problems, but excessive consumption should be avoided.

PROLONGED USE

Prolonged use of flutamide may cause liver damage. Because it is an anti-androgen, the drug also reduces the sperm count.
Monitoring Periodic liver-function tests are usually performed. ECG monitoring may also be performed. Bone density may be monitored annually as osteoporotic bone fractures are more likely if flutamide is used for long periods. Glucose levels/HbA1c may be monitored as the risk of diabetes is higher on combined treatment with flutamide plus GnRH agents such as goserelin.

FLUTICASONE

Brand names AirFluSal, Avamys, Combisal, Cutivate, Dymista, Flixonase, Flixotide, Nasofan, Pirinase, Sereflo, Trelegy Ellipta
Used in the following combined preparations Aerivio, Flutiform, Relvar, Seretide

QUICK REFERENCE

Drug group Corticosteroid (p.78)
Overdose danger rating Low
Dependence rating Low
Prescription needed Yes (except for nasal spray)
Available as generic No

GENERAL INFORMATION

Fluticasone is a corticosteroid drug used to control inflammation in asthma and allergic rhinitis. It does not produce relief immediately, so it is important to take the drug regularly. For allergic rhinitis, treatment with the nasal spray needs to begin 2 to 3 weeks before the hay fever season starts.

Fluticasone should be taken regularly by inhaler to prevent asthma attacks; proper instruction is essential to ensure correct use. It is also prescribed in the form of an ointment or cream to treat dermatitis and eczema (see Topical corticosteroids, p.118).

The drug has few serious adverse effects because it is administered directly into the lungs (by inhaler) or nasal mucosa (by nasal spray). Fungal infection causing irritation of the mouth and throat is a possible side effect of the inhaled form but can be minimized by thoroughly rinsing the mouth and gargling with water after each inhalation.

INFORMATION FOR USERS

Follow instructions on the label. Call your doctor if symptoms worsen.
How taken/used Ointment, cream, inhaler, nasal spray.
Frequency and timing of doses *Allergic rhinitis* 1–2 x daily. *Asthma* 2 x daily.
Adult dosage range *Allergic rhinitis* 1–2 sprays into each nostril per dose. *Asthma* 100–1,000mcg per dose.
Onset of effect 4–7 days (asthma); 3–4 days (allergic rhinitis).
Duration of action The effects can last for several days after stopping the drug.
Diet advice None.
Storage Keep in original container at room temperature out of the reach of children.
Missed dose Take as soon as you remember.
Stopping the drug Do not stop without consulting your doctor; symptoms may recur.
Exceeding the dose An occasional unintentional extra dose is unlikely to be a cause for concern. Adverse effects may occur if the recommended dose is regularly exceeded over a prolonged period.

POSSIBLE ADVERSE EFFECTS

Adverse effects are unlikely. Nasal spray may irritate the nasal passages, and sprays or inhalers may cause cough or lead to easy bruising; if these are severe, consult your doctor. Inhalers may cause fungal infection of the throat and mouth; this can be minimized by rinsing out the mouth, brushing the teeth, or gargling with water after every inhalation.

If you develop sore throat, hoarseness, or nosebleed, discuss with your doctor. If wheezing and breathlessness suddenly worsen after inhaler use (paradoxical bronchospasm), stop the drug and call the doctor immediately.

Cream and ointment do not usually cause adverse effects with short-term use, but long-term use may cause skin changes (see below).

INTERACTIONS

Atazanavir, clarithomycin, ritonavir, telaprevir, and itraconazole may increase blood level of fluticasone and risk of adrenal gland suppression.
Vaccines High-dose fluticasone may cause serious generalized infections if live vaccines are given with it. Discuss with your doctor.
Non-steroidal anti-inflammatory drugs (NSAIDs) such as ibuprofen with fluticasone can cause a small but significant increase in the risk of gastrointestinal bleeding.

SPECIAL PRECAUTIONS

Be sure to tell your doctor if:
- You have chronic sinusitis.
- You have had recent nasal ulcers or nasal surgery.
- You have had tuberculosis or another respiratory infection.
- You are taking other medicines.

Pregnancy Safety in pregnancy not established. Discuss with your doctor.
Breast-feeding Safety in breast-feeding not established. Drug unlikely to pass into breast milk; discuss with doctor.
Infants and children Not recommended under 4 years. Reduced dose needed in older children. Avoid prolonged use of ointment in children.
Over 60 No known problems.
Driving and hazardous work No known problems.
Alcohol No known problems.

PROLONGED USE

Long-term use of topical or inhaled fluticasone can lead to peptic ulcers, muscle weakness, osteoporosis, growth retardation in children, and, rarely, adrenal gland suppression. Rarely, nasal spray may cause glaucoma and cataracts. The incidence of long-term side effects from inhalation can be reduced by use of a spacer. Long-term topical treatment may also lead to skin thinning. Patients on long-term fluticasone should carry a steroid card or wear a MedicAlert bracelet.
Monitoring Periodic checks on adrenal gland function may be required if large doses are being taken. Children should have their height monitored during treatment.

FUROSEMIDE (FRUSEMIDE)

Brand names Froop, Frusol, Lasix, and others
Used in the following combined preparations Co-Amilofruse, Frumil, Lasilactone, and others

QUICK REFERENCE

Drug group Loop diuretic (p.31) and antihypertensive drug (p.34)
Overdose danger rating Low
Dependence rating Low
Prescription needed Yes
Available as generic Yes

GENERAL INFORMATION

Furosemide is a powerful, short-acting loop diuretic. Like other diuretics, it is used to treat oedema (accumulation of fluid in tissue spaces) caused by heart failure, and certain lung, liver, and kidney disorders.

Because it is fast acting, furosemide is often used in emergencies to relieve pulmonary oedema (fluid in the lungs). It is particularly useful for people who have impaired kidney function because these people do not respond well to thiazide diuretics (see p.31).

Furosemide increases potassium loss from the body, which can produce a wide variety of symptoms. For this reason, potassium supplements or a potassium-sparing diuretic may be given with the drug.

INFORMATION FOR USERS

Your drug prescription is tailored for you. Do not alter dosage without checking with your doctor.
How taken/used Tablets, liquid, injection.
Frequency and timing of doses Once daily, usually morning; 4–6 x hourly (high dose therapy).
Adult dosage range 20–80mg daily. Dose may be increased to a maximum of 2g daily if doctor considers it necessary.

Onset of effect Within 1 hour (by mouth); within 5 minutes (by injection).
Duration of action Up to 6 hours.
Diet advice Drug may reduce potassium in the body. Eat plenty of potassium-rich fresh fruits and vegetables, such as bananas and tomatoes, unless you have very impaired renal function or you are on dialysis.
Storage Keep in original container at room temperature out of the reach of children. Protect from light.
Missed dose No cause for concern, but take as soon as you remember. However, if it is late in the day do not take the missed dose, or you may need to get up during the night to pass urine. Take the next scheduled dose as usual.
Stopping the drug Do not stop without consulting your doctor; symptoms may recur.
Exceeding the dose An occasional unintentional extra dose is unlikely to be a cause for concern. But if you notice any unusual symptoms, or if a large overdose has been taken, tell your doctor.

POSSIBLE ADVERSE EFFECTS

Adverse effects are mainly due to the rapid fluid loss from furosemide and the resulting disturbance in body salts and water balance. These effects, which include dizziness, nausea, lethargy, and muscle cramps, tend to diminish as the body adjusts to the drug. If a rash, photosensitivity, or vomiting occur, you should stop taking the drug and contact your doctor.

INTERACTIONS

Non-steroidal anti-inflammatory drugs (NSAIDs) Some of these drugs may reduce the diuretic effect of furosemide.
Lithium Furosemide may increase blood levels of lithium and risk of lithium poisoning.
Digoxin Loss of potassium with furosemide may lead to digoxin toxicity.
Aminoglycoside antibiotics used with furosemide may increase the risks of hearing and kidney problems.
Thiazides taken with furosemide may lead to excessive urination.
ACE inhibitors and angiotensin-2-receptor blockers with furosemide may cause severe hypotension so careful dose adjustment may be needed.
Sucralfate, cholestyramine, and colestipol can decrease the absorption of furosemide. Leave at least 2 hours between taking these drugs and taking furosemide.

SPECIAL PRECAUTIONS

Be sure to tell your doctor if:
- You have long-term liver or kidney problems.
- You have gout.
- You have previously had an allergic reaction to furosemide or sulfonamides.
- You have prostate problems.
- You are taking other medicines.

Pregnancy Safety in pregnancy not established. Discuss with your doctor.
Breast-feeding The drug may reduce milk supply, but the amount in the milk is unlikely to affect the baby. Discuss with your doctor.
Infants and children Reduced dose necessary.
Over 60 Reduced dose may be necessary.
Driving and hazardous work Avoid such activities until you have learned how furosemide affects you because the drug may reduce mental alertness and cause dizziness.
Alcohol Keep consumption low. Furosemide increases the likelihood of dehydration after drinking alcohol, and alcohol can increase the blood-pressure-lowering effect of furosemide.

PROLONGED USE

Serious problems are unlikely, but levels of salts, such as potassium, sodium, magnesium, and calcium, may become depleted. Low blood pressure, palpitations, headaches, problems passing urine, or muscle cramps may develop, particularly in older people.
Monitoring Periodic tests may be performed to check kidney function and levels of body salts.

GABAPENTIN

Brand name Gabapentin Zentiva, Neurontin
Used in the following combined preparations None

QUICK REFERENCE

Drug group Anticonvulsant drug (p.14)
Overdose danger rating Medium
Dependence rating Medium
Prescription needed Yes
Available as generic Yes

GENERAL INFORMATION

Gabapentin is an anticonvulsant drug. It is used to treat partial seizures, and is often prescribed in combination with other drugs when a patient's epilepsy is not being satisfactorily controlled with the other drugs alone. Unlike some of the other anticonvulsants, gabapentin does not need blood level monitoring. In addition, it does not have any significant interactions with other anticonvulsant drugs.

The drug is also used to relieve neuropathic pain, such as the pain experienced after shingles or by some people with diabetes.

Patients with impaired kidney function should be given smaller doses, and diabetic patients taking gabapentin may notice fluctuations in their blood sugar levels.

Gabapentin is a Schedule III (Class C) controlled drug in the UK.

INFORMATION FOR USERS

Your drug prescription is tailored for you. Do not alter dosage without checking with your doctor.

How taken/used Tablets, capsules, oral solution. Tablets should be swallowed whole; do not crush them.

Frequency and timing of doses Dose is gradually built up to 3 x daily as maintenance treatment. Leave no more than 12 hours between doses.

Adult dosage range 900–3,600mg daily; maintenance dose reached gradually over a few days.

Onset of effect The full anticonvulsant effect may not be seen for 48 hours.

Duration of action 6–8 hours.

Diet advice None.

Storage Keep in original container at room temperature out of the reach of children.

Missed dose Take as soon as you remember. If your next dose is due within 4 hours, take a dose now and skip the next.

Stopping the drug Gabapentin should not be stopped abruptly. Gradual withdrawal over at least 7 days is advised to reduce the risk of seizures in those being treated for epilepsy.

Exceeding the dose An occasional unintentional extra dose is unlikely to be a cause for concern. Large overdoses may lead to dizziness, double vision, and slurred speech. Notify your doctor if these symptoms occur.

POSSIBLE ADVERSE EFFECTS

Drowsiness, dizziness, fatigue, and muscle tremor are common adverse effects of gabapentin. Discuss with your doctor if drowsiness or fatigue are severe or if muscle tremor, vision disturbances, indigestion, or weight gain occur. Rarely, the drug causes mood changes, hallucinations, a rash, or respiratory depression; if these symptoms develop, contact your doctor immediately.

INTERACTIONS

Antacids containing aluminium or magnesium may reduce the effect of gabapentin. Do not take gabapentin within 2 hours of antacids.

Morphine May increase gabapentin blood levels and increase risk of respiratory depression.

Urinary protein tests for diabetes False-positive readings have been recorded with some tests. Special procedures are required for people with diabetes who are taking gabapentin.

SPECIAL PRECAUTIONS

Be sure to tell your doctor if:

- You have a kidney problem.
- You have diabetes.
- You have a history of psychiatric illness.
- You have a history of substance misuse.
- You are taking other medicines.

Pregnancy Drug is likely to reach fetus and its effects are unknown. Discuss with doctor.

Breast-feeding The drug passes into the breast milk, and the effects on the baby are unknown. Discuss with your doctor.

Infants and children Rarely used under 6 years. Reduced doses based on body weight are required in children under 12 years.

Over 60 Doses may have to be adjusted to allow for decreased kidney function.

Driving and hazardous work Avoid until you have learned how the drug affects you. Gabapentin may produce drowsiness or dizziness.

Alcohol May increase sedative effects of drug.

PROLONGED USE

No problems expected.

GENTAMICIN

Brand names Cidomycin, Gentacidin, Gentasol, Genticin, Minims gentamicin

Used in the following combined preparation Gentisone HC

QUICK REFERENCE

Drug group Aminoglycoside antibiotic (p.61)

Overdose danger rating Low

Dependence rating Low

Prescription needed Yes

Available as generic Yes

GENERAL INFORMATION

Gentamicin is one of the aminoglycoside antibiotics. The injectable form is usually reserved for hospital treatment of serious lung, urinary tract, bone, joint, wound, and other infections, peritonitis, septicaemia, and meningitis. This form is also used together with a penicillin to prevent and treat heart valve infections (endocarditis). Gentamicin drops are used to treat eye and ear infections.

Gentamicin given by injection can have serious adverse effects on the ears and the kidneys. Damage to the ears may lead to deafness and problems with the balance mechanism in the inner ear. Courses of treatment are, therefore, limited to 7 days when possible. Treatment is monitored by measuring blood levels of gentamicin, especially when high doses are needed or kidney function is poor. Rarely, gentamicin can be associated with histamine-related adverse reactions (see p.56).

INFORMATION FOR USERS

Your drug prescription is tailored for you. Do not alter dosage without checking with your doctor.

How taken/used Injection, eye/ear drops.

Frequency and timing of doses 1–3 x daily (injection); 3–4 x daily or as directed (ear drops); every 2 hours or as directed (eye drops).

Adult dosage range According to condition and response (injection); according to your doctor's instructions (eye and ear drops).

Onset of effect Within 1–2 hours.

Duration of action 8–12 hours.

Diet advice None.

Storage Keep in original container at room temperature out of the reach of children.

Missed dose Apply eye/ear preparations as soon as you remember.

Stopping the drug Complete the course. Even if you feel better, the original infection may still be present and may recur if treatment is stopped too soon.

Exceeding the dose Although overdose by injection is dangerous, it is unlikely because treatment is carefully monitored. For other forms of the drug an occasional unintentional extra dose is unlikely to cause concern, but if you notice any unusual symptoms, tell your doctor.

POSSIBLE ADVERSE EFFECTS

Adverse effects are rare, but those that occur with injections may be serious. If you have severe nausea and vomiting, discuss with your doctor. If you develop dizziness, vertigo (loss of balance), impaired hearing, or bloody or cloudy urine, stop using the drug and notify your doctor promptly. If ear drops are used when the eardrum is perforated, damage to the inner ear may occur. Blurred vision or eye irritation may occur with the eye preparations and should be reported to your doctor if severe. Allergic reactions, including rash and itching, may occur with all preparations that contain gentamicin. If such reactions do occur, stop using the drug and contact your doctor immediately.

INTERACTIONS

General note A wide range of drugs, including furosemide, vancomycin, and cephalosporins, increase the risk of hearing loss and/or kidney failure with gentamicin given by injection.

SPECIAL PRECAUTIONS

Be sure to tell your doctor if:

- You have a long-term kidney problem.
- You have a hearing disorder, especially a perforated eardrum.
- You have myasthenia gravis.
- You have Parkinson's disease.
- You have previously had an allergic reaction to aminoglycosides.
- You are taking other medicines.

Pregnancy No evidence of risk with eye or ear drops. Injections are not prescribed, as they may cause hearing defects in the baby. Discuss with your doctor.

Breast-feeding No evidence of risk with eye or ear preparations. Given by injection, the drug may pass into the breast milk. Discuss with your doctor.

Infants and children Reduced dose necessary for injections.

Over 60 Increased likelihood of adverse effects with gentamicin. Close monitoring of treatment is therefore necessary.

Driving and hazardous work No known problems from preparations for the eye or ear.

Alcohol No known problems.

PROLONGED USE

Gentamicin is not usually given for longer than 7 days. When the drug is given by injection, there is a risk of adverse effects on hearing and balance.

Monitoring Blood levels of the drug are usually checked if it is given by injection. Tests on kidney function are also usually carried out.

GLIBENCLAMIDE

Brand name Gliken, Liamide
Used in the following combined preparations None

QUICK REFERENCE

Drug group Drug for diabetes (p.80)
Overdose danger rating High
Dependence rating Low
Prescription needed Yes
Available as generic Yes

GENERAL INFORMATION

Glibenclamide is an oral antidiabetic drug belonging to the sulfonylurea class. Like other drugs of this type, it stimulates the production and secretion of insulin from the islet cells in the pancreas. This promotes the uptake of sugar into body cells, thereby lowering the blood sugar level.

Glibenclamide is used in the treatment of Type 2 diabetes, in conjunction with exercise and a diet that is low in sugar and fats. In conditions of severe illness, injury, or stress, however, the drug may lose its effectiveness, making insulin injections necessary.

Adverse effects are generally mild. The most common side effect is hypoglycaemia (low blood sugar). Symptoms of poor diabetic control will occur if the dosage of glibenclamide is not appropriate.

INFORMATION FOR USERS

Your drug prescription is tailored for you. Do not alter dosage without checking with your doctor.
How taken/used Tablets.
Frequency and timing of doses 1 x daily in the morning with your first meal.
Adult dosage range 5–15mg daily.
Onset of effect Within 3 hours.
Duration of action 10–15 hours.
Diet advice An individualized diabetic diet must be maintained in order for the drug to be fully effective. Follow the advice of your doctor.
Storage Keep in original container at room temperature out of the reach of children. Protect from light.
Missed dose Take with next meal; do not double the dose to account for missed dose.
Stopping the drug Do not stop the drug without consulting your doctor; stopping the drug may lead to worsening of your diabetes.

OVERDOSE ACTION

Seek immediate medical advice in all cases. If any warning symptoms of excessively low blood sugar (such as faintness, dizziness, headache, confusion, sweating, or tremor) occur, eat or drink something sugary. Take emergency action if seizures or loss of consciousness occur.

POSSIBLE ADVERSE EFFECTS

Serious adverse effects are rare with glibenclamide. Symptoms such as faintness, confusion, weakness, tremor, and sweating may be signs of low blood sugar due to lack of food or too high a dose of the drug. If any such symptoms occur, eat or drink something sugary immediately and seek medical assistance. Other possible adverse effects include nausea, vomiting, rash, itching, and weight changes. Discuss with your doctor if these occur or if you have severe constipation or diarrhoea. If jaundice develops, consult your doctor without delay.

INTERACTIONS

General note A variety of drugs may reduce the effect of glibenclamide and so raise blood sugar levels. They include corticosteroids, oestrogens, diuretics, and rifampicin. Others increase the risk of low blood sugar. These include warfarin, aspirin, sulfonamides and other antibacterials, antifungals, NSAIDs, and ACE inhibitors.
Beta blockers may mask symptoms of hypoglycaemia, especially non-cardioselective beta blockers such as propranolol.

SPECIAL PRECAUTIONS

Be sure to tell your doctor if:

- You have long-term liver or kidney problems.
- You are allergic to sulfonylurea drugs.
- You have thyroid problems.
- You have porphyria or glucose-6-phosphate
- dehydrogenase (G6PD) deficiency.
- You have ever had problems with your adrenal glands.
- You are taking other medicines.

Pregnancy Not usually prescribed. Insulin is generally substituted in pregnancy because it gives better diabetic control.
Breast-feeding The drug passes into breast milk and may cause low blood sugar in the baby.
Infants and children Not prescribed.
Over 60 Reduced dose may be necessary due to greater risk of low blood sugar with drug.

Driving and hazardous work Usually no problems, but avoid these activities if you have warning signs of low blood sugar.
Alcohol Avoid. Alcohol may upset diabetic control, increasing the risk of hypoglycaemia.
Surgery and general anaesthetics Notify your doctor or dentist that you have diabetes before undergoing any surgery.
Sunlight and sunbeds Take care with exposure to sunlight and tanning beds as the drug may increase the skin's sensitivity to ultraviolet light.

PROLONGED USE
No problems expected.
Monitoring Regular testing of blood sugar control is required. Periodic assessment of the eyes, heart, and kidneys may also be advised.

GLICLAZIDE

Brand names Bilxona, Dacadis MR, Diamicron (MR), Edicil MR, Laaglyda MR, Nazdol MR, Vamju, Ziclaseg, Zicron (PR)
Used in the following combined preparations None

QUICK REFERENCE
Drug group Drug for diabetes (p.80)
Overdose danger rating High
Dependence rating Low
Prescription needed Yes
Available as generic Yes

GENERAL INFORMATION
Gliclazide is an oral drug for diabetes belonging to the sulfonylurea group. It stimulates the production and secretion of insulin from the pancreas. This promotes the uptake of sugar into body cells, thereby lowering the level of sugar in the blood. The drug is used to treat Type 2 diabetes mellitus, in conjunction with diet, exercise, and weight loss. In severe illness, injury, stress, or surgery, however, it may lose its effectiveness, necessitating the use of insulin injections. Adverse effects are generally mild.

INFORMATION FOR USERS
Your drug prescription is tailored for you. Do not alter dosage without checking with your doctor.
How taken/used Tablets, modified release (MR) tablets.
Frequency and timing of doses 1–2 x daily (in the morning and evening with a meal).
Dosage range 40–320mg daily (doses above 160mg are divided into two doses).
Onset of effect Within 1 hour.
Duration of action 12–24 hours.
Diet advice An individualized diabetic diet must be maintained for the drug to be fully effective. Follow the advice of your doctor.
Storage Keep in original container at room temperature out of the reach of children.
Missed dose Take with next meal; do not double the dose to account for missed dose.
Stopping the drug Do not stop without consulting your doctor; stopping the drug may lead to worsening of the underlying condition.

OVERDOSE ACTION
Seek immediate medical advice in all cases. If early warning symptoms of excessively low blood sugar (such as faintness, dizziness, headache, confusion, sweating, or tremor) occur, eat or drink something sugary. Take emergency action if seizures or loss of consciousness occur.

POSSIBLE ADVERSE EFFECTS
Serious adverse effects are rare with gliclazide. Dizziness, faintness, confusion, weakness, tremor, and sweating may be signs of low blood sugar due to lack of food or too high a dose of the drug. If these symptoms occur, eat or drink something sugary immediately and seek medical assistance. Other possible adverse effects include nausea, vomiting, rash, itching, and weight changes. Discuss with your doctor if they occur or if you have severe constipation or diarrhoea. If jaundice develops, consult your doctor without delay.

INTERACTIONS
General note A variety of drugs may reduce the effect of gliclazide and so raise blood sugar levels. These include corticosteroids, oestrogens, NSAIDs, diuretics, and rifampicin. Other drugs increase the risk of low blood sugar. These include warfarin, sulfonamides and other antibacterials, aspirin, beta blockers, ACE inhibitors, and antifungals (gliclazide should not be used with miconazole in particular).

SPECIAL PRECAUTIONS
Be sure to tell your doctor if:
- You have long-term liver or kidney problems.
- You are allergic to sulfonylurea drugs.
- You have thyroid problems.
- You have porphyria.

◆ You have ever had problems with your adrenal glands.
◆ You are taking other medicines.

Pregnancy Not recommended. May cause abnormally low blood sugar in the newborn baby. Insulin is generally substituted in pregnancy because it gives better diabetic control.
Breast-feeding The drug passes into the breast milk and may cause low blood sugar in the baby. Discuss with your doctor.
Infants and children Not prescribed.
Over 60 Signs of low blood sugar may be more difficult to recognize in older adults. Reduced dose may be necessary.
Driving and hazardous work Avoid until you know how gliclazide affects you because it can cause dizziness, drowsiness, and confusion.
Alcohol Avoid. Alcohol may upset diabetic control, increasing the risk of hypoglycaemia.
Surgery and general anaesthetics Notify your doctor or dentist that you have diabetes before undergoing any surgery.
Sunlight and sunbeds Avoid exposure to the sun and do not use a sunlamp or sunbed.

PROLONGED USE
No problems expected.
Monitoring Regular testing of blood sugar control is required. Periodic assessment of the eyes, heart, and kidneys may also be advised.

GLUCAGON

Brand name GlucaGen
Used in the following combined preparations None

QUICK REFERENCE
Drug group Drug for diabetes (p.80)
Overdose danger rating Low
Dependence rating Low
Prescription needed Yes
Available as generic No

GENERAL INFORMATION
Glucagon is a hormone produced by the pancreas. A synthetic injectable form is used as an emergency treatment for low blood sugar (hypoglycaemia) in unconscious diabetic patients on insulin. In contrast to insulin, it raises blood sugar by mobilizing liver stores of glycogen, which is released into the blood as glucose. Glucagon will not work when glycogen stores are depleted, as in starvation or extreme fasting, alcohol-induced hypoglycaemia, or impaired adrenal function. Glucagon blocks the activity of smooth muscle in the intestines, so may be used to test bowel motility. It can also stimulate contraction of heart muscle so may be used to treat severe beta-blocker overdoses, and it can be used to investigate adult growth hormone deficiency.

Although it is usually given by medical personnel, glucagon packs may be given to some people with diabetes for emergency use.

INFORMATION FOR USERS
Your drug prescription is tailored for you. Do not alter dosage without checking with your doctor.
How taken/used Injection.
Frequency and timing of doses *Hypoglycaemia* 1 x intramuscular or subcutaneous injection. *Bowel motility testing* 1 x intravenous injection.
Adult dosage range *Hypoglycaemia* 1mg. *Bowel motility testing* 0.2–1.0mg.
Onset of effect Within 10 minutes.
Duration of action Up to 40 minutes (intramuscular/subcutaneous injection) or 20 minutes (intravenous injection).
Diet advice If used for hypoglycaemia, carbohydrates should be eaten as soon as possible after the injection to prevent further hypoglycaemia.
Storage Store at 2–8°C; do not freeze, protect from light, and keep out of the reach of children. The drug should be reconstituted from its powder form just before administration. Packs for personal use in emergencies will last up to 18 months.
Missed dose Not applicable as the drug is for one-off use only.
Stopping the drug Not applicable as the drug is for one-off use only.
Exceeding the dose If the drug is used under medical supervision, overdosage is unlikely. In other situations, exceeding the dose is unlikely to cause major problems, but call your doctor promptly if you have nausea or vomiting.

POSSIBLE ADVERSE EFFECTS
Adverse effects of glucagon vary according to its use. If used as an emergency treatment for hypoglycaemia in a person with diabetes, it may cause nausea and vomiting or, less commonly, abdominal pain; tell your doctor if any of these symptoms are severe. If a rash or swelling of the lips or tongue occur, the drug should be stopped and immediate medical

help sought. If used for diagnostic purposes, adverse effects are rare but may include symptoms of hypoglycaemia (such as faintness, dizziness, headache, confusion, sweating, or tremor), low blood pressure, and palpitations. If any of these symptoms occur, tell the doctor immediately; the drug should be stopped.

INTERACTIONS

Insulin counteracts the effects of glucagon.
Indomethacin may reduce the effectiveness of glucagon.
Warfarin Glucagon may increase the effects of warfarin.
Beta blockers may cause brief rise in blood pressure and heart rate after glucagon given.

SPECIAL PRECAUTIONS

Be sure to tell your doctor if:
- You have heart problems.
- You have a phaeochromocytoma (a rare tumour of the adrenal gland).
- You have an insulinoma or glucagonoma (rare tumours of the pancreas).
- You are allergic to glucagon or lactose.
- You are taking other medicines.

Pregnancy No evidence of risk.
Breast-feeding No evidence of risk.
Infants and children Reduced dose necessary.
Over 60 Increased likelihood of adverse effects.
Driving and hazardous work If drug used to treat hypoglycaemia, avoid such activities until all signs of hypoglycaemia have gone. If drug used diagnostically, avoid such activities until after carbohydrates have been consumed.
Alcohol Avoid until blood sugar levels normal.

PROLONGED USE

Glucagon is not used long term.

GLYCERYL TRINITRATE

Brand names Deponit, Minitran, Nitrocine, Nitro-Dur, Nitrolingual, Nitronal, Percutol, Rectogesic, Transiderm-Nitro, and others
Used in the following combined preparations None

QUICK REFERENCE

Drug group Anti-angina drug (p.33)
Overdose danger rating Medium
Dependence rating Low
Prescription needed No (most preparations); yes (injection)
Available as generic Yes

GENERAL INFORMATION

Glyceryl trinitrate is a type of vasodilator called a nitrate and is used to relieve the pain of angina attacks. It is available in short-acting forms (sublingual or buccal tablets, ointment, and spray) and long-acting forms (slow-release tablets and patches). The short-acting forms act very quickly to relieve angina. The drug is given by injection or infusion in hospital for severe angina, heart failure, and to control high blood pressure. It may also be used topically to treat anal fissures.

Glyceryl trinitrate may cause a variety of minor adverse effects, such as flushing and headache; however, most of these can be controlled by adjusting the dosage. It is best taken for the first time while sitting, as fainting may follow the drop in blood pressure caused by the drug.

INFORMATION FOR USERS

Follow instructions on the label. Call your doctor if symptoms worsen.
How taken/used Buccal tablets, sublingual tablets, injection, infusion, ointment, gel, skin patches, spray.
Frequency and timing of doses *Angina prevention* 3 x daily (buccal tablets); every 3–4 hours (ointment); once daily (patches). *Angina relief* Use buccal or sublingual tablets, ointment, or spray at the onset of an attack or immediately prior to exercise. Dose may be repeated within 5 minutes if further relief required. *Anal fissure* Every 12 hours for up to 8 weeks.
Adult dosage range *Angina prevention* 2–15mg daily (buccal tablets); 5–15mg daily (patches); as directed (ointment). *Angina relief* 0.3–1mg per dose (sublingual tablets); 1–3mg per dose (buccal tablets); 1–2 sprays per dose (spray). *Anal fissure* 3mg daily in 2 equal doses.
Onset of effect *Angina* 1–3 minutes (buccal and sublingual tablets and spray); 30–60 minutes (patches and ointment). *Anal fissure* 12 hours.
Duration of action 20–30 minutes (sublingual tablets and spray); 3–5 hours (buccal tablets and ointment); up to 24 hours (patches); up to 12 hours (anal fissure preparations).
Diet advice None.
Storage Keep sublingual tablets in an airtight glass container fitted with a foil-lined, screw-on cap in a cool, dry place out of the reach of children. Protect from light. Do not expose to heat. Discard tablets within 8 weeks of

opening. Check label of other preparations for storage conditions.

Missed dose If your next dose is due within 6 hours, skip the missed dose and take your next scheduled dose as usual (buccal tablets); otherwise, take as soon as you remember, or when needed. If your next dose is due within 2 hours, take a single dose now and skip the next (other preparations).

Stopping the drug Do not stop taking the drug without consulting your doctor.

Exceeding the dose An occasional unintentional extra dose is unlikely to cause problems. Large overdoses may cause symptoms such as dizziness, vomiting, severe headache, sweating, seizures, or loss of consciousness. Notify your doctor.

POSSIBLE ADVERSE EFFECTS

The most serious adverse effect is lowered blood pressure, which may cause dizziness, fainting, or collapse. If dizziness occurs, discuss with your doctor; if fainting or collapse occur, stop taking the drug and consult your doctor without delay. Other effects, such as headache and flushing, usually decrease in severity after regular use and can also be controlled by adjusting the drug dosage. If these are severe, discuss with your doctor.

INTERACTIONS

Antihypertensive drugs and other anti-angina drugs These drugs increase the possibility of lowered blood pressure or fainting when taken with glyceryl trinitrate.

Sildenafil, tadalafil, and vardenafil The hypotensive effect of glyceryl trinitrate is increased significantly by these drugs; they should not be used with glyceryl trinitrate.

SPECIAL PRECAUTIONS

Be sure to consult your doctor or pharmacist before taking this drug if:

- You have any other heart condition.
- You have a lung condition.
- You have long-term liver or kidney problems.
- You have any blood disorders.
- You have glaucoma.
- You have thyroid disease.
- You have low blood pressure.
- You have anaemia.
- You have a recent head injury or stroke.
- You are taking other medicines.

Pregnancy Safety in pregnancy not established. Discuss with your doctor.

Breast-feeding It is not known whether the drug passes into the breast milk. Discuss with your doctor.

Infants and children Not usually prescribed.

Over 60 No special problems.

Driving and hazardous work Avoid until you have learned how glyceryl trinitrate affects you because the drug can cause dizziness.

Alcohol Avoid excessive intake. Alcohol may increase the risk of lowered blood pressure, causing dizziness and fainting.

PROLONGED USE

The drug's effects usually grow slightly weaker during prolonged use as the body adapts. Timing of the doses may be changed to prevent this effect. Preparations for anal fissures should not be used for more than 8 weeks.

Monitoring Periodic checks on blood pressure are usually required when glyceryl trinitrate is used for angina.

GOSERELIN

Brand names Zoladex, Zoladex LA

Used in the following combined preparations None

QUICK REFERENCE

Drug group Anticancer drug (p.94)

Overdose danger rating Low

Dependence rating Low

Prescription needed Yes

Available as generic No

GENERAL INFORMATION

Goserelin is a synthetic analogue of the hormone gonadorelin (now more commonly called gonadotrophin-releasing hormone, or GnRH). Like GnRH, the drug stimulates the release of other hormones from the pituitary gland, which in turn control the production of sex hormones.

Goserelin reduces testosterone levels in men and oestrogen levels in pre-menopausal women, and is used to treat prostate cancer in men and breast cancer in women. At the start of treatment for prostate cancer, it is often given with an anti-androgen drug (see p.85) to control an initial growth spurt of the tumour – known as "tumour flare". The drug is also used in the management of endometriosis and fibroids in women, and in assisted reproduction. The first dose is normally given during menstruation to avoid the possibility that the patient may be pregnant. Women of child-bearing age are advised to use barrier methods of contraception during treatment.

Loss of bone density is an important side effect in women. Therefore, repeat courses of the drug are given only for cancers.

INFORMATION FOR USERS

Your drug prescription is tailored for you. Do not alter dosage without checking with your doctor.
How taken/used Implant injection, long-acting (LA) implant injection.
Frequency and timing of doses *Endometriosis* Every 28 days, maximum of a single 6-month course only (implant). *Fibroids* Every 28 days, maximum 3 months' treatment (implant). *Breast and prostate cancer* Every 28 days. *Prostate cancer* Every 12 weeks (LA implant).
Adult dosage range *Endometriosis/fibroids/breast and prostate cancer* 3.6mg (implant) every 28 days; 10.8mg (LA implant) every 3 months.
Onset of effect *Endometriosis/fibroids/breast cancer* Within 24 hours; *Prostate cancer* 1–2 weeks after tumour flare.
Duration of action 28 days (implant); 12 weeks (LA implant).
Diet advice None.
Storage Not applicable. Not for home use.
Missed dose No cause for concern. Treatment can be resumed when possible.
Stopping the drug Do not stop treatment without consulting your doctor.
Exceeding the dose Overdosage is unlikely since treatment is not self-administered.

POSSIBLE ADVERSE EFFECTS

Symptoms similar to those of the menopause in women or orchidectomy (removal of the testes) in men are common. They include hot flushes, sweating, reduced libido, erectile dysfunction (in men), and breast enlargement and tenderness. There may also be bone pain, and some women have vaginal bleeding early in treatment. Discuss with your doctor if these are severe. More rarely, goserelin may cause rash, wheezing, a reaction at the injection site, dizziness, fainting, leg weakness or numbness, and ovarian cysts (in women). Report any such effects to your doctor straight away.

INTERACTIONS

Antidiabetic drugs Goserelin may reduce the blood-sugar-lowering effect of these drugs.

SPECIAL PRECAUTIONS

Be sure to tell your doctor if:
- ◆ You have osteoporosis.
- ◆ You have diabetes.
- ◆ You may be pregnant.
- ◆ You have previously been treated with goserelin (or another gonadorelin analogue) for endometriosis or fibroids.
- ◆ You have polycystic ovarian disease.
- ◆ You are allergic to gonadorelin analogues.
- ◆ You are taking other medicines.

Pregnancy Not prescribed. Risk of harm to the fetus.
Breast-feeding Not recommended. Discuss with your doctor.
Infants and children Not recommended.
Over 60 No special problems.
Driving and hazardous work No special problems.
Alcohol No special problems.

PROLONGED USE

Goserelin is only used in the long term for treatment of prostate or breast cancer. Bone density may be lost, and medication to counteract this may be given.
Monitoring Women are usually monitored for changes in bone density.

HALOPERIDOL

Brand names Haldol, Halkid
Used in the following combined preparations None

QUICK REFERENCE

Drug group Butyrophenone antipsychotic drug (p.13)
Overdose danger rating Medium
Dependence rating Low
Prescription needed Yes
Available as generic Yes

GENERAL INFORMATION

Introduced in the 1960s, haloperidol is an antipsychotic drug used to treat schizophrenia and other psychoses, to control mania, and to reduce agitation and violent behaviour. Haloperidol is also used in the short term to treat severe anxiety. It does not cure the underlying disorder but relieves the distressing symptoms. The drug is also used in the control of

Tourette's syndrome and to treat intractable hiccups and vomiting.

The main drawback of haloperidol is that it can produce the side effect of abnormal, involuntary facial movements and stiffness of the limbs. As a result, it is no longer recommended for first-line treatment of schizophrenia.

INFORMATION FOR USERS

Your drug prescription is tailored for you. Do not alter dosage without checking with your doctor.

How taken/used Tablets, capsules, liquid, injection, depot injection.

Frequency and timing of doses 2–4 x daily.

Adult dosage range *Mental illness* 3–10mg daily initially, up to a maximum of 20mg daily. *Severe anxiety* 1mg daily.

Onset of effect 2–3 hours (by mouth); 20–30 minutes (by injection).

Duration of action 6–24 hours (by mouth); 2–4 hours (injection); up to 4 weeks (depot injection).

Diet advice None.

Storage Keep in original container at room temperature out of the reach of children.

Missed dose Take as soon as you remember. If your next dose is due within 3 hours, take a single dose now and skip the next.

Stopping the drug Do not stop the drug without consulting your doctor; symptoms may recur.

Exceeding the dose An occasional unintentional extra dose is unlikely to cause problems. Larger overdoses may cause unusual drowsiness, muscle weakness or rigidity, and/or faintness. Notify your doctor.

POSSIBLE ADVERSE EFFECTS

Various minor anticholinergic symptoms (see p.7), such as dry mouth and blurred vision, can occur, but these often diminish with time. Drowsiness, lethargy, insomnia, and sexual dysfunction may also occur; discuss with your doctor if these are severe. The most significant adverse effect of haloperidol is abnormal facial movements and limb stiffness (parkinsonism). Discuss these effects with your doctor; they may be controlled by adjusting the dosage. The drug may also sometimes cause palpitations, breathlessness, or sweating; if this happens, discuss with your doctor. Rarely, haloperidol may cause a high fever or confusion; if so, you should stop taking it and consult your doctor immediately.

INTERACTIONS

Sedatives Sedatives are likely to increase the sedative properties of haloperidol.

Rifampicin and anticonvulsants These drugs may reduce the effects of haloperidol, the dosage of which may need to be increased.

Lithium This drug may increase the risk of parkinsonism and effects on the nerves.

Methyldopa This drug may increase the risk of parkinsonism and low blood pressure.

Anticholinergic drugs Haloperidol may increase the side effects of these drugs.

Drugs that can affect heart rhythm (e.g. antidepressants, antifungals, antiarrhythmics, antibiotics, and antihistamines) There is an increased risk of irregular heart rhythms when these drugs are used with haloperidol.

SPECIAL PRECAUTIONS

Be sure to tell your doctor if:

- You have long-term liver or kidney problems.
- You have heart or circulation problems or have had a stroke.
- You have had epileptic seizures.
- You have Parkinson's disease or other movement disorders.
- You are taking other medicines.

Pregnancy Short-term nervous system problems may occur in babies when haloperidol is taken during the third trimester. The drug is occasionally used under psychiatric supervision. Discuss with your doctor.

Breast-feeding The drug passes into the breast milk and may affect the baby. Discuss with your doctor.

Infants and children Rarely required. Reduced dose necessary.

Over 60 Reduced dose may be necessary.

Driving and hazardous work Avoid such activities until you have learned how haloperidol affects you because the drug may cause drowsiness and slowed reactions.

Alcohol Avoid. Alcohol may increase the sedative effect of this drug.

PROLONGED USE

Use of this drug for more than a few months may lead to tardive dyskinesia (abnormal, involuntary movements of the eyes, face, and tongue). Occasionally, jaundice may occur. In older people with dementia who take haloperidol, a small increase in strokes, blood clots, seizures, and death has been reported.

HEPARIN/LOW MOLECULAR WEIGHT HEPARINS

Brand names [dalteparin] Fragmin, [enoxaparin] Clexane, Inhixa, [tinzaparin] Innohep

Used in the following combined preparations None

QUICK REFERENCE

Drug group Anticoagulant drug (p.37)

Overdose danger rating High

Dependence rating Low

Prescription needed Yes

Available as generic Yes (both heparin and LMWH)

GENERAL INFORMATION

Heparin is an anticoagulant drug used to prevent formation of blood clots and aid in their dispersion. Because the drug acts quickly, it is particularly useful in emergencies to prevent further clotting when a clot has already reached the lungs or the brain, for instance. People undergoing open heart surgery or kidney dialysis are given heparin to prevent clotting. A low dose is sometimes given following surgery to prevent the development of deep vein thrombosis (clots in the leg veins). Heparin is often given in conjunction with other slower-acting anticoagulants, such as warfarin. It is also used to treat unstable angina.

The most serious adverse effect, as with all anticoagulants, is excessive bleeding, so the blood's clotting ability is monitored very carefully. In addition, bruising may occur around the injection site.

Several types of heparin, called low molecular weight heparins (LMWH), do not have to be administered in hospital.

INFORMATION FOR USERS

Heparin is given only under medical supervision and is not for self-administration.

How taken/used Injection, intravenous infusion.

Frequency and timing of doses Every 8–12 hours or continuous intravenous infusion (unfractionated heparin); once daily (LMWH).

Dosage range Dosage is determined by nature of the condition being treated or prevented.

Onset of effect Within 15 minutes.

Duration of action 4–12 hours after end of treatment; 24 hours after treatment stops (LMWH).

Diet advice None.

Storage Keep in original container at room temperature out of the reach of children.

Missed dose Notify your doctor.

Stopping the drug Do not stop taking the drug without consulting your doctor. Stopping the drug may lead to clotting of blood.

OVERDOSE ACTION

Seek immediate medical advice in all cases. Take emergency action if bleeding, severe headache, or loss of consciousness occur.

POSSIBLE ADVERSE EFFECTS

Bleeding is the most common adverse effect; the risk is increased in people with impaired kidney function. Inform your doctor immediately if bleeding or bruising occur. Less common effects include hair loss, aching bones, breathing difficulties, jaundice, vomiting blood, and rash. Consult your doctor if hair loss or aching bones occur. If you develop breathing difficulties, rash, or jaundice, or vomit blood, notify your doctor immediately; you should also stop the drug if you develop a rash.

INTERACTIONS

Aspirin and other NSAIDs may increase the anticoagulant effect of heparin and the risk of bleeding in the intestines or joints. Do not take these drugs with heparin.

ACE inhibitors and potassium supplements taken with heparins may increase the risk of high blood potassium.

Clopidogrel, ticlopidine, and dipyridamole These drugs may increase the anticoagulant effect of heparin. The dosage of heparin may need to be adjusted accordingly.

SPECIAL PRECAUTIONS

Be sure to tell your doctor if:

- You have long-term liver or kidney problems.
- You have high blood pressure.
- You bleed easily or are currently bleeding.
- You have any allergies.
- You have peptic ulcers.
- You have diabetes.
- You have had a previous reaction to heparin.
- You have had a recent stroke, injury, or surgery.
- You are taking other medicines.

Pregnancy Careful monitoring is necessary in pregnancy as heparin may cause the mother to bleed excessively if taken near delivery. Discuss with your doctor.

Breast-feeding No evidence of risk.

Infants and children Reduced dose necessary according to age and weight.

Over 60 No special problems, but older people may be more prone to bleeding.

Driving and hazardous work Avoid risk of injury, as excessive bruising and bleeding may occur.

Alcohol No special problems.

Surgery and general anaesthetics Heparin may need to be stopped beforehand. Discuss with your doctor or dentist before any surgery.

PROLONGED USE

Osteoporosis and hair loss may occur very rarely with long-term use; tolerance to heparin may also develop.

Monitoring Periodic blood and liver function tests will be required.

HYDROCHLOROTHIAZIDE

Brand names None

Used in the following combined preparations
Acezide, Capozide, Co-amilozide, Cozaar Comp, Dyazide, Moduretic, and others

QUICK REFERENCE

Drug group Thiazide diuretic (p.31)

Overdose danger rating Low

Dependence rating Low

Prescription needed Yes

Available as generic No

GENERAL INFORMATION

Hydrochlorothiazide belongs to the thiazide group of diuretic drugs, which remove excess water from the body and reduce oedema (fluid retention) in people with congestive heart failure, kidney disorders, cirrhosis of the liver, and premenstrual syndrome. It is also used in combination with other antihypertensives (see p.34) to treat high blood pressure; in the UK, it is only available in combination with other antihypertensives. The drug increases potassium loss in the urine, which can cause a variety of symptoms (see p.31), and increases the likelihood of irregular heart rhythms, particularly in patients who are taking drugs such as digoxin. For this reason, potassium supplements or potassium-sparing diuretics are often given with hydrochlorothiazide.

INFORMATION FOR USERS

Your drug prescription is tailored for you. Do not alter dosage without checking with your doctor.

How taken/used Tablets.

Frequency and timing of doses Once daily, or every 2 days, early in the day.

Adult dosage range *Hypertension* 25–50mg daily. *Oedema* 25–100mg daily.

Onset of effect Within 2 hours.

Duration of action 6–12 hours.

Diet advice Use of this drug may reduce potassium in the body. Eat plenty of fresh fruit and vegetables. Discuss with your doctor the advisability of reducing your salt intake.

Storage Keep in original container at room temperature out of the reach of children. Protect from light.

Missed dose No cause for concern, but take as soon as you remember. However, if it is late in the day do not take the missed dose, or you may have to get up during the night to pass urine. Take the next scheduled dose as usual.

Stopping the drug Do not stop the drug without consulting your doctor; symptoms may recur.

Exceeding the dose An occasional unintentional extra dose is unlikely to be a cause for concern. But if you notice any unusual symptoms, or if a large overdose has been taken, tell your doctor.

POSSIBLE ADVERSE EFFECTS

Adverse effects are generally rare, and most are caused by excessive loss of potassium in the urine. They include muscle cramps, lethargy, dizziness, headache, nausea, vomiting, constipation, and temporary erectile dysfunction (impotence). Speak to your doctor if you have nausea, vomiting, or constipation, or if the other effects are severe; they can usually be corrected by taking a potassium supplement. Rarely, gout may occur in susceptible people, and certain forms of diabetes may become more difficult to control. If you develop new skin lesions, tell your doctor. If a rash occurs, stop the drug and call your doctor promptly.

INTERACTIONS

Non-steroidal anti-inflammatory drugs (NSAIDs) Some NSAIDs may reduce the diuretic effect of hydrochlorothiazide, so its dosage may need to be adjusted.

Anti-arrhythmic and digitalis drugs increase the risk of toxicity from low blood potassium with hydrochlorothiazide.

Corticosteroids further increase loss of potassium from the body if taken with hydrochlorothiazide, and may reduce its diuretic effect.
Lithium Hydrochlorothiazide may increase lithium levels in the blood, leading to a risk of serious adverse effects.

SPECIAL PRECAUTIONS

Be sure to tell your doctor if:
- You have long-term liver or kidney problems.
- You have had gout.
- You have diabetes.
- You are taking other medicines.

Pregnancy Safety in pregnancy not established. Discuss with your doctor.
Breast-feeding The drug passes into the breast milk, but normal doses are unlikely to affect the baby adversely. Discuss with your doctor.
Infants and children Not usually prescribed. Reduced dose necessary.
Over 60 Increased likelihood of adverse effects.
Driving and hazardous work Avoid until you have learned how drug affects you as it may reduce mental alertness and cause dizziness.
Alcohol Keep intake low. Hydrochlorothiazide increases the likelihood of dehydration and hangovers after consumption of alcohol.

PROLONGED USE

Excessive loss of potassium and imbalances of other salts may result. The drug increases skin sensitivity to sunlight. Long-term use increases the risk of non-melanoma skin cancers. See your doctor if you find any new skin lesions.
Monitoring Blood tests may be performed periodically to check kidney function and levels of potassium and other salts.

HYDROCORTISONE

Brand names Corlan, Dioderm, Efcortelan, Efcortesol, Hydrocortistab, Hydrocortone, Mildison, Solu-Cortef
Used in the following combined preparations Alphaderm, Anusol Plus HC, Xyloproct, and many others

QUICK REFERENCE

Drug group Corticosteroid (p.78)
Overdose danger rating Low
Dependence rating Low
Prescription needed Yes (except for some topical preparations)
Available as generic Yes

GENERAL INFORMATION

Hydrocortisone is chemically identical to the hormone cortisol, which is produced by the adrenal glands, and is therefore prescribed to replace natural hormones in adrenal insufficiency (Addison's disease). Its main use is in treating a variety of allergic and inflammatory conditions. In topical preparations, it gives prompt relief from inflammation of the skin, eye, and outer ear. It is also used orally or by injection to relieve asthma, inflammatory bowel disease, and many rheumatic and allergic disorders. Injected directly into the joints, the drug relieves pain and stiffness (see p.51).

Overuse of skin preparations can lead to permanent thinning of the skin. Taken by mouth, long-term treatment with high doses may cause serious side effects.

INFORMATION FOR USERS

Your drug prescription is tailored for you. Do not alter dosage without checking with your doctor.
How taken/used Tablets, lozenges, injection, rectal foam, cream, ointment, eye/ear ointment/drops.
Frequency and timing of doses Varies according to condition and preparation.
Dosage range Varies according to condition and preparation.
Onset of effect Within hours. Full effect may not be felt for several days.
Duration of action Up to 12 hours.
Diet advice Salt intake may need to be restricted if the drug is taken by mouth. It may also be necessary to take potassium supplements.
Storage Keep in original container at room temperature out of the reach of children.
Missed dose Take as soon as you remember. If your next dose is due within 2 hours, take a single dose now and skip the next.
Stopping the drug Do not stop without consulting your doctor, particularly after prolonged treatment with oral hydrocortisone – sudden cessation may be harmful. Your doctor will supervise a gradual reduction in dosage.
Exceeding the dose An occasional unintentional extra dose is unlikely to be a cause for concern. But if you notice any unusual symptoms, or if a large overdose has been taken, tell your doctor.

POSSIBLE ADVERSE EFFECTS

Taken by mouth, hydrocortisone may cause indigestion, weight gain, and acne. Discuss with your doctor if any of these are severe. It may also cause fluid retention, and high doses may cause muscle weakness, mood changes, and menstrual irregularities; consult your doctor if any of these symptoms occur. Long-term use of high doses, especially when taken by mouth, may cause various serious adverse effects (see Prolonged use). These are carefully monitored during treatment.

INTERACTIONS

Barbiturates, anticonvulsants, and rifampicin reduce the effectiveness of hydrocortisone.
Antidiabetic drugs Hydrocortisone reduces the action of these drugs.
Antihypertensive drugs Hydrocortisone reduces the effects of these drugs.
Vaccines Severe reactions can occur if certain vaccines are given with hydrocortisone.
Aspirin and other NSAIDs Increased risk of peptic ulcer and bleeding from the stomach with hydrocortisone.

SPECIAL PRECAUTIONS

Be sure to tell your doctor if:
- You have liver or kidney problems.
- You have had a peptic ulcer.
- You have had a mental illness or epilepsy.
- You have glaucoma.
- You have had tuberculosis.
- You have diabetes or heart problems.
- You are taking other medicines.

Pregnancy No evidence of risk with topical preparations. Oral doses may adversely affect the developing baby. Discuss with your doctor.
Breast-feeding The drug passes into the breast milk and may affect the baby. Discuss with your doctor.
Infants and children Reduced dose necessary.
Over 60 Reduced dose may be necessary.
Driving and hazardous work No special problems.
Alcohol Avoid. Alcohol may increase the risk of peptic ulcer when this drug is taken by mouth.
Surgery and general anaesthetics Notify your doctor; you may need to have hydrocortisone by injection in hospital.
Infection Avoid exposure to chickenpox, shingles, or measles if having systemic treatment.

PROLONGED USE

Prolonged high dosage can lead to peptic ulcers, glaucoma, muscle weakness, osteoporosis, and growth retardation in children. People on long-term treatment should carry a steroid treatment card.
Monitoring Periodic checks on blood pressure and blood sugar levels are usually required (oral forms).

HYOSCINE

Brand names Boots Travel Calm, Buscopan, Joy-Rides, Kwells, Scopoderm TTS
Used in the following combined preparation Papaveretum and Hyoscine Injection

QUICK REFERENCE

Drug group Drug for irritable bowel syndrome (p.43), drug affecting the pupil (p.114), and anti-emetic drug (p.19)
Overdose danger rating Medium
Dependence rating Low
Prescription needed No (for most preparations)
Available as generic Yes

GENERAL INFORMATION

Originally derived from the henbane plant (*Hyoscyamus niger*), hyoscine is an anticholinergic drug (p.7) that has both an antispasmodic effect on the intestine and a calming action on the nerve pathways that control nausea and vomiting. By its anticholinergic action, hyoscine also dilates the pupil.

The drug is produced in two forms. Hyoscine butylbromide is prescribed to reduce spasm of the gastrointestinal tract in irritable bowel syndrome and, sometimes with other drugs, to treat dysmenorrhoea (painful menstruation). The other form, hyoscine hydrobromide, is used to control motion sickness and the giddiness and nausea caused by disturbances of the inner ear (see Vertigo and Ménière's disease, p.20) and can be given as tablets and skin patches. Eye drops containing this form are used to dilate the pupil during eye examinations and eye surgery. The hydrobromide form is also used as a premedication to dry secretions before operations.

INFORMATION FOR USERS

Follow instructions on the label. Call your doctor if symptoms worsen.
How taken/used Tablets, injection, skin patches.
Frequency and timing of doses *Irritable bowel syndrome* Up to 4 x daily, as required, by mouth (tablets). *Motion sickness* Up to 3 x daily (tablets); every 3 days as required (patches).

Adult dosage range *Irritable bowel syndrome* 30–80mg daily (hyoscine butylbromide). *Motion sickness* 0.3mg per dose (tablets); 1 mg over 72 hours (hyoscine hydrobromide patches).
Onset of effect Within 1 hour.
Duration of action Up to 6 hours (by mouth); up to 72 hours (patches).
Diet advice None.
Storage Keep in original container at room temperature out of the reach of children. Protect from light.
Missed dose Take when you remember. Adjust the timing of your next dose accordingly.
Stopping the drug Can be safely stopped as soon as you no longer need it.
Exceeding the dose An occasional unintentional extra dose is unlikely to cause problems. Large overdoses may cause drowsiness or agitation. Notify your doctor.

POSSIBLE ADVERSE EFFECTS

Administered by mouth or injection, hyoscine has a strong anticholinergic effect, causing various minor symptoms, such as dry mouth, drowsiness, and constipation. Discuss with your doctor if these are severe; they can sometimes be minimized by a reduction in dosage. The butylbromide form of hyoscine is less likely to cause these side effects. Other possible adverse effects of hyoscine include blurred vision, difficulty in passing urine, and an increased heart rate. Consult your doctor if you experience any of these symptoms.

INTERACTIONS

Anticholinergic drugs Many drugs have anticholinergic effects, such as dry mouth, difficulty in passing urine, and constipation. The risk of such side effects is increased with hyoscine.
Sedatives All drugs with a sedative effect on the central nervous system, including anti-anxiety and sleeping drugs, antidepressants, opioid analgesics, and antipsychotics, are likely to increase the sedative properties of hyoscine.
Sublingual tablets Hyoscine can cause a dry mouth and may reduce the effectiveness of sublingual tablets.

SPECIAL PRECAUTIONS

Be sure to consult your doctor or pharmacist before taking this drug if:

- ◆ You have long-term liver or kidney problems.
- ◆ You have heart problems.
- ◆ You have epilepsy.
- ◆ You have megacolon or intestinal obstruction problems.
- ◆ You have had glaucoma.
- ◆ You have prostate trouble or urinary retention.
- ◆ You have porphyria.
- ◆ You are taking other medicines.

Pregnancy Safety not established. Discuss with your doctor.
Breast-feeding Safety not established. Discuss with your doctor.
Infants and children Not recommended under 4 years for motion sickness. Patches not recommended under 10 years. Other uses not recommended under 6 years. Reduced dose necessary in older children.
Over 60 Reduced dose may be necessary.
Driving and hazardous work Avoid until you know how hyoscine affects you because the drug can cause drowsiness and blurred vision.
Alcohol Avoid. Alcohol may increase the sedative effect of this drug.

PROLONGED USE

Use of this drug for longer than a few days is unlikely to be necessary.

IBUPROFEN

Brand names Anadin Ultra, Brufen, Calprofen, Fenbid, Hedex, Ibugel, Ibuleve, Ibumousse, Nurofen, and others
Used in the following combined preparations Nurofen Plus, Nuromol, Solpadeine Migraine, and others

QUICK REFERENCE

Drug group Analgesic (p.7) and non-steroidal anti-inflammatory drug (p.48)
Overdose danger rating Low
Dependence rating Low
Prescription needed No (some preparations)
Available as generic Yes

GENERAL INFORMATION

Ibuprofen is a non-steroidal anti-inflammatory drug (NSAID). Like other drugs in this group, it reduces pain, stiffness, fever, and inflammation. It is an effective treatment for the symptoms of osteoarthritis, rheumatoid arthritis, and gout. In the treatment of rheumatoid arthritis, ibuprofen may be prescribed with slower-acting drugs. Other uses include relief of mild to moderate headache (including migraine), juvenile arthritis, menstrual and dental pain, ankylosing spondylitis, pain from soft tissue injuries, or pain following an operation. It has fewer side effects (especially at low doses) than many other NSAIDs, and a lower risk of gastrointestinal bleeding and ulcers.

Ibuprofen is also available as a cream or gel that can be applied to the skin for muscular aches and sprains.

INFORMATION FOR USERS

Follow instructions on the label. Call your doctor if symptoms worsen.

How taken/used Tablets, slow release (SR) tablets, capsules, SR capsules, liquid, granules, cream, mousse, gel.

Frequency and timing of doses 1–2 x daily (SR preparations); 3–4 x daily (topical forms and other oral preparations). Take all oral preparations with or after food.

Dosage range *Adults* 600mg–2.4g daily. *Children* Dosage varies according to age and/or body weight.

Onset of effect Pain relief begins in 15 minutes–2 hours. Full anti-inflammatory effect in arthritic conditions may take up to 2 weeks.

Duration of action 5–10 hours.

Diet advice None.

Storage Keep in original container at room temperature out of the reach of children.

Missed dose Take as soon as you remember. If your next dose is due within 2 hours, take a single dose now and skip the next.

Stopping the drug When taken for short-term pain relief, the drug can be safely stopped as soon as you no longer need it. If it is given for long-term treatment of arthritis, seek medical advice before stopping it.

Exceeding the dose An occasional unintentional extra dose is unlikely to be a cause for concern. But if you notice any unusual symptoms, or if a large overdose has been taken, tell your doctor.

POSSIBLE ADVERSE EFFECTS

Gastrointestinal problems, such as heartburn, indigestion, nausea, and vomiting, are common. More rarely, ibuprofen may cause headache, dizziness, drowsiness, swelling of the feet or legs, and weight gain. Discuss with your doctor if any of these effects are severe. If a rash or itching occur, you should stop taking the drug and consult your doctor. If you experience wheezing, breathlessness, or black or bloodstained faeces, you should stop the drug and contact your doctor without delay.

INTERACTIONS

General note Ibuprofen interacts with a wide range of other drugs, including aspirin, other NSAIDs, oral anticoagulants, corticosteroids, and SSRI antidepressants, to increase the risk of bleeding and/or peptic ulcers.

Ciprofloxacin Ibuprofen increases risk of seizures with this drug and related antibiotics.

Antihypertensive drugs and diuretics The beneficial effects of these drugs may be reduced by ibuprofen; rarely, diuretics can also increase the risk of adverse effects on the kidneys.

Ciclosporin and tacrolimus increase the risk of adverse effects on the kidneys.

SPECIAL PRECAUTIONS

Be sure to consult your doctor or pharmacist before taking this drug if:

- You have long-term kidney or liver problems.
- You have high blood pressure, heart problems, or coronary artery disease, or have had a previous stroke.
- You have had a peptic ulcer, oesophagitis, or acid indigestion.
- You are allergic to aspirin or other NSAIDs.
- You have asthma.
- You are taking other medicines.

Pregnancy The drug may increase the risks of adverse effects on the baby's heart and may prolong labour if taken in the third trimester. Discuss with your doctor.

Breast-feeding The drug passes into the breast milk, but normal doses are unlikely to affect the baby adversely. Discuss with your doctor.

Infants and children Reduced dose necessary.

Over 60 Reduced dose may be necessary.

Driving and hazardous work No problems expected.

Alcohol Avoid. Alcohol may increase the risk of stomach disorders with ibuprofen.

Surgery and general anaesthetics Ibuprofen may prolong bleeding. Discuss with your doctor or dentist before any surgery.

PROLONGED USE

Prolonged use of ibuprofen increases the risk of bleeding from peptic ulcers and in the bowel. It also carries a small risk of a heart attack or stroke. To minimize these risks, the lowest effective dose is given for the shortest time.

IMATINIB

Brand name Glivec
Used in the following combined preparations None

QUICK REFERENCE

Drug group Anticancer drug (p.94)
Overdose danger rating Medium
Dependence rating Low
Prescription needed Yes
Available as generic No

GENERAL INFORMATION

Imatinib belongs to an expanding class of anticancer drugs called tyrosine kinase inhibitors. They act by blocking a specific enzyme (tyrosine kinase) in certain cancer cells, thus halting their growth and replication. Because of this targeted action, the drugs have relatively little effect on non-cancerous cells (unlike many older anticancer drugs). Imatinib is used principally against chronic myeloid leukaemia (CML) but may also be used to treat some other bone marrow cancers and some rare gastrointestinal tumours. It can be used alone or in combination with other anticancer drugs.

Imatinib generally produces fewer adverse effects than older anticancer drugs. However, it does not usually provide a long-term cure because the cancer cells eventually mutate to become resistant to its effects.

INFORMATION FOR USERS

Your drug prescription is tailored for you. Do not alter dosage without checking with your doctor.
How taken/used Tablets.
Frequency and timing of doses 1–2 x daily with food, at the same time every day.
Adult dosage range 100–800mg daily.
Onset of effect The drug starts inhibiting the enzyme within hours, but effect on cancer cells may take days to weeks to become detectable.
Duration of action Several days.
Diet advice None.
Storage Store in original packaging below 30°C out of the reach of children.
Missed dose Take as soon as you remember that day. If you do not remember that day, omit the missed dose and take the next dose as scheduled. Do not double your next dose.
Stopping the drug Do not stop the drug without consulting your doctor because this may lead to a worsening of the underlying condition.
Exceeding the dose An occasional unintentional extra dose is unlikely to cause major problems. But if you notice any unusual symptoms or if a large overdose has been taken, tell your doctor.

POSSIBLE ADVERSE EFFECTS

Imatinib can cause a variety of adverse effects: commonly gastrointestinal symptoms such as nausea, vomiting, and diarrhoea, as well as headache, dizziness, lightheadedness, and muscle pain. Discuss with your doctor if any of these effects are severe. Oedema (fluid build-up), which may cause rapid weight gain, and rash are also common; discuss with your doctor. Imatinib may affect the blood count, giving rise to easy bruising, bleeding, and signs of infection, such as fever, sore throat, or mouth ulcers; report these symptoms to your doctor without delay. More rarely, it may cause chest pain, palpitations, cough, jaundice, or severe abdominal pain; notify your doctor promptly if any of these symptoms occur.

INTERACTIONS

General note A wide range of drugs (including over-the-counter and herbal remedies) may affect levels of imatinib in the body, so you need to check with your doctor or pharmacist before taking any new medication or remedy.
Thyroxine Imatinib can increase the breakdown of thyroxine so the thyroxine dose may need adjustment.
Warfarin Imatinib may affect the level of warfarin; this may require adjustment of the warfarin dose or you may be switched to heparin.

SPECIAL PRECAUTIONS

Be sure to tell your doctor if:
- ◆ You have liver, kidney, or heart problems.
- ◆ You have a history of hepatitis B.
- ◆ You have had your thyroid gland removed and are taking thyroxine.
- ◆ You are taking other medicines.

Pregnancy Safety not established. Discuss with your doctor.
Breast-feeding Not recommended.
Infants and children Used only by specialist children's doctors.
Over 60 No special problems.
Driving and hazardous work Avoid until you have learned how the drug affects you. It may cause dizziness or blurred vision.
Alcohol No special problems.

PROLONGED USE
Imatinib tends to cause fewer adverse effects than many other anticancer drugs when used long term. However, the cancer cells may become resistant to the drug's effects, in which case treatment will be stopped.
Monitoring Regular monitoring is carried out to check your blood count and the function of organs such as the liver and kidney. Blood tests are also performed to monitor the response of the cancer to imatinib. Children who are being treated with imatinib should have their growth regularly monitored.

IMIPRAMINE

Brand name None
Used in the following combined preparations None

QUICK REFERENCE
Drug group Antidepressant (p.12) and drug for urinary disorders (p.110)
Overdose danger rating High
Dependence rating Low
Prescription needed Yes
Available as generic Yes

GENERAL INFORMATION
Imipramine belongs to the tricyclic class of antidepressant drugs. It is used mainly for long-term treatment of depression, to elevate mood, improve appetite, increase physical activity, and restore interest in everyday life. Because it is less sedating than some other tricyclic antidepressants, it is particularly useful when a depressed person has become withdrawn or apathetic. The drug is also prescribed to treat night-time enuresis (bedwetting) in children.

The most common adverse effects of imipramine are the result of the drug's anticholinergic action (p.7). In overdose, imipramine may cause coma and abnormal heart rhythms.

INFORMATION FOR USERS
Your drug prescription is tailored for you. Do not alter dosage without checking with your doctor.
How taken/used Tablets, liquid.
Frequency and timing of doses 1–3 x daily.
Dosage range *Adults* Usually 75–200mg daily (up to maximum 300mg in hospital patients). *Children* Reduced dose according to age and weight. Usual starting dose 25mg daily in children aged 6–7 years.
Onset of effect Some benefits and effects may appear within hours, but full antidepressant effect may not be felt for 2–6 weeks.
Duration of action After prolonged treatment, antidepressant effect may persist for up to 6 weeks, common adverse effects for 1–2 weeks.
Diet advice None.
Storage Keep in original container at room temperature out of the reach of children.
Missed dose Take as soon as you remember. If your next dose is due within 3 hours, take a single dose now and skip the next.
Stopping the drug Do not stop without consulting your doctor, who will supervise a gradual reduction in dosage. Stopping abruptly may cause withdrawal symptoms.

OVERDOSE ACTION
Seek immediate medical advice in all cases. Take emergency action if palpitations are noted or consciousness is lost.

POSSIBLE ADVERSE EFFECTS
The possible adverse effects of imipramine are mainly the result of its anticholinergic action and its effect on the normal rhythm of the heart. Common effects include sweating, flushing, dry mouth, constipation, and weight gain; discuss with your doctor if these are severe. Contact your doctor in any case of blurred vision, dizziness, or drowsiness. If you develop difficulty in passing urine, confusion, or palpitations, stop taking the drug; if you have palpitations, call the doctor immediately.

INTERACTIONS
Anti-arrhythmic drugs increase the risk of abnormal heart rhythms.
Sedatives and warfarin Imipramine may increase the effects of these drugs.
Antihypertensives and anticonvulsants The effects of these are reduced by imipramine.
Monoamine oxidase inhibitors (MAOIs) These drugs are prescribed with imipramine only under strict supervision due to the possibility of a serious interaction.
Some selective serotonin reuptake inhibitors (SSRIs) can increase levels of imipramine.

SPECIAL PRECAUTIONS
Be sure to tell your doctor if:
- You have had heart problems.
- You have long-term liver or kidney problems.

- You have had epileptic seizures.
- You have porphyria.
- You have had glaucoma.
- You have prostate problems.
- You have had mania or a psychotic illness.
- You are taking other medicines.

Pregnancy Avoid becoming pregnant if possible. Discuss with your doctor.

Breast-feeding The drug passes into the breast milk, but normal doses are unlikely to affect the baby adversely. Discuss with your doctor.

Infants and children Not recommended under 6 years. Reduced dose needed in older children.

Over 60 Increased likelihood of adverse effects. Reduced dose may therefore be necessary.

Driving and hazardous work Avoid such activities until you have learned how imipramine affects you because the drug can cause reduced alertness and blurred vision.

Alcohol Avoid. Alcohol may increase the sedative effect of imipramine.

Surgery and general anaesthetics Imipramine may need to be stopped before you have a general anaesthetic. Discuss with your doctor or dentist before any operation.

PROLONGED USE

No problems expected. Imipramine is not usually prescribed for children as a treatment for bedwetting for longer than 3 months.

INDAPAMIDE

Brand names Alkapamid, Cardide SR, Indipam, Lorvacs XL, Natrilix, Natrilix SR, Rawel, Tensaid XL

Used in the following combined preparation Coversyl Plus

QUICK REFERENCE

Drug group Diuretic (p.30)
Overdose danger rating Low
Dependence rating Low
Prescription needed Yes
Available as generic Yes

GENERAL INFORMATION

Indapamide is closely related to thiazide diuretics in its effects but is mainly used to treat hypertension (high blood pressure). The drug increases secretion of salt by the kidneys in the same way as thiazide diuretics. This causes more water to be lost from the body, which reduces the total blood volume and lowers blood pressure. Indapamide is sometimes combined with other antihypertensive drugs but not with other diuretics.

The drug's diuretic effects are slight at low doses, but susceptible people need to have their blood levels of potassium and uric acid monitored. These include older people, those taking digitalis drugs, or people who have gout or hyperaldosteronism (overproduction of the hormone aldosterone). Unlike the thiazides, indapamide does not affect control of diabetes at low doses.

INFORMATION FOR USERS

Your drug prescription is tailored for you. Do not alter dosage without checking with your doctor.

How taken/used Tablets, slow release (SR) tablets.

Frequency and timing of doses Once daily in the morning.

Adult dosage range 1.5–2.5mg.

Onset of effect 1–2 hours, but the full effect may take several months.

Duration of action 12–24 hours.

Diet advice None.

Storage Keep in original container at room temperature out of the reach of children.

Missed dose Take as soon as you remember. If your next dose is due within 4 hours, take a single dose now and skip the next.

Stopping the drug Do not stop taking the drug without consulting your doctor; high blood pressure may return.

Exceeding the dose An occasional unintentional extra dose is unlikely to cause problems. But if you notice any unusual symptoms, or if a large overdose has been taken, notify your doctor.

POSSIBLE ADVERSE EFFECTS

Indapamide usually causes few adverse effects. The most common problems are rashes and mild disruptions in blood chemistry (due to loss of electrolytes, such as potassium, in the urine), which may cause fatigue and muscle cramps. If you have a rash, or severe cramps or fatigue, discuss with your doctor. More rarely, indapamide may cause headache, dizziness, diarrhoea or constipation, and nausea; consult your doctor if these are severe. Notify your doctor in all cases if you develop palpitations, fainting, tingling or pins and needles, or erectile dysfunction (impotence).

INTERACTIONS

Loop diuretics There is a risk of imbalance of salts in the blood if taken with indapamide.
Anti-arrhythmic and digitalis drugs Loss of potassium with indapamide use may lead to toxicity with these drugs.
Lithium Blood levels of lithium are increased when it is taken with indapamide.

SPECIAL PRECAUTIONS

Be sure to tell your doctor if:
- You have liver or kidney problems.
- You have diabetes.
- You have gout.
- You have hyperaldosteronism or hyperparathyroidism.
- You are allergic to sulfonamide drugs.
- You are taking other medicines.

Pregnancy Safety not established. Discuss with your doctor.
Breast-feeding Safety not established. Discuss with your doctor.
Infants and children Not prescribed.
Over 60 No special problems.
Driving and hazardous work No special problems.
Alcohol No special problems.

PROLONGED USE

Long-term use of indapamide may lead to potassium loss.
Monitoring Blood potassium and uric acid levels may be checked periodically.

INFLIXIMAB

Brand names Flixabi, Inflectra, Remicade, Remsima, Zessly
Used in the following combined preparations None

QUICK REFERENCE

Drug group Drug for inflammatory bowel disease (p.44) and disease-modifying antirheumatic drug (p.49)
Overdose danger rating Low
Dependence rating Low
Prescription needed Yes
Available as generic Yes

GENERAL INFORMATION

Infliximab is a monoclonal antibody (see p.95) that can modify the activity of the immune system and so lessen inflammation. It reduces the activity in the body of a substance called tumour necrosis factor alpha (TNF-alpha), which drives several inflammatory conditions, such as psoriasis, rheumatoid arthritis, Crohn's disease, ankylosing spondylitis, and ulcerative colitis; it can therefore be used to treat these conditions. The drug is given by intravenous infusion, generally into the arm.

Infections, most often affecting the upper respiratory tract and the urinary tract, occur more commonly with infliximab treatment.

INFORMATION FOR USERS

The drug is given only under medical supervision and is not for self-administration.
How taken/used Intravenous infusion.
Frequency and timing of doses Every 6–8 weeks, although doses may be more frequent at the start of treatment. Infusion time is generally over a 2-hour period.
Adult dosage range Dosing is based on body weight; 3mg/kg to 5mg/kg per dose.
Onset of effect 1 hour; full beneficial effect may take several weeks to develop.
Duration of action 2–8 weeks.
Diet advice None.
Storage Not applicable. The drug is not normally kept in the home.
Missed dose As infliximab is given every 6–8 weeks, it is important to adhere to the dosing schedule arranged by your doctor. Missed doses should be rectified as soon as possible.
Stopping the drug No adverse effects are reported when stopping infliximab abruptly.
Exceeding the dose Unlikely, as infliximab is given in hospital under close supervision.

POSSIBLE ADVERSE EFFECTS

Infusion reactions commonly occur during or within 1–2 hours after treatment, particularly with the first or second treatment. Delayed reactions, including muscle and joint pain, fever, and rash, may occur 3–12 days after infusion. If you have reaction to the infusion, or severe nausea, vomiting, diarrhoea, headache, back pain, or dizziness, discuss with your doctor. Susceptibility to infection is a rarer adverse effect; discuss any instance with your doctor. If you have swelling of the tongue, wheezing, or a rash, you should stop the drug and seek immediate medical attention.

INTERACTIONS

Anakinra and abatacept should not be combined with infliximab as there is an increased risk of reactions and serious infections.

Vaccines Infliximab may affect the efficacy of vaccines.

SPECIAL PRECAUTIONS

Infliximab is given only under close medical supervision, but be sure to tell your doctor if:

◆ You have active tuberculosis or any other current infection.

◆ You have any signs of infection (e.g. fever, malaise, wounds, dental problems).

◆ You are having surgery or dental treatment

◆ You have liver or kidney problems.

◆ You have a central nervous system disorder such as multiple sclerosis.

◆ You have recently received, or are scheduled to receive, a vaccine.

◆ You have had heart failure.

◆ You are taking other medicines.

Pregnancy Limited clinical data on effects. Used only if essential.

Breast-feeding Not recommended during treatment or for 6 months after last dose.

Infants and children Not recommended.

Over 60 No special problems.

Driving and hazardous work Avoid until you have learned how infliximab affects you because it can cause fatigue and dizziness.

Alcohol No special problems.

PROLONGED USE

Increased risk of infections (e.g. tuberculosis). A rare type of lymphoma has been reported in a few patients, but no causal relationship with infliximab has been established.

Monitoring Periodic blood and liver-function tests may be carried out. Body temperature, heart rate, and blood pressure may be monitored during the first infusion.

INSULIN

Brand names Abasaglar (glargine), Actrapid, Apidra, Fiasp, Humalog, Human Mixtard, Humulin, Hypurin, Hypurine porcine, Insulatard, Insuman, Lantus, Levemir, Lyumjev, Novomix, NovoRapid, Suliqua, Toujeo, Tresiba, Xultophy, and others

QUICK REFERENCE

Drug group Drug for diabetes (p.80)
Overdose danger rating High
Dependence rating Low
Prescription needed Yes
Available as generic No

GENERAL INFORMATION

Insulin is a hormone that is made by the pancreas and is vital to the body's ability to use sugar. It is given by injection to supplement or replace natural insulin in treating diabetes mellitus. It is the only effective treatment in Type 1 diabetes and may also be prescribed in Type 2 diabetes. Insulin should be used with a carefully controlled diet. Illness, vomiting, or changes in diet or exercise levels may require dosage adjustment.

Insulin is available in short-, medium-, or long-acting forms; combinations of types are often given. People using insulin should carry a warning card or tag. They should watch out for signs of hypoglycaemia (low blood sugar), as defined below, and should eat something sugary if these do develop.

INFORMATION FOR USERS

Your drug prescription is tailored for you. Do not alter dosage without checking with your doctor.

How taken/used Injection, infusion pump, pen injection.

Frequency and timing of doses 1–5 x daily, injected under skin via insulin syringe. Usually given 15–30 minutes before meals (short-acting); some forms given directly before or after eating. Exact timing of injections and longer-acting preparations tailored to individual needs; follow instructions given.

Dosage range Exact timing of doses is tailored to individual needs. Follow manufacturer's instructions.

Onset of effect 10–60 minutes (short-acting); within 2 hours (medium-acting); 2–4 hours (long-acting).

Duration of action 2–8 hours (short-acting); 18–26 hours (medium-acting); 28–36 hours (long-acting).

Diet advice A special diabetes diet is necessary. Follow your doctor's advice.

Storage Refrigerate, but once opened the drug may be stored at room temperature for 1 month. Do not freeze. Follow the instructions on the container.

Missed dose Discuss with your doctor. Appropriate action depends on the dose and the type of insulin.

Stopping the drug Do not stop taking the drug without consulting your doctor; confusion and coma may occur.

OVERDOSE ACTION

Seek immediate medical advice. If warning signs of low blood sugar (e.g. faintness, dizziness, headache, confusion, sweating, or tremor) occur, have a sugary food or drink. Take emergency action if seizures or loss of consciousness occur.

POSSIBLE ADVERSE EFFECTS

The most common side effect of insulin is hypoglycaemia (low blood sugar). If symptoms occur (see Overdose action, above), eat or drink something sugary and seek immediate medical advice. Irritation or lump formation at the injection site is also common; other, less common adverse effects include dimpling of the skin at the injection site and eyesight problems. Discuss with your doctor if any of these occur. Serious allergic reactions (itchy rash, facial swelling, and breathing difficulties) are rare; if they occur, you should seek urgent medical attention.

INTERACTIONS

General note 1 Many drugs, including some antibiotics, monoamine oxidase inhibitors (MAOIs; see p.12), and oral antidiabetic drugs, increase the risk of low blood sugar.

General note 2 Check with your doctor or pharmacist before taking any other medications; some contain sugar and may upset control of diabetes.

Corticosteroids, growth hormone, oestrogens, thyroxine, and diuretics may oppose the effect of insulin.

Beta blockers may affect insulin needs and mask signs of low blood sugar.

SPECIAL PRECAUTIONS

Be sure to tell your doctor if:

◆ You have had a previous allergic reaction to insulin.

◆ You are taking other medicines, or your other drug treatment is changed.

Pregnancy No evidence of risk to the developing baby from insulin, but poor control of diabetes increases the risk of birth defects. Careful monitoring is required because insulin requirements may change.

Breast-feeding No evidence of risk. Adjustment in dose may be necessary while breast-feeding.

Infants and children Reduced dose necessary.

Over 60 No special problems.

Driving and hazardous work You must inform the DVLA you are taking insulin. You must check your blood sugar before driving and follow DVLA guidelines. Avoid driving or dangerous activities if you have signs of low blood sugar.

Alcohol Avoid. Alcoholic drinks upset diabetic control.

Surgery and general anaesthetics Insulin requirements may increase during surgery, and blood glucose levels will need to be monitored during and after an operation. Notify your doctor or dentist that you are diabetic before any surgery.

PROLONGED USE

Insulin can affect fat tissue under the skin, causing lumps or dimples that may affect absorption. Rotation of the injection sites within the injection area can help to prevent these reactions. No other problems expected.

Monitoring Regular monitoring of blood sugar levels is required.

INTERFERON

Brand names Avonex, Betaferon, Extavia, Flixabi, Immukin, IntronA, Pegasys, PegIntron, Rebif, Roferon-A, Viraferon

Used in the following combined preparations None

QUICK REFERENCE

Drug group Antiviral drug (p.67) and anticancer drug (p.94)

Overdose danger rating Medium

Dependence rating Low

Prescription needed Yes

Available as generic Yes

GENERAL INFORMATION

Interferons are a group of substances normally produced in cells that have been infected with viruses or stimulated by other substances. They are thought to promote resistance to several types of viral infection (p.67). Three main types of interferon (alfa, beta, and gamma) are used to treat a range of diseases. Interferon alfa is used for leukaemias, other cancers, and chronic hepatitis B and C. Interferon beta reduces the frequency and severity of relapses in multiple sclerosis. Interferon gamma is prescribed in conjunction with antibiotics for patients with chronic granulomatous disease or severe malignant osteopetrosis (a rare inherited condition in which the bones become abnormally dense).

Interferons commonly cause flulike side effects, and they may also cause more severe adverse effects (see below).

INFORMATION FOR USERS

This drug is given only under medical supervision and is not for self-administration.

How taken/used Injection.

Frequency and timing of doses Once daily 3 times a week, depending on product and condition being treated.

Adult dosage range Depends on product and condition being treated. Dosage may be calculated from body surface area or weight.

Onset of effect Active in body within 1 hour, but effects may not be noted for 1–2 months.

Duration of action Immediate effects last for about 12 hours.

Diet advice None.

Storage Store in a refrigerator at 2–8°C. Do not let it freeze, and protect from light. Keep out of the reach of children.

Missed dose Not applicable. This drug is usually given only in hospital under close medical supervision.

Stopping the drug Discuss with your doctor.

Exceeding the dose Overdosage is unlikely since treatment is carefully monitored.

POSSIBLE ADVERSE EFFECTS

Headache, lethargy, depression, dizziness, drowsiness, digestive disturbances, chills, fever, muscle aches, poor appetite, and weight loss are common adverse effects of interferon. Hair loss, vision problems, and shortness of breath or cough are rarer effects. Notify your doctor of all severe or unusual symptoms without delay; some may be dose-related, requiring a reduction in dosage.

INTERACTIONS

General note Numerous drugs increase the risk of adverse effects on the blood, heart, or nervous system; the doctor will take account of this when prescribing them with interferon.

Vaccines Interferon may reduce effectiveness.

Theophylline/aminophylline The effects of this drug may be increased by interferon.

Sedatives All drugs that have a sedative effect on the central nervous system are likely to increase the sedative properties of interferon. Such drugs include opioid analgesics, anti-anxiety and sleeping drugs, antihistamines, antidepressants, and antipsychotics.

SPECIAL PRECAUTIONS

Interferon is prescribed only under close medical supervision, taking account of your present condition and medical history, but be sure to tell your doctor if:

- You have long-term liver or kidney problems.
- You have heart disease.
- You have very abnormal blood lipid levels.
- You have diabetes.
- You have depression or suicidal thoughts.
- You have had epileptic seizures, asthma, eczema, psoriasis, or previous drug allergies.
- You are taking other medicines, including complementary remedies.

Pregnancy Not usually prescribed, but some interferons may be considered if necessary. Discuss with your doctor.

Breast-feeding Some types can be used during breast-feeding. Discuss with your doctor.

Infants and children Not usually used in infants. Some types may be used in children.

Over 60 Increased likelihood of adverse effects. Reduced dose may be necessary.

Driving and hazardous work Not applicable.

Alcohol Avoid. Alcohol may increase the sedative effects of this drug.

PROLONGED USE

May increase risk of liver damage. Blood cell production in the bone marrow may be reduced. Repeated large doses are associated with lethargy, fatigue, collapse, and coma.

Monitoring Frequent tests are done to monitor blood composition and liver function. With interferon alfa, monitoring of thyroid function, blood lipids, and vision are also necessary.

IPRATROPIUM BROMIDE

Brand names Atrovent, Iprovent, Rinatec

Used in the following combined preparations Combivent, Duovent, Otrivine Extra Dual Relief

QUICK REFERENCE

Drug group Bronchodilator (p.21)

Overdose danger rating Low

Dependence rating Low

Prescription needed Yes

Available as generic Yes

GENERAL INFORMATION

Ipratropium bromide is an anticholinergic bronchodilator that relaxes the muscles surrounding the bronchioles (the airways in the lungs). The drug is used primarily in the maintenance of airways in reversible airway disorders, particularly chronic obstructive pulmonary disease (COPD). It is given only by inhaler or via a nebulizer for these conditions. It is also used in treating acute attacks of asthma, especially severe attacks in hospital. In these cases, it is usually used together with sympathomimetic bronchodilators, such as salbutamol (p.396). In addition, ipratropium bromide is prescribed as a nasal spray to treat a continually runny nose due to allergy.

Unlike with other anticholinergic drugs, side effects are rare. The drug must be used with caution by people with glaucoma, but problems are unlikely at normal doses and if an inhaler or nebulizer is used correctly.

INFORMATION FOR USERS

Your drug prescription is tailored for you. Do not alter dosage without checking with your doctor.

How taken/used Inhaler, liquid for nebulizer, nasal spray.

Frequency and timing of doses 3–4 x daily (inhaler); 2 sprays into each nostril 2–3 x daily (nasal spray).

Adult dosage range 80–320mcg daily (inhaler); 400–2,000mcg daily (nebulizer); 1–2 puffs to the affected nostril 2–3 x daily (nasal spray).

Onset of effect 3–30 minutes.

Duration of action Up to 8 hours.

Diet advice None.

Storage Keep in original container at room temperature out of the reach of children. Do not puncture or burn containers.

Missed dose Take as soon as you remember. If your next dose is due within 2 hours, take a single dose now and skip the next.

Stopping the drug Do not stop without consulting your doctor; symptoms may recur.

Exceeding the dose An occasional unintentional extra dose is unlikely to be a cause for concern. But if you notice any unusual symptoms or have taken a large overdose, notify your doctor.

POSSIBLE ADVERSE EFFECTS

Side effects are rare; the most common are dry mouth or throat, nausea, headache, and a cough. Constipation and difficulty in passing urine may also occur. If any of these symptoms are severe or if you experience palpitations or a fast heart rate, discuss with your doctor. If you develop a rash or facial swelling, stop taking the drug and consult your doctor. Rarely, eye pain or altered vision may occur if the drug comes into contact with the eyes during use with an inhaler or nebulizer, or wheezing or breathlessness may worsen immediately after inhaler use (paradoxical bronchospasm); if any of these symptoms occur, stop using the drug and contact your doctor immediately.

INTERACTIONS

Pasireotide may increase the risk of bradycardia (abnormally slow heart rate) when used with ipratropium bromide.

SPECIAL PRECAUTIONS

Be sure to tell your doctor if:

- You have glaucoma.
- You have prostate problems.
- You have difficulty in passing urine.
- You have cystic fibrosis.
- You are taking other medicines.

Pregnancy No evidence of risk, but discuss with your doctor before using in the first 3 months of pregnancy.

Breast-feeding No evidence of risk, but discuss with your doctor.

Infants and children Reduced dose necessary.

Over 60 No special problems.

Driving and hazardous work Avoid such activities until you know how the drug affects you because it may cause blurred vision or dizziness, especially if administered by nebulizer.

Alcohol No known problems.

PROLONGED USE

No special problems.

IRBESARTAN

Brand name Aprovel, Ifirmasta

Used in the following combined preparation CoAprovel

QUICK REFERENCE

Drug group Vasodilator (p.30) and antihypertensive drug (p.34)

Overdose danger rating Medium

Dependence rating Low

Prescription needed Yes

Available as generic No

GENERAL INFORMATION

Irbesartan is a member of the group of vasodilators (drugs that widen blood vessels) called angiotensin II blockers (p.30) and is used to treat hypertension (high blood pressure). It is also used to protect the kidneys in people with Type 2 diabetes who have hypertension and impaired kidney function.

Unlike ACE inhibitors (p.30), irbesartan does not cause a persistent dry cough. The drug is also available in combination with a diuretic (CoAprovel), which may increase its blood-pressure-lowering effect.

INFORMATION FOR USERS

Your drug prescription is tailored for you. Do not alter dosage without checking with your doctor.

How taken/used Tablets.

Frequency and timing of doses Once daily.

Adult dosage range 150mg (maintenance dose), increased to 300mg if needed; 75mg may be used in people over 75 years and those who are on haemodialysis.

Onset of effect Within 1 hour. Blood pressure is lowered within 1–2 weeks, and maximum beneficial effect occurs 4–6 weeks from start of treatment.

Duration of action 24 hours.

Diet advice None.

Storage Keep in original container at room temperature out of the reach of children.

Missed dose Take as soon as you remember. If your next dose is due within 8 hours, take a single dose now and skip the next.

Stopping the drug Do not stop without consulting your doctor. Stopping the drug may lead to worsening of the underlying condition.

Exceeding the dose An occasional unintentional extra dose is unlikely to be a cause for concern. Large overdoses may cause dizziness, fainting, and a faint pulse or slow heart rate. Notify your doctor.

POSSIBLE ADVERSE EFFECTS

Adverse effects are usually mild and transient. Common ones include dizziness, fatigue, flushing, and nausea. Discuss with your doctor if these are severe. More rarely, there may be headache or muscle or joint pains; talk to your doctor if these are severe or if you develop a rash. If you develop swelling of the lips or face, stop taking the drug and contact your doctor promptly. An exaggerated drop in blood pressure may occur if you take the drug when you are dehydrated.

INTERACTIONS

Diuretics Risk of a sudden fall in blood pressure if these are being taken when irbesartan treatment is started. They may also affect sodium and potassium levels in the blood.

Potassium supplements, potassium-sparing diuretics, and ciclosporin used with irbesartan may raise levels of potassium in the blood.

Antihypertensive drugs increase the effects of irbesartan.

Lithium Irbesartan increases the blood levels and toxicity of lithium.

Non-steroidal anti-inflammatory drugs (NSAIDs) Some may reduce the blood-pressure-lowering effects of irbesartan, and there is a risk that they may worsen kidney function.

ACE inhibitors (e.g. enalapril, captopril, lisinopril, or ramipril) and potassium salts may increase potassium levels when taken with irbesartan. However, these drugs are not routinely prescribed with irbesartan.

SPECIAL PRECAUTIONS

Be sure to tell your doctor if:

- You have heart problems, including heart failure.
- You have kidney problems or stenosis of the kidney's arteries.
- You have lactose/galactose intolerance or glucose/galactose malabsorption.
- You are taking other medicines.

Pregnancy Not prescribed. If you become pregnant during treatment, consult your doctor without delay.

Breast-feeding Safety not established. Discuss with your doctor.

Infants and children Not prescribed.

Over 60 Increased risk of adverse effects. Reduced dose may therefore be necessary.

Driving and hazardous work Avoid until you know how irbesartan affects you because the drug can cause dizziness and fatigue.

Alcohol Regular intake of excessive alcohol may raise the blood pressure and reduce the effectiveness of irbesartan.

PROLONGED USE

No special problems.

Monitoring Periodic checks on blood potassium levels and kidney function may be performed.

ISONIAZID

Brand names Cemidon, Tebesium [solutions for injection]
Used in the following combined preparations Rifater, Rifinah, Rimstar, Voractiv

QUICK REFERENCE

Drug group Antituberculous drug (p.65)
Overdose danger rating High
Dependence rating Low
Prescription needed Yes
Available as generic Yes

GENERAL INFORMATION

Isoniazid (also known as INAH or INH) has been in use since the 1950s and is still an effective drug for tuberculosis. It is given alone to prevent tuberculosis and in combination with other drugs to treat the disease. Treatment usually lasts for 6 months. However, courses lasting 9 months or a year may sometimes be prescribed.

Although isoniazid usually causes few adverse effects, one side effect is the increased loss of pyridoxine (vitamin B6) from the body. This effect, which is more likely with high doses, is rare in children but common among people with poor nutrition. Since pyridoxine deficiency can lead to irreversible nerve damage, supplements are usually given.

INFORMATION FOR USERS

Your drug prescription is tailored for you. Do not alter dosage without checking with your doctor.
How taken/used Tablets, injection.
Frequency and timing of doses Normally once daily.
Dosage range *Adults* 300mg daily. *Children* According to age and weight.
Onset of effect Over 2–3 days.
Duration of action Up to 24 hours.
Diet advice Take 30 minutes before food because food decreases absorption of isoniazid.
Storage Keep in original container at room temperature out of the reach of children. Protect from light.
Missed dose Take as soon as you remember. If your next dose is scheduled within 8 hours, take a single dose now and skip the next.
Stopping the drug Take the full course. Even if you feel better the infection may still be present and may recur if treatment is stopped too soon.

OVERDOSE ACTION

Seek immediate medical advice in all cases. Take emergency action if breathing difficulties, seizures, or loss of consciousness occur.

POSSIBLE ADVERSE EFFECTS

Serious problems are uncommon, but all adverse effects should receive prompt medical attention because of the possibility of nerve or liver damage; such damage is more likely with long-term use (see Prolonged use). Adverse effects include nausea, vomiting, fatigue, weakness, numbness, tingling, rash, and mood changes. If you develop blurred vision, jaundice, twitching, or muscle weakness, stop the drug and consult your doctor without delay.

INTERACTIONS

Alcohol and rifampicin Large quantities of alcohol may reduce the effectiveness of isoniazid. If the two are taken together, the likelihood of liver damage is increased; if rifampicin is also being taken, the risk of liver damage is increased further.
Theophylline Isoniazid may increase levels and effects of theophylline.
Anticonvulsants The effects of these drugs may be increased with isoniazid.
Antacids These drugs may reduce the absorption of isoniazid.
Ketoconazole Isoniazid reduces the blood concentration of ketoconazole.

SPECIAL PRECAUTIONS

Be sure to tell your doctor if:
- You have long-term liver or kidney problems.
- You have had liver damage following isoniazid treatment in the past.
- You have problems with drug or alcohol misuse.
- You have diabetes.
- You have porphyria.
- You have HIV infection.
- You have had epileptic seizures.
- You are taking other medicines.

Pregnancy No evidence of risk. Discuss with your doctor.
Breast-feeding The drug passes into the breast milk and may affect the baby. The infant should be monitored for signs of toxic effects. Discuss with your doctor.
Infants and children Reduced dose necessary.
Over 60 Increased likelihood of adverse effects.

Driving and hazardous work No special problems.
Alcohol Avoid excessive amounts.

PROLONGED USE

Pyridoxine (vitamin B6) deficiency may occur with prolonged use and lead to nerve damage. Supplements are usually prescribed. There is also a risk of serious liver damage.
Monitoring Periodic blood tests are usually performed to monitor liver function.

ISOSORBIDE DINITRATE/ MONONITRATE

Brand names [dinitrate] Isoket Retard; [mononitrate] Chemydur, Elantan, Imdur, Isib, Ismo, Isodur, Isotard, Modisal, Monomax, Monomil XL, Monosorb XL, Zemon
Used in the following combined preparations None

QUICK REFERENCE

Drug group Nitrate vasodilator (p.30) and anti-angina drug (p.33)
Overdose danger rating Medium
Dependence rating Low
Prescription needed No (some preparations); yes (other preparations and injection)
Available as generic Yes

GENERAL INFORMATION

Isosorbide dinitrate and isosorbide mononitrate are vasodilator drugs similar to glyceryl trinitrate (p.264). They are usually used to treat patients with angina, and are also used in some cases of heart failure.

Unlike glyceryl trinitrate, however, both of these drugs are stable and can be stored for long periods without losing their effectiveness.

The effectiveness of both drugs is reduced if the drugs are taken continuously. To minimize this, formulations are often designed to give a drug-free period when taken once daily.

INFORMATION FOR USERS

Follow instructions on the label. Call your doctor if symptoms worsen.
How taken/used *Dinitrate* Tablets, slow release (SR) tablets, injection, spray. *Mononitrate* Tablets, SR tablets, SR capsules.
Frequency and timing of doses *Relief of angina attacks* As required (spray). *Heart failure/ prevention of angina* 2–4 x daily; 1–2 x daily (SR tablets, capsules).
Adult dosage range *Prevention of angina* 30–120mg daily (in divided doses). *Treatment of angina* 1–3 doses under the tongue (spray). *Heart failure* 40–240mg daily (in divided doses).
Onset of effect 2–3 minutes (spray); 20–30 minutes (SR tablets, capsules).
Duration of action 4–6 hours (dinitrate tablets); 8–10 hours (mononitrate tablets); up to 17 hours (SR tablets); up to 10 hours (SR capsules); 1–2 hours (spray).
Diet advice None.
Storage Keep in original container at room temperature out of the reach of children. Protect from light.
Missed dose Take as soon as you remember. If your next dose is due within 2 hours, take a single dose now and skip the next.
Stopping the drug Do not stop taking the drug without consulting your doctor; stopping may lead to worsening of the underlying condition.
Exceeding the dose An occasional unintentional extra dose is unlikely to cause problems. Large doses may cause dizziness, headache, or shortness of breath. Notify your doctor.

POSSIBLE ADVERSE EFFECTS

Headache, flushing, and dizziness are common side effects of isosorbide dinitrate and isosorbide mononitrate in the early stages of treatment. Consult your doctor if you have dizziness or severe headache or flushing; small doses in the initial stages can help to minimize these symptoms. The most serious adverse effect is excessively lowered blood pressure, which may cause fainting or weakness as well as dizziness, and may need to be monitored regularly. If these symptoms occur or if your heart rate is unusually fast or slow, consult your doctor. Regular use of the drug and/or dosage adjustment may lessen adverse effects.

INTERACTIONS

Sildenafil, tadalafil, and vardenafil significantly enhance the blood-pressure-lowering effect of nitrates; they should not be used together.
Antihypertensives cause further lowering of blood pressure when taken with nitrates.

SPECIAL PRECAUTIONS

Be sure to consult your doctor or pharmacist before taking this drug if:

- ◆ You have long-term liver or kidney problems.
- ◆ You have any blood disorders or anaemia.

◆ You have glaucoma.
◆ You have low blood pressure.
◆ You have ever had a heart attack.
◆ You have an underactive thyroid.
◆ You have glucose-6-phosphate dehydrogenase (G6PD) deficiency.
◆ You have had a recent head injury.
◆ You are taking other medicines.

Pregnancy Safety in pregnancy not established. Discuss with your doctor.
Breast-feeding Safety not established. Discuss with your doctor.
Infants and children Not usually prescribed.
Over 60 No special problems.
Driving and hazardous work Avoid such activities until you have learned how isosorbide dinitrate or mononitrate affects you because these drugs can cause dizziness.
Alcohol Avoid. Alcohol may further lower blood pressure, depressing the heart and causing dizziness and fainting.

PROLONGED USE

The initial adverse effects may disappear with prolonged use, but the effects of the drug become weaker as the body adapts. This may be overcome by a change in the dose to allow a drug-free period during each day.

ISOTRETINOIN

Brand names Reticutan, Roaccutane
Used in the following combined preparations None

QUICK REFERENCE

Drug group Drug for acne (p.121)
Overdose danger rating Medium
Dependence rating Low
Prescription needed Yes
Available as generic Yes

GENERAL INFORMATION

Isotretinoin, a drug chemically related to vitamin A, is prescribed for severe acne that has not responded to other treatments. It reduces production of the skin's natural oils (sebum) and of the horny protein (keratin) in the skin's outer layers; this action also makes it useful in conditions such as ichthyosis, in which the skin thickens abnormally, causing scaling.

A single 16-week course of isotretinoin treatment often clears the acne. The skin may be very dry, flaky, and itchy at first, but this usually improves with continued use. Serious adverse effects include liver damage and bowel inflammation.

INFORMATION FOR USERS

Your drug prescription is tailored for you. Do not alter dosage without checking with your doctor.
How taken/used Capsules.
Frequency and timing of doses 1–2 x daily (take with food or milk).
Adult dosage range Dosage is determined individually.
Onset of effect 2–4 weeks. Acne may worsen initially in some people but usually improves in 7–10 days.
Duration of action Effects persist for several weeks after the drug is stopped. Acne is usually completely cleared.
Diet advice None.
Storage Keep in original container at room temperature out of the reach of children. Protect from light.
Missed dose Take as soon as you remember. If your next dose is due within 4 hours, take a single dose now and skip the next.
Stopping the drug Can be safely stopped as soon as you no longer need it, but best results are achieved when the course of treatment is completed as prescribed.
Exceeding the dose An occasional unintentional extra dose is unlikely to cause problems. Large overdoses may cause headaches, vomiting, abdominal pain, facial flushing, incoordination, and dizziness. Notify your doctor.

POSSIBLE ADVERSE EFFECTS

Dry, flaking skin and lips, dry nose or nosebleeds, muscle or joint pain, and dry or inflamed eyes often occur. Skin pigmentation changes and temporary loss or increase of hair may also occur. Consult your doctor if you have eye problems or if these other symptoms are severe. If you have headache, nausea, vomiting, blood in the faeces, impaired vision, rash, mood changes, or unusual bruising, consult your doctor promptly. If abdominal pain or diarrhoea occur, stop taking the drug and consult your doctor immediately.

INTERACTIONS

Tetracycline antibiotics increase the risk of high pressure in the skull, leading to headaches, nausea, and vomiting.

Skin-drying preparations Medicated cosmetics, soaps, and toiletries, and anti-acne or abrasive skin preparations increase the likelihood of skin dryness and irritation with isotretinoin.
Vitamin A supplements increase the risk of adverse effects from isotretinoin and should be avoided.
Progestogen-only contraceptive pills work poorly during isotretinoin treatment. Women should use an alternative method of contraception (see below) for 1 month before, during, and 1 month after treatment.

SPECIAL PRECAUTIONS

Do not donate blood during or after taking isotretinoin. Be sure to tell your doctor if:

- You have long-term liver or kidney problems.
- You have diabetes, arthritis, or gout.
- You have a history of depression.
- You have fructose intolerance or are allergic to soya or peanuts.
- You have high blood fat levels.
- You wear contact lenses.
- You are pregnant or planning a pregnancy.
- You are taking other medicines.

Pregnancy Must not be prescribed. The drug causes fetal abnormalities. Women of child-bearing age must use at least one user-independent hormonal form of contraception or two barrier methods for 1 month before, during, and 1 month after treatment.
Breast-feeding Not recommended. Likely to pass into breast milk and may affect the baby.
Infants and children Not prescribed to children under 12 years.
Over 60 Not usually prescribed.
Driving and hazardous work Avoid until you know how the drug affects you because it can cause vision problems in dim light.
Alcohol Regular heavy drinking may raise blood fat levels and increase the risk of hepatitis with isotretinoin.
Sunlight, sunbeds, and skin care To avoid skin damage, use a sunscreen or sunblock; do not use a sunlamp or sunbed. Avoid wax depilation, laser treatment, and dermabrasion for 6 months after treatment.

PROLONGED USE

Treatment rarely exceeds 16 weeks. Prolonged use may raise blood fat levels, and increase the risk of heart and blood vessel disease. Bone changes may occur.
Monitoring Liver function tests and checks on blood fat levels are performed.

KETOCONAZOLE

Brand names Boots Anti-Dandruff Ketoconazole Shampoo, Daktarin Gold, Dandrazol, Nizoral
Used in the following combined preparations None

QUICK REFERENCE

Drug group Antifungal drug (p.71)
Overdose danger rating Low
Dependence rating Low
Prescription needed Yes (except for some shampoos)
Available as generic Yes

GENERAL INFORMATION

Ketoconazole was previously used to treat severe, internal systemic fungal infections by mouth, but this application has been discontinued due to the risk of severe liver damage. However, the drug is still available as a topical cream to treat fungal skin and vaginal infections, and as a shampoo for scalp infections and seborrhoeic dermatitis. Used in this way, it is extremely safe because very little is absorbed into the blood – in fact, blood levels of the drug are usually undetectably low.

Side effects of ketoconazole are uncommon. However, the drug may occasionally alter the colour of the hair or cause itching, skin rashes, or in rare cases, hair loss.

INFORMATION FOR USERS

Your drug prescription is tailored for you. Do not alter dosage without checking with your doctor.
How taken/used Cream, shampoo.
Frequency and timing of doses 1–2 x daily (cream); 1–2 times weekly (shampoo for seborrhoeic dermatitis); 1 x daily for 5 days (shampoo for tinea versicolor).
Dosage range As directed.
Onset of effect Within a few hours; full beneficial effect may take several days (or weeks in severe infections).
Duration of action Up to 24 hours.
Diet advice None.
Storage Keep in original container at room temperature out of the reach of children.
Missed dose No cause for concern, but apply the missed dose as soon as you remember.
Stopping the drug Apply the full course. Even if you feel better, the original infection may still

be present and may recur if treatment is stopped too soon.

Exceeding the dose An occasional unintentional extra application is unlikely to be a cause for concern.

POSSIBLE ADVERSE EFFECTS

Applied to the skin or hair, ketoconazole is extremely safe. However, it may rarely affect hair colour, cause itching or a rash, or cause hair loss (alopecia). If changes to hair colour are severe, consult your doctor. If itching, rash, or hair loss occur, stop using the drug and consult your doctor.

INTERACTIONS

None known.

SPECIAL PRECAUTIONS

Be sure to tell your doctor or pharmacist before taking this drug if:

◆ You have previously had an allergic reaction to antifungal drugs.

◆ You are taking other medicines.

Pregnancy No evidence of risk.

Breast-feeding No evidence of risk. The drug does not pass into the breast milk in detectable amounts.

Infants and children No special problems.

Over 60 No special problems.

Driving and hazardous work No special problems.

Alcohol No known problems.

PROLONGED USE

No problems expected. However, ketoconazole is usually used only until the infection has cleared up.

KETOPROFEN

Brand names Orudis, Oruvail, Powergel, Valket, and many others

Used in the following combined preparations None

QUICK REFERENCE

Drug group Non-steroidal anti-inflammatory drug (p.48)

Overdose danger rating Medium

Dependence rating Low

Prescription needed Yes (except for some topical preparations)

Available as generic Yes

GENERAL INFORMATION

Ketoprofen is a non-steroidal anti-inflammatory (NSAID) drug. Like other NSAIDs, it relieves pain and reduces inflammation and stiffness in rheumatoid arthritis, osteoarthritis, and ankylosing spondylitis. The drug does not cure the underlying disease, however.

Ketoprofen is also given to relieve mild to moderate pain associated with menstruation and soft tissue injuries, and to ease the pain that occurs following operations.

The most common adverse reactions to ketoprofen, as with all NSAIDs, are gastrointestinal disturbances such as nausea and indigestion. Switching to another NSAID may be recommended by your doctor if unwanted effects are persistent or troublesome.

INFORMATION FOR USERS

Follow instructions on the label. Call your doctor if symptoms worsen.

How taken/used Capsules, slow release (SR) capsules, suppositories, gel.

Frequency and timing of doses Once daily (SR capsules) or 2–4 x daily (capsules) with food; 4 x daily for up to 3 days (injection); 2 x daily (suppositories).

Adult dosage range 100–200mg daily.

Onset of effect Pain relief may be felt in 30 minutes to 2 hours. Full anti-inflammatory effect may not be felt for up to 2 weeks.

Duration of action Up to 8–12 hours.

Diet advice None.

Storage Keep in original container at room temperature out of the reach of children.

Missed dose Take as soon as you remember. If your next dose is due within 4 hours, take a single dose now and skip the next.

Stopping the drug Seek medical advice before stopping the drug.

Exceeding the dose An occasional unintentional extra dose is unlikely to be a cause for concern. Large overdoses may cause vomiting, confusion, or irritability. Notify your doctor.

POSSIBLE ADVERSE EFFECTS

Gastrointestinal disturbances such as indigestion, heartburn, nausea, and vomiting are common with oral forms; suppositories may cause rectal irritation. Less common effects include headache, drowsiness, dizziness, swollen feet or legs, and weight gain. Discuss with your doctor if these symptoms are severe. If you develop rash or itching, stop taking the drug. If you have wheezing or breathlessness, or notice black or bloodstained faeces, stop the drug and notify your doctor promptly. Topical forms of ketoprofen may cause photosensitivity, so treated areas of skin should be protected from sunlight.

INTERACTIONS

General note Ketoprofen interacts with a wide range of drugs, such as aspirin and other NSAIDs, oral anticoagulants, and corticosteroids, to increase the risk of bleeding and/or stomach ulcers.

Lithium, digoxin, and methotrexate Ketoprofen may raise blood levels of these drugs to an undesirable extent.

Phenytoin Ketoprofen may enhance the effects of phenytoin.

Quinolone antibiotics Ketoprofen may increase the risk of seizures if taken with these drugs.

Antihypertensive drugs Ketoprofen may reduce the beneficial effects of these drugs.

SPECIAL PRECAUTIONS

Be sure to tell your doctor or pharmacist before taking this drug if:

- You have long-term liver or kidney problems.
- You have heart problems.
- You have high blood pressure.
- You have asthma.
- You have had a peptic ulcer, oesophagitis, or acid indigestion.
- You have bleeding problems.
- You are allergic to aspirin or other NSAIDs.
- You are taking other medicines.

Pregnancy The drug may increase the risk of adverse effects on the baby's heart and may prolong labour if taken in the third trimester. Discuss with your doctor.

Breast-feeding The drug passes into the breast milk and may affect the baby. Discuss with your doctor.

Infants and children Not recommended for children under 12 years.

Over 60 Increased likelihood of adverse effects. Reduced dose may therefore be necessary.

Driving and hazardous work Avoid such activities until you have learned how ketoprofen affects you because the drug can cause dizziness and drowsiness.

Alcohol Avoid. Alcohol may increase the risk of stomach disorders with ketoprofen.

Surgery and general anaesthetics Ketoprofen may prolong bleeding. Discuss with your doctor or dentist before any surgery.

PROLONGED USE

There is an increased risk of bleeding from peptic ulcers and in the bowel with prolonged use of ketoprofen. There is also a small risk of a heart attack or stroke. To minimize these risks, the lowest effective dose is given for the shortest duration.

LACTULOSE

Brand names Duphalac, Lactugal

Used in the following combined preparations None

QUICK REFERENCE

Drug group Laxative (p.43)

Overdose danger rating Low

Dependence rating Low

Prescription needed No

Available as generic Yes

GENERAL INFORMATION

Lactulose is an effective laxative that softens faeces by increasing the amount of water in the large intestine. It is used to relieve constipation and faecal impaction, especially in older people. It is less likely than some of the other laxatives to disrupt normal bowel action.

Lactulose is also used for preventing and treating a form of brain disturbance associated with liver failure – a condition known as hepatic encephalopathy.

Because lactulose acts locally in the large intestine and is not absorbed into the body, it is safer than many other laxatives. However, the drug can cause stomach cramps and flatulence, especially at the start of treatment.

INFORMATION FOR USERS

Follow instructions on the label. Call your doctor if symptoms worsen.

How taken/used Liquid, powder.

Frequency and timing of doses *Chronic constipation* 2 x daily; *Liver failure* 3–4 x daily.

Adult dosage range *Chronic constipation* 15–30ml daily; *Liver failure* 90–150ml daily.

Onset of effect 24–48 hours.

Duration of action 6–18 hours.

Diet advice Adequate fluid intake is important: up to 8 glasses of water daily.

Storage Keep in original container at room temperature out of the reach of children. Do not store after diluting. Do not refrigerate or freeze.
Missed dose Take as soon as you remember. If your next dose is due within 3 hours, take a single dose now and skip the next.
Stopping the drug In the treatment of constipation, the drug can be safely stopped as soon as you no longer need it.
Exceeding the dose An occasional unintentional extra dose is unlikely to be a cause for concern. But if you notice any unusual symptoms, or if a large overdose has been taken, notify your doctor.

POSSIBLE ADVERSE EFFECTS

Adverse effects include flatulence, belching, stomach cramps, or less commonly nausea, vomiting, and abdominal distension. They are rarely serious and often disappear when your body adjusts to the drug, but consult your doctor if they are severe or if you have abdominal distension. If diarrhoea occurs, this may indicate that the dosage is too high and needs to be adjusted; consult your doctor.

INTERACTIONS

Other laxatives Lactulose combined with other laxatives increases the risk of diarrhoea.

SPECIAL PRECAUTIONS

Be sure to consult your doctor or pharmacist before taking this drug if:

- You have severe abdominal pain.
- You have diabetes.
- You have lactose intolerance or galactosaemia.
- You are taking other medicines.

Pregnancy No evidence of risk. Discuss with your doctor.
Breast-feeding No evidence of risk.
Infants and children Reduced dose necessary.
Over 60 No special problems.
Driving and hazardous work No known problems.
Alcohol No known problems.

PROLONGED USE

Prolonged use, overuse, or too high a dosage of lactulose may lead to diarrhoea and disturbances in the balance of body salts. In children, prolonged use may contribute to the development of dental caries (tooth decay).

LAMOTRIGINE

Brand name Lamictal
Used in the following combined preparations None

QUICK REFERENCE

Drug group Anticonvulsant drug (p.14)
Overdose danger rating Medium
Dependence rating Low
Prescription needed Yes
Available as generic Yes

GENERAL INFORMATION

Lamotrigine is an anticonvulsant drug that is prescribed, either alone or in combination with other anticonvulsants, to treat epilepsy. The drug acts by restoring the balance between excitatory and inhibitory neurotransmitters (see p.7) in the brain. Lamotrigine may be less sedating than older anticonvulsants, and there is no need for blood tests to determine the level of the drug in the blood. It may cause a number of minor adverse effects (see below), most of which will respond to an adjustment in dosage.

Lamotrigine is also occasionally used in specialist centres to treat bipolar affective disorder (manic depressive disorder).

INFORMATION FOR USERS

Your drug prescription is tailored for you. Do not alter dosage without checking with your doctor.
How taken/used Tablets, chewable tablets, dispersible tablets.
Frequency and timing of doses 1–2 x daily.
Adult dosage range 100–500mg daily (maintenance) (100–200mg with sodium valproate). Smaller doses are used at start of treatment. Dose may vary if other anticonvulsant drugs are being taken.
Onset of effect Approximately 5 days at a constant dose.
Duration of action Up to 24 hours.
Diet advice None.
Storage Keep in original container at room temperature out of the reach of children.
Missed dose Take as soon as you remember. If your next dose is due within 2 hours, take a single dose now and skip the next.
Stopping the drug Do not stop without consulting your doctor, who will supervise a gradual reduction in dosage. Abrupt cessation increases the risk of rebound seizures.

Exceeding the dose An occasional unintentional extra dose is unlikely to be a cause for concern. Large overdoses may cause sedation, double vision, loss of muscular coordination, nausea, and vomiting. Contact your doctor immediately.

POSSIBLE ADVERSE EFFECTS
Serious adverse effects are rare with lamotrigine. The most common side effects are headache, tiredness, insomnia, blurred or double vision, and poor muscle coordination; discuss with your doctor if headache or tiredness are severe, if any of these other symptoms occur, or if you have severe nausea. A rash is also a common adverse effect and may indicate a serious hypersensitivity reaction, especially when accompanied by mouth ulcers; if you develop a rash, call your doctor immediately. More rarely, lamotrigine may cause flu-like symptoms, sore throat, unusual bruising, or facial swelling; call your doctor at once if any of these symptoms occur.

INTERACTIONS
Sodium valproate increases and prolongs the effectiveness of lamotrigine. A reduced dose of lamotrigine will be used.
Antidepressants, antipsychotics, rifampicin, mefloquine, and chloroquine may counteract the anticonvulsant effect of lamotrigine.
Carbamazepine may reduce lamotrigine blood levels, but lamotrigine may increase the side effects of carbamazepine.
Phenytoin and phenobarbital may decrease blood levels of lamotrigine so a higher dose of lamotrigine may be needed.

SPECIAL PRECAUTIONS
Be sure to tell your doctor if:
- You have long-term liver or kidney problems.
- You have any blood disorder.
- You are taking other medicines.

Pregnancy Safety in pregnancy not established. Discuss with your doctor.
Breast-feeding The drug passes into the breast milk and may affect the baby. Discuss with your doctor.
Infants and children Not recommended under 2 years. Not recommended as a single therapy under 12 years. Doses may be relatively higher than adult doses due to increased metabolism.
Over 60 No special problems.
Driving and hazardous work Your underlying condition, in addition to the possibility of sedation, dizziness, and vision disturbances with lamotrigine, may make such activities inadvisable. Discuss with your doctor.
Alcohol Alcohol may increase the adverse effects of this drug.

PROLONGED USE
No special problems.

LANSOPRAZOLE

Brand names Zoton FasTab
Used in the following combined preparations None

QUICK REFERENCE
Drug group Anti-ulcer drug (p.41)
Overdose danger rating Low
Dependence rating Low
Prescription needed Yes
Available as generic Yes

GENERAL INFORMATION
Lansoprazole belongs to a group of drugs called proton pump inhibitors (p.41). It is used to treat gastro-oesophageal reflux (rising of stomach acid into the oesophagus), to treat Zollinger-Ellison syndrome (production of large quantities of stomach acid, leading to ulceration), and to prevent or treat peptic ulcers. It works by reducing the amount of acid that the stomach produces.

Lansoprazole may be given with antibiotics as a 7-day course to eradicate *Helicobacter pylori* bacteria, the main cause of peptic ulcers.

Because lansoprazole may mask the symptoms of stomach cancer, it is prescribed only when the possibility of this disease has been ruled out.

INFORMATION FOR USERS
Your drug prescription is tailored for you. Do not alter dosage without checking with your doctor.
How taken/used Capsules, dispersible tablets, liquid (suspension).
Frequency and timing of doses Usually once, sometimes twice, daily, taken before food in the morning.
Dosage range *Peptic ulcer/gastro-oesophageal reflux* 30mg daily. *NSAID-induced ulcer* 15–30mg daily. *Acid-related dyspepsia* 15–30mg daily. *Zollinger-Ellison syndrome* 60mg daily

initially, adjusted according to response. *H. pylori-associated ulcer* 60mg daily, half the dose in the morning and half in the evening.
Onset of effect 1–2 hours.
Duration of action 24 hours.
Diet advice None, although spicy foods and alcohol may exacerbate the condition that is being treated.
Storage Keep in original container at room temperature out of the reach of children. Do not refrigerate.
Missed dose Take as soon as you remember. If your next dose is due within 8 hours, take a single dose now and skip the next.
Stopping the drug Do not stop without consulting your doctor; symptoms may recur.
Exceeding the dose An occasional unintentional extra dose is unlikely to be a cause for concern. But if you notice any unusual symptoms or have taken a large overdose, notify your doctor.

POSSIBLE ADVERSE EFFECTS
Common adverse effects include headache, dizziness, diarrhoea or constipation, indigestion, flatulence or abdominal pain, nausea, and vomiting. Discuss with your doctor if these are severe or if you also experience unusual fatigue or malaise. If a rash or itching occur, stop taking the drug and contact your doctor. A sore throat, mouth, or tongue are very rare adverse effects but should be reported to your doctor at once; you should also stop taking the drug if they occur. Long-term use may increase the risk of intestinal infections and of fractures (see below).

INTERACTIONS
Antifungals (ketoconazole and flucanazole) and theophylline Lansoprazole may reduce the effect of these drugs.
Antacids and sucralfate These drugs may reduce the absorption of lansoprazole and should not be taken within an hour of the drug.
Digoxin Lansoprazole may increase blood levels of digoxin.
Cilostazol Lansoprazole may increase the effect of cilostazol; the two drugs should not be taken together.
Tacrolimus Lansoprazole may increase blood levels of tacrolimus.
Atazanavir Lansoprazole may decrease the effect of atazanavir; the two drugs should not be taken together.

SPECIAL PRECAUTIONS
Be sure to tell your doctor if:
- You have liver problems.
- You are taking other medicines.

Pregnancy Safety not established. Discuss with your doctor.
Breast-feeding Safety not established. Discuss with your doctor.
Infants and children Not recommended.
Over 60 No special problems.
Driving and hazardous work No special problems.
Alcohol Avoid. Alcohol irritates the stomach.

PROLONGED USE
Long-term use of lansoprazole may increase the risk of certain intestinal infections (such as *Salmonella* and *Clostridium difficile*) because of the loss of the natural protection against such infections provided by stomach acid. Prolonged use also increases the risk of fractures and may increase the risk of low magnesium levels in the blood.

LATANOPROST

Brand names Fixapost, Medizol, Monopost, Xalatan
Used in the following combined preparation Xalacom

QUICK REFERENCE
Drug group Drug for glaucoma (p.112)
Overdose danger rating Medium
Dependence rating Low
Prescription needed Yes
Available as generic Yes

GENERAL INFORMATION
Latanoprost is a synthetic derivative of the prostaglandin dinoprost, which constricts the smooth muscle lining the blood vessels and airways. Latanoprost is used as eye drops to reduce pressure inside the eye in open angle (chronic) glaucoma (p.113) and to relieve ocular hypertension by increasing the outflow of fluid from the eye. It is used when patients have not responded to or cannot tolerate the drug of first choice, usually a beta blocker (such as timolol, p.426). Sometimes, combined eye drops of latanoprost and timolol may be prescribed when timolol alone is not adequately controlling the pressure.

Latanoprost eye drops can gradually increase the amount of brown pigment in the eye, darkening the iris. This will be particularly noticeable if only one eye needs treatment. Irises of mixed coloration are especially susceptible; pure blue eyes do not seem to be affected. Latanoprost has also been reported to cause darkening, thickening, and lengthening of the eyelashes.

INFORMATION FOR USERS

Your drug prescription is tailored for you. Do not alter dosage without checking with your doctor.
How taken/used Eye drops.
Frequency and timing of doses 1 x daily, in the evening.
Adult dosage range 1 drop per eye, daily.
Onset of effect 3–4 hours.
Duration of action 24 hours.
Diet advice None.
Storage Keep eye drops in the outer cardboard package to protect from light. Store at room temperature, out of the reach of children. Discard unused solution 4 weeks after opening.
Missed dose Use the next dose as normal.
Stopping the drug Do not stop the drug without consulting your doctor; symptoms may recur.
Exceeding the dose An occasional unintentional extra application is unlikely to cause problems. Excessive use may irritate the eye and produce adverse effects in other parts of the body. Notify your doctor.

POSSIBLE ADVERSE EFFECTS

Darkening of the iris is a very common side effect of latanoprost, and changes to the eyelashes occur almost as often, but neither of these affects vision. Eye irritation and blurred vision are also common; discuss with your doctor if either of these is severe or if you have eye pain, bloodshot or swollen eyes, inflamed eyelids, or facial swelling. Stop using the drug and seek medical advice if you develop chest pains, wheezing, or breathing difficulty.

INTERACTIONS

Other eye drops should not be used within 5 minutes of using latanoprost.

SPECIAL PRECAUTIONS

Be sure to tell your doctor if:
- You wear contact lenses.
- You may have an eye infection.
- You are allergic to latanoprost or any of the ingredients in the formulation.
- You have heart problems.
- You have asthma.
- You are taking other medicines.

Pregnancy Safety not established. Prostaglandins may affect the fetus. Discuss with your doctor.
Breast-feeding The drug may pass into the breast milk and may affect the baby. Discuss with your doctor.
Infants and children Not recommended. Safety not established.
Over 60 No special problems.
Driving and hazardous work The eye drops may cause temporary blurring of vision. Avoid driving and hazardous work until vision has returned to normal.
Alcohol No known problems.

PROLONGED USE

No known problems apart from changes to iris pigment and eyelashes. These changes do not affect vision, but they may not diminish once treatment has been stopped.
Monitoring Although there should be no problems with long-term use, your doctor will continue to monitor eye pigmentation as well as control of the glaucoma.

LEVETIRACETAM

Brand names Desitrend, Keppra
Used in the following combined preparations None

QUICK REFERENCE

Drug group Anticonvulsant drug (p.14)
Overdose danger rating Medium
Dependence rating Low
Prescription needed Yes
Available as generic Yes

GENERAL INFORMATION

Levetiracetam is given to treat some forms of epilepsy as it reduces the likelihood of seizures caused by abnormal nerve signals in the brain. It may be used alone or in combination with other anticonvulsants. It is chemically different from other anticonvulsants, and the precise way in which it works is not fully understood.

Compared to other anticonvulsants, levetiracetam usually causes relatively few adverse effects (see Possible adverse effects, below). In addition, it does not interact with other anticonvulsants, which is a significant advantage. As with all anticonvulsant drugs, it is important that levetiracetam is not stopped abruptly without medical advice as this can precipitate an epileptic seizure.

INFORMATION FOR USERS

Your drug prescription is tailored for you. Do not alter dosage without checking with your doctor.

How taken/used Tablets, liquid, injection.

Frequency and timing of doses 1–2 x daily.

Adult dosage range Initially 250mg once daily, increased after 1–2 weeks to 250mg twice daily. If necessary, dosage can be further increased up to maximum of 1.5g twice daily.

Onset of effect Up to 48 hours.

Duration of action 12 hours.

Diet advice None.

Storage Store in original container at room temperature out of reach of children.

Missed dose Take as soon as you remember. If your next dose is due within 4 hours, take a single dose now and skip the next.

Stopping the drug Do not stop without consulting your doctor; symptoms may recur.

Exceeding the dose An occasional unintentional extra dose is unlikely to cause problems. Large overdoses may cause agitation, impaired consciousness, and coma. Notify your doctor immediately.

POSSIBLE ADVERSE EFFECTS

Most people have few adverse effects. The most common are dizziness, headache, drowsiness, and gastrointestinal problems, such as nausea, vomiting, indigestion, and abdominal pain; less commonly, there may be a cough. Discuss with your doctor if any of these are severe. You should also contact your doctor if you have itching, a rash, mood changes, or depression. Rarely, the drug may cause suicidal thoughts; if so, call your doctor immediately.

INTERACTIONS

Antidepressant drugs (MAOIs, tricyclics, and SSRIs) and mefloquine may reduce the anticonvulsant effect of levetiracetam.

St John's wort may reduce the anticonvulsant effect of levetiracetam.

SPECIAL PRECAUTIONS

Be sure to tell your doctor if:

- You have long-term liver or kidney problems.
- You have a psychotic illness.
- You have a depressive illness.
- You are taking other medicines.

Pregnancy Safety not established. Discuss with your doctor.

Breast-feeding Safety not established. The drug passes into breast milk. Discuss with doctor.

Infants and children Reduced dose necessary.

Over 60 No special problems.

Driving and hazardous work Avoid until you know how levetiracetam affects you because the drug can cause drowsiness in some people.

Alcohol Avoid. Alcohol may worsen any drowsiness caused by levetiracetam.

PROLONGED USE

Usually no problems, although very rarely it can cause depression, other mood changes, personality changes, and suicidal thoughts.

LEVODOPA/ CO-BENELDOPA/ CO-CARELDOPA

Brand names None

Used in the following combined preparations

Caramet CR, Duodopa, Madopar, Madopar CR, Sinemet, Sinemet CR, Stalevo

QUICK REFERENCE

Drug group Drug for parkinsonism (p.16)

Overdose danger rating Medium

Dependence rating Low

Prescription needed Yes

Available as generic Yes

GENERAL INFORMATION

The treatment of Parkinson's disease underwent dramatic change in the 1960s with the introduction of levodopa. Since the body can transform levodopa into dopamine, a chemical messenger in the brain whose absence or shortage causes Parkinson's disease (see p.16), rapid improvements in control were obtained (albeit not a cure). However, while levodopa was effective, it was found to cause severe side effects, such as nausea, dizziness, and palpitations. Even when treatment was initiated gradually, it was difficult to balance the benefits against the adverse reactions.

Today levodopa is prescribed, in a combined form, with carbidopa (as co-careldopa) or benserazide (as co-beneldopa); both of these drugs enhance the effects of levodopa in the brain, as well as helping to reduce the side effects. The drug is taken by mouth and, in severe cases, can be administered in the form of intestinal gel.

INFORMATION FOR USERS

Your drug prescription is tailored for you. Do not alter dosage without checking with your doctor.

How taken/used Tablets, modified release (MR) tablets, dispersible tablets, capsules, intestinal gel.

Frequency and timing of doses 2–6 x daily with food or milk.

Adult dosage range 125–500mg initially, increased until the benefits and side effects are balanced.

Onset of effect Within 1 hour.

Duration of action 2–12 hours.

Diet advice None.

Storage Keep in original container at room temperature out of the reach of children. Store gel in a refrigerator. Protect from light.

Missed dose Take as soon as you remember. If your next dose is due within 2 hours, take a single dose now and skip the next.

Stopping the drug Do not stop without consulting your doctor; stopping the drug may lead to severe worsening of the underlying condition.

Exceeding the dose An occasional unintentional extra dose is unlikely to cause problems. Larger overdoses may cause vomiting or drowsiness. Notify your doctor.

POSSIBLE ADVERSE EFFECTS

Adverse effects are related to the dosage level. At the start of treatment, on a low dosage, side effects are likely to be mild, but they may become more severe as the dosage is increased. Common adverse effects include dark urine, digestive disturbances, abnormal movements, nervousness or agitation, confusion, and hallucinations. Rarer adverse effects include dizziness, fainting, fatigue, sudden sleepiness, and compulsive behaviour. All adverse effects should be discussed with your doctor.

INTERACTIONS

Antidepressants Levodopa may interact with monoamine oxidase inhibitors (MAOIs; see p.12) to cause a dangerous rise in blood pressure. It may also interact with tricyclics.

Iron May reduce absorption of levodopa.

Antipsychotic drugs Some of these drugs may reduce the effect of levodopa.

SPECIAL PRECAUTIONS

Be sure to tell your doctor if:

- You have heart problems.
- You have long-term liver or kidney problems.
- You have epilepsy.
- You have had glaucoma.
- You have a peptic ulcer.
- You have diabetes or any other endocrine disorder.
- You have any serious mental illness.
- You are taking other medicines.

Pregnancy Unlikely to be required. Safety not established. Discuss with your doctor.

Breast-feeding Unlikely to be required. May suppress milk production. Discuss with doctor.

Infants and children Not normally used in children (rarely given to patients under 25 years).

Over 60 No special problems.

Driving and hazardous work Your underlying condition, as well as the possibility of levodopa causing fainting, dizziness, and sudden sleep episodes, may make such activities inadvisable. Discuss with your doctor.

Alcohol No known problems, although levodopa may enhance sedative effects of alcohol.

PROLONGED USE

Effectiveness usually declines with time, necessitating increased dosage. Also, adverse effects become severe at the end of one dose and the onset of another, so that the dosage, frequency, or formulation must be fine-tuned for each individual. Ultimately, other antiparkinsonian drugs may need to be substituted.

LEVOFLOXACIN

Brand names Evoxil, Oftaquix, Quinsair, Tavanic
Used in the following combined preparations None

QUICK REFERENCE

Drug group Antibacterial drug (p.64)
Overdose danger rating Medium
Dependence rating Low
Prescription needed Yes
Available as generic Yes

GENERAL INFORMATION

Levofloxacin is a quinolone antibacterial drug used for soft-tissue, respiratory, and urinary tract infections that have not responded to other antibiotics. It is usually given as tablets, but may be given by intravenous infusion to people who have serious systemic infections or cannot take drugs by mouth. It may also be given by nebulizer for respiratory infections.

Like other quinolones, it may occasionally cause tendon inflammation and damage, especially in older people, those with rheumatoid arthritis, and those taking corticosteroids. Report tendon pain or inflammation to your doctor immediately and stop taking the drug. Rest the limbs until symptoms have subsided.

Levofloxacin may also be given as eye drops to treat eye infections. The most common side effects are eye discomfort and blurred vision; there is no risk of tendon problems.

INFORMATION FOR USERS

Your drug prescription is tailored for you. Do not alter dosage without checking with your doctor.

How taken/used Tablets, intravenous infusion, liquid for nebulizer, eye drops.

Frequency and timing of doses 1 x 2 times daily for 7–14 days depending on infection (tablets); variable with other forms.

Adult dosage range 250–1,000mg daily; variable with eye drops.

Onset of effect 1 hour.

Duration of action 12–24 hours.

Diet advice None.

Storage Keep in original container at room temperature out of the reach of children.

Missed dose Take as soon as you remember, then take your next dose when it is due.

Stopping the drug Take the full course. Even if you feel better, the original infection may still be present, and symptoms may recur if treatment is stopped too soon.

Exceeding the dose An occasional unintentional extra dose is unlikely to cause problems. Large overdoses of oral, infused, or inhaled preparations may cause mental disturbances and seizures. Notify your doctor.

POSSIBLE ADVERSE EFFECTS (ORAL/INFUSED/INHALED FORMS)

Infused or inhaled forms may cause palpitations and a fall in blood pressure; oral forms most commonly cause nausea and vomiting, diarrhoea, and abdominal pain. The drug may also cause headache, dizziness, and drowsiness or restlessness. Discuss with your doctor if these are severe. If a rash, itching, jaundice, fever, or an allergic reaction occur, stop the drug and consult your doctor. If confusion, seizures, or painful or inflamed tendons occur, stop the drug and call your doctor immediately. Aortic aneurysm or dissection have occurred in rare cases; for any sudden onset of chest, back, or abdominal pain, seek urgent medical help.

INTERACTIONS (ORAL/INFUSED/INHALED FORMS)

Anticoagulants The effect of these drugs may be increased by levofloxacin.

Ciclosporin used with levofloxacin carries an increased risk of kidney damage.

Non-steroidal anti-inflammatory drugs (NSAIDs) and theophylline increase the risk of seizures if taken with levofloxacin.

Oral iron preparations and antacids containing magnesium or aluminium hydroxide interfere with absorption of levofloxacin. Do not take antacids within 2 hours of levofloxacin tablets.

Corticosteroids may increase the risk of tendon rupture with levofloxacin.

SPECIAL PRECAUTIONS

Be sure to tell your doctor if:

- You have kidney problems.
- You have epilepsy.
- You have porphyria.
- You have myasthenia gravis.
- You have a history of psychotic illness.
- You have had a previous allergic reaction to a quinolone antibacterial.
- You have had a previous tendon problem with a quinolone.
- You are taking other medicines.

Pregnancy Safety not established. Discuss with your doctor.

Breast-feeding Safety not established. Discuss with your doctor.

Infants and children Not recommended.

Over 60 No special problems, except that tendon damage is more likely over the age of 60.

Driving and hazardous work Avoid until you know how levofloxacin affects you because it can cause dizziness, drowsiness, visual disturbances, and hallucinations.

Alcohol Avoid. Alcohol may increase the sedative effects of levofloxacin.

Sunlight and sunbeds Avoid exposure to strong sunlight or artificial ultraviolet rays because photosensitization may occur.

PROLONGED USE

Not usually prescribed for long-term use.

LEVONORGESTREL

Brand names Emerres, Kyleena, Levonelle 1500, Levonelle One Step, Levosert, Logynon, Mirena, Norgeston, Upostelle
Used in the following combined preparations Logynon ED, Microgynon 30, Ovranette, Rigevidon, and others

QUICK REFERENCE

Drug group Female sex hormone (p.86) and oral contraceptive (p.103)
Overdose danger rating Low
Dependence rating Low
Prescription needed Yes (most preparations)
Available as generic No

GENERAL INFORMATION

Levonorgestrel is a synthetic hormone similar to progesterone, a natural female sex hormone. Its primary use is in oral contraceptives. It acts by thickening the mucus at the neck of the uterus (cervix), thereby making it difficult for sperm to enter the uterus.

The drug is available in combined oral contraceptives (COCs) with an oestrogen. A higher dose is given as a progestogen-only pill (POP) for emergency postcoital contraception, available over the counter to women over 16 years. It is also combined with an oestrogen in hormone replacement therapy (HRT) for menopausal symptoms (p.87). It rarely causes serious adverse effects, but if it is used alone, menstrual irregularities, especially mid-cycle "breakthrough" bleeding, may occur.

INFORMATION FOR USERS

Your drug prescription is tailored for you. Do not alter dosage without checking with your doctor.
How taken/used Tablets, intrauterine device (IUD), patches.
Frequency and timing of doses Once daily, at the same time each day (tablets).
Adult dosage range *Progestogen-only contraceptive* 30mcg daily. *Postcoital contraceptive* 1.5mg as a single dose as soon as possible, within 12 hours, but no later than after 72 hours. *HRT and combined oral contraceptive* Dosage varies according to preparation used.
Onset of effect Within 4 hours, but contraceptive protection may not take full effect for 14 days, depending on day of cycle tablets start.
Duration of action 24 hours. Some effects, not including contraception, may persist for up to 3 months after levonorgestrel is stopped.
Diet advice None.
Storage Keep in original container at room temperature out of the reach of children.
Missed dose *Progestogen-only contraceptive* If a tablet is delayed by 3 hours or more, regard it as a missed dose. See What to do if you miss a pill (p.107). *Postcoital contraceptive* If vomiting occurs within 3 hours, take another tablet immediately. If problem persists, speak to your doctor or pharmacist without delay. *Combined oral contraceptive* Depends on preparation used. See what to do if you miss a pill (p.107).
Stopping the drug The drug can be safely stopped as soon as contraceptive protection is no longer required. If used for menopausal symptoms, consult doctor before stopping.
Exceeding the dose An occasional unintentional extra dose is unlikely to be a cause for concern. But if you notice any unusual symptoms, or if a large overdose has been taken, notify your doctor.

POSSIBLE ADVERSE EFFECTS

The most common effects of levonorgestrel alone are menstrual irregularities (blood spotting between periods or absence of menstruation); discuss with your doctor if these occur. Pain in the lower abdomen is a rare effect but may indicate pregnancy, so consult your doctor promptly. Other effects of levonorgestrel-containing drugs include swollen ankles and feet, weight gain, nausea, vomiting, and breast tenderness. Discuss with your doctor if these are severe or if you have headaches or depression. For risks of long-term use, see below.

INTERACTIONS

General note A number of drugs can reduce blood levels of levonorgestrel and hence its contraceptive protection. They include phenytoin, carbamazepine, rifampicin, some HIV drugs, and herbal remedies such as St John's wort. Consult your doctor or pharmacist before taking other medications.

SPECIAL PRECAUTIONS

Be sure to tell your doctor if:
- You have a personal or family history of breast cancer.
- You have liver or kidney problems, heart failure, high blood pressure, diabetes, asthma, epilepsy, porphyria, or sickle cell anaemia.
- You have abnormal vaginal bleeding.

◆ You have ever had migraines, severe headaches, blood clots, or a stroke.
◆ You have a history of depression.
◆ You are taking other medicines.

Pregnancy Not prescribed. May cause abnormalities in the fetus. Discuss with your doctor.
Breast-feeding The drug passes into the breast milk, but normal doses are unlikely to affect the baby adversely. Discuss with your doctor.
Infants and children Not prescribed.
Over 60 Not prescribed.
Driving and hazardous work No known problems.
Alcohol No known problems.
Surgery and general anaesthetics The drug should be stopped before surgery.

PROLONGED USE

In a COC, the drug increases the thrombosis and breast cancer risk but reduces the endometrial and ovarian cancer risk. In a POP, it carries a small increased risk of breast cancer. As part of HRT, it increases the risk of thrombosis and breast cancer. HRT is advised only for short-term use around the menopause.
Monitoring Blood pressure checks, physical examination, and mammograms may be carried out.

LEVOTHYROXINE

Brand name Eltroxin
Used in the following combined preparations None

QUICK REFERENCE

Drug group Thyroid hormone (p.83)
Overdose danger rating Medium
Dependence rating Low
Prescription needed Yes
Available as generic Yes

GENERAL INFORMATION

Levothyroxine is the main hormone produced by the thyroid gland. A deficiency of this hormone causes hypothyroidism, which is associated with symptoms such as weight gain and slowing of body functions. A synthetic preparation is given to replace the natural hormone when it is deficient. It is also sometimes given in combination with carbimazole or propylthiouracil to treat an overactive thyroid gland (Graves' disease). In addition, levothyroxine is given (in higher doses) to people who have had thyroid cancer. Doses are usually increased gradually to help prevent adverse effects, and particular care is required in patients with heart problems such as angina.

INFORMATION FOR USERS

Your drug prescription is tailored for you. Do not alter dosage without checking with your doctor.
How taken/used Tablets, liquid.
Frequency and timing of doses 1 x daily, ideally before breakfast or first meal.
Dosage range *Adults* 25–150mcg daily, increased at 3–4-week intervals as required. The usual maximum dose is 200mcg daily.
Onset of effect Within 48 hours. Full beneficial effects may not be felt for several weeks.
Duration of action 1–3 weeks.
Diet advice None.
Storage Keep in original container at room temperature out of the reach of children. Protect from light.
Missed dose Take as soon as you remember. If your next dose is due within 8 hours, take a single dose now and skip the next.
Stopping the drug Do not stop the drug without consulting your doctor; symptoms may recur.
Exceeding the dose An occasional unintentional extra dose is unlikely to cause problems. Large overdoses may cause palpitations in next few days. Notify your doctor.

POSSIBLE ADVERSE EFFECTS

Adverse effects of levothyroxine are rare and are usually due to overdosage causing thyoid overactivity. They include anxiety, agitation, diarrhoea, weight loss, sweating, flushing, muscle cramps, insomnia, and tremors. These effects diminish as the dose is lowered, but if they occur, discuss with your doctor. If you experience palpitations or chest pain, seek immediate medical advice. Too low a dose may cause signs of hormone deficiency, such as weight gain, constipation, and altered menstrual periods.

INTERACTIONS

Oral anticoagulants Levothyroxine may increase the effect of these drugs.
Colestyramine This drug may reduce the absorption of levothyroxine.
Amiodarone may affect thyroid activity; levothyroxine dosage may need adjustment.
Anticonvulsant drugs These drugs may reduce the effect of levothyroxine.

Antidiabetic agents The doses of these drugs may need increasing once levothyroxine treatment is started.
Calcium/iron preparations and sucralfate may reduce levothyroxine absorption unless the drugs are taken several hours apart.
Antidepressants Levothyroxine may enhance the effects of tricyclic antidepressants.
Oral contraceptives may increase levothyroxine requirements.

SPECIAL PRECAUTIONS

Be sure to tell your doctor if:
◆ You have high blood pressure.
◆ You have heart problems, such as angina, heart rhythm problems, or heart failure.
◆ You have diabetes.
◆ You have an adrenal gland disorder.
◆ You are taking other medicines.

Pregnancy No evidence of risk, but dosage adjustment may be necessary.
Breast-feeding The drug passes into the breast milk, but normal doses are unlikely to affect the baby adversely. Discuss with your doctor.
Infants and children Dosage depends on age and weight.
Over 60 Reduced dose usually necessary, together with careful dose escalation.
Driving and hazardous work No known problems.
Alcohol No known problems.

PROLONGED USE

No special problems.
Monitoring Periodic tests of thyroid function are required.

LISINOPRIL

Brand names Carace, Zestril
Used in the following combined preparations Carace Plus, Lisoretic, Zestoretic

QUICK REFERENCE

Drug group ACE inhibitor (p.30) and antihypertensive drug (p.34)
Overdose danger rating Medium
Dependence rating Low
Prescription needed Yes
Available as generic Yes

GENERAL INFORMATION

Lisinopril is an ACE inhibitor drug used in the treatment of high blood pressure, diabetic nephropathy (kidney disease), heart failure, and following a heart attack. It works by relaxing the muscles in blood vessel walls, allowing them to dilate (widen), thereby easing blood flow. After a heart attack, it reduces the risk of heart failure if taken long term.

Lisinopril can initially cause a rapid fall in blood pressure, especially when taken with a diuretic drug. Therefore, treatment for heart failure is usually started under close medical supervision, in hospital in severe cases. The first dose is usually very small, and should be taken while lying down, preferably at bedtime.

INFORMATION FOR USERS

Your drug prescription is tailored for you. Do not alter dosage without checking with your doctor.
How taken/used Tablets, oral solution.
Frequency and timing of doses 1 x daily.
Adult dosage range *Hypertension* 2.5–10mg (starting dose) up to 80mg. *Heart failure* 2.5mg (starting dose) up to 35mg. *Prevention of further heart attacks* 2.5–5mg (starting dose) up to 10mg. *Diabetic nephropathy* 2.5–20mg.
Onset of effect 1–2 hours; full beneficial effect may take several weeks.
Duration of action 12–24 hours.
Diet advice Your doctor may advise you to reduce your salt intake to help control your blood pressure.
Storage Keep in original container at room temperature out of the reach of children.
Missed dose Take as soon as you remember. If your next dose is due within 8 hours, take a single dose now and skip the next.
Stopping the drug Do not stop without consulting your doctor. Stopping the drug may lead to worsening of the underlying condition.
Exceeding the dose An occasional unintentional extra dose is unlikely to be a cause for concern. Larger overdoses may cause dizziness or fainting. Notify your doctor.

POSSIBLE ADVERSE EFFECTS

Lisinopril may cause various minor adverse effects. All adverse effects should be reported to your doctor as it may be possible to minimize them by adjusting the dosage. The most common adverse effects are a rash and a persistent dry cough. More rarely, the drug may cause sore mouth or mouth ulcers, dizziness, sore throat, and fever. If swelling of the mouth or lips or breathing difficulty occur, stop the drug and seek immediate medical advice.

INTERACTIONS

Potassium supplements, potassium-sparing diuretic drugs, and ciclosporin Taken with lisinopril, these drugs increase the risk of high blood potassium levels.

Non-steroidal anti-inflammatory drugs (NSAIDs) Some may reduce the effect of lisinopril, and the risk of kidney damage is increased.

Immunosuppressants and allopurinol may increase risk of reduced white cell counts.

Vasodilators, diuretics, and other drugs for hypertension These drugs may increase the blood-pressure-lowering effect of lisinopril.

Lithium Lisinopril may increase blood levels.

Insulin and antidiabetic drugs Lisinopril may increase the effect of these drugs.

mTOR inhibitors such as sirolimus with lisinopril may increase risk of angioedema.

SPECIAL PRECAUTIONS

Be sure to tell your doctor if:

- You have long-term kidney or liver problems.
- You have heart problems.
- You have had angioedema or a previous allergic reaction to ACE inhibitors.
- You are or intend to become pregnant.
- You are taking other medicines.

Pregnancy Not prescribed. There is evidence of harm to the developing fetus.

Breast-feeding Safety not established. Discuss with your doctor.

Infants and children Not recommended.

Over 60 Reduced dose may be necessary.

Driving and hazardous work Avoid until you know how lisinopril affects you because the drug can cause dizziness and fainting.

Alcohol Avoid. Alcohol may increase the blood-pressure-lowering and adverse effects of the drug.

Surgery and general anaesthetics Lisinopril may have to be stopped before you have a general anaesthetic. Discuss with your doctor or dentist before any operation.

PROLONGED USE

No problems expected.

Monitoring Periodic checks on potassium levels, white blood cell count, kidney function, and urine are usually performed.

LITHIUM

Brand names Camcolit, Li-liquid, Liskonum, Priadel

Used in the following combined preparations None

QUICK REFERENCE

Drug group Antimanic drug (p.14)

Overdose danger rating High

Dependence rating Low

Prescription needed Yes

Available as generic Yes

GENERAL INFORMATION

Lithium, the lightest known metal, has been used since the 1940s to treat bipolar disorder (manic depressive disorder). It decreases the intensity and frequency of the swings from extreme excitement to deep depression that characterize the disorder.

The drug is sometimes used together with an antidepressant for depression that has not responded to an antidepressant alone. It is also sometimes used to control aggressive or self-harming behaviour. High levels of lithium can cause serious adverse effects, so blood levels must be carefully monitored. Any apparent benefit may take 2 to 3 weeks to appear; an antipsychotic drug is often given with lithium until it takes effect. Lithium cards, with details of side effects, are available from pharmacies.

INFORMATION FOR USERS

Your drug prescription is tailored for you. Do not alter dosage without checking with your doctor.

How taken/used Tablets, slow release (SR) tablets, liquid.

Frequency and timing of doses 1–2 x daily with meals. Always take the same brand of lithium to ensure a consistent effect; change of brand must be closely supervised.

Adult dosage range 0.3–1.6g daily. Dosage may vary according to individual response and blood levels.

Onset of effect Effects may be noticed in 3–5 days, but the full preventative effect may take 6–12 months.

Duration of action 18–36 hours. Some effects may last for several days.

Diet advice Lithium levels in the blood are affected by the amount of salt in the body, so do not suddenly alter the amount of salt in your diet. Be sure to drink plenty of fluids, especially in hot weather.

Storage Keep in original container at room temperature out of the reach of children.
Missed dose Take as soon as you remember. If your next dose is due within 4 hours, take a single dose now and skip the next.
Stopping the drug Do not stop the drug without consulting your doctor; symptoms may recur.

OVERDOSE ACTION
Seek immediate medical advice in all cases. Take emergency action if seizures or loss of consciousness occur.

POSSIBLE ADVERSE EFFECTS
Many adverse effects are signs of a high blood level of lithium. They include increased urine production, thirst, nausea, vomiting, diarrhoea, tremor, weight gain, drowsiness, lethargy, blurred vision, unsteadiness, and slurred speech. Seek prompt medical advice if increased urine output, thirst, or weight gain are severe, or if you notice any of these other symptoms. If drowsiness, lethargy, blurred vison, unsteadiness, or slurred speech occur, you should also stop taking the drug.

INTERACTIONS
General note Many drugs interact with lithium. Do not take any over-the-counter or prescription drugs without consulting your doctor or pharmacist. For everyday pain relief, use paracetamol in preference to other analgesics.
Diuretics, aspirin, and NSAIDs (p.48) can increase lithium to a dangerous level. Blood levels of lithium should be monitored closely.

SPECIAL PRECAUTIONS
Be sure to tell your doctor if:
- You have long-term liver or kidney problems.
- You have heart or circulation problems.
- You have an overactive thyroid gland.
- You have Addison's disease.
- You are taking other medicines.

Pregnancy Not usually prescribed. May cause defects in the fetus. Discuss with your doctor.
Breast-feeding The drug passes into breast milk and may affect the baby. Discuss with doctor.
Infants and children Not recommended.
Over 60 Increased likelihood of adverse effects. Reduced dose may therefore be necessary.
Driving and hazardous work Avoid until you have learned how lithium affects you because the drug can cause reduced alertness.
Alcohol Avoid. Alcohol may increase the sedative effects of this drug.

PROLONGED USE
Prolonged lithium use may lead to kidney and thyroid problems. Treatment for periods of longer than 5 years is not normally advised unless the benefits are significant and tests show no sign of reduced kidney function. When the decision is taken to stop lithium, it should be reduced gradually over a few weeks.
Monitoring Once stabilized, lithium levels should be checked every 3 months. Thyroid function should be checked every 6–12 months. Kidney function should also be monitored regularly.

LOFEPRAMINE

Brand names None
Used in the following combined preparations None

QUICK REFERENCE
Drug group Tricyclic antidepressant drug (p.12)
Overdose danger rating Medium
Dependence rating Low
Prescription needed Yes
Available as generic Yes

GENERAL INFORMATION
Lofepramine is a tricyclic antidepressant used primarily in long-term treatment of depression. It acts to elevate the mood, improve appetite, increase physical activity, and restore interest in everyday pursuits. Less sedating than some other tricyclic antidepressants, the drug is particularly useful when depression is accompanied by lethargy.

The main advantage of lofepramine over similar drugs is that it seems to have a weaker anticholinergic action (p.7) and thus milder side effects. In overdose, it is thought to be less harmful than other tricyclics. However, like them, it lowers the threshold for seizures.

INFORMATION FOR USERS
Your drug prescription is tailored for you. Do not alter dosage without checking with your doctor.
How taken/used Tablets, liquid.
Frequency and timing of doses 2–3 x daily.
Adult dosage range 140–210mg daily.
Onset of effect Sedation can occur within hours; full antidepressant effect may not be felt for 2–6 weeks.

Duration of action Antidepressant effect may last for 6 weeks. Common adverse effects may persist for the first 1–2 weeks.
Diet advice None.
Storage Keep in original container at room temperature out of the reach of children. Protect from light.
Missed dose Take as soon as you remember. If your next dose is due within 3 hours, take a single dose now and skip the next.
Stopping the drug An abrupt stop can cause withdrawal symptoms and a recurrence of the original problem. Consult your doctor, who may supervise a gradual reduction in dosage over at least 4 weeks.
Exceeding the dose An occasional unintentional extra dose is unlikely to be a cause for concern. But if you notice any unusual symptoms, or if a large overdose has been taken, tell your doctor.

POSSIBLE ADVERSE EFFECTS

The adverse effects of lofepramine are mainly due to its mild anticholinergic action and its blocking action on the transmission of signals through the heart. Sweating, flushing, and drowsiness are common; more rarely, constipation and dryness of the mouth may occur. If any of these are severe or if you experience blurred vision or difficulty in passing urine, discuss with your doctor. If dizziness, fainting, or palpitations occur, stop taking the drug and seek immediate medical attention.

INTERACTIONS

Sedatives All drugs that have sedative effects may intensify those of lofepramine.
Anti-arrhythmic drugs and sotalol These may increase the risk of abnormal heart rhythms.
Warfarin Lofepramine may, rarely, increase the effects of warfarin.
Monoamine oxidase inhibitors (MAOIs) Serious interactions are possible. These drugs are only prescribed together with lofepramine under close specialist medical supervision.
Selective serotonin reuptake inhibitors (SSRIs) Some can increase the amount of lofepramine in the body, causing stronger adverse effects.

SPECIAL PRECAUTIONS

Be sure to tell your doctor if:
- ◆ You have heart problems.
- ◆ You have had epileptic seizures.
- ◆ You have long-term liver or kidney problems.
- ◆ You have glaucoma.
- ◆ You have an overactive thyroid gland.
- ◆ You have prostate trouble.
- ◆ You have porphyria.
- ◆ You are taking other medicines.

Pregnancy Safety in pregnancy not established. Discuss with your doctor.
Breast-feeding Drug passes into breast milk and may affect baby. Discuss with your doctor.
Infants and children Not recommended.
Over 60 Reduced dose may be needed as older people are more sensitive to adverse reactions.
Driving and hazardous work Avoid such activities until you have learned how lofepramine affects you because the drug may cause blurred vision and reduced alertness.
Alcohol Avoid. Alcohol may increase the sedative effects of this drug.
Surgery and general anaesthetics Lofepramine may need to be stopped. Discuss with your doctor or dentist before you have any surgery.

PROLONGED USE

No problems expected.

LOPERAMIDE

Brand names Arret, Boots Diareze, Diocalm Ultra, Imodium
Used in the following combined preparations Diocalm Plus, Imodium Plus

QUICK REFERENCE

Drug group Antidiarrhoeal drug (p.42)
Overdose danger rating Medium
Dependence rating Low
Prescription needed No (most preparations)
Available as generic Yes

GENERAL INFORMATION

Loperamide is available as tablets, capsules, or liquid. It reduces the loss of water and salts from the bowel and slows bowel activity; these actions result in the passage of firmer bowel movements at less frequent intervals.

A fast-acting drug, loperamide is widely prescribed for both sudden and recurrent bouts of diarrhoea. However, it is not generally recommended for diarrhoea caused by infection or poisons because it may delay the expulsion of harmful substances from the bowel. It is often prescribed for people who have had a colostomy or an ileostomy, to reduce fluid loss from the stoma (outlet).

Adverse effects are rare. There is no risk of abuse, as there may be with the opium-based antidiarrhoeals, because loperamide is only minimally absorbed from the gut. It can be purchased over the counter in a pharmacy.

INFORMATION FOR USERS

Follow instructions on the label. Call your doctor if symptoms worsen.

How taken/used Tablets, capsules, liquid.

Frequency and timing of doses *Acute diarrhoea* Take a double dose at start of treatment, then a single dose after each loose bowel movement, up to the maximum daily dose. *Chronic diarrhoea* 2 x daily.

Adult dosage range *Acute diarrhoea* 4mg (starting dose), then 2mg after each loose bowel movement (12–16mg daily); usual dose 6–8mg daily. Use for up to 5 days only (3 days only for children 4–8 years), then consult your doctor. *Chronic diarrhoea* 4–8mg daily (up to 16mg daily).

Onset of effect Within 1–2 hours.

Duration of action 6–18 hours.

Diet advice Ensure adequate fluid, sugar, and salt intake during a diarrhoeal illness.

Storage Keep in original container at room temperature out of the reach of children.

Missed dose Do not take the missed dose. Take your next dose if needed.

Stopping the drug Can be safely stopped as soon as you no longer need it.

Exceeding the dose An occasional unintentional extra dose is unlikely to be a cause for concern. Large overdoses may cause constipation, vomiting, or drowsiness, and affect breathing. Notify your doctor.

POSSIBLE ADVERSE EFFECTS

Most adverse effects are rare with loperamide and some are difficult to distinguish from the effects of the diarrhoea it is used to treat. Headache is the most common effect; consult your doctor if it is severe. If symptoms such as bloating, abdominal pain, dry mouth, or fever persist or worsen during treatment, consult your doctor. If drowsiness, dizziness, or constipation occur, stop taking the drug. If you develop itching or a rash, consult your doctor; with a rash, you should also stop the drug.

INTERACTIONS

None.

SPECIAL PRECAUTIONS

Be sure to consult your doctor or pharmacist before taking this drug if:

- ◆ You have long-term liver or kidney problems.
- ◆ You have had recent abdominal surgery.
- ◆ You have an infection or blockage in the intestine, pseudomembranous colitis, or ulcerative colitis.
- ◆ You are taking other medicines.

Pregnancy Safety in pregnancy not established. Discuss with your doctor.

Breast-feeding Drug passes into breast milk and may affect baby. Discuss with your doctor.

Infants and children Not to be given to children under 4 years. Reduced dose necessary in older children. Children can be very sensitive to the effects of this drug so it should only be used in children under 12 on medical advice.

Over 60 No special problems.

Driving and hazardous work Avoid until you know how loperamide affects you because the drug can cause dizziness or drowsiness.

Alcohol No known problems.

PROLONGED USE

Although this drug is not usually taken for long periods (except by those with a medically diagnosed long-term gastrointestinal condition), special problems are not expected.

LOPINAVIR/RITONAVIR

Brand name Kaletra

Used in the following combined preparations None

QUICK REFERENCE

Drug group Drug for HIV and immune deficiency (p.98)

Overdose danger rating Medium

Dependence rating Low

Prescription needed Yes

Available as generic No

GENERAL INFORMATION

Lopinavir and ritonavir are both antiretroviral drugs from a class known as protease inhibitors. Combined as a single drug, they are used in treating HIV infection. They work by interfering with an enzyme used by the virus to produce genetic material (see p.100).

The combination is prescribed with other antiretrovirals, usually two nucleoside analogues, which together slow the production of HIV. The aim of this combination therapy is to reduce the damage done to the immune system by the virus. However, combination antiretroviral therapy is not a cure for HIV. Taken regularly on a long-term basis, it can reduce the level of the virus in the body and improve the outlook for a person with HIV, but the person will remain infectious and will have a relapse if the treatment is stopped.

INFORMATION FOR USERS

Your drug prescription is tailored for you. Do not alter dosage without checking with your doctor.

How taken/used Tablets, oral liquid.

Frequency and timing of doses Every 12 hours, with food.

Adult dosage range 400mg lopinavir with 100mg ritonavir 2 x daily; alternatively 800/200mg 1 x daily (tablets); 5ml (400mg lopinavir with 100mg ritonavir) 2 x daily (liquid).

Onset of effect Within 1 hour.

Duration of action 12 hours.

Diet advice None.

Storage Keep in original container at room temperature (tablets), or refrigerator (liquid) out of the reach of children.

Missed dose Take as soon as you remember. If next dose is due within 2 hours, take a single dose now and skip the next. It is very important not to miss doses regularly as this can lead to the development of drug-resistant HIV.

Stopping the drug Do not stop taking the drug without consulting your doctor.

Exceeding the dose An occasional unintentional extra dose is unlikely to cause problems. But if you notice any unusual symptoms, or if a large overdose has been taken, notify your doctor.

POSSIBLE ADVERSE EFFECTS

Gastrointestinal symptoms (nausea, vomiting, diarrhoea, and loss of appetite) and fatigue are the most common effects; discuss with your doctor if severe. In addition, discuss any changes in body shape, which are more likely to occur with long-term use. If severe abdominal pain occurs, seek prompt medical help.

INTERACTIONS

General note A wide range of drugs may interact with lopinavir and ritonavir, causing either an increase in adverse effects or a reduction in beneficial effects. Check with your doctor or pharmacist before taking new drugs, including those from the dentist and supermarket, and herbal medicines. Ritonavir is known to interact with some recreational drugs, including ecstasy, so you must discuss the use of such drugs with your doctor or pharmacist.

SPECIAL PRECAUTIONS

Be sure to tell your doctor if:

- You have long-term liver or kidney problems.
- You have heart problems.
- You take recreational drugs.
- You have acute porphyria.
- You have haemophilia.
- You are taking other medicines.

Pregnancy Tablets can be used during pregnancy if clinically needed. The oral solution is not recommended. Discuss with your doctor.

Breast-feeding Safety not established. Breast-feeding is not recommended for HIV-positive mothers as virus may be passed to the baby.

Infants and children Not recommended in children under 2 years. Reduced dose recommended in children over 2 years.

Over 60 Reduced dose may be necessary to minimize adverse effects.

Driving and hazardous work No known problems.

Alcohol The liquid form contains a small amount of alcohol, so care should be taken with alcohol consumption.

PROLONGED USE

Changes in body shape may occur, including redistribution of body fat from the arms and/ or legs to the abdomen and back of the neck.

Monitoring Your doctor will take regular blood samples to check the drugs' effect on the virus. Blood will also be tested for changes in lipids, liver function, cholesterol, and sugar levels.

LORATADINE/ DESLORATADINE

Brand names [loratadine] Boots Hayfever and Allergy Relief All Day, Clarityn, Clarityn Allergy; [desloratadine] NeoClarityn

Used in the following combined preparations None

QUICK REFERENCE

Drug group Antihistamine (p.56)

Overdose danger rating Low

Dependence rating Low

Prescription needed No (loratadine); Yes (desloratadine)

Available as generic Yes

GENERAL INFORMATION

Loratadine, a long-acting antihistamine, is used to relieve symptoms of allergic rhinitis, such as sneezing, nasal discharge, and itching and burning of the eyes. Symptoms are normally relieved within an hour of oral administration. The drug is also used to treat allergic skin conditions such as chronic urticaria (hives). An advantage of loratadine over older antihistamines, such as chlorphenamine, is that it has fewer sedative and anticholinergic effects, so it is less likely to cause drowsiness.

Desloratadine is the active breakdown product of loratadine. It is available as a separate product (NeoClarityn) but offers no advantages over loratadine itself.

Loratadine and desloratadine should be discontinued about 4 days prior to skin testing for allergy as they may decrease or prevent the detection of positive results.

INFORMATION FOR USERS

Follow instructions on the label. Call your doctor if symptoms worsen.

How taken/used Tablets, liquid.
Frequency and timing of doses Once daily.
Adult dosage range 10mg daily (loratadine); 5mg daily (desloratadine).
Onset of effect Usually within 1 hour.
Duration of action Up to 24 hours.
Diet advice None.
Storage Keep in original container at room temperature out of the reach of children.
Missed dose Take as soon as you remember. If your next dose is due within 6 hours, take a single dose now and skip the next.
Stopping the drug Can be safely stopped as soon as you no longer need it.
Exceeding the dose An occasional unintentional extra dose is unlikely to be a cause for concern. But if you notice any unusual symptoms, or if a large overdose has been taken, tell your doctor.

POSSIBLE ADVERSE EFFECTS

Adverse effects are rare. They include fatigue, drowsiness, nausea, headache, dry mouth, palpitations, and fainting. If either of the last two occur, consult your doctor.

INTERACTIONS

Cimetidine, clarithromycin, erythromycin, ketoconazole, fluoxetine, fluconazole, quinidine, and fosamprenavir These drugs may increase the blood levels and effects of loratadine and desloratadine, but this has not been found to cause problems.

SPECIAL PRECAUTIONS

Be sure to consult your doctor or pharmacist before taking this drug if:

- ◆ You have liver disease.
- ◆ You are taking other medicines.

Pregnancy Safety in pregnancy not established. Discuss with your doctor.
Breast-feeding Safety not established. The drug passes into breast milk. Discuss with doctor.
Infants and children Not recommended under 2 years (loratadine). Not recommended under 1 year (desloratadine).
Over 60 No problems expected.
Driving and hazardous work Problems are unlikely, but be aware of how the drug affects you before driving or doing hazardous work.
Alcohol Alcohol will increase any sedative effects of loratadine/desloratadine.

PROLONGED USE

No problems expected.

LOSARTAN

Brand name Cozaar
Used in the following combined preparation
Cozaar-Comp

QUICK REFERENCE

Drug group Vasodilator (p.30) and antihypertensive drug (p.34)
Overdose danger rating Medium
Dependence rating Low
Prescription needed Yes
Available as generic Yes

GENERAL INFORMATION

Losartan belongs to a group of vasodilator drugs called angiotensin II blockers. Used to treat hypertension (high blood pressure), it works by blocking the action of angiotensin II, a naturally occurring substance that constricts blood vessels. This action causes the blood vessel walls to relax, so easing blood pressure. Losartan may also be used to treat heart failure and for kidney disease associated with diabetes and hypertension.

Unlike ACE inhibitors, losartan does not cause a persistent dry cough. Adverse effects, which include diarrhoea, dizziness, and headache, do not commonly occur.

INFORMATION FOR USERS

Your drug prescription is tailored for you. Do not alter dosage without checking with your doctor.

How taken/used Tablets, liquid.

Frequency and timing of doses Once daily.

Adult dosage range 50–100mg. People over 75 years, and other groups that are especially sensitive to the effects of the drug, may start on a dose of 25mg.

Onset of effect *Blood pressure* 1–2 weeks, with maximum effect in 3–6 weeks from start of treatment. *Other conditions* Within 1 hour.

Duration of action 12–24 hours.

Diet advice None.

Storage Keep in original container at room temperature out of the reach of children.

Missed dose Take as soon as you remember. If your next dose is due within 8 hours, take a single dose now and skip the next.

Stopping the drug Do not stop without consulting your doctor. Stopping the drug may lead to worsening of the underlying condition.

Exceeding the dose An occasional unintentional extra dose is unlikely to cause problems. Large overdoses may cause dizziness and fainting. Notify your doctor.

POSSIBLE ADVERSE EFFECTS

Side effects are usually mild. The most common are dizziness, headache, and diarrhoea; discuss with your doctor if these are severe. Consult your doctor if you have a cough or muscle, joint, or back pain. If you have wheezing or swelling of the lips or tongue, stop the drug and contact your doctor immediately.

INTERACTIONS

Vasodilators, diuretics, and other antihypertensives These drugs may increase the blood-pressure-lowering effect of losartan.

Potassium supplements, potassium-sparing diuretics, and ciclosporin Losartan increases the effect of these drugs, leading to raised levels of potassium in the blood.

Lithium Losartan may increase the levels and toxicity of lithium.

Non-steroidal anti-inflammatory drugs (NSAIDs) Some may reduce the blood-pressure-lowering effect of losartan and may also increase the risk of kidney problems if used with losartan.

Fluconazole and rifampicin These drugs may significantly reduce the blood level of the active form of losartan.

SPECIAL PRECAUTIONS

Be sure to tell your doctor if:

- You have stenosis of the kidney arteries.
- You have liver or kidney problems.
- You have experienced angioedema.
- You have galactose intolerance.
- You are taking other medicines.

Pregnancy Not prescribed. There is evidence of harm to the developing fetus.

Breast-feeding Not prescribed. Safety in breast-feeding not established.

Infants and children Not prescribed. Safety not established.

Over 60 Reduced dose may be necessary for people over 75 years.

Driving and hazardous work Avoid until you have learned how losartan affects you because the drug can cause dizziness.

Alcohol Avoid. May increase blood-pressure-lowering and adverse effects of losartan.

PROLONGED USE

No special problems.

Monitoring Periodic checks on blood potassium levels and kidney function may be performed.

MAGNESIUM HYDROXIDE

Brand names Cream of Magnesia, Milk of Magnesia

Used in the following combined preparations Carbellon, Maalox, Milpar, Mucogel, and others

QUICK REFERENCE

Drug group Antacid (p.40) and laxative (p.43)

Overdose danger rating Low

Dependence rating Low

Prescription needed No

Available as generic Yes

GENERAL INFORMATION

Magnesium hydroxide is a fast-acting antacid given to neutralize stomach acid. The drug is available in numerous over-the-counter preparations for the treatment of indigestion and heartburn. It also prevents pain caused by stomach and duodenal ulcers, gastritis, and reflux oesophagitis, although other drugs are normally used for these problems nowadays. In addition, it is used as a laxative; it works by drawing salt and water from the wall of the bowel to soften the faeces.

Magnesium hydroxide is not often used alone as an antacid because of its laxative effect. However, this effect is countered when it is used in combination with aluminium hydroxide, which can cause constipation.

INFORMATION FOR USERS

Follow instructions on the label. Call your doctor if symptoms worsen.

How taken/used Tablets, liquid, powder.

Frequency and timing of doses *Antacid* 1–4 x daily as needed with water, preferably 1 hour after food and at bedtime. *Laxative* Once daily, at bedtime.

Adult dosage range *Antacid* 1–2g per dose (tablets); 5–10ml per dose (liquid). *Laxative* 30-45ml per dose (liquid).

Onset of effect *Antacid* within 15 minutes. *Laxative* 2–8 hours.

Duration of action 2–4 hours.

Diet advice None.

Storage Keep in original container at room temperature out of the reach of children.

Missed dose Take as soon as you remember.

Stopping the drug When used as an antacid, the drug can be safely stopped as soon as you no longer need it. When given as ulcer treatment, follow your doctor's advice.

Exceeding the dose An occasional unintentional extra dose is unlikely to be a cause for concern. But if you notice any unusual symptoms, or if a large overdose has been taken, tell your doctor.

POSSIBLE ADVERSE EFFECTS

Diarrhoea is the only common adverse effect of magnesium hydroxide. Dizziness and muscle weakness due to the body's absorption of excess magnesium may occur in people with poor kidney function (see Prolonged use).

INTERACTIONS

General note Magnesium hydroxide interferes with absorption of a wide range of drugs taken by mouth, including tetracycline antibiotics, iron supplements, diflunisal, phenytoin, gabapentin, and penicillamine. Allow 1–2 hours between taking it and taking other drugs.

Enteric-coated tablets As with other antacids, magnesium hydroxide may allow break-up of the enteric coating of tablets, sometimes leading to stomach irritation.

SPECIAL PRECAUTIONS

Be sure to consult your doctor or pharmacist before taking this drug if:

- You have a long-term kidney problem.
- You have liver problems.
- You have a bowel disorder.
- You are taking other medicines.

Pregnancy No evidence of risk, but discuss the most appropriate treatment with your doctor.

Breast-feeding No evidence of risk, but discuss most appropriate treatment with your doctor.

Infants and children Not recommended under 3 years except on the advice of a doctor. Reduced dose necessary for older children.

Over 60 No special problems.

Driving and hazardous work No known problems.

Alcohol Avoid excessive alcohol as it irritates the stomach and may reduce the benefits of the drug.

PROLONGED USE

Magnesium hydroxide is for occasional use and should not be taken for prolonged periods without consulting your doctor, especially if you experience persistent abdominal pain while taking the drug. If you are over 40 years of age and are experiencing long-term indigestion or heartburn, your doctor will probably refer you to a specialist. Prolonged use in people with kidney damage may cause drowsiness, dizziness, and weakness, resulting from accumulation of magnesium in the body.

MALATHION

Brand names Derbac-M

Used in the following combined preparations None

QUICK REFERENCE

Drug group Drug to treat skin parasites (p.120)

Overdose danger rating Low (medium if swallowed)

Dependence rating Low

Prescription needed No

Available as generic No

GENERAL INFORMATION

Malathion is an organophosphate insecticide used to treat lice and mite infestations. It kills parasites by interfering with their nervous system function, causing paralysis and death.

Malathion is applied topically as a shampoo, liquid, or lotion. The lotion is more convenient to use than shampoo, requiring only a single application. It is also more effective because shampoo is diluted in use. Lotions with a high alcohol content are unsuitable for small children or people with asthma, who may be affected by the solvent, or for treating crab lice in the genital area, but the water-based liquid is suitable. Care should be taken to avoid contact of the drug with the eyes or with broken skin.

If resistance occurs during a course of treatment, your practitioner will recommend an alternative insecticide such as permethrin. Malathion will not prevent infestation.

INFORMATION FOR USERS

Follow instructions on the label. Call your doctor if symptoms worsen.

How taken/used Topical liquid, lotion, shampoo.

Frequency and timing of doses *Scabies* 2 doses, 7 days apart (lotion or topical liquid). *Lice* 3 applications 3 days apart (shampoo); 2 doses, 7 days apart (lotion or topical liquid).

Adult dosage range As directed. Family members and close contacts should also be treated.

Onset of effect *Lotion or topical liquid* Leave on for 12 hours (lice), or 24 hours (scabies), before washing off. For treatment of scabies, if hands are washed with soap within 24 hours of an application, another dose should be applied. *Shampoo* Leave on for 5 minutes, rinse off, repeat, then use a fine-toothed comb.

Duration of action Until washed off.

Diet advice None.

Storage Keep in original container at room temperature out of the reach of children. Protect from light.

Missed dose When a repeat application of the shampoo has been missed, it should be carried out as soon as is practicable.

Stopping the drug Malathion should be administered as a single application or as a short course of treatment.

Exceeding the dose An extra application is unlikely to cause problems. Take emergency action if the insecticide has been swallowed.

POSSIBLE ADVERSE EFFECTS

Used correctly, malathion preparations are unlikely to produce adverse effects, although the alcoholic fumes given off by some lotions may cause wheezing in people with asthma. Rarely, malathion may cause skin irritation; consult your doctor if this is severe.

INTERACTIONS

None.

SPECIAL PRECAUTIONS

Be sure to consult your doctor or pharmacist before taking this drug if:

◆ You have severe asthma or eczema.

Pregnancy No evidence of risk. It is unlikely that enough malathion would be absorbed after occasional application to affect the fetus.

Breast-feeding No evidence of risk. It is unlikely that enough malathion would be absorbed after occasional application to affect the baby.

Infants and children No special problems, but seek medical advice for infants under 6 months.

Over 60 No special problems.

Driving and hazardous work No special problems.

Alcohol No special problems.

PROLONGED USE

Malathion is intended for intermittent use only. The lotions should not be used more than once a week for 3 weeks at a time. If there is a need to use malathion more frequently, it is possible that resistance has built up; seek your doctor's advice.

MEBENDAZOLE

Brand names Boots Threadworm Tablets, Ovex, Vermox

Used in the following combined preparations None

QUICK REFERENCE

Drug group Anthelmintic drug (p.76)

Overdose danger rating Low

Dependence rating Low

Prescription needed No (threadworm infection); Yes (other worm infections)

Available as generic Yes

GENERAL INFORMATION

Mebendazole is used to treat various intestinal worm infestations, including threadworms, roundworms, hookworms, and whipworms. Only threadworm infection is common in the UK, but the others can be acquired during travel to countries with poor sanitation. The drug works by paralysing the worms, which are then passed out in the faeces. However, mebendazole does not kill threadworm eggs, which are deposited on the skin around the anus by adult worms, and reinfection may occur by transfer of the eggs from the anus to the mouth. To prevent reinfection, the drug must be combined with hygiene measures (see below), and all members of the family should be treated at the same time.

INFORMATION FOR USERS

Follow instructions on the label and follow hygiene measures for at least 6 weeks. Call your doctor if symptoms do not improve in a few days or if treatment is unsuccessful.

How taken/used Tablets, oral suspension.

Hygiene measures To prevent threadworm reinfection, wash the hands thoroughly and scrub the nails frequently, especially after going to the toilet and before eating; keep the nails short; avoid biting the nails and sucking the fingers; wash bed linen and towels to kill the eggs; do not share towels, flannels, or sponges; bathe or shower every morning; change underwear every morning; regularly vacuum and clean the house to remove any infective eggs. Oro-anal contact during sex can also cause infection or reinfection and should therefore be avoided.

Frequency and timing of doses *Threadworm* Single dose; can be repeated after 2 weeks if reinfection occurs. *Other worms* 2 x daily for 3 days.

Adult dosage range *Threadworm* 100mg. *Other worms* 200mg daily.

Onset of effect Within a few hours.

Duration of action 12–24 hours.

Diet advice None.

Storage Keep in original container at room temperature out of the reach of children.

Missed dose *Threadworm* Take as soon as you remember. *Other worms* Take as soon as you remember, but no more than 2 tablets or 10ml of liquid in 24 hours.

Stopping the drug *Threadworm* The drug is taken as a single dose, repeated only if necessary. It can safely be stopped when no longer needed. *Other worms* The 3-day course should be completed to ensure effective eradication.

Exceeding the dose A larger than recommended dose is unlikely to cause harm. A very large dose may cause dizziness, abdominal discomfort, or diarrhoea in adults. In infants, it may cause seizures. Notify your doctor.

POSSIBLE ADVERSE EFFECTS

The most common adverse effects are gastrointestinal symptoms, such as abdominal pain and diarrhoea, and these are most likely to occur when there is a high level of worm infestation. If these adverse effects are severe, consult a doctor. Rarely, seizures or a rash may occur; if this happens, stop taking the drug and seek prompt medical help.

INTERACTIONS

Cimetidine may increase the blood level of mebendazole and should be avoided.

Metronidazole may increase the risk of serious skin rashes when used with mebendazole. The two drugs should not be used together.

SPECIAL PRECAUTIONS

Be sure to consult your doctor or pharmacist before taking this drug if:

- You have fructose intolerance.

Pregnancy Safety in pregnancy not established. Discuss with your doctor.

Breast-feeding It is not known if the drug passes into the breast milk, so breast-feeding is not recommended. Discuss with your doctor.

Infants and children Not recommended under 2 years.

Over 60 No special problems.

Driving and hazardous work No special problems.

Alcohol No special problems.

PROLONGED USE

Mebendazole is not used long term.

MEBEVERINE

Brand names Aurobeverine, Boots IBS Relief, Colofac, Colofac IBS, Colofac MR

Used in the following combined preparation Fybogel Mebeverine

QUICK REFERENCE

Drug group Drug for irritable bowel syndrome (p.43)

Overdose danger rating Low

Dependence rating Low

Prescription needed No (some preparations)

Available as generic Yes

GENERAL INFORMATION

Mebeverine is an antispasmodic drug used to relieve painful spasms of the intestine (colic), such as those resulting from irritable bowel syndrome and diverticular disease. The drug has a direct relaxing effect on the muscle in the bowel wall, and may also have an anticholinergic action (p.7), which reduces the transmission of nerve signals to the smooth muscle of the bowel wall and thereby prevents spasm. It does not have serious side effects.

As well as being available on its own, mebeverine is also produced in a combined form with ispaghula husk to provide roughage in an easily assimilable formulation. Both mebeverine on its own and the combined form are commonly used to help control the symptoms of irritable bowel syndrome.

INFORMATION FOR USERS

Follow instructions on the label. Call your doctor if symptoms worsen.

How taken/used Tablets, slow release (SR) capsules, liquid, granules.

Frequency and timing of doses 2–3 x daily, 20 minutes before meals. Combined preparations that contain ispaghula should not be taken immediately before going to bed.

Adult dosage range 300–450mg daily.

Onset of effect 30–60 minutes.

Duration of action 6–8 hours.

Diet advice Combined preparations containing ispaghula should be taken with plenty of water.

Storage Keep in original container at room temperature out of the reach of children. Protect from light.

Missed dose Take as soon as you remember, then return to your normal dosing schedule.

Stopping the drug The drug can be stopped as soon as you no longer need it.

Exceeding the dose An occasional unintentional extra dose is unlikely to be a cause for concern. Larger overdoses will probably cause constipation, and may cause central nervous system excitability.

POSSIBLE ADVERSE EFFECTS

Mebeverine rarely produces side effects. Occasionally, it may cause constipation; consult your doctor if this is severe. If you develop a rash or swelling of the lips, stop taking the drug and contact your doctor promptly.

INTERACTIONS

None.

SPECIAL PRECAUTIONS

Be sure to consult your doctor or pharmacist before taking this drug if:

- You have cystic fibrosis.
- You have porphyria.

Pregnancy Safety in pregnancy not established. Discuss with your doctor.

Breast-feeding Safety in breast-feeding not established. Discuss with your doctor.

Infants and children Not used in infants and children under 18 years.

Over 60 No special problems.

Driving and hazardous work No special problems with this drug.

Alcohol No special problems.

PROLONGED USE

No problems expected.

MEDROXYPROGESTERONE

Brand names Climanor, Depo-Provera, Provera, Syana

Used in the following combined preparations Indivina, Premique, Tridestra

QUICK REFERENCE

Drug group Female sex hormone (p.86)

Overdose danger rating Low

Dependence rating Low

Prescription needed Yes

Available as generic No

GENERAL INFORMATION

Medroxyprogesterone is a progestogen, a synthetic female sex hormone similar to the natural hormone progesterone. This drug is used as part of hormone replacement therapy (HRT; p.87) for women who have a uterus and need progesterone in addition to their long-term oestrogen. It is often used to treat endometriosis, in which there is abnormal growth of the uterine-lining tissue in the pelvic cavity. It may also be used to treat certain menstrual disorders, such as secondary amenorrhoea and abnormal bleeding. Depot injections of the drug are used as a contraceptive; however, since they may cause serious side effects, such as persistent uterine bleeding, amenorrhoea, and prolonged infertility, their use is controversial, and they are recommended only under special circumstances. In addition, the drug may be used to treat some types of cancer, such as cancer of the breast, uterus, or kidney.

INFORMATION FOR USERS

Your drug prescription is tailored for you. Do not alter dosage without checking with your doctor.

How taken/used Tablets, injection.

Frequency and timing of doses 1–3 x daily with plenty of water (by mouth); tablets may need to be taken at certain times during your menstrual cycle; follow the instructions you have been given. Every 3 months (depot injection and intramuscular injection).

Adult dosage range *Menstrual disorders* 2.5–10mg daily. *Endometriosis* 30mg daily. *Cancer* 100–1,500mg daily. *Contraception* 150mg 12-weekly injection.

Onset of effect 1–2 months (cancer); 1–2 weeks (other conditions).

Duration of action 1–2 days (by mouth); up to some months (depot injection).

Diet advice None.

Storage Keep in original container at room temperature out of the reach of children.

Missed dose Take as soon as you remember. If your next dose is due within 3 hours, take a single dose now and skip the next.

Stopping the drug Do not stop the drug without consulting your doctor; symptoms may recur.

Exceeding the dose An occasional unintentional extra dose is unlikely to be a cause for concern. But if you notice any unusual symptoms, or if a large overdose has been taken, tell your doctor.

POSSIBLE ADVERSE EFFECTS

Medroxyprogesterone rarely causes serious adverse effects. Fluid retention may lead to weight gain, swollen ankles or feet, and breast tenderness. Consult your doctor if these are severe, if you have severe nausea or headache, or if you have fatigue, depression, altered sleep, or irregular menstruation. If you develop a rash, itching, acne, or jaundice, stop taking the drug and contact your doctor promptly.

INTERACTIONS

Ciclosporin The effects of this drug may be increased by medroxyprogesterone.

Anticoagulants Medroxyprogesterone may reduce the effects of these drugs.

Rifamycin antibiotics, St John's wort, anticonvulsants, griseofulvin, terbinafine, barbiturates may reduce the effects of medroxyprogesterone.

SPECIAL PRECAUTIONS

Be sure to tell your doctor if:

- You have high blood pressure.
- You have had venous thrombosis, a heart attack, or a stroke.
- You have long-term liver or kidney problems.
- You have porphyria.
- You have epilepsy or a history of depression.
- You have breast cancer.
- You have a history of gallstones, migraines, or lupus.
- You have a history of osteoporosis.
- You are taking other medicines.

Pregnancy Not prescribed. May cause defects in the fetus. Discuss with your doctor.

Breast-feeding The drug passes into the breast milk, but normal doses are unlikely to affect the baby adversely. Discuss with your doctor.

Infants and children Not usually prescribed.

Over 60 No special problems.

Driving and hazardous work No known problems.

Alcohol No known problems.

PROLONGED USE

Long-term use may slightly increase the risk of venous thrombosis in the legs, and of osteoporosis and bone fractures. Bone loss is greatest in the first 2–3 years, then stabilizes. Adequate calcium and vitamin D intake should be ensured throughout treatment. Irregular menstrual bleeding or spotting between periods may also occur.

Monitoring Periodic checks on blood pressure, yearly cervical smear tests, and breast examinations are usually required. Bone density and lipids may also be monitored.

MEFENAMIC ACID

Brand name Ponstan, Ponstan Forte

Used in the following combined preparations None

QUICK REFERENCE

Drug group Non-steroidal anti-inflammatory drug (p.48)

Overdose danger rating Medium

Dependence rating Low

Prescription needed Yes

Available as generic Yes

GENERAL INFORMATION

Like other non-steroidal anti-inflammatory drugs (NSAIDs), mefenamic acid relieves pain and inflammation. The drug is an effective painkiller and is used to treat headache, toothache, and menstrual pains (dysmenorrhoea), as well as to reduce excessive menstrual bleeding (menorrhagia). It is also prescribed for long-term relief of pain and stiffness in rheumatoid arthritis and osteoarthritis.

The most common side effects of mefenamic acid are gastrointestinal: abdominal pain, nausea and vomiting, and indigestion. Other, more serious effects include kidney problems and blood disorders.

INFORMATION FOR USERS

Your drug prescription is tailored for you. Do not alter dosage without checking with your doctor.

How taken/used Tablets, capsules, liquid.

Frequency and timing of doses 3 x daily with or after food.

Adult dosage range 1,500mg daily.

Onset of effect 1–2 hours.

Duration of action Up to 8 hours.

Diet advice None.

Storage Keep in original container at room temperature out of the reach of children.

Missed dose Take as soon as you remember. If your next dose is due within 2 hours, take a single dose now and skip the next.

Stopping the drug Can be safely stopped as soon as you no longer need it.

Exceeding the dose An occasional unintentional extra dose is unlikely to be a cause for concern. Large overdoses may cause poor coordination, muscle twitching, or seizures. Notify your doctor.

POSSIBLE ADVERSE EFFECTS

Gastrointestinal disturbances, such as indigestion and diarrhoea, are the most common side effects of mefenamic acid. If diarrhoea or a rash occur, the drug should be stopped and not used again; discuss with your doctor. Other side effects include dizziness, drowsiness, nausea, and vomiting; discuss with your doctor if these are severe or if abdominal pain occurs. If you experience wheezing, breathlessness, or black or bloodstained faeces, you should stop taking the drug and contact your doctor without delay.

Long-term use of mefenamic acid carries an increased risk of certain serious disorders (see Prolonged use).

INTERACTIONS

General note Mefenamic acid interacts with a wide range of drugs to increase the risk of bleeding and/or peptic ulcers. These medications include other non-steroidal anti-inflammatory drugs (NSAIDs) such as aspirin, as well as oral anticoagulant drugs, such as warfarin; certain antidepressant drugs; and corticosteroids.

Lithium, digoxin, phenytoin, and methotrexate Mefenamic acid may raise blood levels of these drugs to an undesirable extent.

Antihypertensive drugs and diuretics The beneficial effects of these drugs may be reduced by mefenamic acid.

Oral antidiabetic drugs Mefenamic acid may increase the blood-sugar-lowering effect of these drugs.

Ciprofloxacin The risk of seizures with this drug and related antibiotics may be increased by mefenamic acid.

SPECIAL PRECAUTIONS

Be sure to tell your doctor if:

- You have liver or kidney problems.
- You have had a peptic ulcer, oesophagitis, or acid indigestion.
- You have inflammatory bowel disease.
- You have asthma.
- You have high blood pressure.
- You are allergic to aspirin.
- You have any heart problems.
- You are taking other medicines.

Pregnancy Not usually prescribed. May cause defects in the unborn baby and, taken in late pregnancy, may affect the baby's cardiovascular system. Discuss with your doctor.

Breast-feeding Not recommended. The drug passes into the breast milk. Discuss with your doctor.

Infants and children Reduced dose necessary.

Over 60 Increased likelihood of adverse effects.

Driving and hazardous work Avoid such activities until you have learned how mefenamic acid affects you because the drug can cause drowsiness and dizziness.

Alcohol Avoid. Alcohol may increase the risk of stomach irritation with mefenamic acid.

Surgery and general anaesthetics The drug may prolong bleeding. Discuss with your doctor or dentist before any surgery.

PROLONGED USE

There is an increased risk of bleeding from peptic ulcers and in the bowel with prolonged use of mefenamic acid. There is also a small risk of a heart attack or stroke. To minimize these risks, the lowest effective dose is given for the shortest duration.

MEFLOQUINE

Brand name Lariam
Used in the following combined preparations None

QUICK REFERENCE

Drug group Antimalarial drug (p.73)
Overdose danger rating High
Dependence rating Low
Prescription needed Yes
Available as generic No

GENERAL INFORMATION

Mefloquine is used to prevent or treat malaria. It is principally recommended for use in areas where malaria is resistant to other drugs. However, its use is limited by the fact that it can, in some patients, cause serious adverse effects such as depression, suicidal tendencies, anxiety, panic, confusion, hallucinations, paranoid delusions, and seizures.

As with all antimalarials, the use of mosquito repellents and a mosquito net at night are as important in preventing malaria as taking the drug itself.

INFORMATION FOR USERS

Your drug prescription is tailored for you. Do not alter dosage without checking with your doctor.
How taken/used Tablets.
Frequency and timing of doses *Prevention* Once weekly, starting 2–3 weeks before entering endemic area, and continuing until 4 weeks after leaving. *Treatment* Up to 3 x daily every 6–8 hours, after food and with plenty of water.
Adult dosage range *Prevention* 187.5–250mg once weekly. *Treatment* 20–25mg/kg body weight up to a maximum dose of 1.5g.
Onset of effect 2–3 days.
Duration of action Over 1 week. Low levels of the drug and any adverse effects may persist for several months.
Diet advice None.
Storage Keep in original container at room temperature out of the reach of children.
Missed dose Take as soon as you remember. If next dose is due within 48 hours (if taken once weekly for prevention), take a single dose now and skip the next. If you vomit within 30 minutes of taking a dose, take another.
Stopping the drug If you feel it necessary to stop, consult your doctor about alternative treatment before the next dose is due.

OVERDOSE ACTION

Seek immediate medical advice in all cases. Take emergency action if collapse or loss of consciousness occurs.

POSSIBLE ADVERSE EFFECTS

Dizziness, vertigo, nausea, vomiting, headache, and abdominal pain are common adverse effects of mefloquine; discuss with your doctor if these are severe. Rarely, serious adverse effects on the nervous system can occur, including anxiety or panic attacks, depression, hallucinations, and paranoid delusions. if any of these occur, or if you develop hearing problems or palpitations, stop taking the drug and consult your doctor promptly.

INTERACTIONS

General note Mefloquine may increase the effects on the heart of drugs such as beta blockers, calcium channel blockers, and digitalis drugs. It may also affect live-vaccine immunization, which should be completed at least 3 days before the first dose of mefloquine.
Anticonvulsant drugs Mefloquine may decrease the effect of these drugs.
Other antimalarial drugs Mefloquine may increase the risk of adverse effects when taken with these drugs.

SPECIAL PRECAUTIONS

Be sure to tell your doctor if:
- You have long-term liver or kidney problems.
- You have had epileptic seizures.
- You have had depression or any other psychiatric illness.
- You have had a previous allergic reaction to mefloquine or quinine.
- You have heart problems.
- You are taking other medicines.

Pregnancy Not usually prescribed. If unavoidable, the drug is given only after the first trimester. Pregnancy must be avoided during and for 3 months after mefloquine use.
Breast-feeding Not prescribed. The drug passes into the breast milk.
Infants and children Not used under 3 months. Reduced dose necessary in older children.
Over 60 Careful monitoring is necessary in people with liver or kidney problems or with heart disease.
Driving and hazardous work Avoid when taking mefloquine for prevention until you know

how the drug affects you. Also avoid during treatment and for 3 weeks afterwards as the drug can cause dizziness or disturb balance.
Alcohol Keep consumption low.

PROLONGED USE

May be taken for prevention of malaria for up to 1 year.

MERCAPTOPURINE

Brand names Hanixol, Puri-Nethol, Xaluprine
Used in the following combined preparations None

QUICK REFERENCE

Drug group Anticancer drug (p.94)
Overdose danger rating Medium
Dependence rating Low
Prescription needed Yes
Available as generic Yes

GENERAL INFORMATION

Mercaptopurine is an anticancer drug that is widely used in the treatment of certain forms of leukaemia. It is usually given in combination with other anticancer drugs.

Nausea and vomiting, mouth ulcers, and loss of appetite are the most common side effects. Such symptoms tend to be milder than those from other cytotoxic drugs, and often disappear as the body adjusts to the drug.

More seriously, mercaptopurine can interfere with blood cell production, resulting in blood clotting disorders and anaemia, and can cause liver damage. The frequency and severity of infections is also increased.

INFORMATION FOR USERS

Your drug prescription is tailored for you. Do not alter dosage without checking with your doctor.
How taken/used Tablets.
Frequency and timing of doses Once daily.
Dosage range Dosage is determined individually according to body weight and response.
Onset of effect 1–2 weeks.
Duration of action Side effects may persist for several weeks after stopping treatment.
Diet advice The drug can be taken with food or on an empty stomach, but this should be kept consistent each day. Dairy products should be avoided from at least 2 hours before taking the tablets to 1 hour afterwards.
Storage Keep in original container at room temperature out of the reach of children. Protect from light.
Missed dose If your next dose is due within 6 hours, take a single dose now and skip the next. Tell your doctor that you missed a dose.
Stopping the drug Do not stop without consulting your doctor; stopping the drug may lead to worsening of your underlying condition.
Exceeding the dose An occasional unintentional extra dose is unlikely to cause problems. Large overdoses may cause nausea and vomiting. Notify your doctor.

POSSIBLE ADVERSE EFFECTS

The most common adverse effects are nausea, vomiting, and loss of appetite; consult your doctor if these are severe or if you have severe abdominal pain. If you have mouth ulcers, call your doctor; if you have easy bruising or bleeding, sore throat, fever, or jaundice, stop the drug and consult your doctor promptly. Because mercaptopurine interferes with the production of blood cells, it may cause anaemia and blood clotting disorders; in addition, infections are more likely.

INTERACTIONS

Allopurinol This drug increases blood levels of mercaptopurine, and the dosages of both drugs should be adjusted.
Warfarin The effects of warfarin may be decreased by mercaptopurine.
Febuxostat This drug should not be used with mercaptopurine; the combination may lead to reduced levels of white blood cells.
Methotrexate This drug increases blood levels of mercaptopurine. Reduced dose of mercaptopurine may be needed.
Ribavirin Increased risk of drug toxicity when ribavirin is used with mercaptopurine. The two drugs should not be used together.
Co-trimoxazole, trimethoprim, mesalazine, olsalazine, and sulfasalazine These drugs increase the risk of blood problems with mercaptopurine.
Vaccines Mercaptopurine may affect your body's response to live vaccines. Discuss with your doctor before having a vaccine.

SPECIAL PRECAUTIONS

Be sure to tell your doctor if:
- You have long-term liver or kidney problems.
- You have gout.

◆ You have recently had any infection.
◆ You are taking other medicines.

Pregnancy Not usually prescribed. Discuss with your doctor.

Breast-feeding Not advised. The drug passes into the breast milk and may affect the baby adversely. Discuss with your doctor.

Infants and children No special problems.

Over 60 Reduced dose may be necessary. Increased risk of adverse effects.

Driving and hazardous work No known problems.

Alcohol Avoid. Alcohol may increase the adverse effects of this drug.

PROLONGED USE

Long-term use of mercaptopurine may reduce bone marrow activity, leading to a reduction of all types of blood cell. Some people have a genetic susceptibility to this effect. There is also a small increase in the risk of developing certain cancers, such as skin cancer, sarcoma, and lymphoma.

Monitoring Regular blood checks, including tests on liver function, are required.

MESALAZINE

Brand names Asacol, Mesren MR, Mezavant XL, Octasa, Pentasa, Salofalk, Zintasa

Used in the following combined preparations None

QUICK REFERENCE

Drug group Drug for inflammatory bowel disease (p.44)

Overdose danger rating Low

Dependence rating Low

Prescription needed Yes

Available as generic Yes

GENERAL INFORMATION

Mesalazine is prescribed for ulcerative colitis and is sometimes used for Crohn's disease, which affects the ileum and large intestine. It is given to relieve symptoms in an acute attack and is also taken as a preventative measure. When used to treat severe cases, it is often taken with other drugs such as corticosteroids.

When the drug is taken as tablets, the active component is released in the large intestine, where its local effect relieves the inflamed mucosa. Always stick to the same brand of tablet. Enemas and suppositories are also available and are particularly useful when the disease affects the rectum and lower colon.

This drug produces fewer side effects than some older treatments, such as sulfasalazine. Patients unable to tolerate sulfasalazine may be able to take mesalazine with no problem. Anyone hypersensitive to salicylates, such as aspirin, should not take mesalazine.

INFORMATION FOR USERS

Your drug prescription is tailored for you. Do not alter dosage without checking with your doctor.

How taken/used Tablets, slow release (SR) tablets, granules, suppositories, enema (foam or liquid).

Frequency and timing of doses 3 x daily, swallowed whole and not chewed (tablets); 3 x daily (suppositories); once daily at bedtime (enema).

Adult dosage range 2.4–4.8g daily (acute attack); 1.2–2.4g daily (maintenance dose). Dose varies with brand used.

Onset of effect Adverse effects may be noticed within a few days, but full beneficial effects may not be felt for a couple of weeks.

Duration of action Up to 12 hours.

Diet advice Your doctor may advise you, taking account of the condition affecting you.

Storage Keep in original container at room temperature out of the reach of children. Protect from light. Keep aerosol container out of direct sunlight.

Missed dose Take as soon as you remember. If your next dose is due within 2 hours, take a single dose now and skip the next.

Stopping the drug Do not stop without consulting your doctor; symptoms may recur.

Exceeding the dose An occasional unintentional extra dose is unlikely to be a cause for concern. But if you notice any unusual symptoms, or if a large overdose has been taken, tell your doctor.

POSSIBLE ADVERSE EFFECTS

Gastrointestinal problems such as nausea, abdominal pain, and diarrhoea are common; discuss with your doctor if severe. If colitis worsens or you develop a rash, stop taking the drug and consult your doctor. If fever, wheezing, spontaneous bruising or bleeding, sore throat, or malaise occur, stop the drug and immediately contact your doctor, who will do a blood test to check for blood disorders.

INTERACTIONS

Lactulose The release of mesalazine at its site of action may be reduced by lactulose.

Warfarin Mesalazine may reduce the effect of warfarin.
Azathioprine and mercaptopurine may increase the risk of blood problems with mesalazine.

SPECIAL PRECAUTIONS

Be sure to tell your doctor if:
- You have long-term liver or kidney problems.
- You have a blood disorder.
- You are allergic to aspirin.
- You are taking other medicines.

Pregnancy Negligible amounts of mesalazine cross the placenta; however, safety is not established. Discuss with your doctor.
Breast-feeding Negligible amounts of the drug pass into the breast milk. However, safety is not established. Discuss with your doctor.
Infants and children Not recommended for children under 5 years.
Over 60 Dosage reduction not normally necessary unless there is kidney impairment.
Driving and hazardous work No special problems.
Alcohol No special problems.

PROLONGED USE

No problems expected.
Monitoring Regular blood tests and checks on kidney function are usually required.

METFORMIN

Brand names Bolamyn SR, Diagemet XL, Glucient SR, Glucophage SR, Meijumet, Metabet SR, Sukkarto SR, Yaltormin SR
Used in the following combined preparations Competact, Eucreas, Janumet, Jentadueto, Komboglyze, Synjardy, Vipdomet, Vokanamet, Xigduo

QUICK REFERENCE

Drug group Drug for diabetes (p.80)
Overdose danger rating High
Dependence rating Low
Prescription needed Yes
Available as generic Yes

GENERAL INFORMATION

Metformin is an antidiabetic drug commonly used to treat Type 2 diabetes, in which some insulin is still produced by the pancreas. It lowers blood sugar levels by delaying absorption of glucose, reducing glucose production in the liver, and helping your body respond better to its own insulin so that cells take up glucose more effectively. The drug is used in conjunction with diet, weight management, and exercise. It can be given with insulin or other antidiabetics but is often used alone in people with Type 2 diabetes who are obese. It is also used for polycystic ovary syndrome.

INFORMATION FOR USERS

Your drug prescription is tailored for you. Do not alter dosage without checking with your doctor.
How taken/used Tablets.
Frequency and timing of doses 2–3 x daily with food.
Adult dosage range 500mg–3000mg daily, with a low dose at the start of the treatment.
Onset of effect Within 2 hours. It may take 2 weeks to achieve control of diabetes.
Duration of action 8–12 hours.
Diet advice An individualized low-fat, low-sugar diet must be maintained for the drug to be fully effective. Follow your doctor's advice.
Storage Keep in original container at room temperature out of the reach of children.
Missed dose Take as soon as you remember. If your next dose is due within 2 hours, take a single dose now and skip the next.
Stopping the drug Do not stop without consulting your doctor; stopping the drug may lead to worsening of the underlying condition.

OVERDOSE ACTION

Seek immediate medical advice in all cases. Take emergency action if seizures or loss of consciousness occur.

POSSIBLE ADVERSE EFFECTS

A metallic taste in the mouth and minor gastrointestinal symptoms, such as nausea, vomiting, and appetite loss, are common and are often helped by taking the drug with food. Diarrhoea may occur; it usually settles after a few days of treatment but should be reported to your doctor. In rare cases, the drug causes dizziness, confusion, weakness, sweating, or a rash; if these occur, contact your doctor. The most serious effect is a potentially fatal build-up of lactic acid in the blood. This is very rare and usually occurs only in people with diabetes who have impaired kidney function.

INTERACTIONS

General note A number of drugs reduce the effects of metformin, including corticosteroids,

oestrogens, and diuretics. Other drugs, notably monoamine oxidase inhibitors (MAOIs) and beta blockers, increase its effects.
Warfarin Metformin may increase the effect of this anticoagulant drug. The dosage of warfarin may need to be adjusted accordingly.

SPECIAL PRECAUTIONS

Be sure to tell your doctor if:
- You have long-term liver or kidney problems.
- You have heart failure.
- You are a heavy drinker.
- You are taking other medicines.

Pregnancy Not usually prescribed. Insulin is usually substituted because it provides better diabetic control. Discuss with your doctor.
Breast-feeding Safety not established. Discuss with your doctor.
Infants and children Not recommended under 10 years.
Over 60 Increased likelihood of adverse effects. Reduced dose may therefore be necessary.
Driving and hazardous work Usually no problems. Avoid such activities if you have warning signs of low blood sugar.
Alcohol Avoid. Alcohol increases the risk of low blood sugar and can cause coma by increasing the acidity of the blood.
Surgery and general anaesthetics Surgery may reduce the response to this drug. Notify your doctor that you are diabetic; insulin treatment may need to be substituted. Tell your doctor if you are to have a contrast X-ray; metformin should be stopped before the procedure.

PROLONGED USE

Prolonged treatment can deplete reserves of vitamin B12; this may rarely cause anaemia.
Monitoring Regular checks on kidney function and blood sugar control are usually required. Vitamin B12 levels may be checked annually.

METHADONE

Brand names Methadose, Metharose, Physeptone
Used in the following combined preparations None

QUICK REFERENCE

Drug group Opioid analgesic (p.8)
Overdose danger rating High
Dependence rating High
Prescription needed Yes
Available as generic Yes

GENERAL INFORMATION

Methadone is a synthetic drug belonging to the opioid analgesic group. It is used in the control of severe pain, and as a cough suppressant in terminal illness, but it is more widely used to replace morphine or heroin in treating dependence. For this, methadone can be given once daily to prevent withdrawal symptoms. In some cases, dosage can be reduced until the drug is no longer needed.

Tolerance to the drug is marked. Although the initial dose for a person not used to opioids is very low, the dose needed by someone who is dependent could be fatal for a non-user.

INFORMATION FOR USERS

Your drug prescription is tailored for you. Do not alter dosage without checking with your doctor.
How taken/used Tablets, liquid, injection.
Frequency and timing of doses *Pain* 3–4 x daily; 2 x daily (prolonged use). *Cough* 4–6 x daily (starting dose); 2 x daily (prolonged use). *Opioid addiction* Once daily.
Adult dosage range *Pain* 5–10mg per dose initially, adjusted according to response. *Cough* 1–2mg per dose. *Opioid addiction* 10–20mg (starting dose); 40–60mg daily (maintenance).
Onset of effect 15–60 minutes.
Duration of action 36–48 hours.
Diet advice None.
Storage Keep in original container at room temperature out of the reach of children. Protect injections and liquids from light.
Missed dose Take as soon as you remember and return to your normal dosing schedule as soon as possible. If you missed the dose because it caused you to vomit, or if you cannot swallow, consult your doctor.
Stopping the drug If the reason for taking methadone no longer exists, the drug can be slowly reduced and safely stopped. Discuss with your doctor.

OVERDOSE ACTION

Seek immediate medical advice in all cases. Take emergency action if symptoms such as slow or irregular breathing, severe drowsiness, or loss of consciousness occur.

POSSIBLE ADVERSE EFFECTS

Nausea, vomiting, and drowsiness are common effects but diminish as the body adapts to the drug. Constipation is also common and may be longer lasting. Discuss with your doctor if any of these are severe. Dizziness and confusion are also fairly common and should be reported to your doctor immediately. If loss of consciousness or slow, difficult breathing occur, the drug should be stopped and immediate medical attention sought.

INTERACTIONS

Phenytoin, carbamazepine, rifampicin, and ritonavir may reduce the effects of methadone.
Monoamine oxidase inhibitors (MAOIs) and selegiline Taken with methadone, these may cause a dangerous rise or fall in blood pressure.
Erythromycin, clarithromycin, fluconazole, cimetidine and ranitidine may increase the effects of methadone.
Sedatives The effects of all drugs that have a sedative effect on the central nervous system are likely to be increased by methadone.

SPECIAL PRECAUTIONS

Be sure to tell your doctor if:
◆ You have heart or circulatory problems.
◆ You have liver or kidney problems.
◆ You have lung problems such as asthma or bronchitis.
◆ You have thyroid disease.
◆ You have a history of epileptic seizures.
◆ You have a phaeochromocytoma (a type of adrenal gland tumour).
◆ You have problems with alcohol misuse.
◆ You are taking other medicines.

Pregnancy Not prescribed in pregnancy if possible. May cause breathing difficulties in the newborn baby. Discuss with your doctor.
Breast-feeding Safety not established. The drug passes into breast milk and may affect the baby adversely. Discuss with your doctor.
Infants and children Not recommended.
Over 60 Reduced dose necessary.
Driving and hazardous work Your underlying condition or the side effects of the drug itself, such as drowsiness, may make such activities inadvisable. Discuss with your doctor.
Alcohol Avoid. Alcohol increases the sedative effects of the drug and may depress breathing.

PROLONGED USE

Treatment with methadone is always closely monitored. If methadone is being taken long term, the dose must be carefully reduced before the drug is stopped.

METHOTREXATE

Brand names Jylamvo, Maxtrex, Methofill, Metoject, Nordimet, Zlatal
Used in the following combined preparations None

QUICK REFERENCE

Drug group Anticancer drug (p.94)
Overdose danger rating High
Dependence rating Low
Prescription needed Yes
Available as generic Yes

GENERAL INFORMATION

Methotrexate is an anticancer drug used, together with other anticancer drugs, in the treatment of leukaemia, lymphoma, and solid cancers such as those of the breast, bladder, head, and neck. It is also used alone to treat inflammatory conditions such as severe uncontrolled psoriasis, rheumatoid arthritis, and Crohn's disease.

As with most anticancer drugs, methotrexate affects both healthy and cancerous cells, so its usefulness is limited by its adverse effects and toxicity. Folic acid supplements may reduce its toxicity; when methotrexate is given in high doses, it is usually given with folinic acid to prevent it from destroying bone marrow cells. Because of the drug's toxicity and adverse effects it is very important that you do not take methotrexate more often than prescribed by your doctor.

INFORMATION FOR USERS

Your drug prescription is tailored for you. Do not alter dosage without checking with your doctor.
How taken/used Tablets, injection, liquid.
Frequency and timing of doses *Cancer* Single dose once weekly or every 3 weeks. *Other conditions* Single dose once weekly.
Adult dosage range *Cancer* Dosage is determined individually according to the nature of the condition, body weight, and response. *Rheumatoid arthritis* 7.5–20mg weekly. *Psoriasis* 10–25mg weekly.
Onset of effect 30–60 minutes.
Duration of action Short-term effects last up to 24 hours.
Diet advice None.
Storage Keep in original container at room temperature out of the reach of children. Wash your hands after handling the tablets.

Missed dose Take as soon as you remember and consult your doctor.
Stopping the drug Do not stop without consulting your doctor. Stopping the drug may lead to worsening of the underlying condition.

OVERDOSE ACTION

Seek immediate medical advice in all cases. Take emergency action if breathing problems or loss of consciousness occur.

POSSIBLE ADVERSE EFFECTS

Common adverse effects of methotrexate include dry cough; chest pain; nausea and vomiting (which may occur within a few hours of taking the drug); and diarrhoea and mouth or gum ulcers (which may occur a few days after starting treatment). Notify your doctor if dry cough or chest pain are severe or you have any of the other effects. If you have mouth ulcers or inflammation, stop the drug and call the doctor immediately. Less common adverse effects include mood changes, confusion, rash, jaundice, sore throat, fever, easy bleeding or bruising, and breathlessness. If you experience mood changes or confusion, notify your doctor. If you develop any of these other less common symptoms, stop taking the drug and contact your doctor without delay.

INTERACTIONS

General note Many drugs, including non-steroidal anti-inflammatory drugs (NSAIDs), diuretics, ciclosporin, phenytoin, and probenecid, may increase the blood levels and toxicity of methotrexate.
Co-trimoxazole, trimethoprim, and certain antimalarial drugs These drugs may enhance the effects of methotrexate.

SPECIAL PRECAUTIONS

Be sure to tell your doctor if:

- You have liver or kidney problems.
- You have porphyria.
- You have a problem with alcohol misuse.
- You have a peptic or other digestive-tract ulcer.
- You are taking other medicines, especially NSAIDs or antibiotics.

Pregnancy Not prescribed. Methotrexate may cause birth defects in the unborn baby.
Breast-feeding Not advised. The drug passes into breast milk and may affect the baby adversely.
Infants and children For cancer treatment only. Reduced dose necessary.
Over 60 Increased likelihood of adverse effects. Reduced doses necessary.
Driving and hazardous work No special problems.
Alcohol Avoid. Alcohol may increase the adverse effects of methotrexate.

PROLONGED USE

Long-term treatment may be needed for rheumatoid arthritis. Once the condition is controlled, the drug is reduced as much as possible to the lowest effective dose. Long-term methotrexate use may occasionally lead to breathing problems due to scarring of the lungs or, rarely, unusual respiratory infections, such as pneumocystis pneumonia.
Monitoring Full blood counts and kidney and liver function tests will be performed before methotrexate treatment starts and at intervals during treatment.

METHYLCELLULOSE

Brand name Celevac
Used in the following combined preparations None

QUICK REFERENCE

Drug group Laxative (p.43) and antidiarrhoeal drug (p.42)
Overdose danger rating Low
Dependence rating Low
Prescription needed No
Available as generic No

GENERAL INFORMATION

Methylcellulose is a laxative used for the treatment of constipation, diverticular disease, and irritable bowel syndrome. Taken by mouth, methylcellulose is not absorbed into the bloodstream but remains in the intestine. It absorbs up to 25 times its volume of water, thereby softening the faeces and increasing their volume. This agent is also used to reduce the frequency and increase the firmness of faeces in chronic watery diarrhoea, and to control the consistency of faeces after colostomies and ileostomies.

Methylcellulose preparations are used with appropriate dieting in some cases of obesity. The bulking agent swells to give a feeling of fullness, thereby encouraging adherence to a reducing diet.

INFORMATION FOR USERS

Follow instructions on the label. Call your doctor if symptoms worsen.

How taken/used Tablets.

Frequency and timing of doses 3–6 tablets 2 x daily. If used as laxative, unless otherwise instructed, break in mouth and swallow with full glass of water; do not take at bedtime.

Adult dosage range 1.5–6g daily.

Onset of effect Within 24 hours.

Duration of action Up to 3 days.

Diet advice If taken as a laxative, drink plenty of fluids, and drink at least 300ml with each dose. If taken for diarrhoea, avoid liquids for 30 minutes before and after each dose.

Storage Keep in original container at room temperature out of the reach of children.

Missed dose Take as soon as you remember. Take the next dose as scheduled.

Stopping the drug Can be safely stopped as soon as you no longer need it.

Exceeding the dose An occasional unintentional extra dose is unlikely to be a cause for concern. But if you notice any unusual symptoms, or if a large overdose has been taken, tell your doctor.

POSSIBLE ADVERSE EFFECTS

Adverse effects are rare, but when taken by mouth methylcellulose may cause abdominal distension and flatulence. Insufficient fluid intake may cause blockage of the oesophagus (gullet) or intestine. Consult your doctor if you have abdominal pain or severe bloating or flatulence, or if you have had no bowel movement for 2 days after taking the drug.

INTERACTIONS

None.

SPECIAL PRECAUTIONS

Be sure to consult your doctor or pharmacist before taking this drug if:

- You have severe constipation and/or abdominal pain.
- You have unexplained rectal bleeding.
- You have difficulty in swallowing.
- You vomit readily.
- You are taking other medicines.

Pregnancy No evidence of risk to developing baby, but discuss with your doctor.

Breast-feeding No evidence of risk.

Infants and children Reduced dose necessary, but discuss with your doctor.

Over 60 No special problems.

Driving and hazardous work No known problems.

Alcohol No known problems.

PROLONGED USE

No problems expected.

METHYLPHENIDATE

Brand names Concerta XL, Delmosart, Equasym XL, Matoride, Medikinet XL, Ritalin, Tranquilyn, Xaggitin XL, Xenidate XL

Used in the following combined preparations None

QUICK REFERENCE

Drug group Nervous system stimulant (p.17)

Overdose danger rating High

Dependence rating Medium

Prescription needed Yes

Available as generic Yes

GENERAL INFORMATION

Methylphenidate is related to amfetamines and shares similar stimulant properties. Paradoxically, however, methylphenidate is used, under specialist supervision, to treat overactivity in children with severe, persistent attention deficit hyperactivity disorder (ADHD). Children with moderate ADHD should only receive it when psychological treatments have been unsuccessful. In all cases, the drug should be part of an overall treatment programme for ADHD. Growth may be retarded in children receiving the drug and should be closely monitored. However, in affected children growth often returns to normal once the drug is stopped. Methylphenidate is also used to treat narcolepsy in adults and children.

INFORMATION FOR USERS

Your drug prescription is tailored for you. Do not alter dosage without checking with your doctor.

How taken/used Tablets, extra-long release (XL) tablets, XL capsules.

Frequency and timing of doses 1 or 2 x daily (an extra bedtime dose may be needed) swallowed whole, not chewed. Take before meals.

Dosage range *ADHD* 2.5–60mg (children), up to 100mg (adults) daily. *Narcolepsy* 10–60mg daily.

Onset of effect 1–2 hours.

Duration of action 3–6 hours (up to 9 hours for XL preparations).

Diet advice None.
Storage Keep in original container at room temperature out of the reach of children.
Missed dose Take next dose at the usual time. Do not take a double dose.
Stopping the drug Do not stop the drug without consulting your doctor; symptoms may recur.

OVERDOSE ACTION

Seek immediate medical advice. Although an occasional unintended dose is unlikely to be a cause for concern, a large overdose can be extremely dangerous. Take emergency action if a seizure occurs.

POSSIBLE ADVERSE EFFECTS

Adverse effects are common but rarely serious. The common side effects include nausea, abdominal discomfort, dry mouth, irritability, agitation, aggression, rash, and palpitations. More rarely, the drug may cause depression. If nausea, abdominal discomfort, or dry mouth are severe, discuss with your doctor. Other side effects should always be discussed with your doctor. In some cases, the side effects may be difficult to interpret because of pre-existing behavioural problems. In each case, a careful assessment should be made by a specialist at regular intervals.

INTERACTIONS

SSRI and tricylcic antidepressants Methylphenidate can increase blood levels of these drugs. Reduced doses may be required.
MAOI antidepressants When taken with methylphenidate, there is a risk of an extreme rise in blood pressure. Concomitant use of these drugs should be avoided.
Phenytoin Methylphenidate increases blood levels of phenytoin. Reduced dose of phenytoin may be required.
Oral anticoagulants (e.g. warfarin) The anticoagulant effect of these drugs is increased by methylphenidate.

SPECIAL PRECAUTIONS

Be sure to tell your doctor if:
- You have a history of heart problems.
- You have a family history of Tourette's syndrome.
- You have a drug dependency.
- You have epilepsy.
- You have psychiatric illness.

Pregnancy Safety in pregnancy not established. Discuss with your doctor.
Breast-feeding Safety in breast-feeding not established. Discuss with your doctor.
Infants and children Dose varies according to age.
Over 60 Not usually prescribed.
Driving and hazardous work Avoid until you know how methylphenidate affects you.
Alcohol Avoid. Effects of methylphenidate may be enhanced by alcohol.

PROLONGED USE

No problems expected in adults. Methylphenidate may retard growth in children if used for prolonged periods.
Monitoring Regular monitoring of growth should be carried out when methylphenidate is used for prolonged periods in children.

METOCLOPRAMIDE

Brand names Maxolon, Maxolon High Dose, Maxolon SR, Primperan
Used in the following combined preparations MigraMax, Paramax

QUICK REFERENCE

Drug group Gastrointestinal motility regulator and anti-emetic drug (p.19)
Overdose danger rating Medium
Dependence rating Low
Prescription needed Yes
Available as generic Yes

GENERAL INFORMATION

Metoclopramide has a direct action on the gastrointestinal tract. It is used for conditions in which there is a need to encourage normal propulsion of food through the stomach and intestine. The drug has powerful anti-emetic properties and its most common use is in preventing and treating nausea and vomiting. It is particularly effective for relieving the nausea that sometimes accompanies migraine headaches, and the nausea caused by treatment with anticancer drugs. It is also prescribed to alleviate symptoms of heartburn caused by acid reflux into the oesophagus.

One side effect of the drug, muscle spasm of the head and neck, is more likely to occur in children and young adults under 20 years. Other side effects are not usually troublesome.

INFORMATION FOR USERS

Your drug prescription is tailored for you. Do not alter dosage without checking with your doctor.

How taken/used Tablets, powder, liquid, injection.

Frequency and timing of doses Usually 3 x daily; 2 x daily (slow-release preparations).

Adult dosage range Usually 15–30mg daily; dose may be higher for nausea caused by anti-cancer drugs.

Onset of effect Within 1 hour.

Duration of action 6–8 hours.

Diet advice Fatty and spicy foods and alcohol are best avoided if nausea is a problem.

Storage Keep in original container at room temperature out of the reach of children.

Missed dose Take as soon as you remember. If your next dose is due within 3 hours, take a single dose now and skip the next.

Stopping the drug Can be safely stopped as soon as you no longer need it.

Exceeding the dose An occasional unintentional extra dose is unlikely to be a cause for concern. However, large overdoses may cause drowsiness and muscle spasms. Notify your doctor.

POSSIBLE ADVERSE EFFECTS

Adverse effects are rare with metoclopramide. The main adverse effects are drowsiness and, even less commonly, uncontrolled muscle spasm. Other, very rare, adverse effects include restlessness, diarrhoea, muscle tremors or rigidity, and a rash. Consult your doctor if drowsiness is severe, and for all other effects. If you experience muscle spasms of the head or neck or develop a rash, stop taking the drug and consult your doctor urgently.

INTERACTIONS

Sedatives The sedative properties of metoclopramide are increased by all drugs that have a sedative effect on the central nervous system. These include benzodiazepines, antihistamines, antidepressants, and opioid analgesics.

Lithium Metoclopramide increases the risk of central nervous system side effects.

Ciclosporin Metoclopramide may increase the blood levels of this drug.

Drugs for parkinsonism There is an increased risk of adverse effects if these drugs are taken with metoclopramide.

Antipsychotics Metoclopramide increases the risk of adverse effects from these drugs.

Opioid analgesics and anticholinergic drugs These drugs oppose the gastrointestinal effects of metoclopramide.

Aspirin and paracetamol Metoclopramide increases the rate of absorption of these drugs.

SPECIAL PRECAUTIONS

Be sure to tell your doctor if:

- You have long-term liver or kidney problems.
- You have epilepsy.
- You have Parkinson's disease.
- You have porphyria.
- You have phaeochromocytoma.
- You have had recent gastrointestinal illness or surgery.
- You are taking other medicines.

Pregnancy Safety in pregnancy not established. Discuss with your doctor.

Breast-feeding The drug passes into the breast milk but normal doses are unlikely to affect the baby adversely. Discuss with your doctor.

Infants and children Reduced dose necessary. Restricted use in patients who are younger than 20 years.

Over 60 Reduced dose may be necessary.

Driving and hazardous work Avoid until you have learned how metoclopramide affects you because the drug can cause drowsiness.

Alcohol Avoid. Alcohol may oppose the beneficial effects and increase the sedative effects of this drug.

PROLONGED USE

Not normally used long term, except under specialist supervision for certain gastrointestinal disorders.

METOPROLOL

Brand names Betaloc, Betaloc-SA, Lopresor, Lopresor SR

Used in the following combined preparations None

QUICK REFERENCE

Drug group Beta blocker (p.28)

Overdose danger rating High

Dependence rating Low

Prescription needed Yes

Available as generic Yes

GENERAL INFORMATION

Metoprolol is a cardioselective beta blocker used to prevent the heart from beating too fast in conditions such as angina, arrhythmias, and hyperthyroidism. It is also used to prevent migraine attacks or protect the heart from further damage after a heart attack. In addition, it is used to treat high blood pressure (although not usually to initiate treatment). It is less likely than non-cardioselective beta blockers to cause breathing difficulties. However, it should be avoided in people with asthma. It may slow the body's response to low blood sugar in people with diabetes who take insulin.

INFORMATION FOR USERS

Your drug prescription is tailored for you. Do not alter dosage without checking with your doctor.

How taken/used Tablets, slow release (SR) tablets, injection.

Frequency and timing of doses 1–2 x daily (hypertension); 2–3 x daily (angina/arrhythmias); 4 x daily for 2 days, then 2 x daily (heart attack prevention); 2 x daily (migraine prevention); 4 x daily (hyperthyroidism).

Adult dosage range 100–200mg daily.

Onset of effect 1–2 hours.

Duration of action 3–7 hours.

Diet advice None.

Storage Keep in original container at room temperature out of the reach of children.

Missed dose Take as soon as you remember. If your next dose is due within 2 hours, take a single dose now and skip the next.

Stopping the drug Do not stop without consulting your doctor. Stopping suddenly may lead to worsening of the underlying condition.

OVERDOSE ACTION

Seek immediate medical advice in all cases. Take emergency action if breathing difficulties, collapse, or loss of consciousness occur.

POSSIBLE ADVERSE EFFECTS

The adverse effects of metoprolol are common to most beta blockers and tend to diminish with long-term use. All adverse effects should be reported to your doctor. The most common effects are lethargy, fatigue, and cold hands and feet. Less common adverse effects include nausea, vomiting, nightmares or vivid dreams, rash, dry eyes, and visual disturbances. If you experience palpitations or fainting (which may be a sign that the drug has slowed the heart beat excessively), breathlessness, or wheezing, you should stop taking the drug and seek immediate medical attention.

INTERACTIONS

Antihypertensive drugs Metoprolol may enhance the blood-pressure-lowering effect.

Calcium channel blockers may cause low blood pressure, a slow heartbeat, and heart failure if used with metoprolol.

Non-steroidal anti-inflammatory drugs (NSAIDs) may reduce the antihypertensive effect of metoprolol.

Cardiac glycosides (e.g. digoxin) may increase the heart-slowing effect of metoprolol.

Antidiabetic drugs Taken with metoprolol, these drugs may increase the risk of low blood sugar or mask its symptoms.

Antacids may increase the effects of metoprolol.

SPECIAL PRECAUTIONS

Be sure to tell your doctor if:

- You have liver or kidney problems.
- You have asthma, bronchitis, or emphysema.
- You have heart problems.
- You have diabetes.
- You have psoriasis.
- You have phaeochromocytoma (a type of adrenal gland tumour).
- You are taking other medicines.

Pregnancy Not usually prescribed. May affect the baby. Discuss with your doctor.

Breast-feeding The drug passes into the breast milk, but normal doses are unlikely to affect the baby adversely. Discuss with your doctor.

Infants and children Not recommended.

Over 60 Reduced doses necessary. There may be an increased risk of adverse effects.

Driving and hazardous work Avoid until you know how metoprolol affects you because it can cause fatigue, dizziness, and drowsiness.

Alcohol Avoid excessive intake. Alcohol may increase the blood-pressure-lowering effects of metoprolol.

Surgery and general anaesthetics Occasionally, metoprolol may need to be stopped before you have a general anaesthetic; but only do this after discussion with your doctor or dentist.

PROLONGED USE

No special problems.

In very rare cases, use of metoprolol is associated with Peyronie's disease (growth of abnormal fibrous tissue in the penis) and with retroperitoneal fibrosis (growth of abnormal fibrous tissue around the abdominal organs).

METRONIDAZOLE

Brand names Acea, Anabact, Flagyl, Metrogel, Metrosa, Rosiced, Rozex, Zidoval, Zyomet

Used in the following combined preparations None

QUICK REFERENCE

Drug group Antibacterial drug (p.64) and antiprotozoal drug (p.70)

Overdose danger rating Low

Dependence rating Low

Prescription needed Yes

Available as generic Yes

GENERAL INFORMATION

Metronidazole is prescribed to treat protozoal infections and a variety of bacterial infections. It is widely used for trichomonas infection of the vagina. Because the organism responsible for this disorder is sexually transmitted and may not cause any symptoms, a simultaneous course of treatment is usually advised for the sexual partner. Certain infections of the abdomen, pelvis, and gums also respond well to metronidazole. The drug is used to treat septicaemia and infected leg ulcers and pressure sores, and for *Clostridium difficile* infections associated with antibiotic use. Metronidazole may be given to prevent or treat infections after surgery. Because high doses of the drug can penetrate the brain, it is prescribed to treat abscesses occurring there. Metronidazole is also prescribed for amoebic dysentery and giardiasis, a protozoal infection.

INFORMATION FOR USERS

Your drug prescription is tailored for you. Do not alter dosage without checking with your doctor.

How taken/used Tablets, liquid, injection, suppositories, gel, cream.

Frequency and timing of doses 3 x daily for 5–10 days, depending on condition being treated. Sometimes a single large dose is prescribed. Tablets should be taken after meals and swallowed whole with plenty of water. 1–2 x daily (topical preparations).

Adult dosage range 600–2,000mg daily (by mouth); 3g daily (suppositories); 1.5g daily (injection).

Onset of effect The drug starts to work within an hour or so, but beneficial effects may not be felt for 1–2 days.

Duration of action 6–12 hours.

Diet advice None.

Storage Keep in original container at room temperature out of the reach of children. Protect from light.

Missed dose Take as soon as you remember. If your next dose is due within 2 hours, take a single dose now and skip the next.

Stopping the drug Take the full course. Even if you feel better the infection may still be present and symptoms may recur if treatment is stopped too soon.

Exceeding the dose An occasional unintentional extra dose is unlikely to be a cause for concern. But if you notice unusual symptoms, especially numbness or tingling, or if a large overdose has been taken, notify your doctor.

POSSIBLE ADVERSE EFFECTS

Various minor gastrointestinal symptoms (such as nausea and loss of appetite) are common, but these tend to diminish with time. Metronidazole also often causes darkening of the urine, but this is no cause for concern. More rarely, the drug may cause dry mouth, a metallic taste, headache, or dizziness; if these are severe, discuss with your doctor. More serious adverse effects on the nervous system, causing numbness or tingling, are extremely rare but should be reported to your doctor.

INTERACTIONS

Oral anticoagulants, ciclosporin, phenytoin, and fluorouracil Metronidazole may increase the effects of these drugs.

Lithium Metronidazole increases the levels of lithium and the risk of kidney damage.

Cimetidine This drug may increase the levels of metronidazole in the body.

Phenobarbital This drug may reduce the effects of metronidazole.

SPECIAL PRECAUTIONS

Be sure to tell your doctor if:

- You have long-term liver or kidney problems.
- You have porphyria.
- You are taking other medicines.

Pregnancy Safety in pregnancy not established. Discuss with your doctor.

Breast-feeding The drug passes into breast milk, but normal doses are unlikely to affect the baby adversely. However, the drug may give the milk a bitter taste. Discuss with your doctor.

Infants and children Reduced dose necessary.

Over 60 No special problems.

Driving and hazardous work Avoid until you have learned how metronidazole affects you because the drug can cause drowsiness.

Alcohol Avoid. Taken with metronidazole, alcohol may cause flushing, nausea, vomiting, abdominal pain, and headache.

PROLONGED USE

Not usually prescribed for longer than 10 days. Prolonged treatment may cause loss of sensation in the hands and feet (usually temporary), and may also reduce production of white blood cells.

Monitoring Monitoring of blood counts and liver function may be considered if treatment is given for more than 10 days.

MICONAZOLE

Brand names Daktarin, Gyno-Daktarin, Loramyc

Used in the following combined preparation Daktacort

QUICK REFERENCE

Drug group Antifungal drug (p.74)

Overdose danger rating Low

Dependence rating Low

Prescription needed No (cream, powder); Yes (other preparations)

Available as generic Yes

GENERAL INFORMATION

Miconazole is an antifungal drug used to treat *Candida* (yeast) infections of the mouth, *Candida* and bacterial infections of the vagina and gut, and various other fungal infections of the skin. For oral infections, the drug is available as a gel to be used on dentures. Cream, dusting powder, or ointment are used for skin infections, and a variety of vaginal preparations is available. Side effects usually only occur with oral preparations, because miconazole is absorbed in only very small quantities from topical or vaginal application. Pessaries, vaginal capsules, and vaginal cream damage latex condoms and diaphragms.

INFORMATION FOR USERS

Follow instructions on the label. Call your doctor if symptoms worsen.

How taken/used Buccal tablets, pessaries, vaginal cream, vaginal capsules, cream, ointment, oral gel, spray powder.

Frequency and timing of doses 1 x daily in morning (buccal tablets); 4 x daily after food (oral gel); 1–2 x daily (vaginal/skin preparations).

Adult dosage range *Vaginal infections* 1 x 5g applicatorful (cream); 1 x 100mg pessary; 1 x 1.2g vaginal capsule. *Oral/skin infections* As directed.

Onset of effect 2–3 days.

Duration of action Up to 12 hours.

Diet advice None.

Storage Keep in original container at room temperature out of the reach of children.

Missed dose No cause for concern, but take or apply missed dose as soon as you remember.

Stopping the drug Apply the full course. Even if you feel better, the original infection may still be present and may recur if treatment is stopped too soon.

Exceeding the dose An occasional unintentional extra dose is unlikely to cause problems. But if you notice any unusual symptoms or if a large amount has been swallowed, tell your doctor.

POSSIBLE ADVERSE EFFECTS

Adverse effects are rare and usually occur only with oral forms. The main effects include skin irritation or a rash, nausea, and vomiting, any of which should be reported to your doctor if severe, and vaginal irritation, which should be reported to your doctor in all cases.

INTERACTIONS

Oral anticoagulants, ciclosporin, phenytoin, antidiabetics, quinidine, and pimozide Miconazole oral gel and buccal tablets may increase the effects and toxicity of these drugs.

Carbamazepine, phenytoin, calcium channel blockers, and sirolimus, tacrolimus Miconazole oral gel and buccal tablets may increase the effects and toxicity of these drugs.

Simvastatin There is an increased risk of muscle damage if this drug is taken with miconazole. Avoid using together.

SPECIAL PRECAUTIONS

Be sure to consult your doctor or pharmacist before taking this drug if:

- ◆ You have porphyria.
- ◆ You have liver problems.
- ◆ You are taking other medicines.

Pregnancy No evidence of risk with topical preparations. Safety not established for other preparations. Discuss with your doctor.

Breast-feeding Safety not established. Discuss with your doctor.
Infants and children Reduced dose necessary (oral gel).
Over 60 No special problems.
Driving and hazardous work No special problems.
Alcohol No special problems.

PROLONGED USE
No problems expected. Most types of miconazole are not usually prescribed for long-term use, but oral gel may cause diarrhoea if used for a long time.

MINOCYCLINE

Brand names Aknemin, Dexcel Acnamino, Minocin MR, Sebomin MR
Used in the following combined preparations None

QUICK REFERENCE
Drug group Tetracycline antibiotic (p.61)
Overdose danger rating Low
Dependence rating Low
Prescription needed Yes
Available as generic Yes

GENERAL INFORMATION
Minocycline is a tetracycline antibiotic but has a longer duration of action than tetracycline itself (p.421). The drug is most commonly used to treat acne. It may also be given to treat pneumonia or to prevent infection in people with chronic bronchitis, and to treat sexually transmitted infections such as gonorrhoea and non-gonococcal urethritis. In addition, it is used to treat chronic gum disease in adults.

The most frequent side effects are nausea, vomiting, and diarrhoea. The drug also interferes with the balance mechanism in the ear, producing nausea, dizziness, and unsteadiness, but these generally disappear after it is stopped. However, it is safer than other tetracyclines for people with poor kidney function.

INFORMATION FOR USERS
Your drug prescription is tailored for you. Do not alter dosage without checking with your doctor.
How taken/used Tablets, capsules, modified release (MR) capsules, gel.
Frequency and timing of doses 1–2 x daily.
Dosage range *Adults* 100–200mg daily. *Children* Reduced dose according to age and weight.
Onset of effect 4–12 hours.
Duration of action Up to 24 hours.
Diet advice Milk products may impair absorption; avoid from 1 hour before to 2 hours after taking a dose.
Storage Keep in original container at room temperature out of the reach of children.
Missed dose Take as soon as you remember. If your next dose is due within 4 hours, take a single dose now and skip the next.
Stopping the drug Use the full course. Even if you feel better, the original infection may still be present and symptoms may recur if treatment is stopped too soon.
Exceeding the dose An occasional unintentional extra dose is unlikely to be a cause for concern. But if you notice any unusual symptoms, or if a large overdose has been taken, notify your doctor.

POSSIBLE ADVERSE EFFECTS
Minocycline may cause nausea, vomiting, or diarrhoea; consult your doctor if these are severe. Other adverse effects include dizziness and vertigo (loss of balance), and less commonly rashes, itching, increased sensitivity of the skin to sunlight, headache, and blurred vision. If any of these less common effects occur, stop taking the drug and consult your doctor promptly. Long-term use may occasionally cause additional adverse effects (see Prolonged use).

INTERACTIONS
Oral anticoagulants Minocycline may increase the anticoagulant action of these drugs.
Retinoids Taken with minocycline, these drugs may increase the risk of benign intracranial hypertension (high pressure in the skull) leading to headaches, nausea, and vomiting.
Oral contraceptives Minocycline can reduce the effectiveness of these drugs.
Penicillin antibiotics Minocycline interferes with the antibacterial action of these drugs.
Iron may interfere with the absorption of minocycline and may reduce its effectiveness.
Antacids, zinc preparations, and milk interfere with the absorption of minocycline and may reduce its effectiveness. Doses should be separated by 1–2 hours.
Strontium ranelate may reduce the absorption of minocycline. The two drugs should not be used together.

SPECIAL PRECAUTIONS

Be sure to tell your doctor if:
- ◆ You have liver or kidney problems.
- ◆ You have previously had an allergic reaction to a tetracycline antibiotic.
- ◆ You have myasthenia gravis, acute porphyria, or systemic lupus erythematosus.
- ◆ You are taking other medicines.

Pregnancy Not prescribed. May cause birth defects and may damage the teeth and bones of the developing baby, as well as the mother's liver. Discuss with your doctor.

Breast-feeding Not recommended. The drug passes into the breast milk, and may damage developing bones and discolour the baby's teeth. Discuss with your doctor.

Infants and children Not recommended under 12 years. Reduced dose necessary in older children. May discolour developing teeth.

Over 60 No special problems.

Driving and hazardous work Avoid such activities until you have learned how minocycline affects you because it can cause dizziness.

Alcohol No known problems.

How to take your tablets To prevent minocycline from sticking in your throat, take a small amount of water before, and a full glass of water after, each dose. Take this medication while sitting or standing, and do not lie down immediately afterwards.

PROLONGED USE

Prolonged use of minocycline may occasionally cause skin darkening and discoloration of the teeth. Very rarely, it may cause systemic lupus erythematosus.

Monitoring Regular blood tests should be carried out to assess liver function, especially if treatment lasts over 6 months.

MINOXIDIL

Brand names Boots Hair Loss Treatment, Loniten, Regaine

Used in the following combined preparations None

QUICK REFERENCE

Drug group Antihypertensive drug (p.34) and treatment for hair loss (p.125)

Overdose danger rating Medium

Dependence rating Low

Prescription needed Yes (except for scalp lotions)

Available as generic No

GENERAL INFORMATION

Minoxidil is a vasodilator drug (p.30) that works by relaxing the muscles of artery walls and dilating blood vessels. It is effective in controlling dangerously high blood pressure that is rising very rapidly. Because minoxidil is stronger-acting than many other antihypertensive drugs, it is particularly useful for people whose blood pressure is not controlled by other treatment.

Minoxidil causes significant fluid retention and increased heart rate, so it should be prescribed together with a diuretic and a beta blocker to increase effectiveness and to counteract its side effects. Unlike many other drugs in the antihypertensive group, minoxidil rarely causes dizziness and fainting. Its major drawback is that, if it is taken for more than 2 months, it increases hair growth, especially on the face. Although this effect can be controlled by shaving or depilatories, some people find the abnormal growth distressing. This effect is put to use, however, to treat baldness in men and women, and for this purpose minoxidil is applied locally as a solution.

INFORMATION FOR USERS

Your drug prescription is tailored for you. Do not alter dosage without checking with your doctor.

How taken/used Tablets, topical solution.

Frequency and timing of doses Once or twice daily.

Adult dosage range 5mg daily initially, increasing gradually to a maximum of 100mg daily.

Onset of effect *Blood pressure* Within 1 hour (tablets). *Hair growth* Up to 1 year (solution).

Duration of action Up to 24 hours. Some effect may last for 2–5 days after stopping the drug.

Diet advice None.

Storage Keep in original container at room temperature out of the reach of children.

Missed dose Take as soon as you remember (tablets). If next dose is due within 5 hours, take a single dose now and skip the next. If used topically for baldness, any regained hair will be lost when the drug is stopped.

Stopping the drug Do not stop without consulting your doctor; stopping the drug may lead to worsening of the underlying condition.

Exceeding the dose An occasional unintentional extra dose is unlikely to cause problems. Large overdoses may cause nausea, vomiting, palpitations, or dizziness. Notify your doctor.

POSSIBLE ADVERSE EFFECTS

Fluid retention is a common adverse effect of minoxidil, which may lead to ankle swelling and an increase in weight; diuretics are often prescribed to control this effect. Increased growth of hair on the head and body is another common effect. Discuss with your doctor if these effects are severe. More rarely, there may be nausea, breast tenderness, dizziness, lightheadedness, or a rash; consult your doctor if any of these occur. If you experience palpitations, stop taking the drug and notify your doctor immediately. In some cases, allergic and irritant dermatitis may occur with minoxidil lotion.

INTERACTIONS

Antidepressant drugs The hypotensive effects of minoxidil may be enhanced by antidepressant drugs.

Other antihypertensives These drugs may increase the effects of minoxidil.

Oestrogens and progestogens (including those in some contraceptive pills) may reduce the effects of minoxidil.

SPECIAL PRECAUTIONS

Be sure to tell your doctor if:

- You have a long-term kidney problem.
- You have heart problems.
- You have porphyria.
- You are taking other medicines.

Pregnancy Safety in pregnancy not established. Discuss with your doctor.

Breast-feeding The drug passes into the breast milk, but normal doses are unlikely to affect the baby adversely. Discuss with your doctor.

Infants and children Reduced dose necessary.

Over 60 Reduced dose may be necessary.

Driving and hazardous work Avoid such activities until you have learned how minoxidil affects you because the drug can cause dizziness and lightheadedness.

Alcohol Avoid. Alcohol may further reduce blood pressure.

Surgery and general anaesthetics Minoxidil treatment may need to be stopped before you have a general anaesthetic. Discuss this with your doctor or dentist before any surgery.

PROLONGED USE

Prolonged use of this drug may lead to swelling of the ankles and increased hair growth.

MIRTAZAPINE

Brand names None in UK

Used in the following combined preparations None

QUICK REFERENCE

Drug group Antidepressant drug (p.12)

Overdose danger rating Medium

Dependence rating Low

Prescription needed Yes

Available as generic Yes

GENERAL INFORMATION

Mirtazapine is an antidepressant drug that works by increasing two naturally occurring chemicals in the brain: serotonin and norepinephrine (noradrenaline). It is used in treating major depression, the symptoms of which may include feelings of worthlessness, anxiety, and increased or decreased appetite.

The drug may be given at a low dose initially and increased gradually according to the response of the user. If there is no response to mirtazapine at the maximum dose within 2 to 4 weeks, the treatment may be discontinued.

Mirtazapine is available as tablets, orosoluble tablets (placed on the tongue and allowed to dissolve), and an oral solution. Because it has little anticholinergic action (p.7), it is better tolerated than tricyclic antidepressants.

INFORMATION FOR USERS

Your drug prescription is tailored for you. Do not alter dosage without checking with your doctor.

How taken/used Tablets, orosoluble tablets, liquid (oral solution).

Frequency and timing of doses Usually once daily at bedtime.

Adult dosage range 15mg (initial dose) increased gradually to 45mg, according to response.

Onset of effect Within 1–2 weeks, but full beneficial effect may not be felt for 2–4 weeks.

Duration of action At least 24 hours.

Diet advice None.

Storage Keep in original container at room temperature out of the reach of children.

Missed dose Take as soon as you remember, then return to your normal dosing schedule. Do not take an extra dose to make up.

Stopping the drug Do not stop without consulting your doctor, who will supervise a gradual reduction in dosage. Stopping abruptly can lead to withdrawal symptoms.

Exceeding the dose An occasional unintentional extra dose is unlikely to cause problems. Larger overdoses may cause drowsiness and disorientation. Notify your doctor.

POSSIBLE ADVERSE EFFECTS

Some of the adverse effects are similar to symptoms of the illness. Mirtazapine has few anticholinergic effects, but causes sedation at the start of treatment. Other common effects include dizziness, increased appetite and weight gain, fatigue, and swollen ankles and feet due to fluid accumulation. Notify your doctor if you experience ankle or foot swelling or if these other effects are severe. Less commonly, the drug may cause restlessness, headache, and vivid dreams or nightmares; consult your doctor if these are severe. If you develop jaundice, fever, or a sore throat, stop taking the drug and consult your doctor immediately.

INTERACTIONS

Monoamine oxidase inhibitors (MAOIs) should not be taken with or within 2 weeks of stopping mirtazapine, and vice versa.

Warfarin Mirtazapine increases the anticoagulant effect of warfarin.

Antimalarials (artemether with lumefantrine) should not be taken with mirtazapine.

Carbamazepine and phenytoin may reduce blood levels of mirtazapine.

SPECIAL PRECAUTIONS

Be sure to tell your doctor if:

- ◆ You have epilepsy.
- ◆ You have liver or kidney problems.
- ◆ You have angina or you have had a recent heart attack.
- ◆ You have hypertension.
- ◆ You have diabetes.
- ◆ You have a psychiatric illness or bipolar disorder.
- ◆ You have any eye diseases such as glaucoma.
- ◆ You have had a previous allergic reaction to mirtazapine.
- ◆ You are taking other medicines.

Pregnancy Not recommended. Safety not established. Discuss with your doctor.

Breast-feeding Small amounts of the drug pass into the breast milk, but safety not established. Discuss with your doctor.

Infants and children Not recommended.

Over 60 Not recommended.

Driving and hazardous work Avoid until you have learned how mirtazapine affects you because the drug can cause initial sedation and impaired alertness and concentration.

Alcohol Avoid. Mirtazapine may increase the sedative effects of alcohol.

PROLONGED USE

No known problems.

Monitoring Periodic tests of liver function are usually carried out.

MISOPROSTOL

Brand name Cytotec, Mysodelle, Topogyne

Used in the following combined preparations Arthrotec, Napratec

QUICK REFERENCE

Drug group Anti-ulcer drug (p.41)

Overdose danger rating Low

Dependence rating Low

Prescription needed Yes

Available as generic No

GENERAL INFORMATION

Misoprostol reduces acid secretion in the stomach and promotes the healing of gastric and duodenal ulcers. These types of ulcer may be caused by aspirin (p.142) and non-steroidal anti-inflammatory drugs (NSAIDs, p.48), which block the body's synthesis of naturally occurring chemicals called prostaglandins. Misoprostol is a synthetic prostaglandin that acts as a substitute for some of the natural prostaglandins produced by the gut wall to prevent ulceration of the lining. It usually causes ulcers to heal in a few weeks, although it has been largely superseded by proton-pump inhibitors in this role. In some cases, misoprostol is given during treatment with aspirin or NSAIDs as a preventative measure, and combined preparations are available to reduce the likelihood of ulcers occurring.

The most common adverse effects are diarrhoea and indigestion; if these are severe, it may be necessary to stop taking the drug.

Misoprostol also causes the uterus to contract. This may lead to premature labour, so the drug must not be used in pregnancy. However, because of this effect, it may be used in medical termination of pregnancy. The information below relates only to anti-ulcer use.

INFORMATION FOR USERS

Your drug prescription is tailored for you. Do not alter dosage without checking with your doctor.

How taken/used Tablets.

Frequency and timing of doses 2–4 x daily, with or after food.

Adult dosage range 400–800mcg daily.

Onset of effect Within 24 hours.

Duration of action Up to 24 hours; some effects may be longer lasting.

Diet advice None.

Storage Keep in original container at room temperature out of the reach of children.

Missed dose Take as soon as you remember. If your next dose is due within 3 hours, take a single dose now and skip the next.

Stopping the drug Do not stop the drug without consulting your doctor; symptoms may recur.

Exceeding the dose An occasional unintentional extra dose is unlikely to be a cause for concern. But if you notice any unusual symptoms, or if a large overdose has been taken, tell your doctor.

POSSIBLE ADVERSE EFFECTS

The most common side effects are diarrhoea and indigestion. These may be reduced by spreading the doses out during the day. Taking the drug with food may be recommended. If diarrhoea or indigestion are severe, or if you experience severe nausea and vomiting, discuss with your doctor. More rarely, misoprostol may cause vaginal bleeding or bleeding between menstrual periods, abdominal pain, dizziness, or a rash. If any of these occur, consult your doctor; you should also stop taking the drug if you develop a rash.

INTERACTIONS

Magnesium-containing antacids may increase the severity of diarrhoea caused by misoprostol.

SPECIAL PRECAUTIONS

Be sure to tell your doctor if:

- You are or plan to become pregnant.
- You have had a stroke.
- You have heart problems.
- You have high blood pressure.
- You have bowel problems.
- You are taking other medicines.

Pregnancy Misoprostol should not be taken by women of childbearing age. In exceptional cases, it may be prescribed on the condition that effective contraception is used. If taken during pregnancy, the drug can cause the uterus to contract before the baby is due.

Breast-feeding Safety not established. Discuss with your doctor.

Infants and children Not recommended.

Over 60 No special problems.

Driving and hazardous work Avoid until you have learned how misoprostol affects you because the drug can cause dizziness.

Alcohol No problems expected, but excessive amounts may undermine the desired effect of the drug.

PROLONGED USE

No problems expected, but the drug is rarely required long term.

MODAFINIL

Brand name Provigil

Used in the following combined preparations None

QUICK REFERENCE

Drug group Nervous system stimulant (p.17)

Overdose danger rating Medium

Dependence rating Medium

Prescription needed Yes

Available as generic No

GENERAL INFORMATION

Modafinil is a nervous system stimulant used to relieve the excessive sleepiness associated with narcolepsy, obstructive sleep apnoea, and chronic shift work. It has some features in common with amfetamines, including a potential for dependence and abuse, but the risk of these issues is much lower with modafinil than with amfetamines. However, treatment should be initiated by a doctor with a specialist interest in sleep disorders and only after other efforts have been made to treat the underlying condition. The drug should not be given to people with severe or poorly controlled high blood pressure or heart disease.

INFORMATION FOR USERS

Your drug prescription is tailored for you. Do not alter dosage without checking with your doctor.

How taken/used Tablets.

Frequency and timing of doses Single dose in the morning; or twice daily, in the morning and at midday.

Adult dosage range 200–400 mg daily.

Onset of effect Within a few hours.
Duration of action 12–24 hours.
Diet advice None.
Storage Keep in original container at room temperature out of the reach of children.
Missed dose Take as soon as you remember if needed for relief of symptoms. If not needed, do not take the missed dose, and return to your normal dose schedule when necessary.
Stopping the drug Do not stop the drug without consulting your doctor; symptoms may recur.
Exceeding the dose An occasional unintentional extra dose is unlikely to cause problems. Large overdoses may cause insomnia, restlessness, confusion, high blood pressure, and fast heart rate. Notify your doctor immediately.

POSSIBLE ADVERSE EFFECTS

The most common adverse effect is headache. Other side effects include palpitations, a fast heart rate, dizziness, blurred vision, nausea, abdominal pain, decreased appetite, nervousness, and insomnia. Contact your doctor if any of these are severe or if chest pain, depression, or a rash occur; in the case of a rash, you should also stop taking the drug. If modafinil causes suicidal thoughts, stop taking the drug and contact your doctor immediately. There is also a risk of developing new mental health problems, or worsening existing ones, such as anxiety, depression (including suicidal thoughts), aggressive behaviour, or psychosis.

INTERACTIONS

Ciclosprin Modafinil reduces blood levels of ciclosporin.
Oral contraceptives Modafinil reduces the effectiveness of oestrogen-containing contraceptive pills; additional contraceptive methods should be used during treatment and for 2 months afterwards.
Phenytoin Modafinil may increase blood levels of phenytoin.
Antidepressants Modafinil may increase blood levels of antidepressants, so a lower dose of antidepressant may be required.
Warfarin Modafinil may increase warfarin's effects, so lower warfarin dose may be needed.

SPECIAL PRECAUTIONS

Be sure to tell your doctor if:
- You have a liver or kidney problem.
- You have high blood pressure.
- You have a heart problem.
- You have had a psychiatric illness.
- You have a history of alcohol or illicit substance misuse.
- You are taking any other medicine.

Pregnancy Not prescribed in pregnancy as the drug may cause birth defects. Discuss with your doctor.
Breast-feeding Safety not established. Discuss with your doctor.
Infants and children Not prescribed for children under 18 years.
Over 60 Increased likelihood of adverse effects. Reduced dose may therefore be necessary.
Driving and hazardous work Discuss with your doctor. Your underlying condition, and the risk of side effects such as blurred vision or dizziness, may make such activities inadvisable.
Alcohol No special problems.

PROLONGED USE

No special problems.
Monitoring If you have high blood pressure, regular blood pressure monitoring may be carried out.

MOMETASONE

Brand names Asmanex, Elocon, Nasonex
Used in the following combined preparations None

QUICK REFERENCE

Drug group Corticosteroid (p.78)
Overdose danger rating Low
Dependence rating Low
Prescription needed Yes
Available as generic Yes

GENERAL INFORMATION

Mometasone is a corticosteroid drug used as an inhaler to prevent asthma attacks and as a nasal spray to relieve the symptoms of allergic rhinitis. It is also used topically for the treatment of severe inflammatory skin disorders and in conditions such as eczema that have not responded to other corticosteroids (see Topical corticosteroids, p.118).

Serious adverse effects are rare if the drug is used for short periods or in small amounts, but prolonged or excessive topical use may cause local side effects such as thin skin and systemic side effects such as osteoporosis, muscle weakness, and peptic ulcers.

Fungal infections causing irritation of the mouth and throat are a possible side effect of inhaling mometasone. These can be avoided to some degree by rinsing the mouth and gargling with water after each inhalation.

INFORMATION FOR USERS

Your drug prescription is tailored for you. Do not alter dosage without checking with your doctor.
How taken/used Cream, ointment, scalp lotion, inhaler, powder for inhalation, nasal spray.
Frequency and timing of doses 1 x 2 times daily (inhaler); once daily (other forms).
Adult dosage range *Inhaler* 200–800mcg. *Nasal spray* 100mcg (2 puffs) into each nostril. *Topical preparations* As directed, applied thinly.
Onset of effect 12 hours. Full beneficial effect after 48 hours.
Duration of action 24 hours. Effects can last for several days after the drug is stopped.
Diet advice None.
Storage Keep in original container at room temperature out of the reach of children.
Missed dose Take as soon as you remember. If your next dose/application is due within 8 hours, take a single dose or apply the usual amount now and skip the next.
Stopping the drug Do not stop the drug without consulting your doctor; symptoms may recur.
Exceeding the dose An occasional unintentional extra dose/application may not be a cause for concern, but if you notice any unusual symptoms, notify your doctor.

POSSIBLE ADVERSE EFFECTS

Serious adverse effects are unlikely when the drug is used at low doses and/or for short periods. With the inhaler or nasal spray, the most common side effects are irritation of the nasal lining, cough, and bruising. Discuss with your doctor if these are severe or if you develop a sore throat, hoarseness, or nosebleeds. More serious side effects, such as permanent skin changes, may occur with long-term use of the cream or ointment, which should not normally be used on the face. Discuss with your doctor if you notice any such changes. Long-term use of any form of mometasone may cause various disorders (see Prolonged use).

INTERACTIONS

Ketoconazole and itraconazole may increase the systemic effects of mometasone.
HIV protease inhibitors may increase the effect of mometasone.
Macrolides (clarithromycin) may increase the effect of mometasone.
Desmopressin with mometasone may increase the risk of low sodium levels.

SPECIAL PRECAUTIONS

Be sure to tell your doctor if:
- You have had tuberculosis or another respiratory infection.
- You have any other nasal or skin infection.
- You have had recent nasal ulcers or nasal surgery.

Pregnancy Safety not established. Discuss with your doctor.
Breast-feeding No evidence of risk. Discuss with your doctor.
Infants and children Only used for very short courses in children.
Over 60 No special problems.
Driving and hazardous work No special problems.
Alcohol No special problems.

PROLONGED USE

Long-term use can lead to peptic ulcers, glaucoma, muscle weakness, osteoporosis, growth retardation in children, and, rarely, adrenal gland suppression. Prolonged use of topical treatment may also lead to skin thinning. Patients on long-term treatment should carry a steroid card or wear a MedicAlert bracelet.
Monitoring Periodic checks on adrenal gland function may be required if large doses are being taken. Children should have their height monitored.

MONTELUKAST

Brand name Singulair
Used in the following combined preparations None

QUICK REFERENCE

Drug group Anti-allergy drug (p.56)
Overdose danger rating Low
Dependence rating Low
Prescription needed Yes
Available as generic Yes

GENERAL INFORMATION

Montelukast belongs to the leukotriene receptor antagonist (blocker) group of anti-allergy drugs and is used in preventing asthma and allergic rhinitis. It is thought that stimulation of leukotriene receptors by naturally occurring leukotrienes from the mast cells (p.56) plays a part in causing asthma. Montelukast works by blocking these receptors.

The drug is given as an additional medication for asthma when combined treatment with corticosteroids and bronchodilators does not give adequate control. It is given by mouth as chewable tablets or granules.

Montelukast is not a bronchodilator and cannot be used to treat an acute asthma attack.

INFORMATION FOR USERS

Your drug prescription is tailored for you. Do not alter dosage without checking with your doctor.

How taken/used Chewable tablets, granules.

Frequency and timing of doses Once daily at bedtime.

Adult dosage range 10mg.

Onset of effect 2 hours.

Duration of action 24 hours.

Diet advice None.

Storage Keep in original container at room temperature out of the reach of children. Protect from light.

Missed dose Take as soon as you remember. If your next dose is due within 8 hours, take a single dose now and skip the next.

Stopping the drug Do not stop without consulting your doctor as symptoms may recur.

Exceeding the dose An occasional unintentional extra dose is unlikely to be a cause for concern. But if you notice any unusual symptoms, or if a large overdose has been taken, tell your doctor.

POSSIBLE ADVERSE EFFECTS

The most common adverse effects of montelukast are abdominal pain and headache. The drug may also cause nausea, vomiting, diarrhoea, dizziness, agitation, and weakness. Discuss with your doctor if any of these are severe. You should also consult your doctor if you have a fever or flulike symptoms, or if you develop a productive cough, rash, numbness or tingling, or worsening chest symptoms. Severe effects are very rare, but neuropsychiatric reactions including speech impairment and obsessive-compulsive symptoms have been reported. Very rarely, patients taking montelukast have developed features of an inflammatory condition called Churg-Strauss syndrome, which can mimic asthma.

INTERACTIONS

Phenytoin, rifampicin, carbamazepine, and phenobarbital reduce blood levels of montelukast.

Clopidogrel, gemfibrozil, and leflunomide increase blood levels of montelukast.

SPECIAL PRECAUTIONS

Be sure to tell your doctor if:

- You have phenylketonuria.
- You have galactose intolerance.
- You have lactose intolerance.
- You are taking other medicines.

Pregnancy Safety not established. Discuss with your doctor.

Breast-feeding Safety not established. Discuss with your doctor.

Infants and children Reduced dose necessary.

Over 60 No special problems.

Driving and hazardous work Avoid until you know how montelukast affects you because the drug can cause dizziness and drowsiness.

Alcohol No special problems.

PROLONGED USE

No special problems.

MORPHINE/DIAMORPHINE

Brand names Filnarine SR, Morphgesic SR, MST Continus, MXL, Oramorph, Oramorph SR, Sevredol, Zomorph

Used in the following combined preparations Cyclimorph, J. Collis Browne's Mixture, Kaolin and Morphine Mixture

QUICK REFERENCE

Drug group Opioid analgesic (p.7)

Overdose danger rating High

Dependence rating High

Prescription needed Yes (except low-dose antidiarrhoea and cough medicines)

Available as generic Yes

GENERAL INFORMATION

Morphine and diamorphine are opioid analgesics. They are used to relieve severe pain from heart attack, injury, surgery, or chronic diseases such as cancer. They are also sometimes given as premedication before surgery, or to ease breathlessness in patients with pulmonary oedema (fluid on the lungs) or who are terminally ill. Their painkilling effect wears off quickly, so they may be given in a slow-release (long-acting) form for continous severe pain.

These drugs are habit-forming, and dependence and addiction can occur. However, most patients who take them for pain relief over brief periods do not become dependent and are able to stop taking them without difficulty.

Very small amounts of morphine are also included in some over-the-counter medicines for treating diarrhoea and suppressing coughs. These uses are not covered in the information given below.

INFORMATION FOR USERS

Your drug prescription is tailored for you. Do not alter dosage without checking with your doctor.

How taken/used Tablets, slow release (SR) tablets, capsules, SR capsules, liquid, SR granules, injection, suppositories, SR suppositories.

Frequency and timing of doses Every 4 hours; every 12–24 hours (SR preparations).

Adult dosage range 2.5–25mg per dose; however, some patients may need 75mg or more per dose. Doses vary considerably for each user.

Onset of effect Within 1 hour; within 4 hours (SR preparations).

Duration of action 4 hours; up to 24 hours (SR preparations).

Diet advice None.

Storage Keep in original container at room temperature out of the reach of children.

Missed dose Take as soon as you remember. Return to your normal dosing schedule as soon as possible.

Stopping the drug If the reason for taking the drug no longer exists, you may stop the drug and notify your doctor.

OVERDOSE ACTION

Seek immediate medical advice in all cases. Take emergency action if symptoms such as slow or irregular breathing, severe drowsiness, or loss of consciousness occur.

POSSIBLE ADVERSE EFFECTS

Nausea, vomiting, and constipation are common, especially with high doses; anti-nausea drugs or laxatives may be needed to counteract these symptoms. Drowsiness, dizziness, headache, confusion, and itching are also common. Consult your doctor if you have severe digestive problems, drowsiness, or any of these other effects. If breathing difficulties or impaired consciousness occur, stop taking the drug and contact your doctor immediately.

INTERACTIONS

Monoamine oxidase inhibitors (MAOIs) may produce a severe rise in blood pressure when taken with morphine and diamorphine.

Esmolol Effects may be increased by these drugs.

Sedatives Drugs increase risk of respiratory depression with alcohol, antidepressants, antipsychotics, sleeping drugs, and antihistamines.

Buprenorphine and pentazocine increase the risk of opiate withdrawal with these drugs.

SPECIAL PRECAUTIONS

Be sure to tell your doctor if:

- You have long-term liver or kidney problems.
- You have heart or circulatory problems.
- You have a lung disorder such as asthma or bronchitis.
- You have thyroid disease.
- You have a history of epileptic seizures.
- You have a history of prostate or urinary problems.
- You are taking other medicines.

Pregnancy Not usually prescribed. May cause breathing difficulties in the newborn baby. Discuss with your doctor.

Breast-feeding The drug passes into the breast milk, but at low doses adverse effects on the baby are unlikely. Discuss with your doctor.

Infants and children Reduced dose necessary.

Over 60 Increased likelihood of adverse effects. Reduced dose may therefore be necessary.

Driving and hazardous work People on morphine unlikely to be well enough for such activities.

Alcohol Avoid. Alcohol may increase the sedative effects of these drugs.

PROLONGED USE

The effects usually become weaker as the body adapts. Dependence may occur if the drugs are used for extended periods, although this is unusual with the correct dose for pain relief.

MOXONIDINE

Brand name Physiotens

Used in the following combined preparations None

QUICK REFERENCE

Drug group Antihypertensive drug (p.34)

Overdose danger rating Medium

Dependence rating Low

Prescription needed Yes

Available as generic Yes

GENERAL INFORMATION

Moxonidine is an antihypertensive drug that is related to clonidine but is more selective and may therefore have fewer side effects. It works by stimulating alpha-receptors (p.7) within the central nervous system, reducing the signals that constrict the blood vessels. Moxonidine also reduces resistance to blood flow in the peripheral blood vessels.

The drug is less likely than clonidine to cause dry mouth, and, unlike clonidine, has no effect on blood fat levels or glucose. However, other side effects, such as headache and dizziness, may still occur.

INFORMATION FOR USERS

Your drug prescription is tailored for you. Do not alter dosage without checking with your doctor.
How taken/used Tablets.
Frequency and timing of doses Once daily in the morning (initially); 1–2 x daily.
Adult dosage range 200mcg daily initially; increasing after 3 weeks to 400mcg daily, if necessary; increasing again after a further 3 weeks to maximum of 600mcg daily in 2 divided doses if necessary.
Onset of effect 30–180 minutes.
Duration of action 12 hours.
Diet advice None.
Storage Keep in original container at room temperature out of the reach of children.
Missed dose Take as soon as you remember. If your next dose is due within 4 hours, take a single dose now and skip the next.
Stopping the drug Do not stop taking the drug without consulting your doctor, who will supervise a gradual reduction in dosage over a period of 2 weeks.
Exceeding the dose An occasional unintentional extra dose is unlikely to cause problems. Large overdoses may cause drowsiness and a fall in blood pressure.

POSSIBLE ADVERSE EFFECTS

Common side effects of moxonidine include dry mouth, headache, weakness, and fatigue. More rarely, the drug may cause dizziness, nausea, sleep disturbance, sedation, and a rash. Side effects that appear at the start of treatment often decrease in frequency and intensity during the course of treatment. Discuss with your doctor if any of the adverse effects are persistent or severe.

INTERACTIONS

Other antihypertensives, thymoxamine, moxisylyte, and muscle relaxants may increase the blood-pressure-lowering effect of moxonidine.
Sedatives and hypnotics The effect of these drugs may be increased by moxonidine.
Tricyclic antidepressants The effects of these drugs may be increased by moxonidine.

SPECIAL PRECAUTIONS

Be sure to tell your doctor if:
◆ You have liver or kidney problems.
◆ You have heart problems, especially affecting your heart rhythm.
◆ You are taking other medicines.

Pregnancy Safety not established. Discuss with your doctor.
Breast-feeding Safety in breast-feeding not established. Discuss with your doctor.
Infants and children Not recommended.
Over 60 No special problems.
Driving and hazardous work Avoid such activities until you have learned how moxonidine affects you because the drug can cause drowsiness and dizziness.
Alcohol Avoid. Alcohol may increase the sedative effects of this drug.

PROLONGED USE

No special problems.

NAFTIDROFURYL

Brand name Praxilene
Used in the following combined preparations None

QUICK REFERENCE

Drug group Vasodilator (p.30)
Overdose danger rating Medium
Dependence rating Low
Prescription needed Yes
Available as generic Yes

GENERAL INFORMATION

Naftidrofuryl is a vasodilator drug used in the treatment of peripheral circulatory disorders such as Raynaud's syndrome or intermittent claudication (cramplike pain). Most of these conditions are caused by blockage of blood vessels due to spasms or sclerosis (hardening) of the vessel walls.

Naftidrofuryl may improve symptoms and mobility in these conditions, but it is not known if it has any influence on their progress. Lifestyle changes such as giving up smoking and taking exercise (and keeping warm in the case of Raynaud's) are often helpful.

The drug has also been used for treating night cramps, but it is not known how it works to reduce them. It has also been tried for circulatory disorders in the brain.

INFORMATION FOR USERS

Your drug prescription is tailored for you. Do not alter dosage without checking with your doctor.

How taken/used Capsules.

Frequency and timing of doses 3 x daily with meals, swallowed whole with at least one glass of water.

Adult dosage range 300–600mg daily.

Onset of effect 1 hour.

Duration of action 8 hours.

Diet advice Drink plenty of water during treatment.

Storage Keep in original container at room temperature out of the reach of children.

Missed dose Take when you remember. If your next dose is due within 2 hours, take a single dose now and skip the next.

Stopping the drug Do not stop without consulting your doctor; symptoms may recur.

Exceeding the dose An occasional unintentional extra dose is unlikely to cause problems. Large overdoses may cause heart problems and seizures. Notify your doctor immediately.

POSSIBLE ADVERSE EFFECTS

Naftidrofuryl is generally well tolerated. Its most common adverse effect is nausea. Rarely, chest pain, rash, jaundice, or seizures may occur. Consult your doctor if you have severe nausea or any of the rarer side effects. If you have jaundice or seizures, stop taking the drug.

INTERACTIONS

None known.

SPECIAL PRECAUTIONS

Be sure to tell your doctor if:

- ◆ You have liver or kidney problems.
- ◆ You are taking other medicines.

Pregnancy Safety not established. Discuss with your doctor.

Breast-feeding Safety not established. Discuss with your doctor.

Infants and children Not recommended.

Over 60 No special problems.

Driving and hazardous work No special problems.

Alcohol No special problems.

PROLONGED USE

Treatment should be reviewed after 3 months to see if the condition is improving, or if the drug should be stopped.

NAPROXEN

Brand names Feminax, Naprosyn, Nexocin, Stirlescent, and others

Used in the following combined preparation Vimovo (with esomeprazole)

QUICK REFERENCE

Drug group Non-steroidal anti-inflammatory drug (p.48) and drug for gout (p.51)

Overdose danger rating Medium

Dependence rating Low

Prescription needed Yes

Available as generic Yes

GENERAL INFORMATION

Naproxen, a non-steroidal anti-inflammatory drugs (NSAID), is used to reduce pain, stiffness, and inflammation. The drug relieves the symptoms of adult and juvenile rheumatoid arthritis, ankylosing spondylitis, and osteoarthritis, although it does not cure the disease. It is used to treat acute attacks of gout, and may sometimes be prescribed to relieve migraine or pain following orthopaedic surgery, dental treatment, strains, and sprains. It is also effective for treating painful menstrual cramps.

Gastrointestinal side effects are fairly common, and there is an increased risk of bleeding. Hence, for long-term use, naproxen is often prescribed with a gastro-protective drug.

INFORMATION FOR USERS

Your drug prescription is tailored for you. Do not alter dosage without checking with your doctor.

How taken/used Tablets, liquid.

Frequency and timing of doses Every 6–8 hours as required (general pain relief); 1–2 x daily (arthritis); every 6–8 hours (gout). All doses should be taken with or after food.

Adult dosage range *Mild to moderate pain, menstrual cramps* 500mg (starting dose), then 250mg every 6–8 hours as required. *Arthritis* 500–1,000mg daily. *Gout* 750mg (starting dose), then 250mg every 8 hours until attack has subsided.

Onset of effect Pain relief begins within 1 hour. Full anti-inflammatory effect may take 2 weeks.

Duration of action Up to 12 hours.

Diet advice None.

Storage Keep in original container at room temperature out of the reach of children. Protect from light.

Missed dose Take as soon as you remember. If your next dose is due within 4 hours, take a single dose now and skip the next.

Stopping the drug When taken for short-term pain relief, naproxen can be safely stopped as soon as you no longer need it. If prescribed for long-term treatment, however, you should seek medical advice before stopping the drug.

Exceeding the dose An occasional unintentional extra dose is unlikely to be a cause for concern. But if you notice any unusual symptoms, or if a large overdose has been taken, tell your doctor.

POSSIBLE ADVERSE EFFECTS

Most adverse effects are not serious and may diminish with time. Indigestion or heartburn, nausea, and vomiting are common. More rarely, headache, drowsiness, dizziness, swelling of the legs or feet, or weight gain may occur. Discuss with your doctor if any of these are severe. If you develop a rash or itching, stop taking the drug and consult your doctor. If you have wheezing or breathlessness, or black or bloodstained faeces, or you vomit blood (which may look like coffee grounds), stop the drug and contact your doctor without delay.

INTERACTIONS

General note Naproxen interacts with a wide range of drugs to increase the risk of bleeding and/or peptic ulcers. It may also increase blood levels of lithium, methotrexate, and digoxin.

Antihypertensive drugs and diuretics The benefit of these drugs may be reduced by naproxen and the risk of kidney damage increased.

Ciclosporin Naproxen increases the risk of kidney impairment with this drug.

SPECIAL PRECAUTIONS

Be sure to tell your doctor if:

◆ You have long-term liver or kidney problems.

◆ You have heart problems or high blood pressure.

◆ You have a bleeding disorder.

◆ You have had a peptic ulcer, oesophagitis, or acid indigestion.

◆ You are allergic to aspirin or other NSAIDs.

◆ You have asthma.

◆ You are taking other medicines.

Pregnancy The drug may increase the risks of adverse effects on the baby's heart and may prolong labour if taken in the third trimester. Discuss with your doctor.

Breast-feeding The drug passes into the breast milk, but normal doses are unlikely to affect the baby adversely. Discuss with your doctor.

Infants and children Prescribed only to treat juvenile arthritis. Reduced dose necessary.

Over 60 Increased likelihood of adverse effects. Reduced dose may therefore be necessary.

Driving and hazardous work Avoid such activities until you have learned how naproxen affects you because the drug may reduce your ability to concentrate.

Alcohol Avoid. Alcohol may increase the risk of stomach irritation with naproxen.

Surgery and general anaesthetics Naproxen may prolong bleeding. Discuss with your doctor or dentist before surgery.

PROLONGED USE

There is an increased risk of bleeding from peptic ulcers and in the bowel with prolonged use of naproxen. There is also a small risk of a heart attack or stroke. To minimize these risks, the lowest effective dose is given for the shortest duration.

NICORANDIL

Brand name Ikorel

Used in the following combined preparations None

QUICK REFERENCE

Drug group Anti-angina drug (p.33)

Overdose danger rating Medium

Dependence rating Low

Prescription needed Yes

Available as generic No

GENERAL INFORMATION

Nicorandil is the only generally available member of a group of drugs known as potassium channel openers. It is used to treat angina pectoris.

The symptoms of angina result from the failure of narrowed coronary blood vessels to deliver sufficient oxygen to the heart. Nicorandil acts to widen blood vessels. It works by a different mechanism to other anti-angina drugs, and is notable because it widens both veins and arteries. As a result of this action, more oxygen-carrying blood reaches the heart muscle, and the heart's workload is reduced since the resistance against which it has to pump is decreased.

Nicorandil is as effective as other drugs used to treat angina, and when used in combination with others may add to their effects.

INFORMATION FOR USERS

Your drug prescription is tailored for you. Do not alter dosage without checking with your doctor.
How taken/used Tablets.
Frequency and timing of doses 2 x daily.
Adult dosage range 10–80mg daily.
Onset of effect Within 1 hour.
Duration of action Approximately 12 hours.
Diet advice None.
Storage Keep in original container at room temperature out of the reach of children.
Missed dose Take as soon as you remember. If your next dose is due within 4 hours, take a single dose now and skip the next.
Stopping the drug Do not stop without consulting your doctor; stopping the drug may lead to worsening of the underlying condition.
Exceeding the dose An occasional unintentional extra dose is unlikely to cause problems, but large overdoses may cause unusual dizziness and dangerously low blood pressure. Notify your doctor.

POSSIBLE ADVERSE EFFECTS

Adverse effects of nicorandil are generally minor and usually wear off with continued treatment, although a dose reduction may be necessary in some cases. Headache, flushing, nausea, and vomiting are common; discuss with your doctor if these are severe. If you develop mouth, genital, or anal ulcers, dizziness, weakness, jaundice, facial swelling, or rash, contact your doctor; in the case of a rash, you should also stop taking the drug. If you experience palpitations, stop taking the drug and contact your doctor immediately.

INTERACTIONS

Antihypertensive drugs Nicorandil may increase the effects of these drugs.
Sildenafil, tadalafil, and vardenafil increase the effects of nicorandil on blood pressure and should not be used with nicorandil.
MAOI and tricyclic antidepressant drugs may increase the effects of nicorandil on blood pressure, resulting in dizziness.

SPECIAL PRECAUTIONS

Be sure to tell your doctor if:
- You have low blood pressure.
- You have other heart problems.
- You have a history of angioedema.
- You are taking other medicines.

Pregnancy Safety in pregnancy not established. Discuss with your doctor.
Breast-feeding Safety not established. Discuss with your doctor.
Infants and children Not recommended.
Over 60 Reduced dose may be necessary.
Driving and hazardous work Avoid such activities until you have learned how nicorandil affects you because the drug can cause dizziness as a result of lowered blood pressure.
Alcohol Avoid until you are accustomed to the effect of nicorandil. Alcohol may further reduce blood pressure, causing dizziness or other symptoms.

PROLONGED USE

No problems expected.

NICOTINE

Brand names NicAssist, Nicorette, Nicotinell, NiQuitin
Used in the following combined preparations None

QUICK REFERENCE

Drug group Smoking cessation aid
Overdose danger rating Medium
Dependence rating Low
Prescription needed No
Available as generic Yes

GENERAL INFORMATION

Smoking is a difficult habit to stop due to the addiction to nicotine and the psychological aspects of smoking. Taking nicotine in a different form can help the smoker deal with both aspects.

Nicotine is supplied as chewing gum, nasal spray, sublingual tablets, skin patches, lozenges, and inhalator for the relief of withdrawal symptoms. Patches should be applied every

24 hours to unbroken, dry, non-hairy skin on the trunk or the upper arm. Replacement patches should be applied to a different area, and the previous area avoided for several days. The strength of the patch is gradually reduced until abstinence is achieved. The lozenges, chewing gum, nasal spray, and inhalator are used when the urge to smoke occurs.

Electronic cigarettes (e-cigarettes) containing nicotine are also available, and there is evidence that they can help you stop smoking. However, there are none licensed as medicines in the UK, so they are not covered below.

INFORMATION FOR USERS

Follow instructions on the label.

How taken/used Sublingual tablets, lozenges, chewing gum, skin patches, nasal spray, inhalator.

Frequency and timing of doses Hourly (tablets and lozenges); every 24 hours, removing the patch after 16 hours (patches); when the urge to smoke is felt (gum, inhalator, or spray).

Adult dosage range Will depend upon previous smoking habits. 7–22mg per day (patches); 1 x 2mg piece to 15 x 4mg pieces per day (gum); up to 64 x 0.5mg puffs (spray).

Onset of effect A few hours (patches); within minutes (other forms).

Duration of action Up to 24 hours (patches); 30 minutes (other forms).

Diet advice None.

Storage Keep in original container at room temperature out of the reach of children.

Missed dose Change your patch as soon as you remember, and keep the new patch on for the required amount of time before removing it.

Stopping the drug The dose of nicotine is normally reduced gradually.

Exceeding the dose Application of several nicotine patches at the same time could result in serious overdosage. Remove the patches and seek immediate medical help. Overdosage with the tablets, lozenges, gum, or spray can occur only if tablets or lozenges are taken more often than every hour, if many pieces of gum are chewed simultaneously, or if the spray is used more than 4 times an hour. Seek immediate medical help.

POSSIBLE ADVERSE EFFECTS

Nicotine replacement preparations commonly cause local irritation. Patches may cause a skin reaction (which usually disappears in a couple of days); the oral or inhaled forms may cause irritation of the nose or throat, affect taste, and cause a dry mouth. All forms commonly cause headache, dizziness, nausea, indigestion, cold- or flulike symptoms, and insomnia; discuss with your doctor if any of these symptoms are severe. More rarely, chest pains or palpitations may occur; if so, you should consult your doctor immediately.

INTERACTIONS

General note Stopping smoking may increase blood levels of some drugs (such as warfarin, theophylline/aminophylline, and antipsychotic drugs). Discuss with your doctor or pharmacist. Nicotine patches, chewing gums, and nasal spray should not be used with other nicotine-containing products, including cigarettes and e-cigarettes.

SPECIAL PRECAUTIONS

Be sure to consult your doctor or pharmacist before taking this drug if:

- You have long-term liver or kidney problems.
- You have diabetes mellitus.
- You have thyroid disease.
- You have or have had any heart problems, including hypertension and stroke.
- You have a history of peptic ulcers.
- You have phaeochromocytoma.
- You are taking other medicines.

Pregnancy Nicotine should be avoided altogether in pregnancy, but tobacco withdrawal using nicotine replacement may be recommended for pregnant smokers unable to quit.

Breast-feeding Nicotine is found in breast milk, but using nicotine replacement to stop smoking is less hazardous than continuing to smoke while breast-feeding.

Infants and children Nicotine is extremely toxic to small children and may even sometimes be fatal. They should therefore not be exposed to it, and nicotine replacement products should be disposed of very carefully.

Over 60 No special problems.

Driving and hazardous work Usually no problems with nicotine.

Alcohol No special problems.

PROLONGED USE

Nicotine replacement therapy should not normally be used for more than 3 to 6 months.

NIFEDIPINE

Brand names Adalat, Adipine, Coracten, Fortipine LA, Hyolar Retard 20, Nifedipress MR, Tensipine MR, Valni, and others

Used in the following combined preparations Beta-Adalat, Tenif

QUICK REFERENCE

Drug group Anti-angina drug (p.33) and antihypertensive drug (p.34)

Overdose danger rating Medium

Dependence rating Low

Prescription needed Yes

Available as generic Yes

GENERAL INFORMATION

Nifedipine belongs to a group of drugs known as calcium channel blockers. Their main effect is to relax smooth muscle in the arteries supplying the heart muscle and other parts of the body. This improves blood supply to the heart and lowers blood pressure.

The drug is given on a regular basis to help prevent angina attacks but is not used to treat acute attacks. It can be used safely by people with asthma, unlike some other anti-angina drugs (such as beta blockers). It is also widely used to reduce high blood pressure and is often helpful in improving circulation to the limbs in disorders such as Raynaud's disease.

Like other drugs of its class, it may cause blood pressure to fall too low, and occasionally causes disturbances of heart rhythm. In rare cases, it may cause angina to worsen.

INFORMATION FOR USERS

Your drug prescription is tailored for you. Do not alter dosage without checking with your doctor.

How taken/used Tablets, capsules, slow release (SR) tablets, SR capsules.

Frequency and timing of doses 3 x daily; 1–2 x daily (SR preparations).

Adult dosage range 15–90mg daily.

Onset of effect 20–60 minutes.

Duration of action 6–24 hours.

Diet advice Nifedipine should not be taken with grapefruit juice.

Storage Keep in original container at room temperature out of the reach of children. Protect from light.

Missed dose Take as soon as you remember, or when needed. If your next dose is due within 3 hours, take a single dose now and skip the next one.

Stopping the drug Do not stop taking the drug without consulting your doctor; sudden withdrawal may make angina worse.

Exceeding the dose An occasional unintentional extra dose is unlikely to cause problems, but large overdoses may cause dizziness. Notify your doctor.

POSSIBLE ADVERSE EFFECTS

Common side effects include headache; flushing; dizziness, especially on rising, which may be due to reduced blood pressure; ankle swelling; palpitations; heartburn; and nausea. More rarely, there may be diarrhoea, bloating, frequency in passing urine, and a rash. If any of these effects are severe, discuss with your doctor. The severity or frequency of angina attacks may increase. If this happens to you, tell your doctor; you may need an adjustment in dosage or a change of drug.

INTERACTIONS

General note Nifedipine may interfere with the beneficial effects of drugs such as carbamazepine, ciclosporin, magnesium (by injection), tacrolimus, and theophylline.

Antihypertensive drugs Nifedipine may increase the effects of these drugs.

Phenytoin and rifampicin These drugs may reduce the effects of nifedipine.

Digoxin Nifedipine may increase the effects and toxicity of digoxin.

Erythromycin, fluoxetine, some anti-HIV drugs, and antifungals may increase levels of nifedipine.

Grapefruit juice may block the breakdown of nifedipine, increasing its effects.

SPECIAL PRECAUTIONS

Be sure to tell your doctor if:

- You have liver or kidney problem.
- You have heart failure.
- You have had a recent heart attack.
- You have aortic stenosis or obstructive hypertrophic cardiomyopathy.
- You have diabetes.
- You have porphyria.
- You are taking other medicines.

Pregnancy May inhibit labour, but the small risk to the baby has to be weighed against the risk to the mother of uncontrolled hypertension. Discuss with your doctor.

Breast-feeding The drug passes into the breast milk, but only in amounts that are probably too small to harm your baby. Discuss with your doctor.
Infants and children Not recommended.
Over 60 Increased risk of adverse effects. Reduced dose may therefore be necessary.
Driving and hazardous work Avoid such activities until you have learned how nifedipine affects you because the drug can cause dizziness as a result of lowered blood pressure.
Alcohol Avoid. Alcohol may increase the blood-pressure-lowering effects of nifedipine.
Surgery and general anaesthetics Nifedipine may interact with some general anaesthetics, causing a fall in blood pressure. Discuss this with your doctor or dentist before any surgery.

PROLONGED USE
No problems expected.

NITRAZEPAM

Brand names Mogadon
Used in the following combined preparations None

QUICK REFERENCE
Drug group Benzodiazepine sleeping drug (p.10)
Overdose danger rating Medium
Dependence rating High
Prescription needed Yes
Available as generic Yes

GENERAL INFORMATION
Nitrazepam is a benzodiazepine drug used for the short-term treatment of insomnia. Benzodiazepines relieve tension and nervousness, relax muscles, and encourage sleep.

Nitrazepam is long-acting, so when it is taken at night it often produces "hangover" effects the next day. When taken every night, its effects steadily accumulate. Therefore, short courses of 1 or 2 weeks are usually prescribed. Long-term use of the drug leads to daytime sedation, tolerance, and dependence.

Stopping nitrazepam after prolonged use produces rebound insomnia, anxiety, and a withdrawal syndrome that may include confusion, toxic psychosis, and seizures. In this situation, the dosage may need to be tapered off over a period of many weeks.

It is recommended that benzodiazepines should be used to treat insomnia only when the problem is short-term and severe, disabling, or very distressing.

INFORMATION FOR USERS
Your drug prescription is tailored for you. Do not alter dosage without checking with your doctor.
How taken/used Tablets, liquid.
Frequency and timing of doses Once daily, at bedtime.
Adult dosage range 5–10mg daily.
Onset of effect 1–2 hours.
Duration of action 24 hours or more.
Diet advice None.
Storage Keep in original container at room temperature out of the reach of children.
Missed dose If you fall asleep without having taken a dose and wake some hours later, do not take the missed dose. If necessary, return to your normal schedule the following night.
Stopping the drug If you have taken the drug for 2 weeks or less, it can be safely stopped. If you have been taking the drug for longer, consult your doctor, who may supervise a gradual reduction in dosage. Stopping abruptly may lead to withdrawal symptoms.
Exceeding the dose An occasional unintentional extra dose is unlikely to be a cause for concern. Large overdoses may cause unusual drowsiness. Notify your doctor.

POSSIBLE ADVERSE EFFECTS
The main adverse effects of nitrazepam are related mainly to its sedative and tranquillizing properties. The most common include drowsiness the next day, confusion, forgetfulness, uncoordinated walking, dizziness, and double vision. More rarely, the drug may cause headache or vertigo. If any of these effects are severe, or if you experience mood changes or restlessness, discuss with your doctor.

INTERACTIONS
Sedatives All drugs that have a sedative effect on the central nervous system are likely to increase the sedative properties and risk of respiratory depression with nitrazepam. They include alcohol, other sleeping drugs, anti-anxiety drugs, antihistamines, opioid analgesics, antidepressants, and antipsychotics.
Rifampicin reduces the effect of nitrazepam.
Anticonvulsants The side effects and toxicity of these drugs may be increased by nitrazepam.
Ritonavir may raise blood level of nitrazepam.

SPECIAL PRECAUTIONS

Be sure to tell your doctor if:

- You have severe respiratory disease.
- You have kidney or liver problems.
- You have myasthenia gravis.
- You have sleep apnoea.
- You have acute porphyria.
- You are taking other medicines.

Pregnancy Safety not established. Known to affect the developing fetus. The baby may be born with dependence and have withdrawal symptoms. Discuss with your doctor.

Breast-feeding Avoid. Nitrazepam passes into the breast milk.

Infants and children Not recommended

Over 60 Older people are more likely to have adverse effects. Reduced dose and treatment duration are necessary.

Driving and hazardous work Do not drive. The drug's effects persist during the day after taking a dose. It reduces alertness, slows reactions, impairs concentration, and causes drowsiness.

Alcohol Avoid. Alcohol will add to the sedative effects of the drug.

PROLONGED USE

Not recommended. Produces tolerance and dependence.

NORETHISTERONE

Brand names Micronor, Noriday, Noristerat, Primolut N, Utovlan

Used in the following combined preparations Brevinor, Climagest, Elleste Duet, Loestrin, Norinyl, Synphase, and others

QUICK REFERENCE

Drug group Female sex hormone (p.86)

Overdose danger rating Low

Dependence rating Low

Prescription needed Yes

Available as generic Yes

GENERAL INFORMATION

Norethisterone is a synthetic hormone similar to the natural female sex hormone progesterone. A major use of the drug is as an oral contraceptive (p.103), either on its own or with an oestrogen; it is also available in an injectable form. Other uses include postponing menstruation and treating menstrual disorders (p.102) such as endometriosis and dysmenorrhoea. When used for these disorders, it is taken only on certain days of the menstrual cycle. In combination with oestrogens, it is also prescribed as hormone replacement therapy (HRT), which is usually only advised for short-term use around the menopause (p.87), and in the treatment of certain breast cancers.

Adverse effects are rare, but oral contraceptives may cause breakthrough bleeding between menstrual periods (see below).

INFORMATION FOR USERS

Your drug prescription is tailored for you. Do not alter dosage without checking with your doctor.

How taken/used Tablets, injection, skin patch.

Frequency and timing of doses 1–3 x daily (tablets); once every 8 weeks (injection); 2 x weekly (skin patch).

Adult dosage range *Menstrual disorders* 10–15mg daily; *Postponing menstruation* 15mg daily; *Progestogen-only contraceptives* 350mcg daily; *HRT* 700mcg–1mg daily; *Cancer* 30–60mg daily.

Onset of effect Within a few hours.

Duration of action 24 hours (tablets); about 3.5 days (patch); 8 weeks (injection).

Diet advice None.

Storage Keep in original container at room temperature out of the reach of children. Protect from light.

Missed dose Take as soon as you remember. If you are taking the drug for contraception, see What to do if you miss a pill (p.107).

Stopping the drug The drug can be safely stopped as soon as contraceptive protection is no longer required. If prescribed for an underlying disorder, do not stop without consulting your doctor. When the drug is used to treat menstrual disorders, a normal period should occur 2 to 3 days after it is stopped.

Exceeding the dose An occasional unintentional extra dose is unlikely to be a cause for concern. But if you notice any unusual symptoms, or if a large overdose has been taken, tell your doctor.

POSSIBLE ADVERSE EFFECTS

Adverse effects are rarely troublesome and are generally typical of progestogens. The most common is breakthrough bleeding, which should be discussed with your doctor. More rarely, the drug may cause swelling of the ankles or feet, breast tenderness, weight gain, acne, and discoloration of the skin. Discuss with your doctor if these are severe or if you have headaches or depression. If you experience pain or tightness in the chest, or disturbances of vision or hearing, stop taking the drug and contact your doctor immediately. Rarely, prolonged treatment may cause jaundice due to liver damage; if jaundice occurs, stop taking the drug and contact your doctor. However, prolonged use is not generally recommended due to the increased health risks.

INTERACTIONS

General note Norethisterone may interfere with the beneficial effects of many drugs, including oral anticoagulants, anticonvulsants, antihypertensives, and drugs for diabetes. Many other drugs may reduce the contraceptive effect of norethisterone-containing pills. They include anticonvulsants, antituberculous drugs, certain antivirals, antibiotics, and St John's wort. Be sure to inform your doctor that you are taking norethisterone before taking additional prescribed medication.

Ciclosporin Levels of ciclosporin may be raised by norethisterone.

SPECIAL PRECAUTIONS

Be sure to tell your doctor if:

- ◆ You have liver or kidney problems.
- ◆ You have diabetes.
- ◆ You have had epileptic seizures.
- ◆ You have migraine.
- ◆ You have acute porphyria.
- ◆ You have heart or circulatory problems, especially a history of venous thrombosis.
- ◆ You are taking other medicines.

Pregnancy Not usually prescribed. May cause defects in the baby. Discuss with your doctor.

Breast-feeding The drug passes into the breast milk, but normal doses are unlikely to affect the baby adversely. Discuss with your doctor.

Infants and children Not prescribed.

Over 60 Not usually prescribed.

Driving and hazardous work No special problems.

Alcohol No special problems.

Surgery and general anaesthetics Tell the doctor or dentist that you take norethisterone. They will tell you when to stop prior to surgery.

PROLONGED USE

As part of HRT, norethisterone is usually only advised for use around the menopause. It is not normally recommended for long-term use or to treat osteoporosis. HRT increases the risks of venous thrombosis and breast cancer. The breast cancer risk reduces after stopping the drug, disappearing after 10 years.

Monitoring Blood-pressure checks and physical examination, including regular mammograms, may be performed.

NYSTATIN

Brand name Nystan

Used in the following combined preparations Nystaform HC, Timodine

QUICK REFERENCE

Drug group Antifungal drug (p.74)

Overdose danger rating Low

Dependence rating Low

Prescription needed Yes

Available as generic Yes

GENERAL INFORMATION

Nystatin is an antifungal drug named after the New York State Institute of Health, where it was developed in the early 1950s.

The drug has been used effectively against candidiasis (thrush), an infection caused by the *Candida* yeast. Available in a variety of forms, it is given to treat infections of the skin, mouth, throat, oesophagus, and intestinal tract. However, because it is poorly absorbed into the bloodstream from the digestive tract, it is ineffective against systemic infections. It is not given by injection as it would be too toxic in this form. Nystatin rarely causes adverse effects and can be used during pregnancy to treat candidiasis.

INFORMATION FOR USERS

Your drug prescription is tailored for you. Do not alter dosage without checking with your doctor.

How taken/used Liquid, cream, ointment.

Frequency and timing of doses *Mouth or throat infections* 4 x daily. Take after food and hold in the mouth for several minutes before swallowing (liquid). *Intestinal infections* 4 x daily. *Skin infections* 2–4 x daily.

Adult dosage range 2–4 million units daily (by mouth); as directed (skin preparations).

Onset of effect Full beneficial effect may not be felt for 7–14 days.

Duration of action Up to 6 hours.

Diet advice None.

Storage Keep in original container at room temperature out of the reach of children. Protect from light.
Missed dose Take as soon as you remember. Take your next dose as usual.
Stopping the drug Take the full course, and continue treatment for at least 48 hours after symptoms have disappeared. Even if the affected area seems to be cured, the original infection may still be present, and symptoms may recur if treatment is stopped too soon.
Exceeding the dose An occasional unintentional extra dose is unlikely to be a cause for concern. But if you notice any unusual symptoms or a large overdose has been taken, tell your doctor.

POSSIBLE ADVERSE EFFECTS

Adverse effects are uncommon and are usually mild and transient. Nausea and vomiting may occur when high doses are taken by mouth. Diarrhoea and a rash are other rare side effects. Consult your doctor if you develop a rash or if any of the other effects are severe.

INTERACTIONS

None.

SPECIAL PRECAUTIONS

Be sure to tell your doctor if:
- ◆ You are taking other medicines.

Pregnancy No evidence of risk to the fetus.
Breast-feeding No evidence of risk.
Infants and children Reduced dose necessary.
Over 60 No special problems.
Driving and hazardous work No known problems.
Alcohol No known problems.

PROLONGED USE

No problems expected. Usually given as a course of treatment until infection is cured.

OLANZAPINE

Brand names Zalasta, ZypAdhera, Zyprexa, Zyprexa Velotab
Used in the following combined preparations None

QUICK REFERENCE

Drug group Antipsychotic drug (p.13)
Overdose danger rating Medium
Dependence rating Low
Prescription needed Yes
Available as generic Yes

GENERAL INFORMATION

Olanzapine is an atypical antipsychotic drug prescribed to treat schizophrenia and mania and for long-term treatment of bipolar disorder. It works by blocking several chemical transmitters in the brain (p.7), including dopamine, histamine, and serotonin. In schizophrenia, the drug can be used to treat both "positive" symptoms (delusions, hallucinations, and thought disorders) and "negative" symptoms (blunted affect, emotional and social withdrawal). In mania, olanzapine can be used alone or in combination with other drugs.

Olanzapine by injection is used short term for its calming effects in agitation associated with schizophrenia or mania.

INFORMATION FOR USERS

Your drug prescription is tailored for you. Do not alter dosage without checking with your doctor.
How taken/used Tablets, dispersible tablets, injection.
Frequency and timing of doses Once daily (tablets); 1–2 x daily (injection).
Adult dosage range *Schizophrenia* 10mg (starting dose). *Mania* 15mg if used alone or 10mg if used in combination with other drugs (starting dose). For all conditions, the dose can be adjusted between 5mg and 20mg daily (tablets) and 5mg and 10mg daily (injection).
Onset of effect 4–8 hours (tablets); 15–45 minutes (injection).
Duration of action 30–38 hours.
Diet advice None.
Storage Keep in original container at room temperature out of the reach of children. Protect from light.
Missed dose Take as soon as you remember. If your next dose is due within 8 hours, take a single dose now and skip the next.
Stopping the drug Do not stop the drug without consulting your doctor; symptoms may recur.
Exceeding the dose An occasional unintentional extra dose is unlikely to cause problems. Large overdoses may cause unusual drowsiness, depressed breathing, and low blood pressure, or agitation, a rapid pulse, altered speech, and abnormal movements. Notify your doctor.

POSSIBLE ADVERSE EFFECTS

Unusual drowsiness, increased appetite, and weight gain are the most common adverse effects of olanzapine. Dry mouth, reduced libido, and erectile dysfunction are also common. Discuss with your doctor if any of these are severe. Other common adverse effects include dizziness, fainting, and a rash; if any of these occur, notify your doctor. Rarely, difficulty in urinating, or breast tenderness or discharge, may occur; if so, discuss with your doctor. Long-term use may cause movement problems (see Prolonged use).

INTERACTIONS

Sedatives All drugs that have a sedative effect on the central nervous system may increase the sedative effects of olanzapine.
Carbamazepine and smoking These can reduce the effects of olanzapine.
Diabetic medication Olanzapine can affect diabetic control. Dosage of diabetic medications may need to be adjusted.
Ciprofloxacin This can increase the effects of olanzapine.

SPECIAL PRECAUTIONS

Be sure to tell your doctor if:
- You have kidney or liver problems.
- You have diabetes.
- You have glaucoma.
- You have epilepsy.
- You have Parkinson's disease or dementia.
- You have had, or are at risk of, a stroke.
- You are taking other medicines.

Pregnancy Safety not established. Discuss with your doctor.
Breast-feeding Safety not established. The drug passes into the breast milk and may affect your baby. Discuss with your doctor.
Infants and children Not recommended.
Over 60 Reduced dose may be necessary. Increased risk of stroke with long-term use.
Driving and hazardous work Avoid such activities until you have learned how olanzapine affects you because the drug can cause unusual drowsiness.
Alcohol Avoid. Alcohol increases the sedative effects of this drug.

PROLONGED USE

Prolonged use of olanzapine may rarely cause tardive dyskinesia, in which there are involuntary movements of the tongue and face. There is also an increased risk of raised blood lipid levels or of developing diabetes or worsening existing diabetes. With long-term use in older patients, olanzapine also carries a greater risk of stroke than some other antipsychotic drugs.
Monitoring Blood count, blood sugar and lipid levels, heart function (ECG), and liver function may be regularly monitored.

OLAPARIB

Brand names Lynparza
Used in the following combined preparation None

QUICK REFERENCE

Drug group Anticancer drug (p.94)
Overdose danger rating Medium
Dependence rating Low
Prescription needed Yes
Available as generic No

GENERAL INFORMATION

Olaparib is a type of "targeted therapy" for cancer. It is part of an expanding class of drugs called PARP (poly ADP ribose polymerase) inhibitors. PARP is involved in DNA repair, so when it is inhibited by olaparib, cancer cells cannot easily repair the DNA damage that occurs normally in dividing cells. This action is even more critical in cancer cells with a faulty BRCA gene, a common genetic cause of cancer risk. BRCA genes also act in DNA repair, so if both repair mechanisms are impaired, the cancer cells are very likely to die.

The drug is used in metastatic cancers such as ovarian, breast, pancreatic and prostate, especially those with faulty BRCA genes. Side effects of olaparib range from nausea and fatigue to rare but serious lung and white blood cell disorders.

INFORMATION FOR USERS

Your drug prescription is tailored for you. Do not alter dosage without checking with your doctor.
How taken/used Tablets, capsules.
Frequency and timing of doses 2 x daily. Manufacturer recommends taking the capsules at least 1 hour after food and avoiding food for 2 hours after dose. Tablets are not affected by having or not having food.
Adult dosage range 150–400mg (capsules); 100–300mg (tablets).
Onset of effect PARP inhibition may begin within hours, but both the beneficial effects and the side effects tend to take weeks to become apparent.

Duration of action Adverse effects may last for several weeks after drug cessation.

Diet advice Avoid Seville orange, grapefruit, and grapefruit juices; they may increase exposure to olaparib.

Storage Store in the original package to protect from moisture. Keep out of the reach of children. No special temperature requirements.

Missed dose If you miss a dose, take your next normal dose at its scheduled time.

Stopping the drug Do not stop without direction from your cancer doctor. Stopping the drug without an alternative therapy can lead to cancer growth.

Exceeding the dose An occasional unintentional extra dose is unlikely to cause major problems. But if you notice any unusual symptoms or if a large overdose has been taken, tell your doctor.

POSSIBLE ADVERSE EFFECTS

Common side effects include gastrointestinal problems, upper abdominal pain, low white blood cell count, low red blood cell count (anaemia), and low energy. If you have severe appetite loss, nausea, fatigue, headache, cough, or dizziness, consult your doctor. Major side effects are rare but can be life-threatening. They include white blood cell cancer, severe lung inflammation, and blood clots in the lung (pulmonary embolism). If you have a rash, tell your doctor. For bleeding, shortness of breath, chest pain, or fever, call your doctor promptly.

INTERACTIONS

General note Many drugs, over-the-counter treatments, and herbal remedies (such as St John's wort) can affect levels of olaparib. Check with your doctor or pharmacist.

Calcium antagonists Diltiazem and verapamil may both increase olaparib levels.

Antimicrobials Itraconazole, clarithromycin, erythromycin, and fluconazole can raise levels of olaparib; rifampicin can reduce them.

Anticonvulsants Carbamazepine, phenytoin, and phenobarbital may reduce blood levels and effectiveness of olaparib.

SPECIAL PRECAUTIONS

Be sure to tell your doctor if:

- You have kidney or liver problems.
- You have lung or breathing problems.
- You have abnormal white blood cell or red blood cell counts.
- You have had previous lymphoma or leukaemia.
- You are taking other medicines.

Pregnancy Olaparib should not be used in pregnancy. Two complementary forms of contraception are recommended during therapy and for 3 months after finishing. Discuss with your doctor.

Breast-feeding Do not breast-feed while on olaparib or until at least 1 month after end of treatment. Discuss with your doctor.

Infants and children The effects of the drug in children are not known. Olaparib could be used by specialist children's doctors.

Over 60 No special problems.

Driving and hazardous work Avoid until you have learned how the drug affects you. It may sometimes cause dizziness or malaise.

Alcohol No special problems.

PROLONGED USE

Long-term use can be associated with both white blood cell and red blood cell abnormalities. Hence, full blood counts are usually performed periodically. Long-term use is also associated with changes in kidney function, so this should also be monitored regularly during treatment with olaparib.

OMEPRAZOLE

Brand names Losec, Losec MUPS, Mepradec, Mezzopram
Used in the following combined preparation None

QUICK REFERENCE

Drug group Anti-ulcer drug (p.41)
Overdose danger rating Low
Dependence rating Low
Prescription needed Yes (except some preparations for short-term relief of acid reflux symptoms)
Available as generic Yes

GENERAL INFORMATION

Omeprazole belongs to a group of drugs called proton pump inhibitors (p.41), which reduce stomach acid secretion by blocking the stomach's acid-pumping mechanism. It is used to treat stomach and duodenal ulcers, reflux oesophagitis (in which stomach acid rises into the oesophagus), and Zollinger-Ellison syndrome (in which digestive system tumours cause excess production of stomach acid). Treatment for an ulcer is usually given for 4 to

8 weeks, although it may be given for much longer to prevent ulcers in high-risk patients, such as those taking long-term non-steroidal anti-inflammatory drugs (NSAIDs). The drug may also be given with antibiotics to eradicate the *Helicobacter pylori* bacteria that can cause peptic ulcers. Reflux oesophagitis may be treated for 4 to 12 weeks.

Omeprazole is available over the counter for short-term relief of acid reflux symptoms such as heartburn in adults over 18 years old.

The drug causes few serious side effects. As with other anti-ulcer drugs, it may mask signs of stomach cancer, so it is prescribed only when the possibility of this disease has been ruled out.

INFORMATION FOR USERS

Your drug prescription is tailored for you. Do not alter dosage without checking with your doctor. For over-the-counter preparations, follow the instructions and call your doctor if symptoms worsen.

How taken/used Tablets, capsules, injection, intravenous infusion.

Frequency and timing of doses 1–2 x daily (2 x daily for doses above 80mg).

Adult dosage range 10–40mg daily and sometimes up to 120mg daily.

Onset of effect 2–5 hours.

Duration of action Up to 24 hours.

Diet advice None, although spicy foods and alcohol may exacerbate the underlying condition.

Storage Keep in original container at room temperature out of the reach of children. Omeprazole is very sensitive to moisture. It must not be transferred to another container and must be used within 3 months of opening.

Missed dose Take as soon as you remember. If your next dose is due within 8 hours, take a single dose now and skip the next.

Stopping the drug Do not stop the drug without consulting your doctor; symptoms may recur.

Exceeding the dose An occasional unintentional extra dose is unlikely to be a cause for concern. But if you notice any unusual symptoms, or if a large overdose has been taken, notify your doctor.

POSSIBLE ADVERSE EFFECTS

Adverse effects of omeprazole include headache, diarrhoea, and less commonly nausea or constipation. These are usually mild and often diminish with continued use of the drug; discuss with your doctor if these are severe or persistent. Rarely, a rash may develop; if so, you should stop taking the drug and consult your doctor. Long-term use of omeprazole may increase the risk of intestinal infections and, in women, hip fractures (see Prolonged use).

INTERACTIONS

Warfarin The effects of warfarin may be increased by omeprazole.

Phenytoin The effects of phenytoin may be increased by omeprazole.

Clopidogrel The antiplatelet effect of clopidogrel is reduced by omeprazole.

Ciclosporin and tacrolimus Blood levels of these drugs are raised by omeprazole.

Atazanavir The effects of this drug are reduced by omeprazole.

Ketoconazole and itraconazole Blood levels of these drugs may be reduced by omeprazole.

SPECIAL PRECAUTIONS

Be sure to consult your doctor or pharmacist before taking this drug if:

- You have a long-term liver problem.
- You are taking other medicines.

Pregnancy No evidence of risk, but discuss with your doctor.

Breast-feeding The drug may pass into the breast milk. Safety in breast-feeding not established. Discuss with your doctor.

Infants and children Not usually recommended for infants under 1 year. Reduced dose necessary in older children.

Over 60 No special problems.

Driving and hazardous work No special problems with this drug.

Alcohol Avoid. Alcohol irritates the stomach, which can lead to ulceration and acid reflux.

PROLONGED USE

Long-term use of omeprazole may increase the risk of certain intestinal infections (such as *Salmonella* and *Clostridium difficile* infections) because of the loss of the natural protection against such infections that is provided by stomach acid. Prolonged use also increases the risk of hip fractures in post-menopausal women, and may reduce absorption of vitamin B12 and magnesium in the intestine.

ONDANSETRON

Brand names Demorem, Ondemet, Setofilm, Zofran, Zofram Flexi-amp, Zofran Melt

Used in the following combined preparations None

QUICK REFERENCE

Drug group Anti-emetic drug (p.19)

Overdose danger rating Low

Dependence rating Low

Prescription needed Yes

Available as generic Yes

GENERAL INFORMATION

Ondansetron, an anti-emetic, is used especially for treating the nausea and vomiting associated with radiotherapy and anticancer drugs. It may also be prescribed for the nausea and vomiting that occur after surgery.

The dose given and the frequency will depend on which anticancer drug you are having and its dose. In most instances, you will receive ondansetron, either by mouth or by injection, before infusion of the anticancer agent, then tablets for up to 5 days after treatment has finished. The drug is less effective against the delayed nausea and vomiting that occur several days after chemotherapy than against symptoms that occur soon after treatment. For nausea and vomiting after surgery, one dose is usually given before the surgery, and two doses afterwards.

To enhance the effectiveness of ondansetron, it is usually taken with other drugs, such as dexamethasone. Serious adverse effects are unlikely to occur.

INFORMATION FOR USERS

Your drug prescription is tailored for you. Do not alter dosage without checking with your doctor.

How taken/used Tablets, liquid, injection, suppositories.

Frequency and timing of doses Normally 2 x daily, but the frequency will depend on the reason for which the drug is being used.

Adult dosage range 4–32mg daily depending on the reason for which it is being used.

Onset of effect Within 1 hour.

Duration of action Approximately 12 hours.

Diet advice None.

Storage Keep in original container at room temperature out of the reach of children. Protect from light.

Missed dose Take as soon as you remember. If your next dose is due within 2 hours, take a single dose now and skip the next.

Stopping the drug Can be safely stopped as soon as you no longer need it.

Exceeding the dose An occasional unintentional extra dose is unlikely to be a cause for concern. But if you notice any unusual symptoms, or if a large overdose has been taken, tell your doctor.

POSSIBLE ADVERSE EFFECTS

Ondansetron is considered to be safe and is generally well tolerated. It does not cause the sedation or abnormal muscle movements that occur as adverse effects of some other anti-emetic drugs.

The most common adverse effects of ondansetron include constipation, headache, and a warm feeling in the head or stomach. Discuss with your doctor if these are severe. More rarely, palpitations, chest pain, muscle stiffness, or seizures may occur; if so, consult your doctor promptly. If you develop wheezing, an itchy rash, or swelling of the eyelids, lips, or face, you should stop taking the drug and contact your doctor immediately.

INTERACTIONS

Carbamazepine, phenytoin and rifampicin These drugs may accelerate the breakdown of ondansetron and reduce its effect.

Apomorphine may cause a drop in blood pressure when used with ondansetron; the two drugs should not be taken together.

Vandetanib may increase the risk of heart rhythm abnormalities when used with ondansetron; these two drugs should not be taken together.

Tramadol The effect of this drug may be reduced by ondansetron.

SPECIAL PRECAUTIONS

Be sure to tell your doctor if:

- You have a long-term liver problem.
- You have bowel problems.
- You have heart rhythm problems.
- You are taking other medicines.

Pregnancy Safety in pregnancy not established. Discuss with your doctor.

Breast-feeding The drug may pass into the breast milk. Discuss with your doctor.

Infants and children Reduced dose necessary.

Over 60 No special problems.

Driving and hazardous work No problems expected.
Alcohol No known problems.

PROLONGED USE

Ondansetron is not generally prescribed for long-term treatment.

ORLISTAT

Brand names Alli, Beacita, Xenical
Used in the following combined preparations None

QUICK REFERENCE

Drug group Anti-obesity drug
Overdose danger rating Low
Dependence rating Low
Prescription needed No
Available as generic No

GENERAL INFORMATION

Orlistat blocks the action of stomach and pancreatic enzymes (lipases) that digest fats; hence, less dietary fat is absorbed and more passes out in the faeces. This leads to reduced calorie uptake and helps to produce weight loss. The effectiveness of orlistat varies from person to person, and it should only be used in conjunction with healthy lifestyle measures. The increased fat content makes the faeces become oily, and this can cause flatulence. As fat absorption is reduced, there is a danger of fat-soluble vitamins being lost to the body, and a multivitamin supplement may be needed to compensate (see Diet advice, below).

INFORMATION FOR USERS

Follow instructions on the label. Call your doctor if symptoms worsen.
How taken/used Capsules.
Frequency and timing of doses Just before, during, or up to 1 hour after each main meal (up to 3 x daily). If a meal is omitted or contains no fat, do not take the dose of orlistat.
Adult dosage range Up to 360mg daily.
Onset of effect 30 minutes; excretion of excess faecal fat begins about 24–48 hours after the first dose.
Duration of action Orlistat is not absorbed from the gut, and potentially continues to work as it passes through the intestines. If you stop taking the drug, faecal fat returns to normal in 48–72 hours.
Diet advice Eat a nutritionally balanced diet that does not contain quite enough calories, and that provides about 30 per cent of the calories as fat. Eat lots of fruit and vegetables. The intake of fat, carbohydrate, and protein should be distributed over the three main meals. If a multivitamin supplement is needed, it should be taken at least 2 hours before an orlistat dose or at bedtime.
Storage Keep in original container at room temperature out of the reach of children.
Missed dose No cause for concern. Take the next dose with the next meal.
Stopping the drug The drug can be safely stopped as soon as it is no longer needed.
Exceeding the dose An occasional unintentional extra dose is unlikely to be a cause for concern. But if you notice any unusual symptoms, or if a large overdose has been taken, notify your doctor.

POSSIBLE ADVERSE EFFECTS

Most side effects of orlistat depend on how much fat is eaten, as well as the dose of the drug. Common side effects include liquid, oily stools, faecal urgency, flatulence, abdominal or rectal pain, headache, menstrual irregularities, anxiety, fatigue, nausea, infections (e.g. respiratory infections), and hypoglycaemia (low blood sugar). Discuss with your doctor if these are severe. Rarely, rectal bleeding may occur; if this happens, consult your doctor.

INTERACTIONS

General note Orlistat reduces absorption of fat-soluble vitamins (A, D, E, and K), so a multivitamin supplement may be needed. This is particularly important in growing teenagers.
Ciclosporin, oral anticoagulants, amiodarone, and anticonvulsants, and antiretrovirals Orlistat may reduce the effects of these drugs.
Acarbose Avoid using orlistat with acarbose.
Oral contraceptives Absorption may be reduced by orlistat; an additional method of contraception is advisable.
Levothyroxine Dosage and timing of doses may need to be adjusted.

SPECIAL PRECAUTIONS

Be sure to consult your doctor or pharmacist before taking this drug if:

- You have diabetes.
- You have chronic malabsorption syndrome.

◆ You have gallbladder, kidney, or liver problems.
◆ You are taking lipid-lowering drugs.
◆ You are taking other medicines.

Pregnancy Safety not established. Discuss with your doctor.
Breast-feeding Safety not established. Discuss with your doctor.
Infants and children Should not be used in under-18s except on specialist advice.
Over 60 No special problems.
Driving and hazardous work No special problems.
Alcohol No special problems.

PROLONGED USE

Orlistat treatment should be stopped after 12 weeks if you have not lost 5 per cent of your body weight since the start of treatment. It should also be stopped if you have lost less than 10 per cent of your body weight over the first 6 months. If you have lost more than 10 per cent, then the drug may be continued, for up to a maximum of 2 years, until your target weight is approached. When orlistat treatment is stopped, there may be gradual weight gain.

ORPHENADRINE

Brand names None
Used in the following combined preparations None

QUICK REFERENCE

Drug group Drug for parkinsonism (p.16)
Overdose danger rating High
Dependence rating Low
Prescription needed Yes
Available as generic Yes

GENERAL INFORMATION

Orphenadrine is an anticholinergic drug (p.7) that is prescribed to treat all forms of Parkinson's disease. However, it is less effective against the idiopathic form of the disease than other drugs (such as levodopa) and can cause confusion. It is particularly valuable for relieving the tremor and muscle rigidity that often occur with Parkinson's disease, but it is less helpful for improving the slowing of movement that also commonly occurs. It also helps reduce the excessive salivation or dribbling that can occur with Parkinson's disease and is widely used to treat the parkinson-like side effects of antipsychotic drugs. The effects may become less noticeable after orphenadrine has been taken for a long time.

The drug also possesses muscle-relaxant properties and is occasionally used to treat muscle pain and restless leg syndrome.

INFORMATION FOR USERS

Your drug prescription is tailored for you. Do not alter dosage without checking with your doctor.
How taken/used Liquid.
Frequency and timing of doses 2–3 x daily.
Adult dosage range 150–400mg daily.
Onset of effect Within 60 minutes.
Duration of action 8–12 hours.
Diet advice None.
Storage Keep in original container at room temperature out of the reach of children. Protect from light.
Missed dose Take as soon as you remember. If your next dose is due within 2 hours, take a single dose now and skip the next.
Stopping the drug Do not stop the drug without consulting your doctor; symptoms may recur.

OVERDOSE ACTION

Seek immediate medical advice in all cases. Take emergency action if palpitations, seizures, or loss of consciousness occur.

POSSIBLE ADVERSE EFFECTS

The adverse effects of orphenadrine are similar to those of other anticholinergic drugs. The more common effects often diminish with a reduction in dosage; they include dry mouth and skin, difficulty in passing urine, constipation, dizziness, and blurred vision. Discuss with your doctor if blurred vision occurs or if the other symptoms are severe. Rarely, confusion or agitation may occur; if so, discuss with your doctor. If you experience palpitations, you should stop taking the drug and contact your doctor immediately.

INTERACTIONS

General note Orphenadrine reduces gastric motility (the spontaneous stomach movements that move stomach contents into the intestine) and so may affect the absorption of other oral drugs.
Anticholinergic drugs (e.g. tiotropium, chlorphenamine, oxybutynin) The anticholinergic effects of orphenadrine are likely to be increased by these drugs.

SPECIAL PRECAUTIONS

Be sure to tell your doctor if:

◆ You have long-term liver or kidney problems.

◆ You have heart problems.

◆ You have had glaucoma.

◆ You have difficulty in passing urine and have an enlarged prostate.

◆ You are taking other medicines.

Pregnancy Safety not established. Discuss with your doctor.

Breast-feeding Safety not established. Discuss with your doctor.

Infants and children Not usually prescribed.

Over 60 Increased likelihood of adverse effects. Reduced dose may therefore be necessary.

Driving and hazardous work Avoid such activities until you have learned how orphenadrine affects you because the drug can cause dizziness, lightheadedness, and blurred vision.

Alcohol Avoid. Alcohol can worsen some of the adverse effects of orphenadrine.

PROLONGED USE

No problems expected. Effectiveness in treating Parkinson's disease may lessen with time.

OSELTAMIVIR

Brand name Tamiflu
Used in the following combined preparations None

QUICK REFERENCE

Drug group Antiviral drug (p.67)
Overdose danger rating Low
Dependence rating Low
Prescription needed Yes
Available as generic No

GENERAL INFORMATION

Oseltamivir is an antiviral drug that is used to prevent or treat influenza (flu), a virus that infects and multiplies within the lungs. As well as being given for regular seasonal flu, it is also effective against the avian (bird) flu and swine flu strains of the influenza virus. The drug acts by blocking the entry of the virus into body cells. This prevents or alleviates the typical symptoms of flu, including sudden onset of fever, sweating and shivering, cough, runny or stuffy nose, headache, aching muscles, and extreme fatigue. The drug should be taken within 48 hours of the onset of symptoms; it may reduce their duration by 1–2 days.

Oseltamivir is not a substitute for seasonal flu vaccination and is not recommended for prevention of seasonal flu. However, because it does not alter the flu vaccine's effectiveness, it can be taken even if you have been vaccinated.

INFORMATION FOR USERS

Your drug prescription is tailored for you. Do not alter dosage without checking with your doctor.

How taken/used Capsules, liquid (suspension).

Frequency and timing of doses Once daily (prevention); 2 x daily (treatment).

Dosage range *Adults; adolescents over 13 years* 75mg daily (prevention); 150mg daily (treatment). *Children 1–13 years* 30–75mg daily according to body weight (prevention); 60–150mg daily according to body weight (treatment).

Onset of effect Within 24 hours.

Duration of action 12–24 hours.

Diet advice None.

Storage Keep in original container at room temperature out of the reach of children.

Missed dose Take as soon as you remember. If your next dose is due within 2 hours, take a single dose now and skip the next.

Stopping the drug Do not stop without consulting your doctor; symptoms may recur.

Exceeding the dose An occasional unintentional extra dose is unlikely to cause problems. However, if you have any unusual symptoms, or if a large overdose has been taken, tell your doctor.

POSSIBLE ADVERSE EFFECTS

The most common adverse effects – nausea, vomiting, and abdominal pain – mostly occur following the first dose and usually subside as treatment continues. Taking the drug with food helps to reduce these effects, but consult your doctor if they are severe or persistent. If a rash occurs, stop taking the drug and contact your doctor. If psychosis or hallucinations occur, stop the drug and call your doctor immediately.

INTERACTIONS

Leflunomide and teriflunomide may increase the blood level of oseltamivir.

SPECIAL PRECAUTIONS

Be sure to tell your doctor if:

◆ You have kidney problems.

◆ You have ever had an allergic reaction to oseltamivir.

◆ You are taking other medicines.

Pregnancy Safety in pregnancy not established. Discuss with your doctor.
Breast-feeding Safety in breast-feeding not established. Discuss with your doctor.
Infants and children No problems expected.
Over 60 No special problems.
Driving and hazardous work No known problems.
Alcohol No known problems.

PROLONGED USE

No problems expected. Oseltamivir is not usually prescribed for longer than 5 days (children), 7 days (adults), or 6 weeks (adults, during an epidemic).

OXYBUTYNIN

Brand names Ditropan, Kentera, Lyrinel XL
Used in the following combined preparations None

QUICK REFERENCE

Drug group Drug for urinary disorders (p.110)
Overdose danger rating High
Dependence rating Low
Prescription needed Yes
Available as generic Yes

GENERAL INFORMATION

Oxybutynin is an anticholinergic (p.7) and antispasmodic drug used to treat urinary incontinence and frequency in adults and bed-wetting in children. It acts by reducing bladder contraction, thus allowing the bladder to hold more urine. It stops bladder spasms and delays the desire to empty the bladder. It also has some local anaesthetic effect. However, its usefulness is limited to some extent by its side effects, especially in children and older adults. It can aggravate conditions such as an enlarged prostate or coronary heart disease in older adults. Children are more prone to effects on the central nervous system, such as restlessness, disorientation, hallucinations, and seizures.

INFORMATION FOR USERS

Your drug prescription is tailored for you. Do not alter dosage without checking with your doctor.
How taken/used Tablets, modified release (MR) tablets, liquid, patches.
Frequency and timing of doses 2–4 x daily (tablets, liquid); 1–2 x weekly (patch).
Adult dosage range 10–20mg daily (tablets, liquid); 36mg twice weekly (patch).
Onset of effect 1 hour (tablets, liquid); 24–48 hours (patch).
Duration of action Up to 10 hours (tablets, liquid); 96 hours (patch).
Diet advice None.
Storage Keep in original container at room temperature out of the reach of children. Protect liquid from light.
Missed dose Take as soon as you remember. If next dose is due within 2 hours, take a single dose now and skip the next (tablets and liquid). Apply when you remember (patches).
Stopping the drug Do not stop without consulting your doctor; symptoms may recur.

OVERDOSE ACTION

Seek immediate medical advice in all cases. Take emergency action if symptoms such as breathing difficulty, seizures, or loss of consciousness occur.

POSSIBLE ADVERSE EFFECTS

An adjustment in dosage is necessary in children and older adults to minimize adverse effects of oxybutynin. Common side effects include dry mouth, constipation, nausea, facial flushing, and difficulty in passing urine. More rarely, there may be blurred vision, eye pain, headache, or confusion. Discuss with your doctor if any of these are severe or if you develop dry skin. If a rash occurs, you should stop taking the drug and consult your doctor. Oxybutinin can also trigger glaucoma.

INTERACTIONS

General note Oxybutynin reduces gastric motility (the stomach movements that move stomach contents into the intestine), so may affect the absorption of other oral drugs.
Other anticholinergic drugs If oxybutynin is taken with other drugs that have anticholinergic effects, the risk of anticholinergic side effects is increased.

SPECIAL PRECAUTIONS

Be sure to tell your doctor if:
- You have liver or kidney problems.
- You have heart problems.
- You have an enlarged prostate.
- You have hiatus hernia.
- You have ulcerative colitis.
- You have glaucoma.
- You are taking other medicines.

Pregnancy Safety not established. Discuss with your doctor.
Breast-feeding The drug passes into breast milk and its safety in breast-feeding has not been established. Discuss with your doctor.
Infants and children Not recommended under 5 years. Reduced dose needed in older children.
Over 60 Reduced dose necessary.
Driving and hazardous work Avoid such activities until you have learned how oxybutynin affects you because the drug can cause drowsiness, disorientation, and blurred vision.
Alcohol Avoid. Alcohol increases the sedative effects of oxybutynin.

PROLONGED USE
No special problems. The need for continued treatment may be reviewed after 6 months.
Monitoring Periodic eye tests for glaucoma may be performed.

PARACETAMOL

Brand names Alvedon, Anadin Paracetamol, Calpol, Disprol, Hedex, Mandanol, Panadol, Perfalgan, and many others
Used in the following combined preparations Anadin Extra, Codipar, Kapake, Midrid, Migraleve, Panadeine, Paracodol, Paradote, Paramax, Solpadol, Tramacet, Tylex, Zapain, and many others

QUICK REFERENCE
Drug group Non-opioid analgesic (p.8)
Overdose danger rating High
Dependence rating Low
Prescription needed No
Available as generic Yes

GENERAL INFORMATION
One of a group of drugs known as non-opioid analgesics, paracetamol is a common home remedy to relieve mild pain and reduce fever. It is suitable for children as well as adults. One of the primary advantages of paracetamol is that it does not cause stomach upset or bleeding problems. This makes it particularly useful for people with peptic ulcers or those who cannot tolerate aspirin. It is also safe for occasional use by people taking anticoagulants.

Although safe when used as directed, paracetamol is dangerous in overdose, and is capable of causing serious damage to the liver and kidneys. Even a small excess dose may be toxic in frail, older people, patients with liver damage, those with an eating disorder, or those who are malnourished.

INFORMATION FOR USERS
Follow instructions on the label. Call your doctor if symptoms worsen.
How taken/used Tablets, capsules, liquid, suppositories, injection (given in hospital).
Frequency and timing of doses Every 4–6 hours as necessary, but not more than 4 doses per 24 hours in children.
Dosage range *Adults* 500mg–1g per dose up to 4g daily. *Children* 60mg (3–6 months; 2–3 months for fever after immunization, and for other causes of pain and fever in infants weighing more than 4kg and who were born after 37 weeks – 2 doses only); 120mg per dose (6–24 months); 180mg per dose (2–4 years); 240mg per dose (4–6 years); 250mg per dose (6–8 years); 375mg per dose (8–10 years); 500mg per dose (10–12 years); 500–750mg per dose (12–16 years).
Onset of effect Within 15–60 minutes.
Duration of action Up to 6 hours.
Diet advice None.
Storage Keep in original container at room temperature out of the reach of children.
Missed dose Take as soon as you remember if required to relieve pain. Otherwise do not take the missed dose, and take a further dose only when you are in pain.
Stopping the drug Can be safely stopped as soon as you no longer need it.

OVERDOSE ACTION
Seek immediate medical advice in all cases. Take emergency action if nausea, vomiting, or stomach pain occur.

POSSIBLE ADVERSE EFFECTS
Paracetamol rarely produces side effects when taken as recommended. Nausea may sometimes occur; discuss with your doctor if it is severe. If you develop a rash, stop taking the drug and contact your doctor promptly.

INTERACTIONS
Anticoagulants such as warfarin may need dosage adjustment if taken with regular high doses of paracetamol.
Carbamazepine may increase the rate at which paracetamol is metabolized.

Colestyramine reduces the absorption and possibly the effectiveness of paracetamol.
Metoclopramide and domperidone increase the rate at which the body absorbs paracetamol.
Imatinib Paracetamol should be used at a reduced dosage or avoided with imatinib.
Anticonvulsants (e.g. carbamazepine, phenytoin, barbiturates) increase the rate at which paracetamol is metabolized. This can reduce its effects but raise the risk of toxicity.

SPECIAL PRECAUTIONS

Be sure to consult your doctor or pharmacist before using this drug if:

- You have liver or kidney problems.
- You have cystic fibrosis.
- You have an eating disorder.
- You are taking other medicines.

Pregnancy Not known to be harmful.
Breast-feeding The drug passes into the breast milk but in amounts too small to be harmful.
Infants and children Not suitable for infants under 2 months. For older infants and children, reduced dose necessary up to 16 years of age (see dosage information, above).
Over 60 No special problems.
Driving and hazardous work No special problems.
Alcohol Small amounts probably safe, but regularly exceeding daily allowance can increase the risk of liver damage from paracetamol.

PROLONGED USE

Do not take paracetamol for longer than 48 hours except on the advice of your doctor. If the drug is taken long term as recommended, there is relatively little evidence of harm.

PAROXETINE

Brand name Seroxat
Used in the following combined preparations None

QUICK REFERENCE

Drug group Antidepressant drug (p.12)
Overdose danger rating Low
Dependence rating Low
Prescription needed Yes
Available as generic Yes

GENERAL INFORMATION

Paroxetine is one of the selective serotonin reuptake inhibitor (SSRI) antidepressant class. It is used in treating depression, and helps to control the anxiety that often accompanies it. It is also used to treat generalized anxiety disorder, social phobia, panic disorder, obsessive-compulsive disorders, and post-traumatic stress disorder. Paroxetine is sometimes given to treat severe premenstrual syndrome.

Paroxetine is less likely than the older tricyclic antidepressants to cause anticholinergic side effects such as dry mouth, blurred vision, and difficulty in passing urine, and is much less dangerous in overdose. However, withdrawal symptoms can occur if the drug is not stopped gradually over several weeks.

INFORMATION FOR USERS

Your drug prescription is tailored for you. Do not alter dosage without checking with your doctor.
How taken/used Tablets, liquid.
Frequency and timing of doses Once daily, in the morning.
Dosage range 10–40mg daily.
Onset of effect Onset of therapeutic response, usually occurs within 14 days; full antidepressant effect may not be felt for 6 weeks (or longer for anxiety disorders).
Duration of action Antidepressant effect may last for some time following prolonged use.
Diet advice None.
Storage Keep in original container at room temperature out of the reach of children.
Missed dose Take as soon as you remember.
Stopping the drug Do not stop the drug without consulting your doctor. Stopping abruptly can cause withdrawal symptoms.
Exceeding the dose An occasional unintentional extra dose is unlikely to be a cause for concern. Large doses may cause unusual drowsiness. Notify your doctor immediately.

POSSIBLE ADVERSE EFFECTS

Common adverse effects include nausea, diarrhoea, sweating, tremor, weakness, drowsiness, dizziness, insomnia, sexual dysfunction in both sexes (e.g. lack of orgasm), and abnormal dreams; rarely, nervousness, anxiety, or agitation occur. Consult your doctor if severe. If you have suicidal thoughts or attempts, stop taking the drug and seek urgent medical help.

INTERACTIONS

General note Any drug that affects the breakdown of others in the liver may alter blood levels of paroxetine or vice versa.

Anticoagulants Paroxetine may increase the effects of these drugs.
Antipsychotics and tricyclic antidepressants Paroxetine may increase the levels and toxicity of these drugs.
Monoamine oxidase inhibitors (MAOIs) Avoid paroxetine during or within 14 days of MAOI treatment as serious reactions may occur.
Aspirin and non-steroidal anti-inflammatory drugs (NSAIDS) Increased risk of gastric bleeding when these drugs are used with paroxetine.
Serotonergics such as triptans (for migraine), other SSRIs (eg fluoxetine), tramadol, or even St John's wort, increase the risk of serotonin syndrome with paroxetine. This can be fatal.

SPECIAL PRECAUTIONS

Be sure to tell your doctor if:
- You have long-term liver or kidney problems.
- You have heart problems or bleeding disorders.
- You have glaucoma.
- You have a history of mania, or a history or family history of epilepsy.
- You have had problems withdrawing from other antidepressants.
- You are taking other medicines.

Pregnancy Safety in pregnancy not established. Discuss with your doctor.
Breast-feeding The drug passes into the breast milk. Discuss with your doctor.
Infants and children Not generally recommended under 18 years.
Over 60 Increased likelihood of adverse effects. Reduced dose may be necessary.
Driving and hazardous work Avoid until you have learned how paroxetine affects you because the drug can cause drowsiness.
Alcohol Avoid. Alcohol may increase the sedative effects of this drug.

PROLONGED USE

Withdrawal symptoms may occur if the drug is not stopped gradually over at least 4 weeks. These include dizziness, electric shock sensations, anxiety, nausea, and insomnia. These rarely last for more than 1–2 weeks. There is also a small risk of suicidal thoughts and self-harm in children and adolescents, although the drug is rarely used for this age group.
Monitoring Any person experiencing drowsiness, confusion, muscle cramps, or seizures should be monitored for low sodium levels in the blood. Under-18s should be monitored for suicidal thoughts and self-harm.

PERINDOPRIL

Brand name Coversyl
Used in the following combined preparation Coversyl Plus

QUICK REFERENCE

Drug group ACE inhibitor (p.30) and antihypertensive drug (p.34)
Overdose danger rating Medium
Dependence rating Low
Prescription needed Yes
Available as generic Yes

GENERAL INFORMATION

Perindopril is an ACE inhibitor, one of a group of drugs used to treat high blood pressure and heart failure, and to reduce the risk of cardiac events such as heart attack in certain heart conditions. The drug relaxes the muscles in the blood-vessel walls, allowing the vessels to dilate, thereby easing blood flow. It lowers blood pressure promptly, but may need to be taken for several weeks to achieve maximum effect. For heart failure, it is usually combined with a diuretic. This can give dramatic improvement, relaxing the muscle in blood vessel walls and reducing the heart's workload.

At the start of treatment, ACE inhibitors can cause a very rapid fall in blood pressure. Therefore, the first dose is usually low and is taken at bedtime so that the patient can stay lying down.

Perindopril can cause a persistent dry cough in up to 20 per cent of patients.

INFORMATION FOR USERS

Your drug prescription is tailored for you. Do not alter dosage without checking with your doctor.
How taken/used Tablets.
Frequency and timing of doses Once daily, 30 minutes before food, usually in the morning.
Adult dosage range 4mg initially, then 4–8mg daily.
Onset of effect 30–60 minutes; full beneficial effect may take several weeks.
Duration of action 24 hours.
Diet advice Your doctor may advise you to reduce your salt intake to help control your blood pressure.

Storage Keep in original container at room temperature out of the reach of children.
Missed dose Take as soon as you remember. If next dose is due within the next 8 hours, take a single dose now, and skip the next.
Stopping the drug Do not stop without consulting your doctor; stopping the drug may lead to worsening of the underlying condition.
Exceeding the dose An occasional unintentional extra dose is unlikely to cause problems, but large overdoses may cause dizziness or fainting. Notify your doctor.

POSSIBLE ADVERSE EFFECTS

Perindopril may cause a variety of adverse effects but they are usually mild and disappear soon after treatment has started. It may also cause kidney impairment or affect the blood with long-term use (see Prolonged use). All adverse effects should be reported to your doctor. The most common are a persistent dry cough and a rash. More rarely, there may be mouth ulcers or a sore mouth, dizziness, sore throat, or fever. If swelling of the mouth or lips or breathing difficulties occur, stop taking the drug and contact your doctor immediately.

INTERACTIONS

Lithium Blood levels and toxicity of this drug may be raised by perindopril.
Vasodilators, diuretics, and other antihypertensives These drugs may increase the blood-pressure-lowering effect of perindopril.
Ciclosporin, potassium salts, and potassium-sparing diuretics increase the risk of high blood potassium levels with perindopril and should be avoided.
Non-steroidal anti-inflammatory drugs (NSAIDs) may reduce the effects of perindopril. There is also a risk of kidney damage when they are taken together with perindopril.

SPECIAL PRECAUTIONS

Be sure to tell your doctor if:
- You have long-term kidney or liver problems.
- You have heart problems.
- You have had angioedema or a previous allergic reaction to ACE inhibitors.
- You are taking other medicines.
- You are pregnant or intend to become pregnant.

Pregnancy Not prescribed. There is evidence of harm to the developing fetus.
Breast-feeding Safety not established. Discuss with your doctor.
Infants and children Not recommended.
Over 60 Reduced dose may be necessary.
Driving and hazardous work Avoid until you know how perindopril affects you because the drug can cause dizziness and fainting.
Alcohol Avoid. Alcohol may increase the blood-pressure-lowering and adverse effects of the drug.
Surgery and general anaesthetics Perindopril may have to be stopped before you have a general anaesthetic. Discuss with your doctor or dentist before any operation.

PROLONGED USE

No problems expected.
Monitoring Periodic checks on potassium levels, white blood cell count, kidney function, and urine are usually performed.

PERMETHRIN

Brand name Lyclear
Used in the following combined preparations None

QUICK REFERENCE

Drug group Drug to treat skin parasites (p.120)
Overdose danger rating Low
Dependence rating Low
Prescription needed No
Available as generic Yes

GENERAL INFORMATION

Permethrin is an insecticide used to treat pubic lice (but not head lice) and scabies infestations. The drug works by interfering with the nervous system of the parasites, causing paralysis and death in them. Permethrin is less toxic to humans than some of the other types of insecticide, although it is toxic to some animals, such as cats.

Permethrin is applied topically as a cream to treat pubic lice and scabies infestations. It should not be used on broken or infested skin. In children and older adults, the entire body surface, including the face, scalp, neck, and ears, may have to be covered; adults are treated from the neck downwards. For pubic lice, the entire body should be treated and the permethrin left on overnight. A second treatment 7 days later is needed. For both pubic lice and scabies, all family members should be treated at the same time, to prevent recontamination, and the process repeated after a week.

There are signs that the parasites are developing resistance to permethrin. If the drug does not work for you, your pharmacist should be able to suggest an alternative treatment (e.g. malathion).

Permethrin is also an ingredient of some insect repellents used to impregnate clothing and mosquito nets in malarial regions.

INFORMATION FOR USERS

Follow instructions on the label. Call your doctor if symptoms worsen.

How taken/used Cream.

Frequency and timing of doses Once only, repeating after 7 days (2 years and over); under specialist supervision only (infants and children under 2 years). Avoid contact with eyes and broken or infected skin.

Dosage range As directed.

Onset of effect *Pubic lice* Wash off after 12–24 hours. *Scabies* Wash off after 8–12 hours.

Duration of action Until washed off.

Diet advice None.

Storage Keep in original container at room temperature out of the reach of children. Protect from light.

Missed dose Timing of the second application is not rigid; use as soon as you remember.

Stopping the drug Not applicable.

Exceeding the dose An occasional extra application is unlikely to cause problems. If drug is accidentally swallowed, take emergency action.

POSSIBLE ADVERSE EFFECTS

In general, permethrin is well tolerated on the skin, although mild irritation is common, with stinging, itching, and redness. Rarely, a rash may develop. Discuss with your doctor if any of these effects are severe.

INTERACTIONS

Corticosteroids Any eczemalike reactions to permethrin should not be treated with corticosteroid drugs, as these drugs may lower the immune response to the mites.

SPECIAL PRECAUTIONS

Be sure to tell your doctor if:

◆ You are taking other medicines.

Pregnancy Safety not established. Discuss with your doctor.

Breast-feeding Safety not established. Discuss with your doctor.

Infants and children Under specialist supervision only under 2 years. No special problems in older children.

Over 60 No special problems, but consult your doctor or a health professional.

Driving and hazardous work No special problems.

Alcohol No special problems.

Safety hazard Risk of burns if treated skin or contaminated clothing is exposed to open flames, due to alcohol content of preparations.

PROLONGED USE

Permethrin should not be used topically for prolonged periods; it is intended for intermittent use only. Prolonged use of permethrin to impregnate clothing and netting is not known to cause serious toxic effects.

PHENELZINE

Brand name Nardil

Used in the following combined preparations None

QUICK REFERENCE

Drug group Antidepressant drug (p.12)

Overdose danger rating High

Dependence rating Low

Prescription needed Yes

Available as generic No

GENERAL INFORMATION

Phenelzine is a monoamine oxidase inhibitor (MAOI) antidepressant. It works by blocking the enzyme monoamine oxidase, which normally breaks down neurotransmitters (mainly serotonin and noradrenaline) in the brain and elsewhere in the body (p.7). Low levels of these neurotransmitters in the brain are a causative factor in depression, and the effect of MAOIs is to increase their levels. Due to its potentially serious adverse effects and interactions with other drugs and foodstuffs, use of phenelzine is reserved for people for whom other antidepressants have been ineffective or those whose depression occurs together with anxiety, phobia, hysteria, or hypochondria.

INFORMATION FOR USERS

Your drug prescription is tailored for you. Do not alter dosage without checking with your doctor.

How taken/used Tablets.

Frequency and timing of doses Initially, 3–4 x daily. After satisfactory response has been achieved, dose may be gradually reduced to once daily or once every other day.

Adult dosage range 15–60mg daily. Patients treated in hospital may have up to 90mg daily.

Onset of effect Effectiveness may not be felt for up to 4 weeks.

Duration of action Antidepressant effect may last for months or longer after prolonged use.

Diet advice Avoid foods containing tyramine, such as cheese, meat or yeast extracts, fermented soya bean extracts, pickled herrings, hung game, and alcoholic (including low-alcohol) drinks. Discuss with your doctor.

Storage Store between 2–8°C in a refrigerator. Keep out of the reach of children.

Missed dose Take as soon as you remember. If next dose is due within 12 hours, skip missed dose and take the next dose as scheduled.

Stopping the drug Do not stop the drug without consulting your doctor. Stopping abruptly may cause withdrawal symptoms and a recurrence of depression.

OVERDOSE ACTION

Seek immediate medical advice in all cases. An overdose may be fatal. Take emergency action if breathing problems or loss of consciousness occur.

POSSIBLE ADVERSE EFFECTS

Side effects are common, and some are potentially serious. Common effects are dizziness, drowsiness, nausea, vomiting, constipation, sleep disturbance, blurred vision, and twitching or jerking movements. Discuss with your doctor if any of these are severe. More rarely, a rash, fever, muscle tightness, jaundice, or suicidal thoughts may occur. If the rash is severe, contact your doctor promptly. If any of the other rare symptoms occur, stop taking the drug and consult your doctor immediately.

INTERACTIONS

General note Phenelzine interacts with a wide range of drugs, and some interactions may be dangerous. Consult your doctor before taking any other medication.

Tyramine Phenelzine interacts with tyramine-containing food and drinks (see Diet advice, above) to cause a potentially life-threatening rise in blood pressure.

SPECIAL PRECAUTIONS

Be sure to tell your doctor if:

- You have high blood pressure or heart disease.
- You have had a stroke.
- You have liver disease.
- You have a blood disorder.
- You have diabetes.
- You have epilepsy.
- You have porphyria.
- You have phaeochromocytoma.
- You are taking any other medicines, including over-the-counter cough or cold remedies or illicit drugs.

Pregnancy Safety not established. Discuss with your doctor.

Breast-feeding Safety not established. Discuss with your doctor.

Infants and children Not recommended for children under 16 years old.

Over 60 Increased likelihood of adverse effects. Reduced dose may be necessary.

Driving and hazardous work Avoid until you know how phenelzine affects you; it may cause dizziness, drowsiness, and blurred vision.

Alcohol Avoid. Many alcoholic drinks contain tyramine, which may interact with phenelzine. The drug also enhances the effects of alcohol.

Surgery and general anaesthetics Owing to a potentially dangerous interaction with general anaesthetics, phenelzine should be stopped 2 weeks before any procedure requiring general anaesthesia. Discuss with your doctor or dentist.

PROLONGED USE

Withdrawal symptoms may occur if the drug is not stopped gradually over at least 4 weeks. Such symptoms include nausea, vomiting, malaise, nightmares, and agitation.

PHENOBARBITAL (PHENOBARBITONE)

Brand name None

Used in the following combined preparations None

QUICK REFERENCE

Drug group Barbiturate anticonvulsant drug (p.14)

Overdose danger rating High

Dependence rating High

Prescription needed Yes

Available as generic Yes

GENERAL INFORMATION

Phenobarbital is a barbiturate drug. It is used mainly in treating epilepsy, although this use is steadily declining. It was also used as a sleeping drug and sedative before the development of safer drugs. For epilepsy, phenobarbital is usually given together with another anticonvulsant such as phenytoin (p.360).

The main disadvantage of the drug is that it often causes unwanted sedation. However, tolerance develops within a week or two, and most patients have no problem in long-term use. In children and older adults, it may occasionally cause excessive excitement. Because of their sedative effects, phenobarbital and other barbiturates are sometimes misused.

INFORMATION FOR USERS

Your drug prescription is tailored for you. Do not alter dosage without checking with your doctor.

How taken/used Tablets, liquid, injection.

Frequency and timing of doses Once daily, usually at night.

Dosage range Adults 60–180mg daily.

Onset of effect 30–60 minutes (by mouth).

Duration of action 24–48 hours (some effect may persist for up to 6 days).

Diet advice People taking the drug long term should eat plenty of fresh green vegetables to prevent possible deficiency of vitamins A, D, K, and folic acid.

Storage Keep in original container at room temperature out of the reach of children.

Missed dose Take as soon as you remember. If the next dose is due within 10 hours, take a single dose now and skip the next.

Stopping the drug Do not stop taking the drug without consulting your doctor, who may supervise a gradual reduction in dosage. Stopping abruptly may cause seizures or lead to restlessness, trembling, and insomnia.

OVERDOSE ACTION

Seek immediate medical attention in all cases. Take emergency action if unsteadiness, severe weakness, confusion, or loss of consciousness occur.

POSSIBLE ADVERSE EFFECTS

Most of the adverse effects of phenobarbital result from its sedative effect. They can sometimes be minimized by a medically supervised reduction in dosage. Common side effects include drowsiness, clumsiness, unsteadiness, dizziness, and fainting. Discuss with your doctor if these are severe. More rarely, the drug may cause confusion, mood changes, or memory problems. Consult your doctor if any of these occur. If you develop a rash, localized swellings, or mouth ulcers, you should stop taking the drug and contact your doctor immediately. Rarely, phenobarbital may cause suicidal thoughts; if this occurs, seek immediate medical help.

INTERACTIONS

General note Phenobarbital interacts with a wide range of other drugs. Consult your doctor or pharmacist before taking any new drugs, including herbal remedies.

Sedatives All such drugs are likely to increase the sedative properties of phenobarbital.

Anticoagulants, corticosteroids, oral contraceptives, and protease inhibitors Their effect may be decreased by phenobarbital.

Antipsychotics, antidepressants, mefloquine, chloroquine, and St John's wort may reduce the anticonvulsant effect of phenobarbital.

SPECIAL PRECAUTIONS

Be sure to tell your doctor if:

- You have long-term liver or kidney problems.
- You have heart problems.
- You have poor circulation.
- You have porphyria.
- You have breathing problems.
- You have depression.
- You are taking other medicines.

Pregnancy The drug may affect the fetus and increase the tendency of bleeding in newborn babies. Discuss with your doctor.

Breast-feeding The drug passes into the breast milk and could cause drowsiness in the baby. Discuss with your doctor.

Infants and children Reduced dose necessary.

Over 60 Increased likelihood of confusion. Reduced dose may therefore be necessary.

Driving and hazardous work Your underlying condition, in addition to the possibility of reduced alertness while taking phenobarbital, may make such activities inadvisable. Discuss with your doctor.

Alcohol Never drink alcohol while under treatment with phenobarbital. Alcohol may interact dangerously with this drug.

PROLONGED USE

With prolonged use, tolerance to the drug's sedative effects may develop. Dependence may also result, and withdrawal symptoms may occur if the drug is stopped suddenly. Long-term use may also lead to deficiency of vitamins A, D, K, and folic acid.

Monitoring Blood samples may be taken periodically to test blood levels of the drug.

PHENOXYMETHYLPENICILLIN

Brand name None

Used in the following combined preparations None

QUICK REFERENCE

Drug group Penicillin antibiotic (p.60)

Overdose danger rating Low

Dependence rating Low

Prescription needed Yes

Available as generic Yes

GENERAL INFORMATION

Phenoxymethylpenicillin, also known as penicillin V, is a synthetic penicillin-type antibiotic prescribed for a wide range of infections. It is only given by mouth and was the first orally active penicillin to be synthesized.

Various commonly occurring respiratory tract infections, such as some types of tonsillitis and pharyngitis, as well as ear infections, often respond well to this drug. Phenoxymethylpenicillin is also used to treat less common infections caused by the *Streptococcus* bacterium, such as scarlet fever and erysipelas (a skin infection). It is used long term to prevent the recurrence of rheumatic fever, a rare but potentially serious condition. It is also used long term to prevent infections following removal of the spleen or in sickle cell disease.

As with other penicillin antibiotics, the most serious, although rare, adverse effect is an allergic reaction that may cause collapse, wheezing, and a rash in susceptible people.

INFORMATION FOR USERS

Your drug prescription is tailored for you. Do not alter dosage without checking with your doctor.

How taken/used Tablets, liquid.

Frequency and timing of doses 4 x daily, at least 30 minutes before food.

Dosage range *Adults* 2–4g daily. *Children* Reduced dose according to age.

Onset of effect Within a few hours.

Duration of action Up to 12 hours.

Diet advice None.

Storage Keep in original container at room temperature out of the reach of children.

Missed dose Take as soon as you remember. If your next dose is due within 2 hours, take a single dose now and skip the next.

Stopping the drug Take the full course. Even if you feel better, the original infection may still be present and may recur if the treatment is stopped too soon.

Exceeding the dose An occasional unintentional extra dose is unlikely to be a cause for concern. But if you notice any unusual symptoms, or if a large overdose has been taken, tell your doctor.

POSSIBLE ADVERSE EFFECTS

Most users do not have any serious adverse effects. Common effects are nausea and vomiting; diarrhoea may also occur. Discuss with your doctor if these are severe. Rarely, however, phenoxymethylpenicillin may provoke a serious allergic reaction called anaphylaxis. If you develop a rash, itching, wheezing or breathing difficulties, stop taking the drug and seek immediate medical attention.

INTERACTIONS

Warfarin Phenoxymethylpenicillin potentially alters the anticoagulant effect of warfarin.

Typhoid vaccine Penicillins may inactivate oral typhoid vaccine if taken together with vaccine.

Probenecid increases the level of phenoxymethylpenicillin in the blood.

Neomycin reduces the level of phenoxymethylpenicillin in the blood.

Methotrexate Excretion of this drug may be greatly reduced by phenoxymethylpenicillin, leading to toxicity.

SPECIAL PRECAUTIONS

Be sure to tell your doctor if:

- You have a long-term kidney problem.
- You have had a previous allergic reaction to a penicillin or cephalosporin antibiotic.
- You are taking other medicines.

Pregnancy No evidence of risk.

Breast-feeding The drug passes into the breast milk, but normal doses are unlikely to affect the baby adversely. Discuss with your doctor.

Infants and children Reduced dose necessary.

Over 60 No special problems.

Driving and hazardous work No known problems.
Alcohol No known problems.

PROLONGED USE

Prolonged use may increase the risk of *Candida* infections and diarrhoea.

PHENYTOIN/ FOSPHENYTOIN

Brand name [phenytoin] Epanutin; [fosphenytoin] Pro-Epanutin
Used in the following combined preparations None

QUICK REFERENCE

Drug group Anticonvulsant drug (p.14)
Overdose danger rating High
Dependence rating Low
Prescription needed Yes
Available as generic Yes

GENERAL INFORMATION

Phenytoin is used to treat epilepsy. It decreases the likelihood of convulsions by reducing abnormal electrical activity in the brain. Fosphenytoin is given by injection for severe seizures. Phenytoin has also been used for other disorders, such as migraine, trigeminal neuralgia, and certain abnormal heart rhythms. The dose must be adjusted according to blood levels of the drug. Patients are advised to keep to one brand. Some adverse effects are more severe in children, so other options are preferred. Phenytoin powerfully activates liver enzymes that metabolize other drugs, so it can often trigger significant interactions.

INFORMATION FOR USERS

Your drug prescription is tailored for you. Do not alter dosage without checking with your doctor.
How taken/used Tablets, chewable tablets, capsules, liquid, injection.
Frequency and timing of doses 1–2 x daily with food or plenty of water.
Dosage range *Adults* 200–500mg daily (usually as a single dose). *Children* According to age and weight. Note: a small increase in the dose can cause a disproportionately high drug level in the blood.
Onset of effect Full anticonvulsant effect may not be felt for 7–10 days.
Duration of action 24 hours.
Diet advice Folic acid and vitamin D deficiency may occasionally occur. Make sure you eat a balanced diet containing fresh, green vegetables and dairy products.
Storage Keep in original container at room temperature out of the reach of children.
Missed dose Take as soon as you remember.
Stopping the drug Do not stop the drug without consulting your doctor; seizures may recur.

OVERDOSE ACTION

Seek immediate medical advice in all cases. Take emergency action if unsteadiness, severe weakness, confusion, or loss of consciousness occur.

POSSIBLE ADVERSE EFFECTS

Many of the adverse effects appear only after prolonged use. Dizziness, headache, nausea, vomiting, and insomnia are common. More rarely, increased body hair or overgrowth of the gums may occur. Discuss with your doctor if any of these become severe; the doctor may prescribe a different anticonvulsant. If you have confusion or unsteadiness, or develop a rash, fever, sore throat, or mouth ulcers, contact your doctor at once. Long-term use of phenytoin may cause other adverse effects (see Prolonged use).

INTERACTIONS

General note Many drugs may interact with phenytoin, causing an increase or a reduction in the blood level of phenytoin. The dosage of phenytoin may need to be adjusted. Consult your doctor or pharmacist.
Oral contraceptives Phenytoin may reduce their effectiveness.
Antidepressants, antipsychotics, mefloquine, chloroquine, and St John's wort These preparations may reduce the effect of phenytoin.
Warfarin The anticoagulant effect of this drug may be altered. An adjustment in its dosage may be necessary.

SPECIAL PRECAUTIONS

Be sure to tell your doctor if:
- You have long-term liver or kidney problems.
- You have heart problems.
- You have diabetes.
- You have porphyria.
- You are taking other medicines.

Pregnancy The drug may be associated with malformation and a tendency to bleeding in

the newborn baby. The mother should take folic acid supplements. Discuss with doctor.
Breast-feeding The drug passes into the breast milk, but normal doses are unlikely to affect the baby adversely. Discuss with your doctor.
Infants and children Reduced dose necessary. Increased likelihood of overgrowth of the gums and excessive growth of body hair.
Over 60 Reduced dose may be necessary.
Driving and hazardous work Your underlying condition, as well the effects of phenytoin, may make such activities inadvisable. Discuss with your doctor.
Alcohol Avoid. Alcohol increases the sedative effects of this drug.

PROLONGED USE

There is a slight risk that blood abnormalities may occur. Prolonged use may also lead to adverse effects on skin, gums, and bones. In addition, it may disrupt control of diabetes. People of Han Chinese ethnic origin are particularly prone to toxic side effects.
Monitoring Periodic blood tests are performed to monitor levels of the drug in the body, composition of the blood cells and blood chemistry, and blood levels of vitamin D.

PILOCARPINE

Brand names Minims Pilocarpine, Salagen
Used in the following combined preparations None

QUICK REFERENCE

Drug group Drug for glaucoma (p.112)
Overdose danger rating Medium
Dependence rating Low
Prescription needed Yes
Available as generic Yes

GENERAL INFORMATION

Pilocarpine is a miotic drug that is used to treat chronic glaucoma and severe glaucoma prior to surgery. The eye drops are fast-acting, but have to be reapplied every 4 to 8 hours. Pilocarpine frequently causes blurred vision; spasm of the eye muscles may cause headaches, particularly at the start of treatment. However, serious adverse effects are rare. Pilocarpine tablets are used to treat dry mouth following radiotherapy to the head and neck, and dry mouth and eyes due to Sjögren's syndrome (an autoimmune disease).

INFORMATION FOR USERS

Your drug prescription is tailored for you. Do not alter dosage without checking with your doctor.
How taken/used Tablets, eye drops.
Frequency and timing of doses *Eye drops* 4 x daily (chronic glaucoma); 5-minute intervals until condition is controlled (acute glaucoma). *Tablets* 3–4 x daily after food with plenty of water.
Adult dosage range According to formulation and condition. In general, 1–2 eye drops are used per application. *Tablets* 15–30mg daily.
Onset of effect 15–30 minutes.
Duration of action 4–8 weeks for maximum effect (tablets); 3–8 hours (eye drops).
Diet advice None.
Storage Keep tablets/eye drops in original container at room temperature out of the reach of children. Discard drops 1 month after opening.
Missed dose Use as soon as you remember. If less than 2 hours before your next dose, skip the missed dose and take the next dose now.
Stopping the drug Do not stop the drug without consulting your doctor; symptoms may recur.
Exceeding the dose An occasional unintentional extra application is unlikely to cause problems. Excessive use may cause facial flushing, an increase in the flow of saliva, and sweating. If accidentally swallowed, seek medical attention immediately.

POSSIBLE ADVERSE EFFECTS

The adverse effects vary according to the form of the drug. Eye drops commonly cause headache or brow ache (which usually wear off after a few days), blurred vision, poor night vision, sweating, chills, and eye pain or irritation. More rarely, they may cause red, watery eyes or twitching of the eyelids. If you have eye pain or irritation, consult your doctor immediately; discuss other symptoms with your doctor if they are severe. Pilocarpine tablets commonly cause nausea, diarrhoea, blurred vision, dizziness, headache, and frequent urination. Discuss with your doctor if these are severe. If wheezing occurs, stop the drug and contact your doctor immediately.

INTERACTIONS

General note A wide range of drugs may enhance the effects of pilocarpine tablets, including antihistamines (e.g. chlorphenamine), tricyclic antidepressants, and phenothiazines (e.g. chlorpromazine).

Beta blockers These drugs may reduce the effects of pilocarpine and make conduction disturbances in the heart more likely.
Calcium channel blockers may increase the systemic effect of pilocarpine.

SPECIAL PRECAUTIONS

Be sure to tell your doctor if:
◆ You have asthma.
◆ You have inflamed eyes.
◆ You wear contact lenses.
◆ You have heart, liver, or gastrointestinal problems.
◆ You are taking other medicines.

Pregnancy Avoid unless potential benefit outweighs risk. Safety of tablets and eye drops not established. Discuss with your doctor.
Breast-feeding Not known whether pilocarpine is excreted into breast milk, and safety has not been established. Discuss with your doctor.
Infants and children Information is limited, but no significant safety issues have been reported.
Over 60 Reduced night vision is particularly noticeable; no dosage adjustment required.
Driving and hazardous work Avoid such activities, especially in poor light, until you have learned how pilocarpine affects you because it may cause short sight and poor night vision.
Alcohol No known problems.

PROLONGED USE

The effect of the drug may occasionally wear off as the body adapts, but may be restored by changing temporarily to another drug.
Monitoring Pressure inside the eye and the visual fields should be monitored in patients with glaucoma who are using pilocarpine.

PIOGLITAZONE

Brand names Actos, Glidipion
Used in the following combined preparation Competact

QUICK REFERENCE

Drug group Drug for diabetes (p.80)
Overdose danger rating High
Dependence rating Low
Prescription needed Yes
Available as generic Yes

GENERAL INFORMATION

Pioglitazone is an oral antidiabetic drug of the thiazolidinedione type, used to treat Type 2 diabetes. It works by reducing insulin resistance in body tissues, which leads to a reduction of blood glucose levels. The effects appear gradually and reach their full extent in about 8 weeks. Pioglitazone may be used alone but is often used with metformin and/or a sulfonylurea; it is available as a combined preparation with metformin. It works better in obese people with diabetes, although it often causes weight gain. It may also be used with insulin in people with Type 2 diabetes, although this may increase the risk of heart failure. Bone fractures are another possible adverse effect.

INFORMATION FOR USERS

Your drug prescription is tailored for you. Do not alter dosage without checking with your doctor.
How taken/used Tablets.
Frequency and timing of doses 1 x daily.
Adult dosage range 15–45mg daily.
Onset of effect 60 minutes; it can take 8 weeks for full effects to appear.
Duration of action 12–24 hours.
Diet advice An individualized diabetic diet must be maintained for the drug to be fully effective. Follow your doctor's advice.
Storage Keep in original container at room temperature out of the reach of children.
Missed dose Take as soon as you remember. If your next dose is due within 2 hours, take a single dose now and skip the next.
Stopping the drug Do not stop without consulting your doctor; stopping the drug may lead to worsening of the underlying condition.

OVERDOSE ACTION

Seek immediate medical advice in all cases. If you have warning signs of low blood sugar (such as faintness, dizziness, headache, confusion, sweating, or tremor), eat or drink something sugary. Take emergency action if loss of consciousness occurs.

POSSIBLE ADVERSE EFFECTS

Fatigue and weakness (due to anaemia) and weight gain (even on a strict diabetic diet) are common side effects, as are indigestion, flatulence, nausea, abdominal pain, and headache. More rarely, the drug may cause dark urine, dizziness, pins and needles, bone pain in the arms, hands, and feet, oedema (water retention), breathlessness, and a cough. Discuss with your doctor if indigestion or flatulence are severe or if you have any of the other side effects. If jaundice occurs, stop taking the drug and contact your doctor immediately. Pioglitazone has also been associated with heart failure, and long-term use carries an increased risk of fractures (see Prolonged use).

INTERACTIONS

Diazoxide, corticosteroids, diuretics, and progesterones may reduce the effects of pioglitazone.
Gemfibrozil reduces the metabolism of pioglitazone, so a reduced dose may be necessary.
Non-steroidal anti-inflammatory drugs (NSAIDs) may increase the risk of fluid retention.
Rifampicin reduces the blood level of pioglitazone, so an increased dose may be necessary.

SPECIAL PRECAUTIONS

Be sure to tell your doctor if:
- You have liver problems.
- You are anaemic.
- You have a history of heart failure, angina, heart attack, or stroke.
- You have severe kidney failure.
- You have osteoporosis.
- You are taking other medicines.

Pregnancy Safety not established. Discuss with your doctor.
Breast-feeding Safety not established. Discuss with your doctor.
Infants and children Not recommended.
Over 60 No special problems, but older people may be more susceptible to side effects.
Driving and hazardous work No known problems.
Alcohol Avoid excessive intake. Alcohol can increase the effects of pioglitazone.

PROLONGED USE

Pioglitazone, like other antidiabetic drugs, can be used indefinitely but should be discontinued if there is no evidence of an adequate response. Heart failure signs are more common in patients on pioglitazone, although not mortality from heart failure. Long-term use increases the risk of bone fractures in the arms, hands, and feet, and there is a small risk of developing bladder cancer.
Monitoring Initial and periodic blood tests of liver function will be performed. Weight will be measured at intervals. Blood sugar levels should be monitored regularly. You should tell your doctor if you pass blood in your urine while taking the drug.

PIROXICAM

Brand names Feldene, Feldene Melt
Used in the following combined preparations None

QUICK REFERENCE

Drug group Non-steroidal anti-inflammatory drug (p.48) and drug for gout (p.51)
Overdose danger rating Medium
Dependence rating Low
Prescription needed Yes
Available as generic Yes

GENERAL INFORMATION

Piroxicam is a non-steroidal anti-inflammatory drug (NSAID) that, like others in this group, reduces pain, stiffness, and inflammation. It is used for osteoarthritis, rheumatoid arthritis, acute attacks of gout, and ankylosing spondylitis; it relieves symptoms of arthritis, although it does not cure the disease. The drug is sometimes prescribed in conjunction with slow-acting drugs in rheumatoid arthritis to relieve pain and inflammation while these drugs take effect. It may also be given for pain relief after sports injuries, for conditions such as tendinitis and bursitis, and following minor surgery.

Blood levels of piroxicam remain high for many hours after an oral dose, so it needs to be taken only once daily.

Piroxicam is one of the NSAIDs most likely to cause gastrointestinal side effects.

INFORMATION FOR USERS

Your drug prescription is tailored for you. Do not alter dosage without checking with your doctor.
How taken/used Tablets, capsules, melts, gel.
Frequency and timing of doses 1–3 x daily with food or plenty of water (oral doses). 3-4 x daily (gel).
Adult dosage range 10–20mg daily.
Onset of effect 3–4 hours (pain relief); full effect develops over 2–4 weeks (arthritis) or 4–5 days (gout).
Duration of action Up to 2 days; 7–10 days after treatment stops.
Diet advice None.
Storage Keep in original container at room temperature out of the reach of children. Protect from light.
Missed dose Take as soon as you remember. If your next dose is due within 4 hours, take a single dose now and skip the next.

Stopping the drug When taken for short-term pain relief, the drug can be safely stopped as soon as you no longer need it. If prescribed for the long-term treatment of arthritis, however, seek medical advice before stopping the drug.
Exceeding the dose An occasional unintentional extra dose is unlikely to be a cause for concern. Large overdoses may cause nausea and vomiting. Notify your doctor.

POSSIBLE ADVERSE EFFECTS
The most common adverse effects are gastrointestinal: heartburn, indigestion, nausea, and vomiting. Less commonly, the drug may cause headache, dizziness, drowsiness, swelling of the legs or feet, and weight gain. Discuss with your doctor if any of these are severe. If you develop a rash or itching, stop taking the drug and contact your doctor. If you have wheezing or breathlessness, or have black or blood-stained faeces, stop the drug and call your doctor immediately. Long-term use increases the risk of certain disorders (see below).

INTERACTIONS
General note Piroxicam interacts with a wide range of drugs, including other NSAIDs, corticosteroids, and oral anticoagulants, increasing the risk of bleeding and/or peptic ulcers.
Lithium and methotrexate Piroxicam may raise blood levels of these drugs.
Antihypertensives and diuretics Beneficial effects of these drugs may be reduced by piroxicam.
Ciprofloxacin, norfloxacin, and ofloxacin Piroxicam may increase the risk of seizures when taken with these drugs.
Ritonavir increases blood levels of piroxicam.

SPECIAL PRECAUTIONS
Be sure to tell your doctor if:
- You have liver or kidney problems.
- You have heart problems or high blood pressure.
- You have had a peptic ulcer, oesophagitis, or acid indigestion.
- You have porphyria.
- You have asthma.
- You are allergic to aspirin or other NSAIDs.
- You are taking other medicines.

Pregnancy The drug may increase the risks of adverse effects on the baby's heart and may prolong labour if taken in the third trimester. Discuss with your doctor.
Breast-feeding The drug passes into the breast milk but normal doses are unlikely to affect the baby adversely. Discuss with your doctor.
Infants and children Not recommended under 6 years. Reduced dose necessary.
Over 60 Increased likelihood of adverse effects. Reduced dose may therefore be necessary.
Driving and hazardous work Avoid such activities until you have learned how piroxicam affects you; the drug can cause dizziness.
Alcohol Avoid. Alcohol may increase the risk of stomach disorders with piroxicam.
Surgery and general anaesthetics Piroxicam may prolong bleeding. Discuss with your doctor or dentist before any surgery.

PROLONGED USE
There is an increased risk of bleeding from peptic ulcers and in the bowel with prolonged use of piroxicam. There is also a small risk of a heart attack or stroke. To minimize these risks, the lowest effective dose is given for the shortest duration.

PIZOTIFEN

Brand name None
Used in the following combined preparations None

QUICK REFERENCE
Drug group Drug for migraine (p.18)
Overdose danger rating Medium
Dependence rating Low
Prescription needed Yes
Available as generic Yes

GENERAL INFORMATION
Pizotifen is an antihistamine with a chemical structure similar to that of the tricyclic antidepressants (p.12), and has similar anticholinergic effects (p.7). It is thought to work by blocking histamine and serotonin, chemicals that act on blood vessels in the brain. The drug is prescribed to prevent migraine headaches in people who have frequent, disabling attacks; however, it is not effective in relieving migraine attacks once they have started.

The main disadvantage with prolonged use of pizotifen is that it stimulates the appetite and, as a result, often causes weight gain. It is usually prescribed only for people in whom other measures for migraine prevention, such as avoidance of trigger factors, have failed.

The sweetener used in the liquid medication is hydrogenated glucose syrup, and this may affect levels of blood sugar.

INFORMATION FOR USERS

Your drug prescription is tailored for you. Do not alter dosage without checking with your doctor.

How taken/used Tablets, liquid (available only by special order).

Frequency and timing of doses Once a day (at night) or 3 x daily.

Adult dosage range 1.5–4.5mg daily. Maximum single dose 3mg.

Onset of effect Full beneficial effects may not be felt for several days.

Duration of action Effects of this drug may last for several weeks.

Diet advice People who have migraine may be advised to avoid foods that trigger headaches in their case.

Storage Keep in original container at room temperature out of the reach of children. Protect from light.

Missed dose Take as soon as you remember. If your next dose is due within 4 hours, take a single dose now and skip the next.

Stopping the drug Do not stop the drug without consulting your doctor; symptoms may recur.

Exceeding the dose An occasional unintentional extra dose is unlikely to cause problems. Large overdoses may cause drowsiness, nausea, palpitations, seizures, and coma; tell your doctor.

POSSIBLE ADVERSE EFFECTS

Drowsiness is a common adverse effect that can often be minimized by starting with a low dose and then gradually increasing it. Weight gain, increased appetite, fatigue, nausea, and dizziness are also common. More rarely, pizotifen may cause muscle pains, dry mouth, blurred vision, anxiety, and depression. Consult your doctor if you experience anxiety or depression or if any of the other adverse effects are severe.

INTERACTIONS

Anticholinergic drugs The weak anticholinergic effects of pizotifen may be increased by other anticholinergic drugs, including tricyclic antidepressants.

Antihypertensive drugs The blood-pressure-lowering effects of guanethidine and debrisoquine are reduced by pizotifen.

Sedatives All drugs with a sedative effect on the central nervous system are likely to increase the sedative properties of pizotifen. These include alcohol, sleeping drugs, anti-anxiety drugs, opioid analgesics, and antihistamines.

SPECIAL PRECAUTIONS

Be sure to tell your doctor if:

- You have a long-term kidney problem.
- You have glaucoma.
- You have urinary retention.
- You have prostate problems.
- You have galactose intolerance.
- You have epilepsy.
- You are taking other medicines.

Pregnancy Safety in pregnancy not established. Discuss with your doctor.

Breast-feeding The drug passes into the breast milk, but normal doses are unlikely to affect the baby adversely. Discuss with your doctor.

Infants and children Reduced dose usually necessary. Not recommended under 5 years.

Over 60 No special problems.

Driving and hazardous work Avoid until you know how pizotifen affects you because the drug can cause drowsiness and blurred vision.

Alcohol Avoid. Alcohol may increase the sedative effects of this drug.

PROLONGED USE

Pizotifen often causes weight gain during long-term use. Treatment is usually reviewed every 6 months.

PRAVASTATIN

Brand name Lipostat

Used in the following combined preparations None

QUICK REFERENCE

Drug group Lipid-lowering drug (p.35)

Overdose danger rating Medium

Dependence rating Low

Prescription needed Yes

Available as generic Yes

GENERAL INFORMATION

Pravastatin belongs to the statin group of lipid-lowering drugs. It may be used for people with hypercholesterolaemia (high levels of cholesterol in the blood) who have not responded to other treatments, such as a special diet, and who are at risk of developing heart disease or stroke. However, it has been largely superseded by newer, more potent statins, such as atorvastatin and rosuvastatin. Pravastatin works by blocking the action of an enzyme that is needed for the manufacture of cholesterol, mainly in the liver. As a result, blood levels of cholesterol are lowered, which can help to prevent heart disease and stroke.

Side effects are usually mild and often wear off over time. Pravastatin is concentrated in the liver and may raise levels of liver enzymes, but this does not usually indicate serious liver damage. Rarely, it may cause muscle damage; any unexpected muscle tenderness, pain, or weakness should be reported to your doctor.

INFORMATION FOR USERS

Your drug prescription is tailored for you. Do not alter dosage without checking with your doctor.

How taken/used Tablets.

Frequency and timing of doses Once daily at night.

Adult dosage range 10–40mg daily, changed after intervals of at least 4 weeks.

Onset of effect Within 2 weeks. Full beneficial effect may be felt within 4 weeks.

Duration of action 24 hours.

Diet advice A low-fat diet is usually recommended.

Storage Keep in original container at room temperature out of the reach of children. Protect from light.

Missed dose Take as soon as you remember. If next dose is due within 8 hours, do not take the missed dose, but take next dose as usual.

Stopping the drug Do not stop without consulting your doctor; stopping the drug may lead to worsening of the underlying condition.

Exceeding the dose An occasional unintentional extra dose is unlikely to cause problems. Large overdoses may cause liver problems. Notify your doctor.

POSSIBLE ADVERSE EFFECTS

Most adverse effects are mild and usually disappear with time. Common effects include abdominal pain, constipation, diarrhoea, nausea, flatulence, sleep disturbance, and headache; discuss with your doctor if any of these are severe. If you develop a rash, stop taking the drug. If you have muscle pains, tenderness, weakness, or jaundice, stop taking the drug and call your doctor immediately.

INTERACTIONS

Antifungals Itraconazole, ketoconazole, and possibly other antifungals may increase risk of muscle damage if taken with pravastatin.

Orlistat This drug increases the blood levels and toxicity of pravastatin.

Clarithromycin and erythromycin These drugs increase blood levels of pravastatin.

Other lipid-lowering drugs (fibrates) May increase risk of muscle damage if used with pravastatin.

Ciclosporin and other immunosuppressant drugs Increased risk of muscle damage if taken with pravastatin. Not usually prescribed together.

SPECIAL PRECAUTIONS

Be sure to tell your doctor if:

- You have had liver or kidney problems.
- You have had side effects on your muscles from any other lipid-lowering drugs.
- You have an underactive thyroid.
- You have galactose intolerance.
- You are taking other medicines.

Pregnancy Not recommended. May affect fetal development. Inform your doctor if you are or plan to become pregnant.

Breast-feeding The drug passes into breast milk and may affect the baby. Discuss with doctor.

Infants and children Not recommended under 5 years. Reduced dose necessary in older children, under specialist advice.

Over 60 No special problems.

Driving and hazardous work No special problems.

Alcohol Avoid excessive amounts. May increase risk of liver problems with this drug.

PROLONGED USE

Long-term use can affect liver function.

Monitoring Regular blood tests to check liver and muscle function are usually required.

PREDNISOLONE

Brand names Deltacortril, Minims Prednisolone, Pevanti, Pred Forte, and others

Used in the following combined preparation Scheriproct

QUICK REFERENCE

Drug group Corticosteroid (p.78)

Overdose danger rating Low

Dependence rating Low

Prescription needed Yes

Available as generic Yes

GENERAL INFORMATION

Prednisolone, a powerful corticosteroid, is used for a wide range of conditions, including some skin diseases, rheumatic disorders, allergic states, and certain blood disorders. It is used as eye drops to reduce inflammation in conjunctivitis or iritis and may be given as an enema to treat inflammatory bowel disease. It is also prescribed with fludrocortisone for pituitary or adrenal gland disorders.

Prednisolone taken short term, either by mouth or topically, rarely causes serious side effects. However, long-term treatment with high doses can cause systemic effects, such as osteoporosis, fluid retention, indigestion, diabetes, hypertension, and acne. Enteric-coated tablets reduce the local effects of the drug on the stomach but not these systemic effects.

INFORMATION FOR USERS

Your drug prescription is tailored for you. Do not alter dosage without checking with your doctor.

How taken/used Tablets, injection, suppositories, enema, foam, eye and ear drops.

Frequency and timing of doses *Tablets* Usually once daily or on alternate days with food. *Eye/ear drops* 2–4 x daily, more often initially.

Adult dosage range Considerable variation. Follow your doctor's instructions.

Onset of effect 2–4 days.

Duration of action 12–72 hours.

Diet advice A low-sodium diet may be recommended when the oral form is prescribed for extended periods. Follow your doctor's advice.

Storage Keep in original container at room temperature out of the reach of children. Protect from light.

Missed dose Take as soon as you remember. If your next dose is due within 6 hours, take a single dose now and skip the next.

Stopping the drug Do not stop without consulting your doctor. Abrupt cessation of long-term treatment by mouth may be dangerous.

Exceeding the dose An occasional unintentional extra dose is unlikely to be a cause for concern. But if you notice any unusual symptoms, or if a large overdose has been taken, tell your doctor.

POSSIBLE ADVERSE EFFECTS

Common adverse effects are weight gain, acne, indigestion, and mood changes or depression; more rarely, muscle weakness may occur. Discuss with your doctor if weight gain is substantial or if you develop any of these other symptoms. If you have black or blood-stained faeces, stop taking the drug and contact your doctor immediately.

Serious adverse effects occur only with high doses taken by mouth for long periods; the risk increases with dose and duration of treatment. If you are taking prednisolone tablets regularly, avoid close contact with chickenpox, shingles, and measles and seek urgent medical attention if exposed. Prolonged use of prednisolone may cause various disorders (see below).

INTERACTIONS

Anticonvulsant drugs Carbamazepine, phenytoin, and phenobarbital can reduce the effects of prednisolone.

Vaccines Serious reactions can occur if live vaccines are given with prednisolone. Discuss with your doctor.

Antihypertensive and antidiabetic drugs and insulin Larger doses may be needed when taken with prednisolone.

Ciclosporin and tacrolimus may reduce the dose of prednisolone required.

Non-steroidal anti-inflammatory drugs (NSAIDs) There is an increased risk of peptic ulcers when these drugs are taken with prednisolone.

SPECIAL PRECAUTIONS

Be sure to tell your doctor if:

- You have had a peptic ulcer.
- You have glaucoma.
- You have depression or a psychiatric illness.
- You have any infection or have had tuberculosis.
- You have diabetes or osteoporosis.
- You have high blood pressure.
- You have liver or kidney disease.
- You are taking other medicines.

Pregnancy No evidence of risk with eye or ear drops. Taken as tablets in low doses, harm to the fetus is unlikely. Discuss with your doctor.

Breast-feeding No evidence of risk with eye or ear drops. Taken by mouth, the drug passes into breast milk, but low doses are unlikely to harm the baby. Discuss with your doctor.

Infants and children Only given when essential. Alternate-day dosing preferred to prevent growth retardation.

Over 60 Increased likelihood of adverse effects. Reduced dose may be necessary.

Driving and hazardous work No known problems.

Alcohol Keep consumption low. Alcohol may increase the risk of peptic ulcers with prednisolone taken by mouth or injection.
Infection Avoid exposure to chickenpox, shingles, or measles if having systemic treatment.

PROLONGED USE

Prolonged use by mouth can lead to diabetes, peptic ulcers, glaucoma, muscle weakness, osteoporosis, and growth retardation in children. Prolonged topical use may also lead to skin thinning. People on long-term treatment should carry a steroid card.

PROCHLORPERAZINE

Brand names Buccastem, Stemetil
Used in the following combined preparations None

QUICK REFERENCE

Drug group Phenothiazine antipsychotic drug (p.13) and anti-emetic drug (p.19)
Overdose danger rating Medium
Dependence rating Low
Prescription needed Yes (most preparations)
Available as generic Yes

GENERAL INFORMATION

Prochlorperazine belongs to a group of drugs called the phenothiazines, which act on the central nervous system. In small doses, it controls nausea and vomiting, especially when these occur as side effects of medical treatment by drugs or radiation, or of anaesthesia. It is available over the counter for nausea and vomiting associated with migraine. The drug is also used to treat the nausea that occurs with inner-ear disorders such as vertigo. In large doses, prochlorperazine is sometimes used as an antipsychotic to reduce aggression and suppress abnormal behaviour (see p.13) in schizophrenia, mania, and other mental disorders. It does not cure any of these conditions, but it helps to relieve symptoms.

INFORMATION FOR USERS

Your drug prescription is tailored for you. Do not alter dosage without checking with your doctor.
How taken/used Tablets, buccal tablets, liquid, injection.
Frequency and timing of doses 2–3 x daily.
Adult dosage range *Nausea and vomiting* 20mg initially, then 5–10mg per dose (tablets); 12.5mg per dose (injection). *Mental illness* 25–100mg daily. Larger doses may be given.
Onset of effect Within 60 minutes (by mouth); 10–20 minutes (by injection).
Duration of action 3–6 hours.
Diet advice None.
Storage Keep in original container at room temperature out of the reach of children. Protect from light.
Missed dose Take as soon as you remember. If your next dose is due within 2 hours, take a single dose now and skip the next.
Stopping the drug Do not stop the drug without consulting your doctor; symptoms may recur.
Exceeding the dose An occasional unintentional extra dose is unlikely to be a cause for concern. Large overdoses may cause unusual drowsiness and affect the heart. Notify your doctor.

POSSIBLE ADVERSE EFFECTS

Prochlorperazine has a strong anticholinergic effect (p.7) that can cause a variety of minor symptoms, such as dry mouth and constipation; these often diminish with time. The most significant adverse effect with high doses is tremor and muscle rigidity of the face and limbs (parkinsonism) caused by changes in the balance of brain chemicals. If parkinsonism occurs, or if you experience dizziness and fainting, consult your doctor. Other common effects include drowsiness and lethargy; discuss with your doctor if severe. Rarely, a rash or jaundice may occur; if so, stop taking the drug and consult your doctor. If you develop abnormal facial or eye movements, stop the drug and contact your doctor immediately.

INTERACTIONS

Sedatives All drugs with a sedative effect are likely to increase the sedative effects of prochlorperazine.
Drugs for Parkinson's disease Prochlorperazine may block the beneficial effect of these drugs.
Anticholinergic drugs Prochlorperazine may increase the side effects of these drugs.
Antihypertensive drugs Prochlorperazine can increase the effects of these drugs, especially doxazosin.

SPECIAL PRECAUTIONS

Be sure to tell your doctor if:
- You have heart problems.
- You have liver or kidney problems.

- You have had epileptic seizures.
- You have Parkinson's disease.
- You have dementia.
- You have prostate problems.
- You have glaucoma.
- You are taking other medicines.

Pregnancy Safety in pregnancy not established. Discuss with your doctor.

Breast-feeding The drug passes into the breast milk and may affect the baby. Discuss with your doctor.

Infants and children Not recommended in infants less than 10kg or in young children. Reduced dose necessary in older children due to increased risk of adverse effects.

Over 60 Increased likelihood of adverse effects. Reduced dose may therefore be necessary.

Driving and hazardous work Avoid until you know how the drug affects you because it can cause drowsiness and reduced alertness.

Alcohol Avoid. Alcohol may increase and prolong the sedative effects of this drug.

PROLONGED USE

Use of prochlorperazine for more than a few months may lead to the development of involuntary, potentially irreversible, eye, mouth, and tongue movements (tardive dyskinesia). Occasionally, jaundice may occur.

Monitoring Periodic blood tests may be done.

PROCYCLIDINE

Brand names Arpicolin, Kemadrin

Used in the following combined preparations None

QUICK REFERENCE

Drug group Drug for parkinsonism (p.16)

Overdose danger rating High

Dependence rating Low

Prescription needed Yes

Available as generic Yes

GENERAL INFORMATION

Procyclidine is an anticholinergic drug (p.7) to treat Parkinson's disease. It is especially helpful in the early stages for treating muscle tremor. It also helps to reduce excess salivation. However, it has little effect on the shuffling gait and slow muscle movements that characterize Parkinson's disease. Procyclidine is also often used to treat drug-induced parkinsonism from treatment with antipsychotics.

The drug may cause various adverse effects (see below). However, these are rarely serious enough to warrant stopping the treatment.

INFORMATION FOR USERS

Your drug prescription is tailored for you. Do not alter dosage without checking with your doctor.

How taken/used Tablets, liquid, injection.

Frequency and timing of doses 2–3 x daily, preferably after meals. A further dose may be added at bedtime.

Adult dosage range 7.5–30mg daily, exceptionally up to 60mg daily. Dosage is determined individually in order to find the best balance between effective relief of symptoms and the occurrence of adverse effects.

Onset of effect Within 30 minutes.

Duration of action 8–12 hours.

Diet advice None.

Storage Keep in original container at room temperature out of the reach of children.

Missed dose Take as soon as you remember. If your next dose is due within 2 hours, take a single dose now and skip the next.

Stopping the drug Do not stop the drug without consulting your doctor; symptoms may recur.

OVERDOSE ACTION

Seek immediate medical advice in all cases. Take emergency action if palpitations, seizures, or unconsciousness occur.

POSSIBLE ADVERSE EFFECTS

The adverse effects of procyclidine are mainly the result of its anticholinergic action. Dry mouth, constipation, drowsiness, dizziness, and blurred vision are common. Discuss with your doctor if you have blurred vision or if any of the other symptoms are severe as it may be possible to overcome them by adjusting the drug dosage. Difficulty in passing urine is also common; if it occurs, call your doctor immediately. If you develop confusion, or severe nausea, vomiting, nervousness or anxiety, or rash, discuss with your doctor.

INTERACTIONS

Anticholinergic and antihistamine drugs May increase the adverse effects of procyclidine.

Tricyclic antidepressants, paroxetine (but not other SSRI antidepressants), and antipsychotic drugs These drugs may increase the side effects of procyclidine.

SPECIAL PRECAUTIONS

Be sure to tell your doctor if:

◆ You have long-term liver or kidney problems.
◆ You have a personal or family history of glaucoma.
◆ You have high blood pressure.
◆ You have constipation.
◆ You have prostate or urinary tract problems.
◆ You are taking other medicines.

Pregnancy Safety in pregnancy not established. Discuss with your doctor.

Breast-feeding Safety in breast-feeding not established. Discuss with your doctor.

Infants and children Not recommended.

Over 60 Increased risk of adverse effects. Reduced dose may be necessary.

Driving and hazardous work Avoid such activities until you have learned how procyclidine affects you because the drug can cause drowsiness, blurred vision, and mild confusion.

Alcohol Avoid. Alcohol may increase the sedative effect of this drug.

PROLONGED USE

Prolonged use of procyclidine may provoke the onset of glaucoma.

Monitoring Periodic eye examinations are usually advised.

PROGUANIL WITH ATOVAQUONE

Brand name Malarone, MaloffProtect

Used in the following combined preparation
Not applicable

QUICK REFERENCE

Drug group Antimalarial drug (p.73)
Overdose danger rating Medium
Dependence rating Low
Prescription needed Yes
Available as generic Yes

GENERAL INFORMATION

Proguanil is used to prevent the development of malaria. Microbial resistance to its effects can occur, however, and this has led to it being used in combination with other drugs. Atovaquone is an antiprotozoal drug that is also active against the fungus *Pneumocystis jirovecii* (a cause of pneumonia in people with poor immunity). It is less useful on its own for malaria, but when combined with proguanil it rapidly treats the infection. The combination is also used to prevent malaria, especially in areas where resistance to other drugs is present.

For prevention, you should start taking proguanil with atovaquone a day or two before travelling. Continue during your stay, and for 7 days after your return. It is important to take other precautions as well, such as using an insect repellent at all times and a mosquito net at night. If you develop an illness or fever in the year after your return from a malarial zone, and especially in the first 3 months, go to your doctor immediately and tell the doctor where you have been.

INFORMATION FOR USERS

Your drug prescription is tailored for you. Do not alter dosage without checking with your doctor.

How taken/used Tablets.

Frequency and timing of doses *Prevention* Once daily with food or a milky drink, at the same time each day. Start 1–2 days before travel and continue for period of stay (which should not exceed 28 days) and for 7 days after return. *Treatment* Once daily for 3 days, with food or a milky drink.

Adult dosage range *Prevention* 1 tablet. *Treatment* 4 tablets.

Onset of effect After 24 hours.

Duration of action 24–48 hours.

Diet advice None.

Storage Keep in original container at room temperature out of the reach of children.

Missed dose Take as soon as you remember. If your next dose is due at this time, take both doses together.

Stopping the drug Do not stop taking the drug for 1 week after leaving a malaria-infected area, otherwise there is a risk that you may develop the disease.

Exceeding the dose An occasional unintentional extra dose is unlikely to cause problems. Large overdoses may cause abdominal pain and vomiting. Notify your doctor.

POSSIBLE ADVERSE EFFECTS

Adverse effects are generally fairly mild. The most frequent is diarrhoea or a rash; less common effects include nausea, vomiting, abdominal pain or indigestion, and headache. Discuss with your doctor if you develop a rash or if these other symptoms are severe. More rarely, the drug may cause mouth ulcers, hair loss, or jaundice. Consult your doctor if mouth ulcers are severe or if these other symptoms occur. If you develop a sore throat or fever, contact your doctor urgently.

INTERACTIONS

Warfarin The effects of warfarin may be enhanced by proguanil with atovaquone.
Antacids The absorption of proguanil with atovaquone may be reduced by antacids.
Rifampicin, metoclopramide, and tetracycline antibiotics These drugs reduce the effect of proguanil with atovaquone.

SPECIAL PRECAUTIONS

Be sure to tell your doctor if:

- You have a long-term kidney problem.
- You have a liver problem.
- You currently have diarrhoea and vomiting.
- You are taking other medicines.

Pregnancy Safety in pregnancy not established, although benefits are generally considered to outweigh risks. Folic acid supplements must be taken. Discuss with your doctor.
Breast-feeding The drug passes into breast milk and may affect the baby. Breast-feeding is not recommended while you are taking the drug; it will not protect your baby from malaria. Discuss with your doctor.
Infants and children Reduced dose necessary.
Over 60 No known problems.
Driving and hazardous work Avoid such activities until you know how the drug affects you because it may cause dizziness.
Alcohol No special problems.

PROLONGED USE

No known problems.

PROMAZINE

Brand name None
Used in the following combined preparations None

QUICK REFERENCE

Drug group Anti-anxiety drug (p.11) and antipsychotic drug (p.13)
Overdose danger rating Medium
Dependence rating Low
Prescription needed Yes
Available as generic Yes

GENERAL INFORMATION

Promazine belongs to a group of drugs called phenothiazines, which act on the brain to regulate abnormal behaviour. The main use of this drug is to calm agitated and restless behaviour. It is also given as a sedative for the short-term treatment of severe anxiety, especially anxiety occurring in older people and in those who have a terminal illness.

Promazine is less likely to cause the unpleasant side effects that are experienced with other phenothiazine drugs, particularly abnormal movements and shaking of the arms and legs (parkinsonism). The most common adverse effect of promazine is sedation.

INFORMATION FOR USERS

Your drug prescription is tailored for you. Do not alter dosage without checking with your doctor.
How taken/used Tablets, liquid.
Frequency and timing of doses 4 x daily.
Adult dosage range 100–800mg daily (tablets).
Onset of effect 30 minutes–1 hour.
Duration of action 4–6 hours.
Diet advice None.
Storage Keep in original container at room temperature out of the reach of children. Protect from light.
Missed dose Take as soon as you remember. If your next dose is due within 2 hours, take a single dose now and skip the next.
Stopping the drug Do not stop the drug without consulting your doctor; symptoms may recur.
Exceeding the dose An occasional unintentional extra dose is unlikely to be a cause for concern. Large overdoses may cause drowsiness, dizziness, unsteadiness, seizures, and coma. Notify your doctor.

POSSIBLE ADVERSE EFFECTS

The more common adverse effects, such as drowsiness, lethargy, dry mouth, constipation, and blurred vision, may be helped by a reduction in dosage; discuss with your doctor if you have blurred vision or if any of these other symptoms are severe. Less commonly, promazine may cause mood changes, palpitations, parkinsonism (tremor and muscle rigidity of the face and limbs), or jaundice; consult your doctor if palpitations, parkinsonism, or jaundice occur or if mood changes are severe. You should also stop taking the drug if you have jaundice. Rarely, promazine may affect the body's ability to regulate its temperature, especially in older people.

INTERACTIONS

Sedatives All drugs that have a sedative effect are likely to increase the sedative properties of promazine.

Drugs for parkinsonism Promazine may reduce the effectiveness of these drugs and increase the risk of side effects when used with them.

Sotalol increases the risk of heart rhythm abnormalities when used with promazine.

Lithium increases the risk of side effects when used with promazine.

Other antipsychotic drugs There is an increased risk of adverse effects when other antipsychotic drugs are used with promazine; concurrent use should be avoided.

SPECIAL PRECAUTIONS

Be sure to tell your doctor if:

- You have heart problems.
- You have long-term liver or kidney problems.
- You have had epileptic seizures.
- You have prostate problems.
- You have glaucoma.
- You have Parkinson's disease.
- You have myasthenia gravis.
- You have phaeochromocytoma (a tumour of the adrenal glands).
- You are taking other medicines.

Pregnancy Safety in pregnancy not established. Discuss with your doctor.

Breast-feeding Safety in breast-feeding not established. Discuss with your doctor.

Infants and children Not recommended.

Over 60 Increased likelihood of adverse effects. Reduced dose may therefore be necessary.

Driving and hazardous work Avoid such activities until you have learned how promazine affects you because the drug can cause drowsiness and reduced alertness.

Alcohol Avoid. Alcohol may increase the sedative effect of this drug.

PROLONGED USE

Use of this drug for more than a few months may be associated with jaundice and abnormal movements. Sometimes a reduction in dose may be recommended.

Monitoring Periodic blood tests for liver function and a full blood count should be performed.

PROMETHAZINE

Brand names Avomine, Phenergan, Sominex

Used in the following combined preparations Night Nurse, Tixylix

QUICK REFERENCE

Drug group Antihistamine (p.56) and anti-emetic drug (p.19)

Overdose danger rating Medium

Dependence rating Low

Prescription needed No (most preparations); Yes (injection)

Available as generic Yes

GENERAL INFORMATION

Promethazine is one of a class of drugs called phenothiazines, which were developed in the 1950s for their beneficial effect on abnormal behaviour arising from mental illnesses (see Antipsychotics, p.13). However, it was found to have effects more like the antihistamines used to treat allergies (p.56) and some types of nausea and vomiting (see Anti-emetics, p.19). The drug is widely used to reduce itching in a variety of skin conditions including urticaria (hives), chickenpox, and eczema. It can also relieve nausea and vomiting caused by inner ear disturbances such as Ménière's disease and motion sickness. Because of its sedative effect, promethazine is sometimes given for short periods to induce sleep; it is also used to reduce agitation and is given as premedication before surgery.

Promethazine is used in combined preparations together with opioid cough suppressants for the relief of coughs and nasal congestion.

INFORMATION FOR USERS

Follow instructions on the label. Call your doctor if symptoms worsen.

How taken/used Tablets, liquid, injection.

Frequency and timing of doses *Allergy* 1–3 x daily or as a single dose at night. *Motion sickness* Bedtime on night before travelling, repeating following morning if necessary, then every 6–8 hours as necessary. *Nausea and vomiting* Every 4–6 hours as necessary.

Dosage range *Adults* 25–100mg per dose, depending on preparation and use. Allergy: usually 10mg. *Children* Reduced dose according to age.

Onset of effect Within 1 hour. If dose is taken after start of nausea, onset of effect is delayed.

Duration of action 8–16 hours.
Diet advice None.
Storage Keep in original container at room temperature out of the reach of children. Protect from light.
Missed dose No cause for concern, but take as soon as you remember. Adjust the timing of your next dose accordingly.
Stopping the drug Can be safely stopped as soon as symptoms disappear.
Exceeding the dose An occasional unintentional extra dose is unlikely to cause problems. Large overdoses may cause drowsiness or agitation, seizures, hallucinations, unsteadiness, and coma. Notify your doctor.

POSSIBLE ADVERSE EFFECTS

The drug usually causes only minor anticholinergic effects (p.7). Common adverse effects include drowsiness, lethargy, blurred vision, dry mouth, and urinary retention. Discuss with your doctor if you have urinary retention or if any of these other effects are severe. Less commonly, palpitations may occur; if so, consult your doctor. More serious adverse effects often occur only with long-term use or very high doses. They include photosensitivity; avoid bright sunlight while taking promethazine. If you develop a light-sensitive rash, or abnormal movements (see Prolonged use, below), stop taking the drug and contact your doctor. If the drug causes a swollen mouth or severe dizziness, stop taking it and call your doctor immediately.

INTERACTIONS

Pregnancy urine test Promethazine may interfere with this test, giving a false result.
Skin-prick allergen tests Promethazine should be stopped a week before skin-prick testing with allergen extracts as it may produce a false result.
Sedatives All drugs that have a sedative effect are likely to increase the sedative properties of promethazine. Such drugs include alcohol, other antihistamines, benzodiazepines, opioid analgesics, and antipsychotics.

SPECIAL PRECAUTIONS

Be sure to consult your doctor or pharmacist before taking this drug if:
- You have liver or kidney problems.
- You have had epileptic seizures.
- You have heart disease.
- You have glaucoma.
- You have prostate problems.
- You have difficulty in passing urine.
- You are taking other medicines.

Pregnancy The drug is probably safe in pregnancy, although safety has not been definitively established. Discuss with your doctor.
Breast-feeding The drug passes into the breast milk, but normal doses are unlikely to affect the baby adversely. Discuss with your doctor.
Infants and children Not recommended for children under 6 years. Reduced dose necessary for older children.
Over 60 Reduced dose may be necessary.
Driving and hazardous work Avoid until you have learned how promethazine affects you because the drug can cause drowsiness.
Alcohol Avoid. Alcohol may increase the sedative effects of this drug.
Sunlight and sunbeds Avoid exposure to strong sunlight as, rarely, skin reactions may occur.

PROLONGED USE

Long-term use is rarely necessary. There is also a risk that abnormal movements (extrapyramidal effects, tic-type movements, spasms) will develop with long-term use. Discuss with your doctor in all cases.

PROPRANOLOL

Brand name Bedranol
Used in the following combined preparations None

QUICK REFERENCE

Drug group Beta blocker (p.28) and anti-anxiety drug (p.11)
Overdose danger rating High
Dependence rating Low
Prescription needed Yes
Available as generic Yes

GENERAL INFORMATION

Propranolol, a non-cardioselective beta blocker, is mainly used to treat angina and abnormal heart rhythms and is helpful in controlling the symptoms of an overactive thyroid gland. It also helps to reduce the palpitations, sweating, and tremor of severe anxiety and to prevent migraine. In addition, the drug is used to treat hypertension (high blood pressure), but this use is declining as more selective beta blockers are now available.

Propranolol is not given to people with respiratory diseases (especially asthma) because it can cause breathing difficulties. It should be used with caution by people with diabetes because it affects the body's response to low blood sugar.

INFORMATION FOR USERS

Your drug prescription is tailored for you. Do not alter dosage without checking with your doctor.

How taken/used Tablets, slow release (SR) capsules, liquid, injection.

Frequency and timing of doses 2–4 x daily. Once daily (SR capsules).

Adult dosage range *Abnormal heart rhythms* 30–160mg daily. *Angina* 80–240mg daily. *Hypertension* 160–320mg daily. *Migraine prevention; anxiety* 40–160mg daily.

Onset of effect 1–2 hours (tablets); after 4 hours (SR capsules). In hypertension and migraine, it may be several weeks before full benefits are felt.

Duration of action 6–12 hours (tablets); up to 24 hours (SR capsules).

Diet advice None.

Storage Keep in original container at room temperature out of the reach of children. Protect from light.

Missed dose Take as soon as you remember. If your next dose is due within 2 hours (tablets) or 12 hours (SR capsules), take a single dose now and skip the next.

Stopping the drug Do not stop without consulting your doctor. Stopping abruptly may lead to worsening of the underlying condition.

OVERDOSE ACTION

Seek immediate medical advice. Take emergency action if breathing difficulties, collapse, or loss of consciousness occur.

POSSIBLE ADVERSE EFFECTS

Propranolol's adverse effects are common to most beta blockers and tend to diminish with long-term use. All adverse effects should be reported to your doctor. The most common effects are lethargy, fatigue, and cold hands and feet. Less commonly, there may be nausea, vomiting, vivid dreams or nightmares, and visual disturbances. If you develop visual disturbances, stop taking the drug. If you experience palpitations or fainting (which may indicate that the drug has slowed the heart beat excessively), breathlessness, or wheezing, you should stop taking the drug and contact your doctor immediately.

INTERACTIONS

Antihypertensives Propranolol may enhance their blood-pressure-lowering effect.

Calcium channel blockers may cause low blood pressure, a slow heart beat, and heart failure if used with propranolol.

Non-steroidal anti-inflammatory drugs (NSAIDs) (e.g. indometacin) may reduce the antihypertensive effect of propranolol.

Theophylline/aminophylline Propranolol may increase blood levels of these drugs.

Cimetidine This drug may increase the effects of propranolol.

Cardiac glycosides These may increase the heart-slowing effect of propranolol.

SPECIAL PRECAUTIONS

Be sure to tell your doctor if:

- You have long-term liver or kidney problems.
- You have a breathing disorder such as asthma, bronchitis, or emphysema.
- You have heart problems.
- You have diabetes.
- You have psoriasis.
- You have poor circulation in the legs.
- You are taking other medicines.

Pregnancy May affect the baby. Discuss with your doctor.

Breast-feeding The drug passes into the breast milk, but normal doses are unlikely to affect the baby adversely. Discuss with your doctor.

Infants and children Reduced dose necessary.

Over 60 Increased risk of adverse effects. Reduced starting dose will therefore be necessary.

Driving and hazardous work Avoid such activities until you have learned how the drug affects you because it can cause dizziness.

Alcohol Avoid excessive intake. Alcohol may increase the blood-pressure-lowering effect of propranolol.

Surgery and general anaesthetics Occasionally, propranolol may need to be stopped before you have a general anaesthetic, but you should only do this after discussion with your doctor or dentist.

PROLONGED USE

No problems expected.

PROPYLTHIOURACIL

Brand name None
Used in the following combined preparations None

QUICK REFERENCE

Drug group Drug for thyroid disorders (p.82)
Overdose danger rating Medium
Dependence rating Low
Prescription needed Yes
Available as generic Yes

GENERAL INFORMATION

Propylthiouracil is an antithyroid drug that suppresses formation of thyroid hormones and is used to manage overactivity of the thyroid gland (hyperthyroidism). In Graves' disease (the most common cause of hyperthyroidism), a course of propylthiouracil alone or combined with thyroxine ("block and replace" therapy) – usually given for 6–18 months – may cure the disorder. In other conditions, propylthiouracil is given until other treatments, such as surgery or radioiodine, take effect. If other treatments are not possible or are declined by the patient, the drug can be given long term. It is the treatment of choice for hyperthyroidism in the first trimester of pregnancy. The full effect may take several weeks to develop, and beta blockers may be given during this period to control symptoms.

The most serious adverse effect is a reduction in white blood cells (agranulocytosis), increasing the risk of infection (see Possible adverse effects, below). If you develop a sore throat, mouth ulcers, or a fever, you should see your doctor immediately.

INFORMATION FOR USERS

Your drug prescription is tailored for you. Do not alter dosage without consulting your doctor.
How taken/used Tablets.
Frequency and timing of doses 1–3 x daily.
Dosage range Initially 200–400mg daily. Usually dose can be reduced to 50–150mg daily.
Onset of effect 10–20 days. Full beneficial effects may not be felt for 6–10 weeks.
Duration of action 6–8 hours.
Diet advice Your doctor may advise you to avoid foods that are high in iodine, such as seafood.
Storage Keep in original container at room temperature out of the reach of children. Protect from light.
Missed dose Take as soon as you remember. If your next dose is due within 3 hours, take a single dose now and skip the next.
Stopping the drug Do not stop the drug without consulting your doctor; stopping may lead to a recurrence of hyperthyroidism.
Exceeding the dose An occasional unintentional extra dose is unlikely to cause problems. Large overdoses may cause nausea, vomiting, and headache. Notify your doctor.

POSSIBLE ADVERSE EFFECTS

The most common adverse effects are nausea, vomiting, joint pain, headache, and a rash. Discuss with your doctor if nausea and vomiting are severe or if any of these other symptoms occur. Less commonly, unusual bruising or bleeding may occur; if so, consult your doctor. The most serious side effects of propylthiouracil are jaundice, dark-coloured urine or light-coloured faeces, and a rare but life-threatening reduction in white blood cells (agranulocytosis), which may be indicated by sore throat, fever, or mouth ulcers. If you develop jaundice or changes in urine or faeces, stop the drug and call your doctor immediately. If you have sore throat, mouth ulcers, or fever, you should call your doctor to have your white blood cell count checked.

INTERACTIONS

Anticoagulants Propylthiouracil may reduce the effects of oral anticoagulants.

SPECIAL PRECAUTIONS

Be sure to tell your doctor if:
- You have long-term liver or kidney problems.
- You are pregnant.
- You are taking other medicines.

Pregnancy Prescribed with caution. Risk of goitre and thyroid hormone deficiency (hypothyroidism) in the newborn infant if too high a dose is used. Discuss with your doctor.
Breast-feeding The drug passes into the breast milk and may affect the baby. Discuss with your doctor.
Infants and children Not recommended for children under 6 years. Reduced dose necessary in older children.
Over 60 No special problems.
Driving and hazardous work No problems expected.
Alcohol No known problems.

PROLONGED USE
Propylthiouracil may rarely cause a reduction in the number of white blood cells. There is also a small risk of liver failure, so a blood count may be done and liver function checked before starting treatment. A blood count and blood clotting tests may also be carried out before any surgical procedures.
Monitoring Periodic tests of thyroid function are usually required. If you have a sore throat, fever, or mouth ulcers, your white blood cell count must be checked.

PYRIDOSTIGMINE

Brand name Mestinon
Used in the following combined preparations None

QUICK REFERENCE
Drug group Drug for myasthenia gravis (p.53)
Overdose danger rating High
Dependence rating Low
Prescription needed Yes
Available as generic Yes

GENERAL INFORMATION
Pyridostigmine is used to treat myasthenia gravis (p.53), an autoimmune disease involving faulty transmission of nerve impulses to the muscles. It improves muscle strength by prolonging nerve signals, although it does not cure the disease. In severe cases, it may be prescribed with corticosteroids or other drugs. Pyridostigmine may also be used to reverse temporary paralysis of the bowel and urinary retention following surgical operations.

Cholinergic adverse effects (p.7), such as nausea, abdominal cramps, increased salivation and sweating, and diarrhoea, usually disappear after the dosage of pyridostigmine is reduced, although occasionally an anticholinergic drug such as propantheline is needed to counteract these effects.

INFORMATION FOR USERS
Your drug prescription is tailored for you. Do not alter dosage without checking with your doctor.
How taken/used Tablets.
Frequency and timing of doses Every 3–4 hours initially. Thereafter, according to the needs of the individual.
Dosage range *Adults* 300mg–1.2g daily (by mouth) according to response and side effects. *Children* Reduced dose necessary according to age and weight.
Onset of effect 30–60 minutes.
Duration of action 3–6 hours.
Diet advice None.
Storage Keep in original container at room temperature out of the reach of children. Protect from light.
Missed dose Take as soon as you remember. If your next dose is due within 2 hours, take a single dose now and skip the next.
Stopping the drug Do not stop the drug without consulting your doctor; symptoms may recur.

OVERDOSE ACTION
Seek immediate medical advice in all cases. You may experience severe abdominal cramps, vomiting, weakness, and tremor. Take emergency action if troubled breathing, unusually slow heart beat, seizures, or loss of consciousness occur.

POSSIBLE ADVERSE EFFECTS
Adverse effects of pyridostigmine are usually dose-related and can be avoided by adjusting the dose. Nausea, vomiting, increased salivation, sweating, abdominal cramps, and diarrhoea are common; discuss with your doctor if you have abdominal cramps or diarrhoea or if any of these other symptoms are severe. Less commonly, the drug may cause watering eyes, small pupils, or a rash (which may result from hypersensitivity to the drug). Consult your doctor if any of these symptoms occur. Muscle twitching or increased muscle weakness may sometimes be due to too large a dose; if these occur, contact your doctor immediately.

INTERACTIONS
General note Drugs that suppress the transmission of nerve signals may oppose the effect of pyridostigmine. These drugs include aminoglycoside antibiotics, clindamycin, digoxin, procainamide, quinidine, lithium, and chloroquine.
Propranolol may decrease the effectiveness of pyridostigmine.

SPECIAL PRECAUTIONS
Be sure to tell your doctor if:
- You have asthma.
- You have a long-term kidney problem.
- You have heart problems.

- You have an overactive thyroid gland.
- You have had epileptic seizures.
- You have difficulty in passing urine.
- You have a peptic ulcer.
- You have Parkinson's disease.
- You are taking other medicines.

Pregnancy No evidence of risk to the developing fetus in the first 6 months. Large doses near the time of delivery may cause premature labour and temporary muscle weakness in the baby. Discuss with your doctor.

Breast-feeding No evidence of risk with breast-feeding, but the baby should be monitored for signs of muscle weakness.

Infants and children Reduced dose necessary, calculated according to age and weight.

Over 60 Reduced dose may need to be given. Increased likelihood of adverse effects.

Driving and hazardous work Your underlying condition may make such activities inadvisable. Discuss with your doctor.

Alcohol No special problems.

Surgery and general anaesthetics Pyridostigmine interacts with some anaesthetics. Discuss with your doctor, dentist, or anaesthetist before undergoing any surgery.

PROLONGED USE

Pyridostigmine has been implicated in "Gulf War syndrome" when taken for long periods. However, there is no evidence of this occurring when the drug is used in people with myasthenia gravis.

PYRIMETHAMINE

Brand name Daraprim

Used in the following combined preparation Fansidar

QUICK REFERENCE

Drug group Antiprotozoal drug (p.70) and antimalarial drug (p.73)

Overdose danger rating Medium

Dependence rating Low

Prescription needed Yes

Available as generic No

GENERAL INFORMATION

Pyrimethamine is a drug used to treat protozoal infections, including malaria. Because malaria parasites have developed resistance to pyrimethamine, it is now always given combined with the antibacterial drug sulfadoxine (Fansidar) and artesunate for the treatment of falciparum malaria. The activity of the combination greatly exceeds that of any of the drugs used alone. Pyrimethamine is not used for the prevention of malaria.

Pyrimethamine is also given with another drug, sulfadiazine, to treat toxoplasmosis in people with lowered immunity. Such treatment must be supervised by an expert.

Blood disorders can sometimes develop during prolonged treatment with pyrimethamine. For this reason, blood counts are monitored regularly and vitamin supplements are given.

INFORMATION FOR USERS

Your drug prescription is tailored for you. Do not alter dosage without checking with your doctor.

How taken/used Tablets.

Frequency and timing of doses Once only, daily, or weekly, depending on disorder being treated.

Dosage range *Adults* Depends on condition being treated. *Children* Reduced dose necessary according to age.

Onset of effect 24 hours.

Duration of action Up to 1 week.

Diet advice Ensure adequate fluid intake when taking the drug.

Storage Keep in original container at room temperature out of the reach of children. Protect from light.

Missed dose If you are being treated for toxoplasmosis, take as soon as you remember. If your next dose is due within 24 hours, take a single dose now and alter the dosing day so that your next dose is 1 week later.

Stopping the drug Do not stop taking the drug without discussing it with your doctor.

Exceeding the dose An occasional unintentional extra dose is unlikely to cause problems. Large overdoses may cause trembling, breathing difficulty, seizures, blood disorders, and vomiting. Notify your doctor.

POSSIBLE ADVERSE EFFECTS

Pyrimethamine may cause a variety of adverse effects, including headache, loss of appetite, insomnia, stomach irritation, and a rash. Discuss with your doctor if headache, loss of appetite, or insomnia are severe, or if stomach irritation or a rash develop. Unusual bleeding, bruising, tiredness, weakness, or a sore throat may be signs of a blood disorder and you should notify your doctor promptly if they occur. Breathing problems, fever, signs of a chest infection, or seizures should be reported to your doctor immediately. In the case of seizures, you should also stop taking the drug.

INTERACTIONS

General note Drugs that suppress the bone marrow or cause folic acid deficiency may increase the risk of serious blood disorders if taken with pyrimethamine. They include anticancer and antirheumatic drugs, sulfasalazine, methotrexate, co-trimoxazole, trimethoprim, phenytoin, and phenylbutazone.
Lorazepam may cause liver damage when taken with pyrimethamine.
Alemtuzumab and anakinra can both increase the risk of bone marrow suppression with pyrimethamine.

SPECIAL PRECAUTIONS

Be sure to tell your doctor if:
- You have long-term liver or kidney problems.
- You have had epileptic seizures.
- You have anaemia.
- You are allergic to sulfonamides.
- You have glucose-6-phosphate dehydrogenase (G6PD) deficiency.
- You are taking other medicines.

Pregnancy Pyrimethamine may cause folic acid deficiency in the fetus, so its use is generally avoided in the first trimester. Pregnant women receiving this drug should take a folic acid supplement. Discuss with your doctor.
Breast-feeding The drug enters the breast milk and should be avoided during breast-feeding, especially if combined with sulfonamide drugs.
Infants and children Reduced dose necessary.
Over 60 No special problems.
Driving and hazardous work Problems are unlikely, but the drug may sometimes cause dizziness. If it does so, driving and hazardous activities should be avoided.
Alcohol No known problems.
Sunlight and sunbeds Avoid excessive exposure to sunlight.

PROLONGED USE

Prolonged use may cause folic acid deficiency, leading to serious blood disorders. Folic acid supplements may be recommended (in the form of folinic acid).

Monitoring Regular blood cell counts are required during high-dose or long-term treatment with pyrimethamine.

QUETIAPINE

Brand names Alaquet, Atrolak, Biquelle, Brancico, Mintreleq, Psyquet, Qethartic, Seroquel
Used in the following combined preparations None

QUICK REFERENCE

Drug group Antipsychotic drug (p.13)
Overdose danger rating Medium
Dependence rating Low
Prescription needed Yes
Available as generic Yes

GENERAL INFORMATION

Quetiapine is an atypical antipsychotic prescribed for schizophrenia as well as for mania and depression in bipolar disorder (manic depressive disorder). It can be used to treat both "positive" symptoms (thought disorders, delusions, and hallucinations) and "negative" symptoms (blunted affect and emotional and social withdrawal in schizophrenia).

Older people excrete the drug up to 50 per cent more slowly than the usual adult rate. Therefore, they need to be prescribed much lower doses in order to avoid adverse effects.

INFORMATION FOR USERS

Your drug prescription is tailored for you. Do not alter dosage without checking with your doctor.
How taken/used Tablets.
Frequency and timing of doses 2 x daily, or 1 x daily with slow-release tablets.
Adult dosage range *Schizophrenia* 50mg daily (starting dose). *Mania* 100mg daily (starting dose). Dose increased over several days (both). Usual range is 300–450mg daily, maximum 750mg daily (schizophrenia); 800mg (mania).
Onset of effect 1–7 days.
Duration of action Up to 12 hours.
Diet advice Avoid grapefruit juice as it may increase the drug's effects (see Interactions).
Storage Keep in original container at room temperature out of the reach of children.
Missed dose Take as soon as you remember. If your next dose is due within 4 hours, take a single dose now and skip the next.
Stopping the drug Do not stop the drug without consulting your doctor; symptoms may recur.

Exceeding the dose An occasional unintentional extra dose is unlikely to cause problems. Large overdoses may cause unusual drowsiness, palpitations, and low blood pressure. Notify your doctor.

POSSIBLE ADVERSE EFFECTS

Unusual drowsiness, increased appetite, weight gain, indigestion, constipation, dry mouth, urinary retention, erectile dysfunction, dizziness, and fainting are common adverse effects of quetiapine. Discuss with your doctor if you experience dizziness or fainting or if the other effects are severe. Less commonly, the drug may cause restlessness, a stuffy nose, sore throat, palpitations, breast swelling, or irregular menstrual periods. Consult your doctor if any of these occur. Long-term use of quetiapine may rarely cause abnormal movements and increase the risk of certain disorders (see Prolonged use).

INTERACTIONS

Anticonvulsants Quetiapine may oppose the effect of these drugs. Phenytoin and carbamazepine may reduce the effects of quetiapine.
Sedatives All drugs that have a sedative effect on the central nervous system, including alcohol, are likely to increase the sedative properties of quetiapine.
Erythromycin, clarithromycin, ketoconazole, and fluconazole These drugs may increase the effects of quetiapine.
Grapefruit juice may increase the blood levels and thus the effects of quetiapine.
Protease inhibitors These drugs for HIV/AIDS may increase the blood levels and effects of quetiapine.

SPECIAL PRECAUTIONS

Be sure to tell your doctor if:
- You have epilepsy.
- You have diabetes.
- You have liver or kidney problems.
- You have heart problems.
- You have low blood pressure.
- You have bladder problems.
- You have suicidal thoughts.
- You are taking other medicines.

Pregnancy Safety not established. Discuss with your doctor.
Breast-feeding Safety not established. Discuss with your doctor.
Infants and children Not recommended.
Over 60 Reduced doses necessary. Older people eliminate quetiapine more slowly than younger adults.
Driving and hazardous work Avoid such activities until you have learned how quetiapine affects you; the drug can cause drowsiness.
Alcohol Avoid. Alcohol increases the sedative effects of this drug.

PROLONGED USE

Prolonged use of quetiapine may rarely cause tardive dyskinesia, in which there are involuntary movements of the tongue and face. There is also an increased risk of significant weight gain, developing diabetes, and raised blood lipid levels. With long-term use in older patients, quetiapine also carries a greater risk of stroke than some other antipsychotic drugs.

QUININE

Brand name None
Used in the following combined preparations None

QUICK REFERENCE

Drug group Antimalarial drug (p.73) and muscle relaxant (p.53)
Overdose danger rating High
Dependence rating Low
Prescription needed Yes
Available as generic Yes

GENERAL INFORMATION

Quinine was the earliest antimalarial drug. It often causes side effects but is still given for cases of malaria that are resistant to safer treatments. Because the malaria parasites have become resistant to some of the newer antimalarials, quinine remains the mainstay of treatment, but it is not used as a preventative. It is sometimes given together with an additional drug such as doxycycline or clindamycin for malaria.

At the high doses that are used to treat malaria, quinine may cause ringing in the ears, headaches, nausea, hearing loss, and blurred vision: this group of symptoms is known as cinchonism. In rare cases, quinine may cause bleeding problems.

Quinine is also occasionally used to treat night-time leg cramps, although its effectiveness is limited.

INFORMATION FOR USERS

Your drug prescription is tailored for you. Do not alter dosage without checking with your doctor.

How taken/used Tablets, oral suspension, injection.

Frequency and timing of doses *Malaria* Every 8 hours for 7 days. *Muscle cramps* Once daily at bedtime.

Adult dosage range *Malaria* 1.8g daily. *Muscle cramps* 200–300mg daily.

Onset of effect 1–2 days (malaria); up to 4 weeks (cramps).

Duration of action Up to 24 hours.

Diet advice None.

Storage Keep in original container at room temperature out of the reach of children. Protect from light.

Missed dose Take as soon as you remember. If your next dose is due within 4 hours, skip the missed one and return to your normal dosing schedule thereafter.

Stopping the drug If prescribed for malaria, take the full course. Even if you feel better, the original infection may still be present and may recur if treatment is stopped too soon. If taken for muscle cramps, the drug can safely be stopped as soon as you no longer need it.

OVERDOSE ACTION

Seek immediate medical advice in all cases. Take emergency action if breathing problems, seizures, or loss of consciousness occur.

POSSIBLE ADVERSE EFFECTS

Adverse effects are unlikely with low doses, but all should be reported to your doctor. They include nausea, vomiting, diarrhoea, headache, ringing in the ears, and giddiness. Hearing disturbances, headache, and blurred vision are more common with higher, anti-malarial doses. If a rash, itching, loss of hearing, blurred vision, unusual bruising, or excessive bleeding occur, stop taking the drug and consult your doctor immediately.

INTERACTIONS

Digoxin and flecainide Quinine increases blood levels of these drugs; the dose of digoxin should be reduced. Discuss with your doctor.

Ciclosporin Quinine may reduce the blood level of this drug. Discuss with your doctor.

Cimetidine This drug increases the blood levels of quinine.

Amiodarone and moxifloxacin These drugs should not be used with quinine as this can lead to heart rhythm irregularities.

SPECIAL PRECAUTIONS

Be sure to consult your doctor if:

- You have heart problems, especially rhythm disturbances.
- You have a long-term kidney problem.
- You have tinnitus (ringing in the ears).
- You have optic neuritis.
- You have myasthenia gravis.
- You have glucose-6-phosphate dehydrogenase (G6PD) deficiency.
- You have diabetes.
- You are taking other medicines.

Pregnancy Not usually prescribed. May cause defects in the fetus. Discuss with your doctor.

Breast-feeding The drug passes into the breast milk, but normal doses are unlikely to affect the baby adversely. Discuss with your doctor.

Infants and children Reduced dose necessary.

Over 60 No special problems.

Driving and hazardous work Avoid until you know how quinine affects you as it may cause effects such as visual disturbances and vertigo.

Alcohol No known problems.

PROLONGED USE

Prolonged use of quinine can cause blood disorders. When quinine is used for night cramps, treatment should be reviewed after 4 weeks and stopped if the drug is producing no improvement. If the drug is continued, treatment should be reviewed every 3 months.

RABEPRAZOLE

Brand name Pariet

Used in the following combined preparations None

QUICK REFERENCE

Drug group Anti-ulcer drug (p.41)

Overdose danger rating Low

Dependence rating Low

Prescription needed Yes

Available as generic Yes

GENERAL INFORMATION

Rabeprazole belongs to a class of anti-ulcer drugs called proton pump inhibitors (p.41). Because it inhibits the secretion of gastric acid, it is used to treat gastro-oesophageal reflux disease (GORD), also called heartburn, and to help prevent it from recurring. It can also be used in the treatment of Zollinger-Ellison syndrome (a condition in which the stomach produces extremely large amounts of acid).

Rabeprazole is used to treat active duodenal and peptic ulcers by protecting them from the action of stomach acid, allowing them to heal. The drug is also used in combination with antibiotics to eradicate the *Helicobacter pylori* bacterium in patients with peptic ulcer disease. Rabeprazole is occasionally prescribed to people who experience the gastrointestinal adverse effects associated with non-steroidal anti-inflammatory drugs (NSAIDs) but need to continue NSAID treatment.

INFORMATION FOR USERS

Your drug prescription is tailored for you. Do not alter dosage without checking with your doctor.

How taken/used Tablets.

Frequency and timing of doses Once daily, generally in the morning, before food. Swallow whole; do not crush or chew.

Adult dosage range *Adult dosage* 10–20mg. *Zollinger-Ellison syndrome* 60–120mg.

Onset of effect 2–3 hours. Pain should improve in 2–3 days.

Duration of action Up to 48 hours.

Diet advice None, although spicy foods and alcohol may exacerbate disorder being treated.

Storage Keep in original container at room temperature out of the reach of children.

Missed dose Take as soon as you remember, then return to your normal dosing schedule. Do not take an extra dose to make up.

Stopping the drug The drug can be safely stopped as soon as you no longer need it.

Exceeding the dose An occasional unintentional extra dose is unlikely to be a cause for concern. However, if you notice any unusual symptoms, or if a large overdose has been taken, notify your doctor.

POSSIBLE ADVERSE EFFECTS

Most common effects are mild and usually clear up without the need to stop treatment. They include headache, diarrhoea, abdominal pain, flatulence, and insomnia. Discuss with your doctor if they are severe or if you develop a cough, bronchitis, or sinusitis. Prolonged use increases the risk of intestinal infections and, in women, hip fractures (see below).

INTERACTIONS

Itraconazole and ketoconazole Rabeprazole reduces the effects of these drugs.

Digoxin Rabeprazole may increase the effects of digoxin.

Clopidogrel The antiplatelet effect of clopidogrel may be reduced by rabeprazole.

Warfarin Rabeprazole may increase the anticoagulant effect of warfarin.

Atazanavir Rabeprazole can reduce the blood levels of atazanavir, and the two drugs should not be used together.

SPECIAL PRECAUTIONS

Be sure to tell your doctor if:

- You are allergic to other proton pump inhibitors.
- You think you might be pregnant or you are breast-feeding.
- You have a history of liver disease.
- You are taking other medicines.

Pregnancy Not prescribed; safety not established.

Breast-feeding Not recommended. It is not known whether the drug passes into the breast milk. Discuss with your doctor.

Infants and children Not recommended.

Over 60 No special problems.

Driving and hazardous work Avoid until you have learned how rabeprazole affects you because the drug can cause drowsiness.

Alcohol Avoid. Alcohol irritates the stomach, which can lead to ulceration and acid reflux.

PROLONGED USE

Long-term use of rabeprazole may increase the risk of certain intestinal infections (such as *Salmonella* and *Clostridium difficile* infections) owing to the loss of the natural protection against such infections provided by stomach acid. Prolonged use also increases the risk of hip fractures in women.

RALOXIFENE

Brand name Evista

Used in the following combined preparations None

QUICK REFERENCE

Drug group Drug for bone disorders (p.54)

Overdose danger rating Low

Dependence rating Low

Prescription needed Yes

Available as generic No

GENERAL INFORMATION

Raloxifene is a non-steroidal anti-oestrogen drug (oestrogen is a naturally occurring female sex hormone; see p.86) related to clomifene and tamoxifen. It is prescribed to prevent bone fractures in post-menopausal women who are at increased risk of osteoporosis. It is not a first choice, but is recommended for women who cannot take other drugs for bone disorders.

Raloxifene has no beneficial effect on other menopausal problems such as hot flushes. It is not prescribed to women who might become pregnant because it may harm the unborn baby, and it is not prescribed to men.

There is an increased risk of a thrombosis (blood clot) developing in a leg vein; the risk is similar to that from HRT (p.87). However, owing to this risk, raloxifene is usually stopped if the user becomes immobile or bed-bound, when clots are more likely to form. Treatment is restarted when full activity is resumed.

INFORMATION FOR USERS

Your drug prescription is tailored for you. Do not alter dosage without checking with your doctor.

How taken/used Tablets.

Frequency and timing of doses Once daily.

Adult dosage range 60mg daily.

Onset of effect 1–4 hours.

Duration of action 24–48 hours.

Diet advice Calcium supplements are recommended if dietary calcium is low.

Storage Keep in original container at room temperature out of the reach of children. Protect from light.

Missed dose Take as soon as you remember. If your next dose is due within 8 hours, take a single dose now and skip the next.

Stopping the drug Do not stop without consulting your doctor except under conditions specified in advance, such as immobility, which increases the risk of blood clots forming.

Exceeding the dose An occasional unintentional extra dose is unlikely to be a cause for concern. But if you notice any unusual symptoms, or if a large overdose has been taken, tell your doctor.

POSSIBLE ADVERSE EFFECTS

Hot flushes, leg cramps, swollen ankles or feet, and flulike symptoms are common adverse effects. Headaches are less common. Discuss with your doctor if you have headaches or if any of these other effects are severe. If you develop a rash, stop taking the drug and contact your doctor. Pain, tenderness, swelling, discoloration, or ulceration of the leg may indicate a thrombosis (blood clot) in a leg vein; if these symptoms develop, stop taking the drug and seek immediate medical attention. If a clot occurs elsewhere in the body, there may not be any obvious symptoms.

INTERACTIONS

Anticoagulants Raloxifene reduces the effect of warfarin and acenocoumarol (nicoumalone).

Colestyramine This drug reduces the absorption of raloxifene by the body.

SPECIAL PRECAUTIONS

Be sure to tell your doctor if:

- You have had a blood clot in a vein or a pulmonary embolism.
- You have vaginal bleeding.
- You have liver or kidney problems.
- You are taking other medicines.

Pregnancy Not prescribed to pre-menopausal women.

Breast-feeding Not prescribed to pre-menopausal women.

Infants and children Not prescribed.

Over 60 No special problems.

Driving and hazardous work No special problems.

Alcohol No special problems.

PROLONGED USE

Raloxifene is not normally used for longer than 5 years. It reduces the risk of some types of breast cancer, but this benefit has to be weighed against the increased risk of stroke and venous thrombosis.

Monitoring Liver function tests may be performed periodically.

RAMIPRIL

Brand name Tritace

Used in the following combined preparations Triapin, Triapin mite

QUICK REFERENCE

Drug group ACE inhibitor (p.30) and drug for hypertension (p.34)

Overdose danger rating Medium

Dependence rating Low

Prescription needed Yes

Available as generic Yes

GENERAL INFORMATION

Ramipril belongs to the drug group known as ACE inhibitors. It works by reducing the production of substances that raise blood pressure, making the blood vessels relax and making it easier for the heart to pump blood. The drug is used to treat high blood pressure (p.30), to reduce strain on the heart in patients with heart failure after a heart attack, and to prevent future strokes and heart attacks in patients with established cardiovascular disease. It is also used to treat heart failure from other causes and to preserve kidney function in conditions such as diabetes mellitus. The first dose of an ACE inhibitor can cause blood pressure to drop suddenly, so a few hours' bed rest afterwards is advisable.

Adverse effects are usually mild. Like all ACE inhibitors, ramipril can cause the body to retain potassium. It can also cause a persistent dry cough.

INFORMATION FOR USERS

Your drug prescription is tailored for you. Do not alter dosage without checking with your doctor.

How taken/used Tablets, capsules, oral solution.

Frequency and timing of doses *High blood pressure* Usually once daily. *Heart failure or after heart attack* 1–2 x daily.

Adult dosage range *High blood pressure, heart failure, or after a heart attack* 1.25–10mg daily.

Onset of effect Within 2 hours; full beneficial effect may take several weeks.

Duration of action Up to 24 hours.

Diet advice Your doctor may advise decreasing salt intake to help control blood pressure.

Storage Keep in original container at room temperature out of the reach of children.

Missed dose Take as soon as you remember. If your next dose is due within 6 hours, take a single dose now and skip the next. Subsequently, continue with your usual routine.

Stopping the drug Do not stop without consulting your doctor. Treatment of hypertension and heart failure is normally lifelong, so it may be necessary to substitute alternative therapy.

Exceeding the dose If you notice any unusual symptoms or if a large overdose has been taken, notify your doctor.

POSSIBLE ADVERSE EFFECTS

Most adverse effects from ramipril are mild and transient, but all should be reported to your doctor. A mild rash and a dry cough are common. Sometimes the cough is persistent, which may necessitate withdrawal of the drug. Less commonly, ramipril may cause mouth ulcers, a sore mouth, dizziness, sore throat, or fever. Rarely, it may cause deterioration of kidney function, digestive tract disturbances, a severe rash, or severe swelling of the mouth or lips accompanied by breathing difficulties. If you develop swelling of the mouth or lips and/or breathing difficulties, stop taking the drug and seek immediate medical attention.

INTERACTIONS

Non-steroidal anti-inflammatory drugs (NSAIDs) may reduce blood-pressure-lowering effect of ramipril and increase risk of kidney damage.

Potassium supplements and potassium-sparing diuretics may cause excess levels of potassium in the body.

Ciclosporin and tacrolimus increase the risk of high potassium levels in the blood.

Lithium Ramipril may cause raised blood lithium levels and toxicity.

Vasodilators, diuretics, and other antihypertensive drugs may increase the blood-pressure-lowering effect of ramipril.

SPECIAL PRECAUTIONS

Be sure to tell your doctor if:

- You have long-term liver or kidney problems.
- You have heart problems.
- You have had angioedema or a previous allergic reaction to ACE inhibitors.
- You are taking other medicines.
- You are or intend to become pregnant.

Pregnancy Not prescribed. There is evidence of harm to the developing fetus.

Breast-feeding Safety not established. Discuss with your doctor.

Infants and children Not recommended.

Over 60 Reduced dose may be necessary.

Driving and hazardous work Avoid such activities until you have learned how ramipril affects you because the drug can cause dizziness and fainting.

Alcohol Avoid. Alcohol may increase the blood-pressure-lowering and adverse effects of the drug.

Surgery and general anaesthetics Ramipril may have to be stopped before you have a general anaesthetic. Discuss with your doctor or dentist before any operation.

PROLONGED USE

No problems expected.

Monitoring Periodic checks on potassium levels, white blood cell count, kidney function, and urine are usually performed.

RANITIDINE

Brand names Boots Heartburn Relief Tablets, Gavilast, Ranicalm, Zantac

Used in the following combined preparations None

QUICK REFERENCE

Drug group Anti-ulcer drug (p.41)

Overdose danger rating Low

Dependence rating Low

Prescription needed No (tablets in limited quantities); Yes (other preparations)

Available as generic Yes

GENERAL INFORMATION

Ranitidine is an anti-ulcer drug from the group known as H2 blockers. It reduces acid production by the stomach, allowing ulcers to heal, and is usually given in courses lasting 4 to 8 weeks, with further courses if symptoms recur. In combination with antibiotics, it may be used for ulcers caused by *Helicobacter pylori* infection. It may also be used to protect against ulcers in people taking NSAIDs (p.48), and to reduce discomfort and ulceration in oesophagitis. In medical practice, ranitidine has been largely replaced by newer proton pump inhibitor anti-ulcer drugs, such as omeprazole. It is available over the counter for the short-term treatment of heartburn and indigestion in people over 16 years old.

Unlike the similar drug cimetidine, ranitidine does not increase blood levels of other drugs such as anticoagulants and anticonvulsants. Most people experience no serious side effects during treatment. As ranitidine promotes healing of the stomach lining, there is a risk that it might mask stomach cancer. It is therefore prescribed only when this possibility has been ruled out.

INFORMATION FOR USERS

Your drug prescription is tailored for you. Do not alter dosage without checking with your doctor. For over-the-counter preparations, follow the instructions and call your doctor if symptoms worsen.

How taken/used Tablets, effervescent tablets, liquid, injection.

Frequency and timing of doses Once daily at bedtime or 2–4 x daily.

Adult dosage range 150–600mg daily, depending on the condition being treated. Usual dose is 150mg twice daily.

Onset of effect Within 1 hour.

Duration of action 12 hours.

Diet advice None.

Storage Keep in original container at room temperature out of the reach of children. Protect from light.

Missed dose Take as soon as you remember. If your next dose is due within 3 hours, take a single dose now and skip the next.

Stopping the drug Do not stop the drug without consulting your doctor; symptoms may recur.

Exceeding the dose An occasional unintentional extra dose is unlikely to be a cause for concern. But if you notice any unusual symptoms, or if a large overdose has been taken, tell your doctor.

POSSIBLE ADVERSE EFFECTS

Adverse effects are usually related to dosage level and almost always disappear when treatment finishes. The most common effects are headache and dizziness. Less commonly, nausea, vomiting, constipation, or diarrhoea may occur. Discuss with your doctor if any of these are severe. Rarely, jaundice, agitation, or mental problems may occur; if so, consult your doctor. If you develop a sore throat or fever, contact your doctor immediately.

INTERACTIONS

Ketoconazole Ranitidine may reduce the absorption of ketoconazole. Ranitidine should be taken at least 2 hours after ketoconazole.

Glipizide Ranitidine may increase the absorption of glipizide.

Sucralfate High doses (2g) may reduce the absorption of ranitidine. Sucralfate should be taken at least 2 hours after ranitidine.

Theophylline/aminophylline Ranitidine may increase blood levels of these drugs.

SPECIAL PRECAUTIONS

Be sure to consult your doctor or pharmacist before taking this drug if:

- You have long-term liver or kidney problems.
- You have porphyria.
- You are taking other medicines.

Pregnancy Safety established over several decades of use. May be used in labour and during Caesarian section. Discuss with your doctor.
Breast-feeding The drug passes into the breast milk, but there is no evidence that this is harmful to the baby.
Infants and children Reduced dose necessary.
Over 60 In older and immunocompromised people, ranitidine may increase the risk of pneumonia.
Driving and hazardous work Usually no problems. Dizziness can affect a minority of people.
Alcohol Avoid. Alcohol may aggravate your underlying condition and reduce the beneficial effects of this drug.

PROLONGED USE

Long-term suppression of stomach acid secretion may increase the risk of some types of intestinal infection, such as with salmonella and *Clostridium difficile.*

REPAGLINIDE

Brand name Enyglid, Prandin
Used in the following combined preparations None

QUICK REFERENCE

Drug group Drug for diabetes (p.80)
Overdose danger rating Medium
Dependence rating Low
Prescription needed Yes
Available as generic Yes

GENERAL INFORMATION

Repaglinide is used to treat Type 2 diabetes that cannot be adequately controlled by diet and exercise alone. It acts in a similar way to sulfonylurea drugs by stimulating the release of insulin from the pancreas. Therefore, some of the pancreatic cells need to be functioning in order for it to be effective. It is sometimes given with metformin if that drug is not providing adequate diabetic control.

Repaglinide is fast acting, but its effects last for only about 4 hours. It is best taken just before a meal so that the insulin released by the pancreas can cope with the food. If a meal is likely to be missed, the dose of repaglinide should not be taken. If a tablet has been taken and a meal is not forthcoming, some carbohydrate (as specified by your doctor or dietician) should be eaten as soon as possible.

INFORMATION FOR USERS

Your drug prescription is tailored for you. Do not alter dosage without checking with your doctor.
How taken/used Tablets.
Frequency and timing of doses 1–4 x daily (up to 30 minutes before a meal, and up to 4 meals a day). If you are going to miss a meal, do not take the tablet.
Adult dosage range 500mcg (starting dose), increased at intervals of 1–2 weeks according to response; 4–16mg daily (maintenance dose).
Onset of effect 15–30 minutes.
Duration of action 4–6 hours.
Diet advice Follow the diet advised by your doctor or dietician.
Storage Keep in original container at room temperature out of the reach of children.
Missed dose Do not take tablets between meals. Discuss with your doctor.
Stopping the drug Do not stop taking the drug without consulting your doctor.
Exceeding the dose An overdose will cause low blood sugar, with faintness, dizziness, headache, confusion, sweating, or tremor. Notify your doctor.

POSSIBLE ADVERSE EFFECTS

Gastrointestinal problems, such as nausea, vomiting, abdominal pain, and diarrhoea or constipation, are common at the start of treatment with repaglinide but tend to become less troublesome as treatment continues. Discuss with your doctor if such symptoms are severe or persist. Hypoglycaemia (see Exceeding the dose, above) may also occur; notify your doctor if it is severe. Rarely, repaglinide may cause rash or itching; if so, consult your doctor.

INTERACTIONS

Clarithromycin, itraconazole, ketoconazole, monoamine oxidase inhibitors (MAOIs), trimethoprim, gemfibrozil, ACE inhibitors, salicylates, non-steroidal anti-inflammatory drugs (NSAIDs), and ciclosporin may enhance and/or prolong the hypoglycaemic effect of repaglinide.
Oral contraceptives, thiazide diuretics, corticosteroids, thyroid hormones, danazol, sympathomimetics, rifampicin, barbiturates, and carbamazepine may decrease the effect of repaglinide.
Beta blockers The symptoms of hypoglycaemia may be masked by these drugs, especially by non-cardioselective beta blockers (e.g. propranolol).

SPECIAL PRECAUTIONS

Be sure to tell your doctor if:

- ◆ You have liver or kidney problems.
- ◆ You are taking other medicines.

Pregnancy Safety not established. Discuss with your doctor.

Breast-feeding Safety not established. Discuss with your doctor.

Infants and children Not recommended.

Over 60 No special problems, but safety not established over 75 years.

Driving and hazardous work Avoid if low blood sugar without warning signs is likely.

Alcohol Avoid. Alcohol may upset diabetic control and may increase and prolong the effects of repaglinide.

PROLONGED USE

Repaglinide is usually prescribed indefinitely. No special problems.

Monitoring Periodic monitoring of control of blood glucose levels is necessary.

RIFAMPICIN

Brand names Rifadin, Rimactane

Used in the following combined preparations Rifater, Rifinah, Voractiv

QUICK REFERENCE

Drug group Antituberculous drug (p.65)

Overdose danger rating Medium

Dependence rating Low

Prescription needed Yes

Available as generic Yes

GENERAL INFORMATION

Rifampicin is an antibacterial drug that is highly effective in the treatment of tuberculosis. Taken by mouth, it is widely distributed throughout body tissues including the brain. As a result, it is particularly useful in the treatment of tuberculous meningitis.

The drug is also used to treat leprosy and other serious infections, including brucellosis, Legionnaires' disease, and infections of the bone (osteomyelitis) and of the heart (endocarditis). In addition, it is given to anyone in close contact with meningococcal meningitis in order to prevent infection. Rifampicin is always prescribed with other antibiotics or antituberculous drugs because of rapid development of resistance in some bacteria.

Rifampicin significantly increases the liver's capacity to break down some drugs, and so reduces their effectiveness.

It may impart a harmless red-orange colour to the urine, saliva, and tears, and soft contact lenses may become permanently stained.

INFORMATION FOR USERS

Your drug prescription is tailored for you. Do not alter dosage without checking with your doctor.

How taken/used Tablets, capsules, liquid, injection.

Frequency and timing of doses 1 x daily, 30 minutes before breakfast (leprosy, tuberculosis) or once a month (leprosy); 2 x daily (prevention of meningococcal meningitis); 2–4 x daily, 30 minutes before or 2 hours after meals (other serious infections).

Adult dosage range According to weight; usually 450–600mg daily (tuberculosis, leprosy) or 600mg once a month (leprosy); 600mg–1.2g daily (other serious infections); 1.2g daily for 2 days (meningococcal meningitis).

Onset of effect Over several days.

Duration of action Up to 24 hours.

Diet advice None.

Storage Keep in original container at room temperature out of the reach of children. Protect from light.

Missed dose Take as soon as you remember. If next dose is due within 6 hours, take a single dose now, then return to normal schedule.

Stopping the drug Take the full course. Even if you feel better, the original infection may still be present and symptoms may recur if treatment is stopped too soon. In rare cases stopping the drug suddenly after high-dose treatment can lead to a severe flulike illness.

Exceeding the dose An occasional unintentional extra dose is unlikely to cause problems. Large overdoses may cause liver damage, nausea, vomiting, and lethargy. Notify your doctor immediately.

POSSIBLE ADVERSE EFFECTS

A red-orange discoloration of body fluids normally occurs but is harmless. Headache and breathing difficulties may occur after stopping high-dose treatment. Rarely, rifampicin may cause nausea, vomiting, and diarrhoea; if these are severe, discuss with your doctor. Muscle cramps or aches, rash, itching, or jaundice may occasionally occur; if they do, notify your doctor, promptly in the case of jaundice. If you have a flulike illness or easy bruising or bleeding, stop taking the drug and contact your doctor immediately.

INTERACTIONS

General note Rifampicin may reduce the effectiveness of a wide variety of drugs, such as oral contraceptives (in which case alternative contraceptive methods may be needed), phenytoin, corticosteroids, oral antidiabetic drugs, antiarrhythmics, and warfarin-like anticoagulants. Dosage of these drugs may have to be adjusted at the start or end of rifampicin treatment. Consult your doctor or pharmacist for advice.

SPECIAL PRECAUTIONS

Be sure to tell your doctor if:

- You have long-term liver or kidney problems.
- You have porphyria.
- You wear contact lenses.
- You are taking other medicines.

Pregnancy Safety in pregnancy not established. Discuss with your doctor.

Breast-feeding The drug passes into the breast milk, but normal doses are unlikely to affect the baby adversely. Discuss with your doctor.

Infants and children Reduced dose necessary.

Over 60 Increased risk of adverse effects. Reduced dose may therefore be necessary.

Driving and hazardous work No problems expected.

Alcohol Avoid excessive amounts. Heavy intake may increase the risk of liver damage.

PROLONGED USE

Prolonged use of rifampicin may cause liver damage.

Monitoring Periodic blood tests may be performed to monitor liver function.

RISEDRONATE

Brand names Actonel, Actonel Once a Week

Used in the following combined preparation Actonel Combi

QUICK REFERENCE

Drug group Drug for bone disorders (p.54)

Overdose danger rating Medium

Dependence rating Low

Prescription needed Yes

Available as generic Yes

GENERAL INFORMATION

Risedronate belongs to a group of drugs called bisphosphonates. Used in treating bone disorders such as Paget's disease, it acts directly on the bones by increasing the amount of calcium they absorb, making them stronger. It is also used to prevent or treat osteoporosis in postmenopausal women. Taken as a daily or a weekly dose, it reduces the risk of hip or vertebral fractures. In addition, it is used to treat or prevent corticosteroid-induced osteoporosis.

To reduce the risk of gastrointestinal adverse effects, you should take risedronate first thing in the morning, on an empty stomach and in a standing position, and remain upright for at least 30 minutes afterwards. Risedronate should not be taken at bedtime.

INFORMATION FOR USERS

Your drug prescription is tailored for you. Do not alter dosage without checking with your doctor.

How taken/used Tablets.

Frequency and timing of doses *Paget's disease* Once daily (30mg dose). *Osteoporosis* Once daily (5mg dose); once weekly, on the same day (35mg dose). Swallow whole with water, on rising and before food; or avoid food or drink for at least 2 hours before and after dose.

Adult dosage range *Paget's disease* 30mg daily. *Osteoporosis* 5mg daily; 35mg weekly.

Onset of effect Within 1 month.

Duration of action Some effects may persist for several weeks or months.

Diet advice Avoid calcium-containing products (e.g. milk), vitamin and mineral supplements, and antacids for at least 2 hours before and after dose.

Storage Keep in original container at room temperature out of the reach of children.

Missed dose Take as soon as you remember. Then return to your original dosing schedule. Do not make up for the missed dose (weekly).

Stopping the drug The drug can be safely stopped as soon as you no longer need it.

Exceeding the dose An occasional unintentional dose is unlikely to cause problems. However, if you notice any unusual symptoms, or if a large overdose has been taken, drink a large glass of milk and notify your doctor.

POSSIBLE ADVERSE EFFECTS

Most adverse effects of risedronate are mild to moderate and do not usually necessitate stopping treatment. Common side effects include nausea, diarrhoea or constipation, muscle pain, headache, abdominal pain, and new or worsening heartburn. Notify your doctor if you experience abdominal pain, if heartburn develops or worsens, if any of the other common symptoms are severe, or if you develop jaw pain. If swallowing is difficult or painful or if jaundice occurs, stop taking the drug and contact your doctor. If you develop an allergic rash, itching, or facial swelling, stop taking the drug and seek immediate medical attention.

INTERACTIONS

Antacids, and products containing calcium or iron These products reduce the absorption of risedronate and should be taken at a different time of day.

SPECIAL PRECAUTIONS

Be sure to tell your doctor if:

- ◆ You have kidney problems.
- ◆ You have a history of peptic ulcers or stomach problems.
- ◆ You have low calcium levels in your blood.
- ◆ You are/may be pregnant or you are planning pregnancy.
- ◆ You are breast-feeding.
- ◆ You are unable to sit or stand upright for at least 30 minutes.
- ◆ You have had pain or difficulty in swallowing, or problems with your oesophagus.
- ◆ You are taking other medicines.

Pregnancy Not recommended.
Breast-feeding Not recommended.
Infants and children Not recommended.
Over 60 No special problems.
Driving and hazardous work No special problems.
Alcohol Avoid. May cause further stomach irritation.

PROLONGED USE

In patients with Paget's disease, courses of treatment lasting for longer than 2 months are not usually prescribed, but repeat courses may be required. When used to treat or prevent osteoporosis, risedronate may be taken safely long term.

Monitoring Your doctor may monitor your bone mineral density. Blood and urine tests may be carried out at intervals.

RISPERIDONE

Brand names Risperdal, Risperdal Consta, Risperdal Quicklet
Used in the following combined preparations None

QUICK REFERENCE

Drug group Antipsychotic drug (p.13)
Overdose danger rating Medium
Dependence rating Low
Prescription needed Yes
Available as generic Yes

GENERAL INFORMATION

Risperidone is used to treat people with acute psychiatric disorders and long-term psychotic illnesses such as schizophrenia and mania. By blocking dopamine receptors in the brain, it helps to alleviate, although not cure, "positive" symptoms (such as hallucinations, thought disturbances, and hostility) and "negative" symptoms (such as emotional and social withdrawal). The drug may also help with the depression and anxiety that may occur with schizophrenia. Risperidone is an atypical antipsychotic drug. It is less likely than some other antipsychotics to cause sedation or movement disorders as a side effect. It can also be used for short-term treatment of severe aggression in people with dementia, and may be helpful in autism or Asperger's syndrome.

INFORMATION FOR USERS

Your drug prescription is tailored for you. Do not alter dosage without checking with your doctor.
How taken/used Tablets, dispersible tablets, liquid, injection.
Frequency and timing of doses 1–2 x daily (tablets, liquid).
Adult dosage range *Tablets* 2mg daily (starting dose) increasing to 4–6mg daily (usual maintenance dose); maximum 16mg daily. *Injection* 25mg every 2 weeks (starting dose) increasing to 50mg every two weeks (maximum maintenance dose).
Onset of effect *Tablets* Within 2–3 days, but may take up to 6 weeks before maximum effect is seen. *Injection* Up to 3 weeks before onset of effect.
Duration of action Approximately 2 days.
Diet advice None.
Storage Keep in original container at room temperature (tablets) or in a refrigerator

(injection) out of the reach of children. Protect from light.

Missed dose Take as soon as you remember. If your next dose is due within 3 hours, take a single dose now and skip the next.

Stopping the drug Do not stop without consulting your doctor; symptoms may recur.

Exceeding the dose An occasional unintentional extra dose is unlikely to cause problems. If larger doses have been taken, tell your doctor.

POSSIBLE ADVERSE EFFECTS

Risperidone is generally well tolerated and has a low incidence of causing movement disorders. It is also less sedating than some other antipsychotic drugs. Insomnia, anxiety, agitation, headache, difficulty in concentrating, and weight gain are common; discuss with your doctor if they are severe. Shakiness and tremor are also common and should be discussed with your doctor in all cases. Sexual dysfunction, dizziness, and drowsiness are rare; consult your doctor if sexual dysfunction is severe or if dizziness or drowsiness occur. If you develop a fever, rigid muscles, or confusion, stop taking the drug and contact your doctor immediately.

INTERACTIONS

Sedatives All drugs that have a sedative effect on the central nervous system are likely to increase any sedative effect of risperidone.

Lithium increases the risk of nerve toxicity when used with riseperidone.

Drugs for parkinsonism Risperidone may reduce the effect of these drugs.

Fluoxetine, paroxetine, and verapamil These drugs increase the blood levels of risperidone and the risk of side effects.

Carbamazepine and rifamipicin These drugs reduce the effects of risperidone. Other liver enzyme-inducing drugs (e.g. phenytoin) may have the same effect.

SPECIAL PRECAUTIONS

Be sure to tell your doctor if:

- You have liver, kidney, or bladder problems.
- You have heart or circulation problems.
- You have diabetes or high blood lipid levels.
- You have epilepsy.
- You have Parkinson's disease.
- You have had a stroke, deep vein thrombosis, or pulmonary embolism.
- You have dementia.
- You are taking other medicines.

Pregnancy Short-term nervous system problems may occur in babies when the drug is taken in the third trimester. Discuss with your doctor.

Breast-feeding The drug probably passes into breast milk. Discuss with your doctor.

Infants and children Not recommended under 15 years.

Over 60 Reduced dose may be necessary.

Driving and hazardous work Avoid such activities until you have learned how risperidone affects you because the drug may cause difficulty in concentrating and slowed reactions.

Alcohol Avoid. Alcohol may increase the sedative effects of this drug.

PROLONGED USE

If used long term, permanent movement disorders (tardive dyskinesia) may occur, although they are less likely than with many other antipsychotic drugs. In people with dementia, there may be an increased risk of stroke and death when taking risperidone. Use of the drug may also lead to high levels of prolactin, which may stimulate breast tissue and change the pattern of menstrual periods.

RITUXIMAB

Brand name MabThera, Rixathon, Ruxience, Truxima

Used in the following combined preparations None

QUICK REFERENCE

Drug group Anticancer drug (p.94)

Overdose danger rating Low

Dependence rating Low

Prescription needed Yes

Available as generic Yes

GENERAL INFORMATION

Rituximab is a monoclonal antibody (p.95) that suppresses the immune system and reduces inflammation. It works by reducing the number of B-lymphocytes (a type of white blood cell involved in the production of antibodies). The drug is used with chemotherapy to treat some types of lymphoid cancer, especially B-cell lymphomas and chronic lymphocytic leukaemia, and in combination with methotrexate to treat severe rheumatoid arthritis. It may also be used to treat systemic lupus erythematosus, autoimmune anaemias and platelet disorders, vasculitis, and some skin conditions, such as pemphigus. In addition, it is used to treat acute graft rejection in transplant patients.

Because rituximab suppresses the immune system, serious infections can occur or reactivate with its use. It is important that you tell your doctor if you have previously had hepatitis B or tuberculosis as these disorders may reactivate with rituximab treatment.

INFORMATION FOR USERS

This drug is given only under medical supervision and is not for self-administration.

How taken/used Intravenous infusion.

Frequency and timing of doses Usually 4–8 courses of treatment over a period of up to 2 years, but the precise dosing schedule depends on the condition being treated.

Adult dosage range Each dose: 375–500mg per square metre of body surface area, depending on condition being treated.

Onset of effect Response to rituximab often becomes evident only about 6 weeks after the start of treatment.

Duration of action 6–9 months.

Diet advice None.

Storage Not applicable. The drug is not normally kept at home.

Missed dose The drug is administered in hospital under close medical supervision. If you miss your dose, contact your doctor as soon as possible.

Stopping the drug Discuss with your doctor. Stopping the drug prematurely may lead to worsening of the underlying condition.

Exceeding the dose Overdosage is unlikely since the treatment is carefully monitored and supervised.

POSSIBLE ADVERSE EFFECTS

Fever, chills, shivering, nausea or vomiting, and flushing may occur during the first infusion of rituximab. Abdominal pain or diarrhoea, or, less commonly, allergic reactions (such as wheezing, swelling of the tongue, itchiness, or a rash), may also occur. People with angina may experience worsening of their symptoms. Rarely, forgetfulness, confusion, or paralysis may occur. Rituximab suppresses the immune system, and therefore susceptibility to infection is increased. The drug is given under medical supervision and side effects are monitored. Nevertheless, you should inform the person giving the infusion immediately if you develop an infection or any other adverse effects.

INTERACTIONS

Vaccines Rituximab suppresses the immune system, so live vaccines should not be used while undergoing rituximab treatment. The drug may also make attenuated vaccines less effective. Discuss with your doctor.

Antihypertensive drugs The blood-pressure-lowering effect of antihypertensive drugs may be enhanced when they are taken together with rituximab.

SPECIAL PRECAUTIONS

Be sure to tell your doctor if:

- You have an infection, wound, dental problem, or have had recent surgery.
- You have previously had tuberculosis or hepatitis B.
- You have angina or other heart problems.
- You are, may be, or intend to become pregnant.
- You have recently been vaccinated or are due to be vaccinated.
- You are taking any other medications, especially for high blood pressure.

Pregnancy Safety not established. Discuss with your doctor.

Breast-feeding Not recommended during treatment with rituximab and for 12 months following end of treatment.

Infants and children Not recommended

Over 60 No special problems.

Driving and hazardous work No known problems.

Alcohol No special problems.

PROLONGED USE

Rituximab increases susceptibility to infection, and any infection that develops should be treated promptly. Very rarely, a serious brain infection may develop; you should tell your doctor immediately if you develop memory problems, confusion, difficulty walking, or vision problems.

Monitoring Periodic blood tests may be carried out. Body temperature, blood pressure, and heart rate may be monitored while you receive rituximab infusions.

RIVAROXABAN

Brand name Xarelto
Used in the following combined preparations None

QUICK REFERENCE

Drug group Anticoagulant drug (p.37)
Overdose danger rating High
Dependence rating Low
Prescription needed Yes
Available as generic No

GENERAL INFORMATION

Rivaroxaban is an oral anticoagulant drug with a rapid onset of action. It is used to treat or prevent deep vein thrombosis (blood clots in the leg veins) and pulmonary embolism (blockage of blood vessels in the lungs from clots that have travelled from elsewhere in the body). It is given to prevent strokes and blood clots in the arteries in patients with the heart rhythm problem atrial fibrillation. In combination with antiplatelet drugs, rivaroxaban is also used to prevent coronary thrombosis after a heart attack or severe angina. The most serious side effect of the drug is an increased risk of bleeding. It should not be used in people with damaged or artificial heart valves or those with antiphospholipid syndrome.

INFORMATION FOR USERS

Your drug prescription is tailored for you. Do not alter dosage without checking with your doctor.
How taken/used Tablets.
Frequency and timing of doses 1–2 x daily, with food; tablets may be crushed.
Dosage range 2.5–15mg twice daily, or 20mg once a day.
Onset of effect 1 hour.
Duration of action 12–24 hours.
Diet advice None.
Storage Keep in the original container at room temperature out of the reach of children.
Missed dose Take as soon as you remember. Make up the total daily dose during the day, regardless of gap between dosing (e.g. if on a twice-daily regimen, both doses can be taken at once). However, do not take more than the indicated daily dose.
Stopping the drug Do not stop the drug without consulting your doctor; stopping the drug may lead to worsening of the underlying condition.

OVERDOSE ACTION

Seek immediate medical advice in all cases. Take emergency action if bleeding or loss of consciousness occur.

POSSIBLE ADVERSE EFFECTS

Bleeding is the most common adverse effect of rivaroxaban. If you notice excessive bruising or prolonged bleeding from a minor wound, consult your doctor immediately. You should also call your doctor at once if you develop a rash or itching. If jaundice or swelling of the mouth or tongue occur, call your doctor immediately and stop taking the drug. Other common side effects of rivaroxaban include abdominal pain, faintness, dizziness, nausea, and vomiting. You should discuss with your doctor if any of these occur.

INTERACTIONS

Other anticoagulants, antiplatelet drugs, non-steroidal anti-inflammatory drugs, antibacterial drugs, antifungal drugs, and antiviral drugs There is an increased risk of bleeding if these are used with rivaroxaban.
Anticonvulsant drugs, rifampicin, and St John's wort These may lower the blood level of rivaroxaban and reduce its effectiveness.

SPECIAL PRECAUTIONS

Be sure to tell your doctor if:

- You have liver or kidney problems.
- You have high blood pressure.
- You have a bleeding disorder.
- You have peptic ulcers.
- You have had a brain haemorrhage.
- You have had recent surgery.
- You are taking other medicines.

Pregnancy Safety not established. Discuss with your doctor.
Breast-feeding Safety not established. Discuss with your doctor.
Infants and children Safety not established. Discuss with your doctor.
Over 60 No special problems.
Driving and hazardous work Use caution. Even minor injuries may cause serious bruising and excessive bleeding.
Alcohol Avoid excessive intake.
Surgery and general anaesthetics Rivaroxaban may need to be stopped before you undergo any surgery. Discuss with your doctor or dentist.

PROLONGED USE

No special problems known, but the need for continued treatment should be reviewed. Rivaroxaban is usually used long term only in people with recurrent deep vein thrombosis or pulmonary embolism.

RIVASTIGMINE

Brand names Alzest, Eluden, Exelon, Kerstipon, Nimvastid, Prometax, Rivatev, Voleze
Used in the following combined preparations None

QUICK REFERENCE

Drug group Drug for dementia (p.17)
Overdose danger rating Medium
Dependence rating Low
Prescription needed Yes
Available as generic Yes

GENERAL INFORMATION

Rivastigmine is an inhibitor of the enzyme acetylcholinesterase. This enzyme breaks down the naturally occurring neurotransmitter acetylcholine (p.7) to limit its effects. Blocking the enzyme raises the levels of acetylcholine; in the brain, the effect is to increase alertness, awareness, and memory.

Rivastigmine improves the symptoms of dementia in Alzheimer's disease, and is used to slow the rate of deterioration in that disease. The drug is not recommended for dementia due to other causes. Treatment is initiated under specialist supervision. Those having the treatment are usually assessed at 6-monthly intervals to determine whether the drug is helping. As the disease progresses, the benefit obtained may diminish.

Side effects may include slow heart rate, collapse, agitation, confusion, and depression. The latter three are also possible symptoms of Alzheimer's disease, so may be hard to distinguish from the effects of the disease itself.

INFORMATION FOR USERS

Your drug prescription is tailored for you. Do not alter dosage without checking with your doctor.
How taken/used Capsules, liquid, transdermal patch.
Frequency and timing of doses 2 x daily.
Adult dosage range 3mg daily (starting dose); 6–12mg daily (maintenance dose); 4.6–13.3mg every 24 hours (transdermal patch).
Onset of effect 30–60 minutes. Full effect may take up to 3 months.
Duration of action 9–12 hours.
Diet advice None.
Storage Keep in original container at room temperature out of the reach of children.
Missed dose Take as soon as you remember. If your next dose is due within 4 hours, take a single dose now and skip the next. A carer should oversee the taking of tablets.
Stopping the drug Do not stop the drug without consulting your doctor; symptoms may recur.
Exceeding the dose An occasional unintentional extra dose is unlikely to be a problem. Large overdoses may cause nausea, vomiting, and diarrhoea. Notify your doctor.

POSSIBLE ADVERSE EFFECTS

Common adverse effects include drowsiness, dizziness, weakness, and trembling. Discuss with your doctor if severe. Reduced appetite, weight loss, nausea, abdominal pain, agitation, confusion, urinary incontinence, and infections are also common and should be reported to your doctor in all cases. Mental changes and intestinal problems are usually quite mild. Women may be more susceptible to nausea, vomiting, and weight loss. Rarely, collapse or seizures may occur; if so, stop taking the drug and call your doctor immediately.

INTERACTIONS

Muscle relaxants used in surgery Rivastigmine may increase the effects of some muscle relaxants, but may block the effects of some others.

SPECIAL PRECAUTIONS

Be sure to tell your doctor if:
- You have a heart problem.
- You have liver or kidney problems.
- You have asthma or respiratory problems.
- You have a history of peptic ulcers.
- You have had an epileptic seizure.
- You are taking other medicines.

Pregnancy Not recommended. Safety in pregnancy not established.
Breast-feeding Not recommended.
Infants and children Not recommended.
Over 60 Particular risk of heart problems, low heart rate, and collapse.
Driving and hazardous work Your underlying condition may make such activities inadvisable. Discuss with your doctor.

Alcohol Avoid. Alcohol increases the sedative effects of rivastigmine.
Surgery and general anaesthetics Treatment may need to be stopped before you have a general anaesthetic. Discuss this with your doctor or dentist before any operation.

PROLONGED USE

Rivastigmine treatment may be continued for as long as there is benefit. Stopping the drug leads to a gradual loss of the improvements.
Monitoring Checks at 6-monthly intervals may be performed to test whether the drug is still providing some benefit.

ROPINIROLE

Brand names Adartrel (restless legs only), Aimpart XL, Ralnea XL, Repinex XL, Requip, Requip XL
Used in the following combined preparations None

QUICK REFERENCE

Drug group Drug for parkinsonism (p.16)
Overdose danger rating Low
Dependence rating Low
Prescription needed Yes
Available as generic Yes

GENERAL INFORMATION

Ropinirole mimics dopamine, a neurotransmitter (p.7) in the brain. It is used to treat Parkinson's disease, in which there is a lack of dopamine in the brain. It may be used either alone or combined with levodopa (p.293). Patients taking levodopa alone for several years may experience extremes of activity: overactivity after taking levodopa ("on effect") and underactivity ("off effect") before the next dose of levodopa is due. Used with levodopa, ropinirole helps to reduce these on-off fluctuations. Unlike some other drugs for Parkinson's disease, it does not cause fibrosis (thickening of connective tissue) of the abdomen or heart; however, it may cause excessive sleepiness and a tendency to low blood pressure on standing (postural hypotension). It may also be used for restless legs syndrome (Ekbom's disease).

INFORMATION FOR USERS

Your drug prescription is tailored for you. Do not alter dosage without checking with your doctor.
How taken/used Tablets, modified release (MR) tablets.
Frequency and timing of doses *Parkinson's* 3 x daily (tablets) or 1 x daily (MR tablets). *Restless legs* 1 x daily at night (tablets). In all cases, doses should be taken with or after food.
Adult dosage range *Parkinson's* 750mcg–3mg daily (tablets), 750mcg–24mg (MR tablets). Initially a low dose is given; this is increased until there is a satisfactory response. If given with levodopa, the dose of ropinirole may be reduced. *Restless legs* 250mcg each night, increasing slowly to 4mg maximum.
Onset of effect 1–2 hours.
Duration of action 6–12 hours.
Diet advice None.
Storage Keep in original container at room temperature out of the reach of children.
Missed dose Take as soon as you remember. If your next dose is due within 2 hours, take a single dose now and skip the next.
Stopping the drug Do not stop the drug without consulting your doctor; symptoms may recur.
Exceeding the dose An occasional unintended extra dose is unlikely to be a cause for concern. If you notice any unusual symptoms, or if a large overdose has been taken, tell your doctor.

POSSIBLE ADVERSE EFFECTS

Nausea, drowsiness, and dizziness on standing are common adverse effects. In some cases, drowsiness can be severe, with the sudden onset of sleep during the day. Starting with low doses that are gradually increased helps to reduce the likelihood of side effects. If drowsiness or any of the other common side effects are severe, discuss with your doctor. Rarely, ropinirole may cause confusion, hallucinations, increased sexuality, and compulsive behaviours, such as compulsive gambling. If any of these effects occur, consult your doctor.

INTERACTIONS

Ciprofloxacin The effect of ropinirole may be increased, necessitating dose reduction of ropinirole or use of an alternative antibiotic.
Memantine May enhance the effects of ropinirole. Ropinirole dose may need to be reduced.
Metoclopramide and antipsychotics These drugs reduce the effect of ropinirole and may worsen symptoms.
Smoking reduces blood levels of ropinirole, so stopping smoking may produce side effects resulting from a significant rise in blood levels of ropinirole.

SPECIAL PRECAUTIONS

Be sure to tell your doctor if:

◆ You have postural hypotension or dizziness on standing.

◆ You have changed or intend to change your smoking habit.

◆ You have long-standing kidney or liver problems.

◆ You have had a psychotic illness.

Pregnancy Safety in pregnancy not established. Discuss with your doctor.

Breast-feeding Safety not established, and the drug may suppress lactation. Discuss with your doctor.

Infants and children Unlikely to be required.

Over 60 Reduced dose may be necessary.

Driving and hazardous work Avoid until you know how ropinirole affects you as this drug may cause dizziness and severe drowsiness.

Alcohol No known problems, although ropinirole may enhance the sedative effect of alcohol.

PROLONGED USE

No special problems.

ROSUVASTATIN

Brand name Crestor

Used in the following combined preparations None

QUICK REFERENCE

Drug group Lipid-lowering drug (p.35)

Overdose danger rating Low

Dependence rating Low

Prescription needed Yes

Available as generic No

GENERAL INFORMATION

Rosuvastatin is a statin: a lipid-lowering drug that is used in treating hypercholesterolaemia (high blood cholesterol levels). Cholesterol is a lipid (fat) that is produced naturally in the body and is necessary for the production of many other body chemicals. Rosuvastatin works by inhibiting an enzyme involved in the manufacture of cholesterol in the liver. It is more potent than other statins so can produce lower cholesterol levels than the other statins. It is prescribed to people who have not responded to other forms of therapy, such as a special diet or less potent statins, and who have, or are at risk of developing, coronary artery disease or stroke.

Adverse effects of rosuvastatin are usually mild and wear off with time. However, any unexplained aches or pains or muscle weakness should be reported to your doctor immediately. People of Asian origin are given lower starting doses because the drug works more potently in them.

INFORMATION FOR USERS

Your drug prescription is tailored for you. Do not alter dosage without checking with your doctor.

How taken/used Tablets.

Frequency and timing of doses Once daily at night.

Adult dosage range 5–40mg (5–20mg for patients of Asian origin); 10mg (initial dose), increased to 20mg after 4 weeks, if necessary; a maximum dose of 40mg may be given for severe hypercholesterolaemia.

Onset of effect 2–4 weeks.

Duration of action 24 hours.

Diet advice Low-fat diet usually recommended.

Storage Keep in original container at room temperature, out of the reach of children.

Missed dose Do not take the missed dose. Take the next scheduled dose as usual.

Stopping the drug Do not stop without consulting your doctor. Symptoms may recur.

Exceeding the dose An occasional unintentional extra dose is unlikely to be a cause for concern. But if you notice any unusual symptoms or have taken a large overdose, notify your doctor.

POSSIBLE ADVERSE EFFECTS

Common adverse effects include abdominal pain, constipation or diarrhoea, nausea, flatulence, headache, and sleep disturbance. Most are mild and transient, but discuss with your doctor if they are severe. If you develop a rash, stop taking the drug; if you have jaundice, or muscle tenderness, pain, or weakness, stop the drug and consult your doctor at once.

INTERACTIONS

Ciclosporin This drug increases blood levels of rosuvastatin.

Warfarin Rosuvastatin may enhance the effects of warfarin. The level of anticoagulation (INR) should be monitored.

Erythromycin This drug reduces the effectiveness of rosuvastatin.

Oestrogens Rosuvastatin increases blood levels of some of these drugs.

Gemfibrozil and other lipid-lowering drugs There is an increased risk of adverse effects when these drugs are taken with rosuvastatin.
Antacids may reduce the effectiveness of rosuvastatin.
Anti-HIV drugs may increase the risk of muscle damage when taken with rosuvastatin.

SPECIAL PRECAUTIONS

Be sure to tell your doctor if:
- You have liver or kidney problems.
- You have a personal or family history of muscle problems.
- You have porphyria.
- You are of Asian origin.
- You are taking other medicines.

Pregnancy Not recommended. May affect fetal development. Discuss with your doctor if you are pregnant or intend to become pregnant.
Breast-feeding Not recommended. Safety not established. Discuss with your doctor.
Infants and children Not recommended.
Over 60 Reduced initial dose. Discuss with your doctor.
Driving and hazardous work No special problems.
Alcohol Avoid excessive amounts. Alcohol may increase the risk of developing liver problems with this drug.

PROLONGED USE

Prolonged treatment can adversely affect liver function and may unmask Type 2 diabetes.
Monitoring Periodic blood tests for muscle toxicity and to assess liver function are recommended. If high doses are taken, regular blood tests may also be done to assess renal function.

SACUBITRIL/VALSARTAN

Brand names Entresto
Used in the following combined preparations None

QUICK REFERENCE

Drug group Vasodilator (p.30)
Overdose danger rating Medium
Dependence rating Low
Prescription needed Yes
Available as generic No

GENERAL INFORMATION

Sacubitril/valsartan is a new drug approved for the long-term management of heart failure. It is a combination tablet consisting of sacubitril (an inhibitor of the enzyme neprilysin, which affects the pumping action of the heart) and valsartan (an angiotensin II receptor blocker, or ARB, for lowering blood pressure; see p.34).

Sacubitril/valsartan reduces the strain on the heart in addition to improving the heart's structure and function. Studies show that it provides long-term benefit in patients with symptoms of heart failure. It is administered in conjunction with other therapies for heart failure and in place of other angiotensin II receptor blockers or ACE inhibitors.

Low blood pressure may occur when taking sacubitril/valsartan. Therefore, if you experience light-headedness, dizziness, or headache, you should inform your doctor.

INFORMATION FOR USERS

Your drug prescription is tailored for you. Do not alter dosage without checking with your doctor.
How taken/used Tablets.
Frequency and timing of doses 2 x daily.
Dosage range Adult starting dose either 24/26mg 2 x daily or 49/51mg 2 x daily. Dose may be increased every 2–4 weeks to a maximum of 97/103mg 2 x daily depending upon response.
Onset of effect Effect on blood pressure develops within a few hours. Full beneficial effect on heart failure may take weeks to develop.
Duration of action 12 hours.
Diet advice None.
Storage Keep in original container at room temperature out of the reach of children.
Missed dose Take as soon as you remember. If your next dose is within 6 hours, take a single dose now and skip the next. Continue usual dosing schedule.
Stopping the drug Do not stop without consulting your doctor. Stopping the drug may lead to worsening of the underlying condition.
Exceeding the dose An occasional unintentional extra dose is unlikely to cause problems. Large overdoses may cause dizziness, fainting, and a faint pulse. Notify your doctor.

POSSIBLE ADVERSE EFFECTS

Most effects are minor and disappear soon after treatment starts, but discuss any effects with your doctor. Diarrhoea, nausea, headache, cough, dizziness, and fatigue are common; rash is less common. If you develop wheezing, breathing difficulties, or swollen mouth, lips, or tongue, stop the drug and contact your doctor immediately.

INTERACTIONS

Potassium supplements (including some salt substitutes), potassium-sparing diuretics, and ciclosporin may raise blood levels of potassium.
Statins Blood levels of some statins may increase, making their side effects more likely, especially at higher doses.
Lithium Sacubitril/valsartan may cause raised blood lithium levels and toxicity.
Vasodilators, diuretics, and other antihypertensives may increase the drug's blood-pressure-lowering effect.
Non-steroidal anti-inflammatory drugs (NSAIDs) Some may increase the risk of kidney damage with sacubitril/valsartan.

SPECIAL PRECAUTIONS

Be sure to tell your doctor if:
- You have heart problems, including heart failure.
- You have had angioedema or a previous allergic reaction to an ACE inhibitor or ARB.
- You have long-term liver or kidney problems or stenosis of the kidney's arteries.
- You are or intend to become pregnant.
- You are taking other medicines.

Pregnancy Not prescribed. Discuss with your doctor.
Breast-feeding Safety not established. Discuss with your doctor.
Infants and children Not prescribed.
Over 60 Reduced dose may be necessary.
Driving and hazardous work Avoid such activities until you have learned how sacubitril/valsartan affects you because the drug can cause dizziness, fatigue, and fainting.
Alcohol Avoid. Alcohol may increase the blood-pressure-lowering and adverse effects of the drug.
Surgery and general anaesthetics Sacubitril/valsartan may have to be stopped before you have a general anaesthetic. Discuss with your doctor or dentist.

PROLONGED USE

No special problems. However, periodic checks on serum potassium levels and kidney function are usually performed. Haemoglobin and liver tests may also be carried out.

SALBUTAMOL

Brand names Airomir, Airsalb, Salamol, Salbulin, Ventmax, Ventolin, and others
Used in the following combined preparations Combivent

QUICK REFERENCE

Drug group Bronchodilator (p.21), drug to treat asthma (p.22), and drug used in premature labour (p.109)
Overdose danger rating Low
Dependence rating Low
Prescription needed Yes
Available as generic Yes

GENERAL INFORMATION

Salbutamol is a sympathomimetic bronchodilator used to treat conditions such as asthma, chronic obstructive pulmonary disease (COPD), and bronchospasm, in which the airways become constricted. Although it can be taken by mouth, inhalation is more effective because the drug is delivered directly to the airways, thus giving rapid relief, allowing smaller doses, and causing fewer side effects. If you need to use inhaled salbutamol more than twice a week or have to use it at night, you will probably also be prescribed an inhaled corticosteroid (see Drugs for asthma, p.22) to improve control of your asthma.

Compared to some similar drugs, salbutamol has little stimulant effect on the heart rate and blood pressure, making it safer for people with heart problems or high blood pressure. The drug also relaxes the uterus muscle, so it is used to prevent premature labour (p.109).

INFORMATION FOR USERS

Your drug prescription is tailored for you. Do not alter dosage without checking with your doctor.
How taken/used Tablets, slow release (SR) tablets, SR capsules, liquid, injection, inhaler, nebules for nebulizer, powder for inhalation.
Frequency and timing of doses 3–4 x daily (tablets/liquid); 2 x daily (SR preparations); 1–2 inhalations 3–4 x daily (inhaler); up to 4 x daily (nebules).
Dosage range 8–16mg daily (by mouth); 400–800mcg daily (inhaler); 2.5–20mg daily (nebules).
Onset of effect Within 30–60 minutes (by mouth); within 5–15 minutes (inhaler/nebules).

Duration of action Up to 8 hours (tablets); up to 6 hours (inhaler); up to 12 hours (SR preparations).
Diet advice None.
Storage Keep in original container at room temperature out of the reach of children. Protect from light. Do not puncture or burn inhalers.
Missed dose Take as soon as you remember if you need it. If next dose is due within 2 hours, take a single dose now and skip the next.
Stopping the drug Do not stop the drug without consulting your doctor; symptoms may recur.
Exceeding the dose An occasional unintentional extra dose is unlikely to be a cause for concern. But if you notice any unusual symptoms, or if a large overdose has been taken, tell your doctor.

POSSIBLE ADVERSE EFFECTS

Muscle tremor (particularly of the hands), anxiety, tension, and restlessness are the most common adverse effects. Discuss with your doctor if they are severe or if you develop headache or muscle cramps. If palpitations occur, stop taking the drug and consult your doctor. Rarely, wheezing or breathlessness may worsen immediately after using the inhaler (paradoxical bronchospasm); if so, stop using the drug and contact your doctor immediately.

INTERACTIONS

Theophylline, corticosteroids, and diuretics There is a risk of low potassium levels in the blood if taken with salbutamol.
Other sympathomimetic drugs may increase the effects of salbutamol, thereby also increasing the risk of adverse effects.
Digoxin Salbutamol may cause low potassium levels, increasing the risk of digoxin toxicity. Salbutamol by mouth or injection can reduce digoxin levels.
Beta blockers Drugs in this group may reduce the action of salbutamol.

SPECIAL PRECAUTIONS

Be sure to tell your doctor if:
- You have heart problems.
- You have high blood pressure.
- You have diabetes.
- You have a tendency towards low potassium levels.
- You have an overactive thyroid gland.
- You are taking other medicines.

Pregnancy No evidence of risk when used to treat asthma, or to treat or prevent premature labour. Discuss with your doctor.
Breast-feeding The drug passes into the breast milk, but normal doses are unlikely to affect the baby adversely. Discuss with your doctor.
Infants and children Reduced dose necessary.
Over 60 Increased likelihood of adverse effects. Reduced dose may therefore be necessary.
Driving and hazardous work Avoid until you have learned how salbutamol affects you because the drug can cause tremors.
Alcohol No known problems.

PROLONGED USE

No problems expected, but you should contact your doctor if you find you need to use your salbutamol inhaler more than usual. Failure to respond to the drug may be due to worsening asthma that requires urgent medical attention.
Monitoring Periodic blood tests for potassium may be needed in people on high-dose treatment with salbutamol combined with other asthma drugs and/or diuretics.

SALMETEROL

Brand name Neovent, Serevent, Sereflo, Soltel
Used in the following combined preparation AirFluSal, Combisal, Fusacomb, Seretide, Sirdupla, Stalplex

QUICK REFERENCE

Drug group Bronchodilator (p.21), drug to treat asthma (p.22), and drug used in premature labour (p.109)
Overdose danger rating Low
Dependence rating Low
Prescription needed Yes
Available as generic Yes

GENERAL INFORMATION

Salmeterol is a sympathomimetic bronchodilator used to treat conditions such as asthma, chronic obstructive pulmonary disease (COPD), and bronchospasm, in which the airways inside the lungs become constricted. The advantage of this drug over salbutamol (opposite page) is that it is longer acting.

Salmeterol relaxes the muscle surrounding the airways in the lungs but, because of its slow onset of effect, it is not used for immediate relief of asthma symptoms. It is prescribed to prevent attacks, however, and can be helpful in preventing night-time asthma. Salmeterol should always be used in combination with inhaled or oral corticosteroids. Taken by inhalation, the drug is delivered directly to the airways. This allows smaller doses to be given and reduces the risk of adverse effects.

INFORMATION FOR USERS

Your drug prescription is tailored for you. Do not alter dosage without checking with your doctor.
How taken/used Inhaler, powder for inhalation.
Frequency and timing of doses 2 x daily.
Dosage range 100–200mcg daily.
Onset of effect 10–20 minutes.
Duration of action 12 hours.
Diet advice None.
Storage Keep in original container at room temperature out of the reach of children.
Missed dose Take as soon as you remember. If your next dose is due within 4 hours, take a single dose now and skip the next.
Stopping the drug Do not stop without consulting your doctor; symptoms may recur.
Exceeding the dose An occasional unintentional extra dose is unlikely to be a cause for concern. But if you notice any unusual symptoms, or if a large overdose has been taken, notify your doctor.

POSSIBLE ADVERSE EFFECTS

Side effects of salmeterol are usually mild. Tremor is the most common; discuss with your doctor if it is severe. Palpitations, muscle cramps, or less commonly headache may also occur; consult your doctor in all cases. Rarely, wheezing or breathlessness may suddenly worsen after using the inhaler (paradoxical bronchospasm); if this occurs, stop the drug and call your doctor immediately.

INTERACTIONS

Corticosteroids, theophylline, and diuretics There is an increased risk of low blood potassium levels when high doses of salmeterol are taken with these drugs.
Other sympathomimetics may increase the effects of salmeterol, thereby also increasing the risk of adverse effects.
Triazole antifungal drugs (such as itraconazole and voriconazole) increase the body's exposure to salmeterol.
Digoxin Salmeterol may cause low potasssium levels in the blood, which increases the risk of digoxin toxicity.
Protease inhibitors (e.g. ritonavir, saquinavir, and telaprevir) increase the risk of abnormal heart rhythms when used with salmeterol.

SPECIAL PRECAUTIONS

Be sure to tell your doctor if:
- You have heart problems.
- You have high blood pressure.
- You have an overactive thyroid gland.
- You have diabetes.
- You have a tendency towards low potassium levels.
- You are taking other medicines.

Pregnancy No evidence of risk when used to treat asthma. Benefits of treatment usually outweigh risk that mother's worsening asthma has on fetus. Discuss with your doctor.
Breast-feeding The drug passes into the breast milk, but normal doses are unlikely to affect the baby adversely. Discuss with your doctor.
Infants and children Reduced dose necessary. Not recommended for children under 4 years.
Over 60 No special problems.
Driving and hazardous work No special problems.
Alcohol No known problems.

PROLONGED USE

Salmeterol is intended to be used long term together with an inhaled corticosteroid. The main problem comes from using combinations of anti-asthma drugs, with or without diuretics, leading to low blood potassium levels.
Monitoring Periodic blood tests are usually carried out to monitor potassium levels.

SERTRALINE

Brand name Lustral
Used in the following combined preparations None

QUICK REFERENCE

Drug group Antidepressant drug (p.12)
Overdose danger rating Low
Dependence rating Low
Prescription needed Yes
Available as generic Yes

GENERAL INFORMATION

Sertraline is one of the selective serotonin reuptake inhibitor (SSRI) antidepressants. These tend to cause less sedation than older types of antidepressant, and have different side effects. Sertraline elevates mood, increases physical activity, and restores interest in daily activities. It is used to treat depression, including accompanying anxiety, and obsessive-compulsive disorder (OCD). The drug is also prescribed for post-traumatic stress disorder (PTSD).

Treatment is usually stopped gradually over at least 4 weeks because symptoms such as headache, nausea, and dizziness may occur if the drug is withdrawn suddenly.

INFORMATION FOR USERS

Your drug prescription is tailored for you. Do not alter dosage without checking with your doctor.

How taken/used Tablets.

Frequency and timing of doses Once daily, usually in the morning.

Adult dosage range 25–200mg daily.

Onset of effect Some benefits may appear within 14 days, but full effects may take another 6 weeks; anxiety disorders may take longer.

Duration of action Antidepressant effect may continue for some weeks after prolonged use.

Diet advice None.

Storage Keep in original container at room temperature out of the reach of children.

Missed dose Take as soon as you remember. If your next dose is due within 8 hours, take a single dose now and skip the next.

Stopping the drug Do not stop the drug without consulting your doctor, who may supervise a gradual reduction in dosage.

Exceeding the dose An occasional unintentional extra dose is unlikely to cause problems. Large overdoses may cause adverse effects. Notify your doctor.

POSSIBLE ADVERSE EFFECTS

Common adverse effects include gastrointestinal problems (such as nausea, indigestion, and diarrhoea/loose stools), insomnia or sleepiness, restlessness, anxiety, and sexual dysfunction. Discuss with your doctor if severe. Less commonly, a rash, itching, or skin eruptions may occur; if they do, stop the drug and call your doctor immediately. Rarely, sertraline may cause suicidal thoughts or attempts; if so, stop the drug and seek immediate medical attention.

INTERACTIONS

Anticoagulants The effects of these drugs may be increased by sertraline.

St John's wort There is a danger of increasing the side effects of both substances.

Monoamine oxidase inhibitors (MAOIs) The effects and toxicity of sertraline are greatly increased by MAOIs.

Tramadol and 5HT1 agonists (e.g. sumatriptan) There is an increased risk of adverse effects if these drugs are taken with sertraline.

Antipsychotics Sertraline may increase the levels and effects of some antipsychotics.

SPECIAL PRECAUTIONS

Be sure to tell your doctor if:

- You have long-term liver or kidney problems.
- You have had epileptic seizures.
- You have heart problems.
- You have a history of bleeding disorders.
- You have a history of mania.
- You are taking other medicines.

Pregnancy Safety not established. Discuss with your doctor.

Breast-feeding Safety not established. Discuss with your doctor.

Infants and children Not generally recommended under 18 years.

Over 60 No special problems.

Driving and hazardous work Avoid until you know how sertraline affects you because it can cause drowsiness and visual disturbances.

Alcohol Avoid excessive intake. SSRIs may increase the sedative effects of alcohol.

PROLONGED USE

No known problems in adults. There is a small risk of suicidal thoughts and self-harm in children and adolescents, although the drug is rarely used for this age group.

Monitoring Any person experiencing drowsiness, confusion, muscle cramps, or seizures should be monitored for low sodium levels in the blood. Under-18s should be monitored for suicidal thoughts and self-harm.

SILDENAFIL/TADALAFIL

Brand names [sildenafil] Aronix, Granpidam, Mysildecard, Nipatra, Revatio, Viagra, Vizarsin; [tadalafil] Adcirca, Cialis

Used in the following combined preparations None

QUICK REFERENCE

Drug group Drug for erectile dysfunction (p.108)

Overdose danger rating Medium

Dependence rating Low

Prescription needed Yes (except Viagra for some men)

Available as generic Yes (sildenafil)

GENERAL INFORMATION

Sildenafil and tadalafil are used to treat erectile dysfunction. They do not directly cause an erection, but they prevent the muscle walls of the blood-filled chambers in the penis from relaxing. The drugs are taken only before sexual activity. Sildenafil is also occasionally used to treat pulmonary hypertension (high blood pressure in the arteries supplying the lungs) and Raynaud's disease. Tadalafil may also be used to treat non-cancerous prostate enlargement. Because both drugs are vasodilators, they can lower blood pressure and may increase the effects of antihypertensive drugs. They should not be taken if you are using a nitrate (p.33) because they greatly increase its effects.

Viagra (one brand of sildenafil) is available over the counter to men aged 40–65 who pass a medical check by the pharmacist.

INFORMATION FOR USERS

Your drug prescription is tailored for you. Do not alter dosage without checking with your doctor.

How taken/used Tablets, intravenous injection.

Frequency and timing of doses *Erectile dysfunction* As needed; maximum one dose daily, 1 hour before sexual activity. *Pulmonary hypertension* 3 x daily.

Adult dosage range *Erectile dysfunction* (sildenafil) 25–100mg per dose; (tadalafil) 10–20mg per dose. *Pulmonary hypertension* (sildenafil) 60mg daily (tablets); 30mg (injection).

Onset of effect 30 minutes.

Duration of action 4 hours (sildenafil); up to 36 hours (tadalafil).

Diet advice None, although the drugs take longer to work after a meal, especially a high-fat meal. Grapefruit juice may increase sildenafil levels.

Storage Keep in original container at room temperature out of the reach of children.

Missed dose For erectile dysfunction, use only as needed. For pulmonary hypertension, take as soon as you remember, then take the next dose as scheduled.

Stopping the drug For erectile dysfunction, the drugs can safely by stopped as soon as no longer needed. For pulmonary hypertension, do not stop without consulting your doctor; your condition may worsen.

Exceeding the dose An occasional unintentional extra dose is unlikely to cause problems. Large overdoses may cause headache, dizziness, flushing, and altered vision. Notify your doctor.

POSSIBLE ADVERSE EFFECTS

Adverse effects are common but usually minor. They include headache, flushing, dizziness, indigestion, nasal congestion, blurred vision, altered colour vision, and back pain. Discuss with your doctor if any of these are severe. However, if you develop a persistent, painful erection lasting more than 4 hours (priapism) or chest pain, stop taking the drug and seek immediate medical attention.

INTERACTIONS

Nitrates The effects of these drugs are greatly increased by sildenafil and tadalafil so nitrates are not prescribed together with either of these drugs.

Antihypertensive drugs Sildenafil and tadalafil may enhance the blood-pressure-lowering effect of these drugs.

Cimetidine, erythromycin, nicorandil, ketoconazole (oral), and antiviral drugs These drugs increase the blood levels and the toxicity of sildenafil and tadalafil.

SPECIAL PRECAUTIONS

Be sure to tell your doctor if:

- You have heart problems.
- You have had a stroke or heart attack.
- You have liver or kidney problems.
- You have low or high blood pressure.
- You have sickle cell anaemia, leukaemia, or myeloma.
- You have an inherited eye problem.
- You have an abnormality of the penis.
- You are taking other medicines, especially a nitrate drug.

Pregnancy Not prescribed.

Breast-feeding Not prescribed.

Infants and children Not prescribed for children under 18 years, except rarely for pulmonary hypertension on specialist advice.

Over 60 Reduced dose may be necessary.

Driving and hazardous work Avoid such activities until you have learned how sildenafil or tadalafil affects you because they can cause dizziness and altered vision.

Alcohol No special problems.

PROLONGED USE

No problems expected.

SIMVASTATIN

Brand names Simvador, Zocor

Used in the following combined preparations Cholib, Inegy

QUICK REFERENCE

Drug group Lipid-lowering drug (p.35)

Overdose danger rating Medium

Dependence rating Low

Prescription needed Yes (except low-dose preparations)

Available as generic Yes

GENERAL INFORMATION

One of the statin group of lipid-lowering drugs, simvastatin blocks the action of an enzyme involved in the manufacture of cholesterol in the liver, resulting in lowered blood levels of cholesterol. The drug is prescribed for people with hypercholesterolaemia (high blood cholesterol) who have not responded to other forms of therapy (e.g. a special diet) and who are at risk of developing or have existing coronary heart disease or stroke. Low-dose simvastatin is available over the counter. Side effects are usually mild and wear off with time. In the body, simvastatin is found mainly in the liver, and it may raise the levels of liver enzymes but this does not usually indicate serious liver damage. Rarely, it may cause muscle damage (especially with higher doses), so any unexpected muscle tenderness, pain, or weakness should be reported to your doctor.

INFORMATION FOR USERS

Your drug prescription is tailored for you. Do not alter dosage without checking with your doctor.

How taken/used Tablets.

Frequency and timing of doses Once daily at night.

Adult dosage range 10–80mg daily.

Onset of effect Within 2 weeks; full beneficial effects may not be reached for 4–6 weeks.

Duration of action Up to 24 hours.

Diet advice A low-fat diet is usually recommended. Avoid grapefruit juice.

Storage Keep in original container at room temperature out of the reach of children. Protect from light.

Missed dose Take as soon as you remember. If your next dose is due within 8 hours, do not take the missed dose, but take the next dose on schedule.

Stopping the drug Do not stop without consulting your doctor. Stopping the drug may lead to worsening of the underlying condition.

Exceeding the dose An occasional unintentional extra dose is unlikely to cause problems. Large overdoses may cause liver problems. Notify your doctor.

POSSIBLE ADVERSE EFFECTS

Adverse effects of simvastatin are usually mild and do not last long. The most common are gastrointestinal problems (such as abdominal pain, constipation or diarrhoea, nausea, and flatulence), sleep disturbance, and headache. Discuss with your doctor if these are severe. If a rash develops, stop taking the drug. Rarely, simvastatin may cause jaundice, or muscle pain, tenderness, or weakness. If any of these occur, stop taking the drug and consult your doctor immediately.

INTERACTIONS

Ciclosporin, danazol, fibrates, nicotinic acid, amiodarone, amlodipine, verapamil, diltiazem, ranolazine, itraconazole, ketoconazole, HIV protease inhibitors, macrolide antibiotics, and nefazodone Used with simvastatin, these drugs increase the risk of muscle toxicity. If they are required, simvastatin is withheld temporarily or the dose reduced.

St John's wort reduces blood level of simvastatin.

Anticoagulants (e.g. warfarin) Simvastatin may increase the effect of these drugs. The level of anticoagulation (INR) should be monitored.

Carbamazepine reduces blood levels of simvastatin; simvastatin dose may need to be increased.

Grapefruit juice increases blood levels of simvastatin; avoid regular consumption.

SPECIAL PRECAUTIONS

Be sure to consult your doctor or pharmacist before taking this drug if:

- You have liver or kidney problems.
- You have a personal or family history of muscle problems.
- You have porphyria.
- You are taking other medicines.

Pregnancy Not recommended. May affect fetal development. Discuss with your doctor if you are pregnant or intend to become pregnant.

Breast-feeding The drug passes into the breast milk and may affect the baby. Discuss with your doctor.

Infants and children Not recommended under 5 years. Reduced dose necessary in older children, under specialist advice.
Over 60 No special problems.
Driving and hazardous work No special problems.
Alcohol Avoid excessive amounts. Alcohol may increase the risk of developing liver problems with this drug.

PROLONGED USE

Prolonged treatment can adversely affect liver function.
Monitoring Periodic blood tests to test for muscle toxicity and assess liver function are recommended.

SITAGLIPTIN

Brand name Januvia
Used in the following combined preparation Janumet (with metformin)

QUICK REFERENCE

Drug group Drug for diabetes (p.80)
Overdose danger rating High
Dependence rating Low
Prescription needed Yes
Available as generic No

GENERAL INFORMATION

Sitagliptin is used to treat Type 2 diabetes in combination with diet, exercise, weight control, and often other antidiabetic drugs. It is one of a new class of oral antidiabetics known as DPP-4 inhibitors or gliptins, which block the breakdown of hormones called incretins. Incretins help to increase insulin production, but only when needed, such as after a meal. Gliptins increase the incretin level after a meal, resulting in an increase of insulin, which helps to prevent a blood sugar "high" after eating.

Gliptins are less likely to cause abnormally low blood sugar levels (hypoglycaemia) than other antidiabetic drugs if used on their own. Unlike the sulfonylureas, gliptins do not cause weight gain. Sitagliptin can be used alone or in combination with other antidiabetic drugs, such as metformin or insulin.

INFORMATION FOR USERS

Your drug prescription is tailored for you. Do not alter dosage without checking with your doctor.
How taken/used Tablets.
Frequency and timing of doses Once daily; can be taken with or without food.
Adult dosage range 100mg daily.
Onset of effect Within 1 hour.
Duration of action Up to 24 hours.
Diet advice An individualized diabetic diet must be maintained for the drug to be fully effective. Follow the advice of your doctor.
Storage Store at room temperature away from moisture, heat, and light and out of the reach of children.
Missed dose Take as soon as you remember. Do not take a double dose on the same day.
Stopping the drug Do not stop without consulting your doctor; stopping the drug may lead to worsening of your diabetes control.

OVERDOSE ACTION

The drug is usually safe, but seek immediate medical help if you have early warning signs of low blood sugar (such as faintness, dizziness, headache, confusion, sweating, or tremor), and eat or drink something sugary. Take emergency action if seizures or loss of consciousness occur.

POSSIBLE ADVERSE EFFECTS

Serious side effects are rare with sitagliptin. The most common are stomach discomfort and diarrhoea. Less commonly, it may cause symptoms such as headache, sweating, weakness, tremor, dizziness, faintness, and confusion; these may indicate low blood sugar levels and are more likely to occur when sitagliptin is used in combination with other antidiabetic drugs. If they do occur, eat or drink something sugary and seek immediate medical help. If you develop a severe rash or skin blistering, stop taking the drug and consult your doctor promptly. If you have severe abdominal pain or vomiting, you should stop taking the drug and contact your doctor immediately.

INTERACTIONS

General note Many drugs may interact with sitagliptin to affect blood sugar levels. Some medicines contain sugar and may upset diabetic control. Consult your doctor or pharmacist before taking any other medicines.
Beta blockers may mask symptoms of low blood sugar when taken with sitagliptin.
Digoxin Sitagliptin may increase the blood level of digoxin.

SPECIAL PRECAUTIONS

Be sure to tell your doctor if:

- You have long-term kidney problems.
- You have a history of pancreatitis.
- You are taking other medicines.

Pregnancy Safety not established. Discuss with your doctor.

Breast-feeding Present in breast milk. Safety not established. Discuss with your doctor.

Infants and children Not prescribed.

Over 60 No special problems.

Driving and hazardous work Avoid if you have warning signs of low blood sugar.

Alcohol Avoid. May upset diabetic control.

Surgery and general anaesthetics Notify your doctor or dentist that you have diabetes before you undergo any surgery. Your diabetes medication may need to be altered, and sometimes insulin may need to be substituted.

PROLONGED USE

There is a small increased risk of upper respiratory tract and urinary infections when taking sitagliptin long term.

Monitoring Regular monitoring of your diabetes control is necessary. You may also undergo periodic assessment of the eyes, heart, and kidneys.

SODIUM CROMOGLICATE

Brand names Intal, Nalcrom, Opticrom, Vividrin, and others

Used in the following combined preparations None

QUICK REFERENCE

Drug group Anti-allergy drug (p.56)

Overdose danger rating Low

Dependence rating Low

Prescription needed No (some preparations)

Available as generic Yes

GENERAL INFORMATION

Sodium cromoglicate, introduced in the 1970s, is used primarily to prevent asthma and allergic conditions. When taken by inhaler as a powder (Spinhaler) or spray, it is commonly used to reduce the frequency and severity of asthma attacks, and is also effective in helping to prevent attacks induced by exercise or cold air. The drug has a slow onset of action, and it may be up to 6 weeks before its full anti-asthmatic effect is felt. It is not effective for the relief of an asthma attack.

Sodium cromoglicate is also given as eye drops to prevent or treat allergic conjunctivitis. As a nasal spray, it is used to prevent or treat allergic rhinitis (hay fever). It is also given, in the form of capsules, for food allergy.

Side effects are mild. Coughing and wheezing occurring on inhalation of the drug may be prevented by using a sympathomimetic bronchodilator (p.21) first. Hoarseness and throat irritation can be avoided by rinsing the mouth with water after inhalation.

INFORMATION FOR USERS

Follow instructions on the label. Call your doctor if symptoms worsen.

How taken/used Capsules, inhaler (various types), eye drops, nasal spray.

Frequency and timing of doses *Capsules* 4 x daily before meals, swallowed whole or dissolved in water. *Inhaler, nasal spray* 4–6 x daily. *Eye preparations* 4 x daily (drops).

Adult dosage range 800mg daily (capsules); as directed (inhaler); apply to each nostril as directed (nasal spray); 1–2 drops in each eye per dose (eye drops).

Onset of effect Varies with dosage, form, and condition being treated. Eye conditions and allergic rhinitis may respond after a few days' treatment with drops, while asthma and chronic allergic rhinitis may take 2–6 weeks to show improvement.

Duration of action 4–6 hours. Some effect persists for several days after treatment is stopped.

Diet advice With capsules you may be advised to avoid consuming certain foods. Follow your doctor's advice.

Storage Keep in original container at room temperature out of the reach of children. Protect from light.

Missed dose Take as soon as you remember. If your next dose is due within 2 hours, take a single dose now and skip the next.

Stopping the drug Do not stop without consulting your doctor; symptoms may recur.

Exceeding the dose An occasional unintentional extra dose is unlikely to be a cause for concern. But if you notice any unusual symptoms, or if a large overdose has been taken, tell your doctor.

POSSIBLE ADVERSE EFFECTS

Coughing and hoarseness are common with inhalation of sodium cromoglicate. The nasal spray may cause sneezing. Eye drops may cause eye stinging. These symptoms usually diminish with continued use. Capsules may rarely cause nausea, vomiting, joint pain, or a rash. If any of these occur, call your doctor – immediately in the case of a rash. More rarely, headache, dizziness, wheezing, or breathlessness may occur; discuss with your doctor if you develop wheezing or breathlessness or if headache or dizziness are severe. If wheezing or breathlessness worsens just after inhaler use (paradoxical bronchospasm), stop using the drug and call your doctor immediately.

INTERACTIONS

None known.

SPECIAL PRECAUTIONS

Be sure to tell your doctor if:

◆ You are taking other medicines.

Pregnancy No evidence of risk.

Breast-feeding It is not known whether the drug passes into the breast milk. Discuss with your doctor.

Infants and children Reduced dose necessary.

Over 60 No special problems.

Driving and hazardous work No known problems.

Alcohol No known problems.

PROLONGED USE

No problems expected.

SODIUM VALPROATE (VALPROATE)

Brand names Convulex (valproic acid), Depakim, Depakote, Epilim, Epilim Chrono, Epilim Chronosphere, Episenta, Epival

Used in the following combined preparations None

QUICK REFERENCE

Drug group Anticonvulsant drug (p.14)

Overdose danger rating Medium

Dependence rating Low

Prescription needed Yes

Available as generic Yes

GENERAL INFORMATION

Sodium valproate is an anticonvulsant drug that is effective in treating all forms of epilepsy. The action of sodium valproate is similar to that of other anticonvulsants: reducing electrical discharges in the brain to prevent the excessive build-up of discharges that can lead to epileptic seizures.

The drug is beneficial in long-term treatment and does not usually have a sedative effect. This makes it particularly suitable for children who have either atonic epilepsy (the sudden relaxing of the muscles throughout the body) or absence seizures (during which the person appears to be daydreaming). However, care should be taken if changing from one preparation to a different one.

Sodium valproate is also sometimes used in manic episodes, bipolar disorder, and migraine prevention.

INFORMATION FOR USERS

Your drug prescription is tailored for you. Do not alter dosage without checking with your doctor.

How taken/used Tablets, modified release (MR) tablets, capsules, liquid, injection.

Frequency and timing of doses 1–2 x daily, after food.

Dosage range 600mg–2.5g daily, adjusted as necessary.

Onset of effect Within 60 minutes.

Duration of action 12 hours or more.

Diet advice None.

Storage Keep in original container at room temperature out of the reach of children. Protect from light.

Missed dose Take as soon as you remember. If your next dose is due within 2 hours, take a single dose now and skip the next.

Stopping the drug Do not stop the drug without consulting your doctor, who will supervise a gradual reduction in dosage. Abrupt withdrawal may lead to a recurrence of symptoms.

Exceeding the dose An occasional unintentional extra dose is unlikely to cause problems. Large overdoses may lead to coma. Tell your doctor.

POSSIBLE ADVERSE EFFECTS

Most of the adverse effects of sodium valproate are uncommon, and the most serious ones are rare. They include liver failure, and platelet and bleeding abnormalities. Menstrual periods may become irregular or may cease altogether. The drug may also cause temporary hair loss, weight gain, nausea, and indigestion; discuss with your doctor if any of these are severe. If a rash, drowsiness, jaundice, or unusual bruising or bleeding occur, consult your doctor immediately.

INTERACTIONS

Other anticonvulsant drugs may reduce blood levels of sodium valproate.

Zidovudine When zidovudine and sodium valproate are taken together, the blood levels of zidovudine may increase, leading to increased adverse effects.

Lamotrigine Sodium valproate increases levels of lamotrigine and may lead to increased adverse effects.

Carbapenems These antibacterial drugs reduce the blood level of sodium valproate; concomitant use should be avoided.

Antidepressants, antipsychotics, mefloquine, and chloroquine may reduce the effectiveness of sodium valproate to prevent seizures.

Clarithromycin and erythromycin may increase the effects of sodium valproate.

SPECIAL PRECAUTIONS

Be sure to tell your doctor if:

- You have long-term liver or kidney problems.
- You have porphyria.
- You have any blood disorders.
- You are pregnant or you intend to become pregnant.
- You are taking other medicines.

Pregnancy Not recommended. May cause abnormalities in the fetus. If sodium valproate is essential, extra folic acid supplements must also be taken. Discuss with your doctor.

Breast-feeding The drug passes into the breast milk, but normal doses are unlikely to affect the baby adversely. Discuss with your doctor.

Infants and children Reduced dose necessary. The dose is often based on the weight of the child.

Over 60 Reduced dose may be necessary.

Driving and hazardous work Your underlying condition, as well as the possibility of reduced alertness while taking sodium valproate, may make such activities inadvisable. Discuss with your doctor.

Alcohol Avoid. Alcohol may increase the sedative effects of this drug.

PROLONGED USE

Use of sodium valproate can, very rarely, cause liver damage, which is more likely in the first 6 months of use.

Monitoring Periodic blood tests of liver function and of blood composition may be carried out.

SOTALOL

Brand names Beta-Cardone, Sotacor

Used in the following combined preparations None

QUICK REFERENCE

Drug group Beta blocker (p.28)

Overdose danger rating High

Dependence rating Low

Prescription needed Yes

Available as generic Yes

GENERAL INFORMATION

Sotalol is a non-cardioselective beta blocker (p.28) used in the prevention and treatment of heart rhythm problems, notably ventricular and supraventricular arrhythmias (p.32).

The drug has an additional anti-arrhythmic action compared to other beta blockers. However, it is no longer prescribed for the other conditions for which beta blockers are used (e.g. hypertension). This is due to the risk of a serious but infrequent side effect called "torsades de pointes", a kind of ventricular arrhythmia that can cause loss of consciousness or even sudden death. For this reason, anyone who is prescribed sotalol will be carefully monitored.

INFORMATION FOR USERS

Your drug prescription is tailored for you. Do not alter dosage without checking with your doctor.

How taken/used Tablets.

Frequency and timing of doses 2 x daily.

Dosage range 80mg daily initially, increased at 2–3-day intervals to 160–320mg daily. Higher doses of 480–640mg only under specialist supervision.

Onset of effect 12 hours.

Duration of action 12 hours.

Diet advice None.

Storage Keep in original container at room temperature out of the reach of children. Protect from light.

Missed dose Take as soon as you remember. If your next dose is due within 3 hours, take a single dose now and skip the next.

Stopping the drug Do not stop taking the drug without consulting your doctor, who will supervise a gradual reduction in dosage. Sudden withdrawal may lead to worsening of your condition.

OVERDOSE ACTION

Seek immediate medical advice in all cases of overdose by mouth. Take emergency action if breathing difficulties, palpitations, collapse, or loss of consciousness occur.

POSSIBLE ADVERSE EFFECTS

A very fast heart rate with palpitations could be a symptom of torsades de pointes; if you experience this you should notify your doctor immediately. Lethargy, fatigue, and cold hands and feet are common adverse effects; discuss with your doctor in all cases. If you have nightmares or vivid dreams, rash, dry eyes, or visual disturbances, stop taking the drug and consult your doctor. If you develop fainting, palpitations, breathlessness, or wheezing, stop the drug and call your doctor immediately.

INTERACTIONS

Calcium channel blockers These may cause low blood pressure, a slow heart beat, and heart failure if taken with sotalol.

Diuretics, amphotericin, corticosteroids, and some laxatives may lower blood potassium levels, increasing the risk of torsades de pointes.

Anti-arrhythmics Taking these with sotalol may slow the heart rate and affect heart function.

Cardiac glycosides (e.g. digoxin) These may increase the heart-slowing effect of sotalol.

Antihypertensives Sotalol may enhance the blood-pressure-lowering effect of these drugs.

Phenothiazines, antidepressants, astemizole, moxifloxacin, mizolastine, ivabradine, antipsychotics, and erythromycin These drugs increase the risk of torsades de pointes with sotalol.

SPECIAL PRECAUTIONS

Be sure to tell your doctor if:

◆ You have liver or kidney problems.
◆ You have a breathing disorder such as asthma, bronchitis, or emphysema.
◆ You have heart or heart rhythm problems.
◆ You have diabetes.
◆ You have psoriasis.
◆ You have poor circulation in the legs.
◆ You have lactose intolerance.
◆ You are taking other medicines.

Pregnancy Not usually prescribed. May affect the fetus. Discuss with your doctor.

Breast-feeding The drug passes into the breast milk and may affect the baby. Discuss with your doctor.

Infants and children Not prescribed.

Over 60 Reduced dose may be necessary.

Driving and hazardous work Avoid until you have learned how sotalol affects you because the drug can cause dizziness and fatigue.

Alcohol Avoid excessive intake. Alcohol may increase the blood-pressure-lowering effect of sotalol.

Surgery and general anaesthetics Occasionally, sotalol may need to be stopped before you have a general anaesthetic, but only do this after discussion with your doctor or dentist.

PROLONGED USE

Sotalol may be taken indefinitely for prevention of ventricular arrhythmias.

Monitoring Periodic blood tests are usually performed to monitor levels of potassium and magnesium. The heart beat is usually monitored for any risk of developing torsades de pointes.

SPIRONOLACTONE

Brand name Aldactone

Used in the following combined preparations Aldactide, Lasilactone

QUICK REFERENCE

Drug group Potassium-sparing diuretic (p.31)

Overdose danger rating Low

Dependence rating Low

Prescription needed Yes

Available as generic Yes

GENERAL INFORMATION

Spironolactone belongs to the class of drugs known as potassium-sparing diuretics. It is used either alone or in combination with thiazide or loop diuretics to treat oedema (fluid retention) resulting from congestive heart failure, cirrhosis of the liver, and nephrotic syndrome (a kidney disorder). It is also used to reduce blood pressure, especially in people with Conn's syndrome, a condition caused by a benign tumour in one of the adrenal glands.

The drug is relatively slow to act; its effects may appear only after several days of treatment. As with other potassium-sparing diuretics, there is a risk of unusually high potassium levels in the blood if the kidneys are functioning abnormally. For this reason, it is prescribed with caution to people with kidney failure.

Spironolactone does not worsen gout or diabetes, as do some other diuretics. The major side effect is nausea, but abnormal breast enlargement (gynaecomastia) may occur in men.

INFORMATION FOR USERS

Your drug prescription is tailored for you. Do not alter dosage without checking with your doctor.
How taken/used Tablets, capsules, liquid.
Frequency and timing of doses Once daily, usually in the morning.
Adult dosage range 25–400mg daily.
Onset of effect Within 1–3 days, but full effect may take up to 2 weeks.
Duration of action 2–3 days.
Diet advice Avoid foods that are high in potassium, such as dried fruit and salt substitutes.
Storage Keep in original container at room temperature out of the reach of children. Protect from light.
Missed dose Take as soon as you remember.
Stopping the drug Do not stop the drug without consulting your doctor; symptoms may recur.
Exceeding the dose An occasional unintentional extra dose is unlikely to be a cause for concern. But if you notice any unusual symptoms, or if a large overdose has been taken, tell your doctor.

POSSIBLE ADVERSE EFFECTS

The main problem with spironolactone is the possibility that potassium may be retained by the body, causing muscle weakness and numbness. Consult your doctor if these symptoms occur. The drug commonly causes nausea and vomiting; more rarely, it may cause headache, lethargy, drowsiness, and irregular menstruation. Discuss with your doctor if these are severe. It may also cause breast enlargement or tenderness in both sexes, and erectile dysfunction (impotence) in men; if these occur, consult your doctor. If a rash develops, stop the drug and contact your doctor immediately.

INTERACTIONS

ACE inhibitors, non-steroidal anti-inflammatory drugs (NSAIDs), angiotensin II blockers, ciclosporin, tacrolimus, and potassium salts may increase the risk of raised blood levels of potassium, and can intensify the lowering of blood pressure caused by spironolactone.
Lithium Spironolactone may increase the blood levels of lithium, leading to an increased risk of lithium toxicity.
Digoxin Adverse effects may result from increased digoxin levels.

SPECIAL PRECAUTIONS

Be sure to tell your doctor if:
- You have long-term liver or kidney problems.
- You have porphyria.
- You have Addison's disease.
- You have a metabolic disorder.
- You are taking other medicines.

Pregnancy Not usually prescribed. May have adverse effects on the baby. Discuss with your doctor.
Breast-feeding The drug passes into the breast milk, but normal doses are unlikely to affect the baby adversely. Discuss with your doctor.
Infants and children Reduced dose necessary.
Over 60 Increased likelihood of adverse effects. Reduced dose may therefore be necessary.
Driving and hazardous work Avoid such activities until you have learned how spironolactone affects you because the drug may occasionally cause drowsiness.
Alcohol No known problems.

PROLONGED USE

Long-term use in young people is avoided if possible due to the endocrine effects of the drug; for young patients, eplerenone may be a better alternative.
Monitoring Blood tests may be performed to check kidney function and levels of body salts.

STRONTIUM RANELATE

Brand name None
Used in the following combined preparations None

QUICK REFERENCE

Drug group Drug for bone disorders (p.54)
Overdose danger rating Low
Dependence rating Low
Prescription needed Yes
Available as generic Yes

GENERAL INFORMATION

Strontium ranelate is used to treat severe osteoporosis, to reduce the risk of fractures. The active ingredient is derived from a naturally occurring element, strontium, which acts on cells in bone to increase bone formation and reduce resorption, leading to a rebalance of cell turnover in favour of bone formation.

Because strontium ranelate has been associated with heart disorders, it is used, under specialist supervision, only for those with severe osteoporosis for whom there are no suitable alternative treatments. Apart from the risk of heart disorders and a small increase in the risk of deep vein thrombosis (blood clots in the legs and lungs), the drug generally causes few adverse reactions in those who are prescribed it. Very rarely, some people may develop a serious allergic reaction to it, which may affect other organs in the body.

INFORMATION FOR USERS

Your drug prescription is tailored for you. Do not alter dosage without checking with your doctor.

How taken/used Granules dissolved in water.

Frequency and timing of doses Once daily, usually at night.

Adult dosage range 2g daily.

Onset of effect 3–5 hours. Beneficial effects may take several months to be felt.

Duration of action Up to a week.

Diet advice Food, milk, milk products, and calcium reduce the absorption of strontium ranelate. You should take the drug at bedtime or between meals and allow at least 2 hours before or after food, milk, or milk products or calcium supplements.

Storage Keep in original container below 30°C out of the reach of children. Protect from light.

Missed dose Take the next dose at the time it is due. Do not take a double dose to make up for a missed dose.

Stopping the drug Do not stop without consulting your doctor. Stopping the drug may lead to a worsening of the underlying condition.

Exceeding the dose An occasional unintentional extra dose is unlikely to cause problems. However, if a large overdose has been taken, notify your doctor.

POSSIBLE ADVERSE EFFECTS

In general, people prescribed strontium ranelate experience few adverse effects. The common side effects of nausea and diarrhoea are mild and often settle with continued use; the drug also commonly causes headache and drowsiness. Discuss with your doctor if any of these effects are severe. More rarely, the drug may cause swelling or pain in one leg; if this occurs, consult your doctor promptly. Very rarely, strontium ranelate may cause a serious allergic reaction. If you develop a skin rash, fever, or swollen glands while taking it, you should stop taking the drug and consult your doctor immediately.

INTERACTIONS

Tetracycline and quinolone antibiotics (e.g. tetracycline and ciprofloxacin) Strontium ranelate may reduce absorption of these drugs. It should be stopped when taking a course of these antibiotics.

Antacids and products containing calcium, magnesium, or aluminium These products can reduce the absorption of strontium ranelate so should be given at least 2 hours before or after you take the drug.

SPECIAL PRECAUTIONS

Be sure to tell your doctor if:

- You have ever had a previous adverse reaction to strontium ranelate.
- You have long-term kidney problems.
- You have or have had heart problems.
- You have had a stroke or disease affecting the blood vessels in the brain.
- You have high blood pressure.
- You are being treated or have been treated for blood clots in your legs or lungs.
- You are confined to bed or you are due to have surgery.
- You have phenylketonuria.
- You are taking other medicines.

Pregnancy Not prescribed. In women, the drug is used only after the menopause.

Breast-feeding Not prescribed. In women, the drug is used only after the menopause.

Infants and children Not prescribed. The drug is for use in post-menopausal women only.

Over 60 No special problems.

Driving and hazardous work No specific problems.

Alcohol No special problems.

PROLONGED USE

The long-term safety of strontium ranelate is uncertain, especially regarding the risk of heart disorders. For this reason, it is prescribed only under specialist supervision and when there are no suitable alternatives.

Monitoring Blood and other tests may be carried out to monitor your bone density. Strontium ranelate can interfere with the blood tests used to measure calcium level.

SUCRALFATE

Brand name None
Used in the following combined preparations None

QUICK REFERENCE

Drug group Ulcer-healing drug (p.41)
Overdose danger rating Low
Dependence rating Low
Prescription needed Yes
Available as generic Yes

GENERAL INFORMATION

Sucralfate, a drug partly derived from aluminium, is prescribed to treat gastric and duodenal ulcers. It is particularly used to prevent stress-induced ulcers in patients who are seriously ill. The drug does not neutralize stomach acid, but it forms a protective barrier over the ulcer that protects it from attack by digestive juices, giving it time to heal.

If it is necessary during treatment to take antacids to relieve pain, these should be taken at least half an hour before or after sucralfate.

There are a few reports of seriously ill patients developing bezoars (balls of indigestible material) in the stomach while on sucralfate. The safety of the drug for long-term use has not yet been confirmed. Therefore, courses of more than 12 weeks are not recommended.

INFORMATION FOR USERS

Your drug prescription is tailored for you. Do not alter dosage without checking with your doctor.

How taken/used Tablets, liquid.

Frequency and timing of doses 2–6 x daily, 1 hour before each meal, and at bedtime, at least 2 hours after food. The tablets may be dispersed in a little water before swallowing.

Dosage range 4–8g daily.

Onset of effect Some improvement may be noted after one or two doses, but it takes a few weeks for an ulcer to heal.

Duration of action Up to 5 hours.

Diet advice Your doctor will advise if supplements are needed.

Storage Keep in original container at room temperature out of the reach of children.

Missed dose Do not make up the dose you missed. Take your next dose on your original dosing schedule.

Stopping the drug Do not stop without consulting your doctor; symptoms may recur.

Exceeding the dose An occasional unintentional extra dose is unlikely to be a cause for concern. But if you notice any unusual symptoms, or if a large overdose has been taken, notify your doctor.

POSSIBLE ADVERSE EFFECTS

Most people do not experience any adverse effects with sucralfate. The most common are constipation, which will diminish as your body adjusts to the drug, and indigestion. Rarely, diarrhoea, dry mouth, and headache may occur. Discuss with your doctor if any of these effects are severe. Nausea, rash, itching, dizziness, or vertigo are also rare side effects; you should consult your doctor if they occur.

INTERACTIONS

General note Sucralfate may reduce the absorption and effect of a range of drugs, including ranitidine, digoxin, phenytoin, warfarin, levothyroxine, and antibacterials. Take these and other medications at least 30 minutes before or 2 hours after sucralfate.

Antacids and other indigestion remedies These reduce the effectiveness of sucralfate and should be taken at least 30 minutes before or after sucralfate.

SPECIAL PRECAUTIONS

Be sure to tell your doctor if:

- You have a long-term kidney problem.
- You are taking other medicines.

Pregnancy Safety in pregnancy not established, although so little of the drug is absorbed into the body that it is probably safe. Discuss with your doctor.

Breast-feeding It is not known whether the drug passes into breast milk. Discuss with your doctor.

Infants and children Not usually prescribed.

Over 60 No special problems.

Driving and hazardous work Usually no problems, but sucralfate may cause dizziness in some people.

Alcohol Avoid. Alcohol may counteract the beneficial effect of this drug.

PROLONGED USE

Sucralfate is not usually prescribed for periods longer than 12 weeks at a time. Prolonged use of the drug may lead to deficiencies of vitamins A, D, E, and K.

SULFASALAZINE

Brand names Salazopyrin, Sulazine EC
Used in the following combined preparations None

QUICK REFERENCE

Drug group Drug for inflammatory bowel disease (p.44) and disease-modifying antirheumatic drug (p.49)
Overdose danger rating Low
Dependence rating Low
Prescription needed Yes
Available as generic Yes

GENERAL INFORMATION

Sulfasalazine, a chemical combination of a sulfonamide and a salicylate, is used to treat the inflammatory bowel disorders ulcerative colitis (which mainly affects the large intestine) and Crohn's disease (which usually affects the small intestine). Sulfasalazine is also used to modify, halt, or slow the underlying disease process in severe rheumatoid arthritis.

Adverse effects such as nausea, loss of appetite, and general discomfort are more likely when higher doses are taken. Side effects caused by stomach irritation may be avoided by using a specially coated tablet form of the drug. Allergic reactions such as fever and skin rash may be avoided or minimized by low initial doses, followed by gradual increases. Maintenance of adequate fluid intake is important while taking this drug. In rare cases among men, temporary sterility may occur.

INFORMATION FOR USERS

Your drug prescription is tailored for you. Do not alter dosage without checking with your doctor.
How taken/used Tablets, liquid, suppositories.
Frequency and timing of doses 2–4 x daily after meals with a glass of water (tablets); 2 x daily (suppositories).
Adult dosage range *Crohn's disease/ulcerative colitis* 4–8g daily in acute attacks. *Ulcerative colitis* up to 2g daily for maintenance therapy. *Rheumatoid arthritis* 500mg–3g daily.
Onset of effect Adverse effects may occur within a few days, but full beneficial effects may take 1–3 weeks, depending on the severity of the condition.
Duration of action Up to 24 hours.
Diet advice It is important to drink plenty of liquids (at least 1.5 litres a day) during treatment. Sulfasalazine may reduce absorption of folic acid from the intestine, leading to a deficiency of this vitamin. Eat plenty of green vegetables. Your doctor may also recommend folic acid supplements.
Storage Keep in original container at room temperature out of the reach of children.
Missed dose Take as soon as you remember. If your next dose is due within 2 hours, take a single dose now and skip the next.
Stopping the drug Do not stop without consulting your doctor; symptoms may recur.
Exceeding the dose An occasional unintentional extra dose is unlikely to be a cause for concern. But if you notice any unusual symptoms, or if a large overdose has been taken, notify your doctor.

POSSIBLE ADVERSE EFFECTS

Adverse effects are common with high doses but may disappear with a reduction in dosage. Symptoms such as nausea and vomiting may be helped by taking the drug with food. Orange or yellow discoloration of the urine may occur but is no cause for concern. Other common side effects include malaise, loss of appetite, insomnia, mood changes, headache, and joint pain; discuss with your doctor if headache or joint pain occur or if the other symptoms are severe. Ringing in the ears is rare; discuss with your doctor if it is severe. Fever, a rash, and unusual bruising or bleeding are also rare side effects of sulfasalazine; seek immediate medical attention if they occur.

INTERACTIONS

General note 1 Sulfasalazine may increase the effects of some drugs, including mercaptopurine and azathioprine. With azathioprine, there is also an increased risk of blood count abnormalities.
General note 2 Sulfasalazine reduces the absorption and effect of some drugs, including digoxin, folic acid, and iron.

SPECIAL PRECAUTIONS

Be sure to tell your doctor if:
- You have long-term liver or kidney problems.
- You have asthma or severe allergies.
- You have glucose-6-phosphate dehydrogenase (G6PD) deficiency.
- You have a blood disorder.
- You have porphyria.

◆ You are allergic to sulfonamides or salicylates.
◆ You wear soft contact lenses.
◆ You are taking other medicines.

Pregnancy No evidence of risk to developing fetus. Folic acid supplements may be required. Discuss with your doctor.
Breast-feeding The drug passes into the breast milk and may affect the baby. Discuss with your doctor.
Infants and children Not recommended under 2 years. Reduced dose necessary for older children, according to body weight.
Over 60 No special problems.
Driving and hazardous work No special problems.
Alcohol No known problems.

PROLONGED USE
Blood disorders may occur with prolonged use of this drug. Maintenance dosage is usually continued indefinitely.
Monitoring Periodic tests of blood composition and liver function are usually required as well as periodic urine tests.

SUMATRIPTAN

Brand names Imigran, Imigran Subject
Used in the following combined preparations None

QUICK REFERENCE
Drug group Drug for migraine (p.18)
Overdose danger rating Medium
Dependence rating Low
Prescription needed Yes (injection and nasal spray); No (others)
Available as generic Yes

GENERAL INFORMATION
Sumatriptan is a highly effective drug for migraine, usually given when people fail to respond to analgesics (such as aspirin and paracetamol). The drug is of considerable value in the treatment of acute migraine attacks, whether or not they are preceded by an aura, but is not meant to be taken regularly to prevent attacks. Sumatriptan is also used for the acute treatment of cluster headache (a form of migraine headache). It should be taken as soon as possible after the onset of the attack, although, unlike other drugs used in migraine, it will still be of benefit at whatever stage of the attack it is taken.

INFORMATION FOR USERS
Your drug prescription is tailored for you. Do not alter dosage without checking with your doctor.
How taken/used Tablets, injection, nasal spray.
Frequency and timing of doses Should be taken as soon as possible after the onset of an attack, but it is equally effective at any stage. Do not take a second dose for the same attack, or within 2 hours if migraine recurs.
Adult dosage range *Tablets* 50–100mg per attack, up to maximum of 300mg in 24 hours if another attack occurs. Do not take a second dose for the same attack, or within 2 hours if migraine recurs. *Injection* 6mg per attack, up to maximum of 12mg (two injections) in 24 hours if another attack occurs. Do not take a second dose for the same attack, or within 1 hour if migraine recurs. *Nasal spray* Adults: 1 x 20mg puff into one nostril per attack, to maximum of 40mg (2 puffs) in 24 hours if another attack occurs; age 12 to 17 years: 1 x 10mg puff into one nostril per attack, to maximum of 20mg (2 puffs) in 24 hours if another attack occurs.
Onset of effect 30–45 minutes (tablets); 10–15 minutes (injection); 15 minutes (nasal spray).
Duration of action *Tablets* 2–4 hours. *Injection* 1½–2 hours. *Nasal spray* 1–3 hours.
Diet advice None, unless otherwise advised.
Storage Keep in original container at room temperature out of the reach of children. Protect from light.
Missed dose Not applicable, as drug is taken only to treat a migraine attack.
Stopping the drug Taken only to treat a migraine attack.
Exceeding the dose An occasional unintentional extra tablet or injection is unlikely to cause problems. But if you notice any unusual symptoms, or if a large overdose has been taken, notify your doctor.

POSSIBLE ADVERSE EFFECTS
Many of the adverse effects disappear after about 1 hour as your body adjusts to the drug, but contact your doctor if they are severe or persistent. Common effects include pain at the injection site, flushing, a feeling of tingling or heat, and a feeling of heaviness or weakness. Less commonly, sumatriptan may cause dizziness, fatigue, or drowsiness. If you develop palpitations or chest pain, stop the drug and seek immediate medical attention.

INTERACTIONS

Antidepressants Monoamine oxidase inhibitors (MAOIs) and some others (e.g. fluvoxamine, fluoxetine, paroxetine, sertraline, St John's wort) increase risk of adverse effects with sumatriptan.
Lithium High risk of adverse effects if lithium and sumatriptan are taken together.
Ergotamine must be taken at least 6 hours after sumatriptan, and sumatriptan must be taken at least 24 hours after ergotamine.

SPECIAL PRECAUTIONS

Be sure to consult your doctor or pharmacist before taking this drug if:

- You have liver or kidney problems.
- You have heart problems.
- You have high blood pressure.
- You have had a heart attack or a stroke.
- You have angina.
- You are allergic to some medicines.
- You are taking other medicines.

Pregnancy Safety in pregnancy not established. Discuss with your doctor.
Breast-feeding Safety not established. Discuss with your doctor.
Infants and children Not recommended under 12 years.
Over 60 Not recommended over 65 years.
Driving and hazardous work Avoid until you have learned how sumatriptan affects you because the drug can cause drowsiness.
Alcohol No special problems, but some drinks may provoke migraine in some people.
Surgery and general anaesthetics Notify your doctor or dentist if you have used sumatriptan within 48 hours prior to surgery.

PROLONGED USE

Sumatriptan should not be used continually to prevent migraine but only to treat attacks.

TACROLIMUS

Brand names Adoport, Advagraf, Dailiport, Envarsus, Modigraf, Perixis, Prograf, Protopic
Used in the following combined preparations None

QUICK REFERENCE

Drug group Immunosuppressant drug (p.97)
Overdose danger rating Medium
Dependence rating Low
Prescription needed Yes
Available as generic Yes

GENERAL INFORMATION

Tacrolimus is an immunosuppressant drug used in many types of organ transplant to help prevent rejection. It is usually used in combination with other immunosuppressants. Tacrolimus may also be used topically to treat skin conditions such as eczema and psoriasis when other drugs are inappropriate or have been unsuccessful. As tacrolimus suppresses the immune system when taken by mouth or injected, it increases susceptibility to infection and it can also cause kidney damage. The drug should not be taken by people who are allergic to any macrolide antibiotic. If you are taking oral tacrolimus, it is important to use the same formulation every time as they are not all interchangeable.

INFORMATION FOR USERS

Your drug prescription is tailored for you. Do not alter dosage without checking with your doctor.
How taken/used Capsules, slow release (SR) capsules, granules, liquid, injection, ointment.
Frequency and timing of doses *Oral and injected preparations* 1–2 x daily. Oral preparations should be taken on an empty stomach or 2–3 hours after a meal. *Topical preparation* Initially 1–2 x daily; reduced to 2 x weekly when eczema improves.
Dosage range *Oral and injected preparations* Dosage is calculated on an individual basis. *Topical preparation* 0.1% or 0.03% ointment (adults); 0.03% ointment (children).
Onset of effect Within 12 hours (oral and injection). 1–2 weeks (ointment).
Duration of action 2–4 days.
Diet advice If taking tacrolimus orally, avoid high-potassium foods and grapefruit juice. No special restrictions for other preparations.
Storage Store drug at room temperature and protect from moisture. Keep out of the reach of children.
Missed dose Take as soon as you remember, unless your next dose is due within 12 hours, in which case omit the missed dose and take the next dose as scheduled. Do not double your next dose.
Stopping the drug Do not stop the drug without consulting your doctor. If it is being taken after a transplant, stopping may lead to organ rejection. If the drug is being used for eczema, stopping may lead to recurrence or worsening of symptoms.

Exceeding the dose An occasional unintentional dose is unlikely to cause major problems. Large oral overdoses may cause tremor, headache, vomiting, and kidney damage. Notify your doctor.

POSSIBLE ADVERSE EFFECTS

Used topically, tacrolimus may cause local irritation, rash, or paraesthesia (pins-and-needles); discuss with your doctor if these occur. Taken orally, common side effects include nausea, difficulty in sleeping or drowsiness, diarrhoea, headache, tremor, and paraesthesia; discuss with your doctor if nausea, sleeping problems, or drowsiness are severe or if any of the other symptoms occur. If you experience spontaneous bruising or bleeding, fever, a sore throat, confusion, or seizures, seek immediate medical attention. Tacrolimus may increase the risk of diabetes or worsen diabetic control; it may also cause other adverse effects with long-term use (see Prolonged use).

INTERACTIONS

General note Many drugs may affect the level of tacrolimus. Check with your doctor before taking a new medication or stopping or changing current medication.

Grapefruit juice and St John's wort can affect blood levels of tacrolimus and should be avoided if taking the drug orally or by injection. If tacrolimus is being taken after a transplant, the interaction with St John's wort can cause organ rejection.

Vaccines Tacrolimus may affect your response to vaccines. Discuss with your doctor before having a vaccine.

SPECIAL PRECAUTIONS

Tacrolimus is prescribed only under medical supervision, but be sure to tell your doctor if:

- You have long-term kidney or liver problems.
- You have heart disease or high blood pressure.
- You have lactose intolerance.
- You have a peanut or soya allergy.
- You are pregnant or planning a pregnancy.
- You are taking other medicines.

Pregnancy Safety not established. Discuss with your doctor.

Breast-feeding Safety not established. Discuss with your doctor.

Infants and children Used only by specialist children's doctors.

Over 60 No special problems.

Driving and hazardous work If taking tacrolimus orally, avoid such activities until you know how the drug affects you. It may cause drowsiness. No known problems with topical use.

Alcohol Avoid. Alcohol may increase drowsiness (oral tacrolimus), or cause skin irritation (topical tacrolimus).

Sunlight and sunbeds Avoid prolonged, unprotected exposure as this can increase the risk of skin cancer.

PROLONGED USE

Long-term oral or injected tacrolimus can affect kidney and/or liver function, increases susceptibility to infection, and is linked to an increased risk of some skin and lymphoid cancers. Prolonged use may also increase the risk of high blood pressure or diabetes. Topically, the drug is associated with herpes skin infections (e.g. cold sores); there may also be an increased risk of skin cancer.

Monitoring For oral or injected forms of tacrolimus, regular blood tests, kidney and liver function tests, blood pressure checks, and tests for diabetes should be carried out.

TAMOXIFEN

Brand name Soltamox
Used in the following combined preparations None

QUICK REFERENCE

Drug group Anticancer drug (p.94)
Overdose danger rating Low
Dependence rating Low
Prescription needed Yes
Available as generic Yes

GENERAL INFORMATION

Tamoxifen is an anti-oestrogen drug (oestrogen is a naturally occurring female sex hormone; see p.86). It is used for two conditions: infertility and breast cancer.

When given to treat certain types of infertility, the drug is taken only on certain days of the menstrual cycle.

Used as an anticancer drug for breast cancer, tamoxifen works by blocking the effect of natural oestrogens that stimulate the growth of tumours with oestrogen receptors (oestrogen-receptor-positive tumours). This reduces the risk of tumours recurring after surgical removal of the tumour.

As its effect is specific, tamoxifen has fewer adverse effects than most other drugs used for breast cancer. However, it may cause eye damage if high doses are taken for long periods.

INFORMATION FOR USERS

Your drug prescription is tailored for you. Do not alter dosage without checking with your doctor.

How taken/used Tablets, liquid.

Frequency and timing of doses 1–2 x daily.

Adult dosage range *Breast cancer* 20mg daily. *Infertility* 20–80mg daily.

Onset of effect Side effects may be felt within days, but beneficial effects may take 4–10 weeks.

Duration of action Effects may be felt for several weeks after stopping the drug.

Diet advice None.

Storage Keep in original container at room temperature out of the reach of children. Protect from light.

Missed dose Take as soon as you remember. If your next dose is due within 2 hours, take a single dose now and skip the next.

Stopping the drug Do not stop without consulting your doctor; stopping the drug may lead to worsening of your underlying condition.

Exceeding the dose An occasional unintentional extra dose is unlikely to be a cause for concern. But if you notice any unusual symptoms, or if a large overdose has been taken, tell your doctor.

POSSIBLE ADVERSE EFFECTS

Adverse effects are rarely serious and do not usually need treatment to be stopped. Nausea, vomiting, hot flushes, and hair loss are the most common effects; discuss with your doctor if they are severe. There is a small risk of endometrial cancer (cancer of the womb lining), so you should notify your doctor as soon as possible of any symptoms such as irregular vaginal bleeding or discharge. Rarely, bone or tumour pain, rash, itching, or blurred or reduced vision may occur; if so, consult your doctor. If you experience calf pain or swelling, call your doctor immediately.

INTERACTIONS

Anticoagulants People being treated with anticoagulants such as warfarin usually need a lower dose of the anticoagulant.

SSRI antidepressants These may reduce the effectiveness of tamoxifen.

Anticancer medicines Cytotoxic medicines taken together with tamoxifen may increase the risk of adverse effects, especially the risk of venous thrombosis.

SPECIAL PRECAUTIONS

Be sure to tell your doctor if:

- ◆ You are pregnant or planning a pregnancy.
- ◆ You have cataracts or poor eyesight.
- ◆ You have porphyria.
- ◆ You have a history of venous thrombosis.
- ◆ You are taking other medicines.

Pregnancy Not usually prescribed. May have effects on the fetus. Discuss with your doctor.

Breast-feeding Not usually prescribed. Discuss with your doctor.

Infants and children Not prescribed.

Over 60 No special problems.

Driving and hazardous work Do not drive until you know how tamoxifen affects you because it can cause dizziness and blurred vision.

Alcohol No known problems.

Surgery and general anaesthetics Tell your doctor or anaesthetist that you are taking tamoxifen before you have any surgery. You may be advised to stop taking it 6 weeks beforehand.

PROLONGED USE

There is a risk of damage to the eye with long-term, high-dose treatment. There is also a small increased risk of endometrial cancer and venous thrombosis with long-term tamoxifen treatment, but these risks are outweighed by the benefit of preventing the recurrence of breast cancer.

Monitoring Eyesight may be tested periodically.

TAMSULOSIN

Brand names Contiflo XL, Diffundox XL, Faramsil, Flomaxtra XL, Losinate MR, Tabphyn MR, Tamurex, and many others

Used in the following combined preparations Combodart (with dutasteride), Vesomni (with solifenacin)

QUICK REFERENCE

Drug group Drug for urinary disorders (p.110)

Overdose danger rating Medium

Dependence rating Low

Prescription needed Yes (most preparations)

Available as generic Yes

GENERAL INFORMATION

Tamsulosin is a selective alpha blocker drug used to treat urinary retention due to benign prostatic hypertrophy, or BPH (enlarged prostate gland). The drug, as it passes through the prostate, relaxes the muscle in the wall of the urethra, thereby increasing urine flow.

Tamsulosin is available over the counter for men aged 45–74 years with symptoms of BPH. If symptoms have not improved (or have got worse) within 2 weeks, the drug should be stopped and you should consult your doctor. If symptoms have improved with the drug, you should still see your doctor within 6 weeks to confirm that the symptoms are due to BPH.

Like other alpha blockers, tamsulosin may lower blood pressure rapidly after the first dose. For this reason, the first dose should be taken at home so that, if dizziness or weakness occur, you can lie down until they have disappeared.

INFORMATION FOR USERS

Your drug prescription is tailored for you. Do not alter dosage without checking with your doctor. If taking an over-the-counter preparation, follow the instructions and consult your doctor if symptoms do not improve or worsen.

How taken/used Tablets, modified release (MR) tablets, capsules, MR capsules.

Frequency and timing of doses Once daily, swallowed whole, after breakfast.

Adult dosage range 400mcg.

Onset of effect 1–2 hours.

Duration of action 24 hours.

Diet advice None.

Storage Keep in original container at room temperature out of the reach of children.

Missed dose Take as soon as you remember. If your next dose is due within 4 hours, take a single dose now and skip the next.

Stopping the drug Do not stop taking the drug without consulting your doctor; stopping suddenly may lead to a rise in blood pressure.

Exceeding the dose An occasional unintentional extra dose is unlikely to cause problems. Large overdoses may produce sedation, dizziness, low blood pressure, and rapid pulse. Notify your doctor immediately.

POSSIBLE ADVERSE EFFECTS

Dizziness seems to be the most common adverse effect, but this usually improves after the first few doses. Weakness, fainting, ejaculatory problems, headache, drowsiness, and palpitations are also common. Rarely, nausea, vomiting, and diarrhoea or constipation may occur. Discuss with your doctor if any of these symptoms are severe. If you develop a rash or itching, consult your doctor promptly.

INTERACTIONS

Antidepressants, beta blockers, calcium channel blockers, diuretic drugs, and thymoxamine These drugs are all likely to increase the blood-pressure-lowering effect of tamsulosin.

SPECIAL PRECAUTIONS

Be sure to consult your doctor or pharmacist before taking this drug if:

- You have had low blood pressure.
- You have liver or kidney problems.
- You have heart failure.
- You have a history of depression.
- You are taking drugs for high blood pressure.
- You collapse after passing urine.
- You are taking other medicines.
- You have cataract surgery planned.

Pregnancy Not prescribed.

Breast-feeding Not prescribed.

Infants and children Not prescribed.

Over 60 No special problems.

Driving and hazardous work Avoid until you know how tamsulosin affects you because the drug can cause drowsiness and dizziness.

Alcohol Avoid until you know how tamsulosin affects you because alcohol can further lower blood pressure.

Surgery and general anaesthetics Tamsulosin may need to be stopped before you have any surgery. Discuss with your doctor or dentist.

PROLONGED USE

No special problems.

TEMAZEPAM

Brand name None

Used in the following combined preparations None

QUICK REFERENCE

Drug group Benzodiazepine sleeping drug (p.10)

Overdose danger rating Medium

Dependence rating High

Prescription needed Yes

Available as generic Yes

GENERAL INFORMATION

Temazepam belongs to a group of drugs called benzodiazepines. The actions and adverse effects of this group are described more fully under Anti-anxiety drugs (p.11). Temazepam is used for short-term treatment of insomnia. Because it is short acting compared with other benzodiazepines, the drug is less likely to cause drowsiness and/or lightheadedness the next day. However, temazepam is not usually effective in preventing early morning waking.

Like other benzodiazepine drugs, temazepam can be habit-forming if taken regularly over a long period. Its effects also grow weaker with time. For these reasons, treatment with temazepam is usually only continued for a few days at a time.

INFORMATION FOR USERS

Your drug prescription is tailored for you. Do not alter dosage without checking with your doctor.

How taken/used Tablets, liquid.

Frequency and timing of doses Once daily, 30 minutes before bedtime.

Adult dosage range 10–40mg.

Onset of effect 15–40 minutes, or longer.

Duration of action 6–8 hours.

Diet advice None.

Storage Keep in original container at room temperature out of the reach of children. Protect from light.

Missed dose If you fall asleep without having taken a dose and wake some hours later, do not take the missed dose. If necessary, return to your normal dose schedule the next night.

Stopping the drug If you have been taking the drug continuously for less than 2 weeks, it can be safely stopped as soon as you no longer need it. If you have been taking the drug for longer, consult your doctor, who may supervise a gradual reduction in dosage. Stopping abruptly may lead to withdrawal symptoms (see p.10).

Exceeding the dose An occasional unintentional extra dose is unlikely to be a cause for concern. Large overdoses may cause severe drowsiness and breathing problems. Consult your doctor immediately.

POSSIBLE ADVERSE EFFECTS

The principal adverse effects of temazepam are related to its sedative and tranquillizing properties. These effects usually diminish after the first few days of treatment; however, some people experience a paradoxical increase in impulsivity, anxiety, and hostility. Common adverse effects include daytime drowsiness, headache, forgetfulness, and confusion. Discuss with your doctor if you have significant headache or drowsiness; if forgetfulness or confusion occur, you should also stop taking the drug. More rarely, temazepam may cause dizziness, unsteadiness, and vivid dreams or nightmares. Consult your doctor if you experience any of these rarer effects.

INTERACTIONS

Sedatives All drugs that have a sedative effect on the central nervous system are likely to increase the sedative properties of temazepam, which may potentially be fatal. Such drugs include alcohol and other anti-anxiety and sleeping drugs, opioid analgesics, antidepressants, antihistamines, and antipsychotics.

SPECIAL PRECAUTIONS

Be sure to tell your doctor if:

- You have severe respiratory disease.
- You have porphyria.
- You have liver or kidney problems.
- You have myasthenia gravis.
- You have had problems with alcohol or drug misuse.
- You are taking other medicines.

Pregnancy Not usually recommended; may cause adverse effects on the newborn baby at the time of delivery. Discuss with your doctor.

Breast-feeding The drug passes into the breast milk, and should be avoided during breast-feeding if possible. Discuss with your doctor.

Infants and children Not recommended.

Over 60 Reduced dose may be necessary. Increased likelihood of adverse effects.

Driving and hazardous work Avoid such activities until you have learned how temazepam affects you because the drug can cause reduced alertness and slowed reactions.

Alcohol Avoid. Alcohol may increase the sedative effect of this drug.

PROLONGED USE

Regular use of this drug over several weeks can lead to a reduction in its effect as the body adapts. It may also be habit-forming when taken for extended periods, and withdrawal symptoms may occur when the drug is stopped. Temazepam should not normally be used for longer than 1–2 weeks.

TENOFOVIR

Brand name Viread
Used in the following combined preparations Atripla, Eviplera, Stribild, Truvada

QUICK REFERENCE

Drug group Drug for HIV and immune deficiency (p.98) and antiviral drug (p.67)
Overdose danger rating Medium
Dependence rating Low
Prescription needed Yes
Available as generic No

GENERAL INFORMATION

Tenofovir is an antiviral drug used to treat (although not cure) HIV and hepatitis B infection. It is a nucleotide reverse transcriptase inhibitor, which blocks an enzyme, reverse transcriptase, that viruses need to replicate. In treating HIV infection, tenofovir is usually used in combination with other anti-HIV drugs to reduce production of new viruses before the immune system is irreversibly damaged. This combined therapy is known as antiretroviral therapy, or ART. Tenofovir may also be used alone to treat some cases of chronic hepatitis B infection.

Although tenofovir reduces the viral load in people with HIV or hepatitis B, it does not completely rid the body of these viruses. They may still be transmitted to other people and so it is important to continue taking precautions to avoid infecting others.

INFORMATION FOR USERS

Your drug prescription is tailored for you. Do not alter dosage without checking with your doctor.
How taken/used Tablets, granules.
Frequency and timing of doses Once daily, with food or liquid, at the same time every day. If you vomit within 1 hour of taking a tablet, take another; if more than 1 hour afterwards, do not take another. Granules should be mixed with soft food, swallowed without chewing, and not mixed with liquids.
Adult dosage range 245mg daily (1 tablet, or granules as directed).
Onset of effect May take from many weeks to a year before virus levels reduce significantly.
Duration of action Up to several days.
Diet advice None.
Storage Keep in original container at room temperature and out of the reach of children.
Missed dose Take the missed dose as soon as you remember unless your next dose is due within 12 hours, in which case skip the missed dose and take the next dose as scheduled.
Stopping the drug Do not stop without consulting your doctor; your condition may worsen.
Exceeding the dose An occasional unintentional extra dose is unlikely to cause problems. However, a large overdose may cause serious side effects; notify your doctor immediately.

POSSIBLE ADVERSE EFFECTS

Gastrointestinal side effects are common with tenofovir. As part of ART for HIV infection, the drug may also affect blood sugar and cholesterol levels and cause redistribution of body fat. Common adverse effects include dizziness, headache, nausea, diarrhoea, rash, muscle pain or weakness, tiredness, lethargy, altered distribution of body fat, and joint stiffness or pain. Discuss with your doctor if any of these are severe. Rarely, tenofovir may cause inflammation of the pancreas and bone problems. If you develop severe upper abdominal pain, stop taking the drug and contact your doctor immediately.

INTERACTIONS

General note Various drugs that affect the kidneys may affect blood levels of tenofovir, necessitating an adjustment of its dose. These include antibacterials (e.g. aminoglycosides, pentamidine, and vancomycin); antifungals (e.g. amphotericin B); antivirals (e.g. foscarnet, ganciclovir, adefovir, and cidofovir); immunosuppressants (e.g. tacrolimus); and some anticancer drugs (e.g. interleukin-2).
Other anti-HIV drugs Tenofovir may interact with anti-HIV drugs containing didanosine to increase blood levels of didanosine and reduce CD4 white blood cell counts, which may result in severe inflammation of the pancreas and may sometimes be fatal.

SPECIAL PRECAUTIONS

Be sure to tell your doctor if:
- You have kidney or liver disease.
- You have diabetes.
- You have a high blood cholesterol level.

◆ You have lactose intolerance.
◆ You are or plan to become pregnant.
◆ You are taking other medicines, especially corticosteroids.

Pregnancy Safety not established. Discuss with your doctor.
Breast-feeding It is not known if the drug passes into breast milk. However, the HIV and hepatitis B viruses can be passed on in breast milk so breast-feeding is not recommended.
Infants and children Not recommended.
Over 60 No known problems.
Driving and hazardous work Avoid such activities until you have learned how the drug affects you because it may cause dizziness.
Alcohol Avoid. Alcohol increases the risk of developing serious bone problems.

PROLONGED USE

Long-term use may cause loss of bone density and inflammation of the pancreas. In people with both HIV and hepatitis B or C, tenofovir may cause potentially fatal liver problems. ART including tenofovir may cause redistribution of body fat and abnormal blood sugar and lipid levels.
Monitoring Liver function tests are routine, and people being treated for HIV will have regular checks of blood cell counts (including CD4 counts), viral load, blood sugar and cholesterol levels, and response to treatment.

TERBINAFINE

Brand names Lamisil AT 1% Cream/Gel/Spray, Lamisil Cream, Lamisil Once, Lamisil Tablets
Used in the following combined preparations None

QUICK REFERENCE

Drug group Antifungal drug (p.74)
Overdose danger rating Low
Dependence rating Low
Prescription needed Yes (except for some skin preparations)
Available as generic Yes

GENERAL INFORMATION

Terbinafine is an antifungal drug used to treat fungal infections of the skin and nails, particularly tinea (ringworm). It is also used as a cream for candida (yeast) infections. It has largely replaced older drugs such as griseofulvin because it is more easily absorbed and is therefore more effective. Skin infections are treated in 2 to 6 weeks, but treatment of nail infections may take up to 6 months.

Rare adverse effects include a sore mouth and/or throat, jaundice, a severe skin rash, and bruising and/or bleeding in the mouth. Report any of these to your doctor without delay.

INFORMATION FOR USERS

Your drug prescription is tailored for you. Do not alter dosage without checking with your doctor.
How taken/used Tablets, spray, cream, gel, skin solution.
Frequency and timing of doses Once daily (tablets); 1–2 x daily (cream or gel); once only (solution).
Adult dosage range *Tinea infections* 250mg (tablets or gel). *Candida infections* As directed (cream).
Onset of effect Depends on the type and severity of infection.
Duration of action 24 hours.
Diet advice None.
Storage Keep in original container at room temperature out of the reach of children. Protect from light.
Missed dose Take as soon as you remember. If your next dose is due within 4 hours, take a single dose now and skip the next.
Stopping the drug Take the full course. Even if you feel better, the original infection may still be present and may recur if treatment is stopped too soon.
Exceeding the dose An occasional unintentional extra dose is unlikely to be a cause for concern. But if you notice any unusual symptoms, or if a large overdose has been taken, tell your doctor.

POSSIBLE ADVERSE EFFECTS

Most adverse effects are mild and transient. Nausea, indigestion, bloating, abdominal pain, diarrhoea, and headache are common. Less commonly, terbinafine may cause loss or disturbance of taste, dizziness, tiredness, pins and needles, and muscle or joint pain. Discuss with your doctor if you have muscle or joint pain or if any of these other symptoms are severe. Rarely, it can cause severe toxicity affecting the skin, liver, and bone marrow. If you develop a severe rash; soreness, bruising, or bleeding in the mouth or throat; jaundice; or abnormally dark urine or pale faeces, stop taking it and call your doctor immediately.

INTERACTIONS

Rifampicin This drug may reduce the blood level and effect of terbinafine.

Cimetidine This drug may increase the blood level of terbinafine.

Oral contraceptives Breakthrough bleeding may occur when these are taken with terbinafine.

Ciclosporin Terbinafine may reduce the blood level of ciclosporin.

SPECIAL PRECAUTIONS

Be sure to consult your doctor or pharmacist before taking this drug if:

- You have liver or kidney problems.
- You have psoriasis.
- You have an autoimmune disorder (e.g. systemic lupus erythematosus).
- You are taking other medicines.

Pregnancy Safety in pregnancy not established. Discuss with your doctor.

Breast-feeding Safety not established. Discuss with your doctor.

Infants and children Safety not established. Discuss with your doctor.

Over 60 No special problems.

Driving and hazardous work Avoid such activities until you know how terbinafine affects you because the drug can cause dizziness.

Alcohol No known problems.

PROLONGED USE

Long-term use of oral terbinafine may rarely cause severe liver damage.

Monitoring Periodic blood tests are usually done to check the drug's effect on the liver.

TERBUTALINE

Brand name Bricanyl

Used in the following combined preparations None

QUICK REFERENCE

Drug group Bronchodilator (p.21)

Overdose danger rating Low

Dependence rating Low

Prescription needed Yes

Available as generic Yes

GENERAL INFORMATION

Terbutaline is a sympathomimetic bronchodilator used to treat conditions such as asthma, chronic obstructive pulmonary disease (COPD), and bronchospasm, in which the airways become constricted. Terbutaline is also used to delay premature labour (p.109).

Muscle tremor is common with terbutaline and usually disappears if the dose is reduced or with continued use as the body adapts to the drug. Like other sympathomimetics, it may also cause nervousness and restlessness.

INFORMATION FOR USERS

Your drug prescription is tailored for you. Do not alter dosage without checking with your doctor.

How taken/used Tablets, liquid (syrup), injection, inhaler, nebules for nebulizer.

Frequency and timing of doses 3 x daily (tablets/syrup); as necessary (inhaler).

Dosage range *Adults* 7.5–15mg daily (tablets/syrup); 0.5mg when required, up to 2mg daily (inhaler); as directed by doctor (nebules). *Children* Reduced dose according to age and weight.

Onset of effect Within a few minutes (inhaler); within 1–2 hours (tablets/syrup).

Duration of action 7–8 hours (tablets/syrup).

Diet advice None.

Storage Keep in original container at room temperature out of the reach of children. Protect from light. Do not puncture or burn aerosol containers.

Missed dose Do not take the missed dose. Take your next dose as usual.

Stopping the drug Do not stop the drug without consulting your doctor; symptoms may recur.

Exceeding the dose An occasional unintentional extra dose is unlikely to be a cause for concern. But if you notice any unusual symptoms, or if a large overdose has been taken, tell your doctor.

POSSIBLE ADVERSE EFFECTS

Muscle tremor (particularly in the hands), anxiety, and restlessness are the most common adverse effects. Discuss with your doctor if they are severe or if you have headaches or muscle cramps. Palpitations are also common; if they occur, stop the drug and consult your doctor. Rarely, wheezing or breathlessness may worsen immediately after inhaler use (paradoxical bronchospasm). If this happens, stop the drug and call your doctor immediately.

INTERACTIONS

Other sympathomimetics (see p.7) may add to the effects of terbutaline and vice versa, so increasing the risk of adverse effects.

Monoamine oxidase inhibitors (MAOIs) Terbutaline may interact with these drugs to cause a dangerous rise in blood pressure.
Diuretics, corticosteroids, and theophylline taken with terbutaline may reduce blood levels of potassium, causing muscle weakness.
Beta blockers may reduce the beneficial effects of terbutaline.

SPECIAL PRECAUTIONS

Be sure to tell your doctor if:
- ◆ You have heart problems.
- ◆ You have high blood pressure.
- ◆ You have an overactive thyroid.
- ◆ You have diabetes.
- ◆ You are taking other medicines.

Pregnancy Safety in early pregnancy not established, although drug is used in late pregnancy to prevent premature labour. Discuss with your doctor.
Breast-feeding The drug passes into breast milk but in amounts too small to affect the baby.
Infants and children Reduced dose necessary.
Over 60 Increased likelihood of adverse effects. Reduced dose may therefore be necessary.
Driving and hazardous work Avoid until you have learned how terbutaline affects you because it can cause tremor of the hands.
Alcohol No special problems.

PROLONGED USE

No problems expected. However, contact your doctor if you find you are needing to use your terbutaline inhaler more than usual. Failure to respond to the drug may be due to worsening asthma that requires urgent medical attention.
Monitoring Periodic blood tests for potassium may be needed in people on high-dose treatment with terbutaline combined with other asthma drugs.

TESTOSTERONE

Brand names Nebido, Restandol Testocaps, Sustanon, Testavan, Testim, Testogel, Tostran
Used in the following combined preparations None

QUICK REFERENCE

Drug group Male sex hormone (p.85)
Overdose danger rating Low
Dependence rating Low
Prescription needed Yes
Available as generic Yes

GENERAL INFORMATION

Testosterone is a male sex hormone that is produced by the testes in men and, in small quantities, by the ovaries in women. The hormone encourages bone and muscle growth in both men and women and stimulates sexual development in men.

The drug is used to treat testosterone deficiency (hypogonadism) resulting from pituitary or testicular disorders. It is also used to initiate puberty in male adolescents if this has been delayed due to deficiency of the natural hormone.

Testosterone can interfere with growth or cause overly rapid sexual development in adolescents. High doses in women may cause deepening of the voice, excessive hair growth, or hair loss.

INFORMATION FOR USERS

Your drug prescription is tailored for you. Do not alter dosage without checking with your doctor.
How taken/used Injection, implanted pellets, gel, patch, oral and buccal preparations.
Frequency and timing of doses Varies according to preparation and condition being treated (injection); 5g daily, according to response, to maximum of 10g daily (gel); every 6 months (implant); once daily (patch).
Dosage range Varies with method of administration and the condition being treated.
Onset of effect 2–3 days. Full effect may take several months.
Duration of action 1 week to more than 3 months (injection); approximately 6 months (implant).
Diet advice None.
Storage Keep in original container at room temperature out of the reach of children. Protect from light.
Missed dose No cause for concern, but take as soon as you remember.
Stopping the drug Do not stop taking the drug without consulting your doctor.
Exceeding the dose An occasional unintentional extra dose is unlikely to be a cause for concern. However, if you notice unusual symptoms, or if a large overdose was taken, notify your doctor.

POSSIBLE ADVERSE EFFECTS

Most of the more serious adverse effects are likely to occur only with long-term treatment and may be helped by a reduction in dosage. Acne and skin irritation with gel or patches are common adverse effects. More rarely, hair loss, mood changes, and water retention may occur. Discuss with your doctor if any of these are severe. If you develop jaundice, stop using the drug and contact your doctor promptly. In men, the drug may also cause abnormal erections, breast development, and difficulty in passing urine; if these occur, they should be reported to your doctor. In women, adverse effects include unusual hair growth or hair loss, deepening of the voice, and enlargement of the clitoris; discuss with your doctor if hair loss is severe or if these other changes occur. Those using topical gel formulations should be aware that close contact with gel application sites can transfer significant amounts of the drug to other people. Pregnant women and young children are particularly at risk of adverse effects if such transfer occurs.

INTERACTIONS

Anticoagulants Testosterone may increase the effect of warfarin-like anticoagulants, requiring adjustment of their dosage.

Antidiabetic drugs Testosterone enhances their effects, requiring reduction of their dosage.

SPECIAL PRECAUTIONS

Be sure to tell your doctor if:

- You have long-term liver or kidney problems.
- You have heart problems.
- You have prostate problems.
- You have high blood pressure.
- You have epilepsy or migraine headaches.
- You have diabetes.
- You are taking other medicines.

Pregnancy Not prescribed. Avoid skin-to-skin transfer of testosterone from other people.

Breast-feeding Not prescribed during breast-feeding. Avoid skin-to-skin transfer of testosterone from other people.

Infants and children Not prescribed for infants and young children. Reduced dose necessary in adolescents.

Over 60 Rarely required. Increased risk of prostate problems in older men. Reduced dose may therefore be necessary.

Driving and hazardous work No special problems with this drug.

Alcohol No special problems.

PROLONGED USE

Prolonged use of this drug may lead to reduced growth in adolescents. In older men, it may accelerate prostate disease.

Monitoring Regular blood tests for the effects of treatment are necessary, such as red blood cell count, electrolyte levels, liver function tests, and PSA (prostate-specific antigen) levels.

TETRACYCLINE/ LYMECYCLINE

Brand name Tetralysal 300

Used in the following combined preparation Deteclo

QUICK REFERENCE

Drug group Tetracycline antibiotic (p.61)

Overdose danger rating Low

Dependence rating Low

Prescription needed Yes

Available as generic Yes

GENERAL INFORMATION

Tetracycline and lymecycline are both tetracyclines. This was once a very widely used class of antibiotics, but the rise of drug-resistant bacteria has reduced their effectiveness in many types of infection. Tetracycline and lymecycline are commonly used for acne, rosacea, and diabetic diarrhoea, and to eradicate *Helicobacter pylori* infection, and are still used to treat chronic bronchitis, destructive forms of dental disease, and certain chest and genital infections due to mycoplasma organisms. They remain the treatment of choice for infections due to *Chlamydia* and *Rickettsia*.

Taken by mouth, these drugs can sometimes cause nausea, vomiting, and diarrhoea. Tetracyclines may discolour developing teeth if taken by children or by the mother during pregnancy. People with poor kidney function are not prescribed tetracycline/lymecycline as these drugs can cause further deterioration.

INFORMATION FOR USERS

Your drug prescription is tailored for you. Do not alter dosage without checking with your doctor.

How taken/used Tablets, capsules.

Frequency and timing of doses *By mouth* 2–4 x daily, at least 1 hour before or 2 hours after meals (tetracycline); 1–2 x daily (lymecycline). Always swallow doses with water.

Adult dosage range *Infections* 1–2g daily (tetracycline); 916–1,032mg daily (lymecycline). *Acne* 1g daily (tetracycline); 408mg daily (lymecycline).
Onset of effect 4–12 hours. Improvement in acne may not be noticed for up to 4 weeks.
Duration of action Up to 6 hours.
Diet advice Milk products should be avoided for 1 hour before and 2 hours after taking the drug.
Storage Keep in original container at room temperature out of the reach of children.
Missed dose Take as soon as you remember. If your next dose is due within 2 hours, take a single dose now and skip the next.
Stopping the drug Take the full course. Even if you feel better, the original infection may still be present and may recur if treatment is stopped too soon.
Exceeding the dose An occasional unintentional extra dose is unlikely to be a cause for concern. But if you notice any unusual symptoms, or if a large overdose has been taken, tell your doctor.

POSSIBLE ADVERSE EFFECTS

Swallowing difficulties and/or oesophageal irritation may occur if a dose is taken with insufficient water, and the medication may stick in your throat if you lie down immediately after taking it. Other common adverse effects include nausea, vomiting, and diarrhoea; discuss with your doctor if they are severe. More rarely, the drug may cause a rash (which may sometimes be light-sensitive) and itching; if these occur, you should stop taking the drug and consult your doctor. If jaundice, headache, or visual disturbances occur, you should stop taking the drug and contact your doctor immediately.

INTERACTIONS

Iron This may reduce the effectiveness of tetracycline/lymecycline.
Oral anticoagulants Tetracycline/lymecycline may increase the action of these drugs.
Retinoids may increase the adverse effects of tetracycline/lymecycline.
Diuretics should not be used with lymecycline.
Oral contraceptives Tetracycline/lymecycline may reduce the effectiveness of oral contraceptives.
Antacids and milk These interfere with the absorption of tetracycline/lymecycline and may reduce their effectiveness. Doses should be separated by 1–2 hours.
Methotrexate Tetracycline may increase the risk of methotrexate toxicity.

SPECIAL PRECAUTIONS

Be sure to tell your doctor if:
- You have long-term liver or kidney problems.
- You have previously had an allergic reaction to a tetracycline antibiotic.
- You have myasthenia gravis, acute porphyria, or systemic lupus erythematosus.
- You are taking other medicines.

Pregnancy Not prescribed. May cause birth defects and may damage the teeth and bones of the developing baby as well as the mother's liver. Discuss with your doctor.
Breast-feeding Not recommended. The drugs pass into the breast milk and may damage developing bones and discolour the baby's teeth. Discuss with your doctor.
Infants and children Not recommended under 12 years. Reduced dose necessary in older children. May discolour developing teeth.
Over 60 No special problems.
Driving and hazardous work No known problems.
Alcohol No known problems.
How to take your tablets To prevent the medication from sticking in your throat, take a small amount of water before, and a full glass of water after, each dose. Take this medication while sitting or standing and do not lie down immediately afterwards.

PROLONGED USE

No problems expected.

TEZACAFTOR/IVACAFTOR

Brand name Symkevi
Used in the following combined preparation None

QUICK REFERENCE

Drug group Drug for cystic fibrosis
Overdose danger rating Low
Dependence rating Low
Prescription needed Yes
Available as generic No

GENERAL INFORMATION

Tezacaftor and ivacaftor are drugs used to treat cystic fibrosis. In this genetic disorder, the protein that regulates the flow of fluid in and out of cells lining the lungs (and other organs) is defective due to inherited mutations in the gene containing the code for this protein. The defect causes a build-up of sticky mucus in these organs, which leads to lung infections and affects other organs such as the pancreas. Tezacaftor and ivacaftor are designed to work in tandem to improve the function of the defective protein. This action leads to improved lung function and reduces the aggravated symptoms caused by repeated airway infections.

Tezacaftor and ivacaftor (Symkevi) are licensed for the specific gene mutations that cause the defective protein. The treatment is indicated in a combination regimen with ivacaftor tablets and can only be prescribed by a cystic fibrosis specialist.

INFORMATION FOR USERS

Follow instructions on the label. Call your doctor if symptoms worsen.

How taken/used Tablets

Frequency and timing of doses 1 x Symkevi (tezacaftor and ivacaftor) tablet in the morning, 1 x ivacaftor tablet in the evening, approximately 12 hours apart.

Adult dosage range Symkevi tablet: tezacaftor 100mg/ivacaftor 150mg; ivacaftor tablet: 150mg.

Onset of effect 15 days; full effects may take weeks to appear.

Duration of action Tezacaftor 6–7 days; ivacaftor 9 hours.

Diet advice Take with food containing fats. Avoid food or drink containing grapefruit or Seville oranges during treatment.

Storage Keep in original container at room temperature out of the reach of children. Protect from light.

Missed dose If it is 6 hours or less since a missed morning or evening dose, take the dose as soon as possible and continue the usual schedule. If more than 6 hours have passed, do not take the missed dose but take the next scheduled dose at the usual time. Do not take more than one dose of either tablet at the same time.

Stopping the drug Do not stop without consulting your doctor. Stopping the drug may lead to worsening of the underlying condition.

Exceeding the dose An occasional unintentional extra dose is unlikely to be a cause for concern. But if you notice any unusual symptoms, or if a large overdose has been taken, tell your doctor.

POSSIBLE ADVERSE EFFECTS

Report any adverse effects to your doctor. Headache, nausea, and sinus congestion are frequently reported. Other common effects are nasal or throat irritation, ear problems, dizziness, rash, abdominal pain, and diarrhoea. More rarely, breast problems or a breast mass, or cataracts, may develop.

INTERACTIONS

Rifampicin, rifabutin, phenobarbital, carbamazepine, phenytoin, St. John's wort, and grapefruit may reduce blood levels of tezacaftor and ivacaftor.

Warfarin Increased anticoagulant effect with ivacaftor.

Ketoconazole, itraconazole, posaconazole, voriconazole, fluconazole, telithromycin, clarithromycin, and erythromycin may increase blood levels of tezacaftor and ivacaftor.

SPECIAL PRECAUTIONS

Be sure to tell your doctor if:

- You have long-term kidney or liver problems.
- You are taking other medicines.

Pregnancy Safety in pregnancy not established. Discuss with your doctor.

Breast-feeding Not known if tezacaftor or ivacaftor, or products of their metabolism in body, pass into breast milk. Discuss with doctor.

Infants and children Not recommended under 12 years.

Over 60 Limited information on the drug. No known problems.

Driving and hazardous work No known problems.

Alcohol No known problems.

PROLONGED USE

Monitoring Regular blood tests will be carried out to monitor your liver function.

THALIDOMIDE

Brand name Celgene

Used in the following combined preparations None

QUICK REFERENCE

Drug group Drug for leprosy (p.65) and multiple myeloma

Overdose danger rating Medium

Dependence rating Low

Prescription needed Yes

Available as generic No

GENERAL INFORMATION

Thalidomide was originally introduced in the 1950s as a sedative and became popular for treating morning sickness in pregnancy. By 1961, though, it was clear that the drug caused severe birth defects and it was withdrawn.

Thalidomide was subsequently found to be effective in treating leprosy (also known as Hansen's disease) and in blocking the growth of blood vessels to tumours. Currently in the UK there are strict controls on prescribing the drug; it is used only to treat multiple myeloma (a type of bone marrow cancer) in combination with other drugs, and, very rarely, for leprosy. Because it can cause severe birth defects when taken during pregnancy and can also be present in semen, women of childbearing age and men must ensure that reliable contraception is used. Thalidomide also increases the risk of peripheral nerve damage and venous thromboembolism (deep vein thrombosis and pulmonary embolism).

INFORMATION FOR USERS

Follow instructions on the label. Your drug prescription is tailored for you. Do not alter dosage without checking with your doctor.

How taken/used Capsules.

Frequency and timing of doses Once daily at bedtime for up to 72 weeks.

Adult dosage range 200mg daily.

Onset of effect 2–5 hours.

Duration of action 7–8 hours.

Diet advice None.

Storage Keep in original container out of the reach of children.

Missed dose Take the missed dose as soon as you remember unless your next dose is due within 12 hours, in which case omit the missed dose and take the next dose as scheduled.

Stopping the drug Do not stop without consulting your doctor; your condition may worsen.

Exceeding the dose An occasional unintentional extra dose is unlikely to cause problems. However, a large overdose may cause serious side effects; consult your doctor or go to hospital immediately.

POSSIBLE ADVERSE EFFECTS

Thalidomide often causes drowsiness and nerve damage. The latter may be mild, causing numbness and tingling in the hands or feet, or more severe and painful; in some cases, the nerve damage may be irreversible. If you experience numbness or tingling in your hands and feet, consult your doctor. Other common effects include constipation, headache, dizziness, sleepiness, blurred vision, bruising or bleeding, and leg pain or swelling. Discuss with your doctor if you have headaches or if constipation, sleepiness, or dizziness are severe. If you experience blurred vision, you should stop taking the drug and consult your doctor. If you have unusual bleeding or bruising, rash, blisters, mouth ulcers, palpitations, or cessation of menstrual periods, stop taking the drug and contact your doctor immediately. Thalidomide also carries a significant risk of venous thromboembolism, which may cause pain or swelling in a leg, chest pain, breathlessness, or, rarely, collapse. If any of these occur, stop taking the drug and seek urgent medical help. The risks of nerve damage and thromboembolism are greater with prolonged use (see below).

INTERACTIONS

Sedative drugs Thalidomide increases the drowsiness caused by other sedative drugs, such as antihistamines, anticholinergics, opioids, benzodiazepines, and alcohol.

Beta blockers There is an increased risk of an abnormally low heart rate when beta blockers are used with thalidomide.

SPECIAL PRECAUTIONS

Be sure to tell your doctor if:

- You are sexually active, pregnant, or intending to become pregnant.
- You have lactose intolerance.
- You have kidney or liver problems.
- You have a history of thromboembolism or heart disease.
- You have problems with sensation in your hands or feet.
- You are taking other medicines.

Pregnancy Thalidomide must not be used; it causes severe birth defects. Women of childbearing age must use contraception. The drug is present in semen; men taking it must ensure that they and/or their partner use contraception. Women who think they may have become pregnant should stop the drug and consult their doctor immediately.

Breast-feeding Avoid as it is not known whether thalidomide passes into breast milk.

Infants and children Not recommended under 18 years.
Over 60 Older people are at increased risk of potentially serious adverse effects. Discuss with your doctor.
Driving and hazardous work Avoid such activities if you experience side effects such as dizziness, tiredness, sleepiness, or blurred vision.
Alcohol Avoid. Alcohol increases the sedative effect of thalidomide.

PROLONGED USE

Prolonged use increases the risk of nerve damage and venous thromboembolism. If you are at high risk of thromboembolism, you may be prescribed preventative drugs.
Monitoring You will have regular blood tests and checks of your reflexes and nerve function.

THEOPHYLLINE/ AMINOPHYLLINE

Brand names [theophylline] Uniphyllin; [aminophylline] Phyllocontin
Used in the following combined preparations None

QUICK REFERENCE

Drug group Bronchodilator (p.21)
Overdose danger rating High
Dependence rating Low
Prescription needed No (except for injection)
Available as generic Yes

GENERAL INFORMATION

Theophylline (and aminophylline, which breaks down to theophylline in the body) is used to treat bronchospasm (constriction of the air passages). The drug improves breathing in people with asthma, bronchitis, and emphysema. It is usually taken continuously for prevention, but aminophylline injections are sometimes used for acute attacks.

Slow-release formulations of the drugs produce beneficial effects lasting for up to 12 hours. These preparations may be prescribed twice daily, but they are also useful as a single dose taken at night to prevent night-time asthma and early-morning wheezing.

Treatment with theophylline must be monitored because the effective dose is very close to the toxic dose. Some adverse effects, such as indigestion, nausea, headache, and agitation, can be controlled by regulating the dosage and checking blood levels of the drug.

INFORMATION FOR USERS

Follow instructions on the label. Call your doctor if symptoms worsen.
How taken/used Modified release (MR) tablets, injection.
Frequency and timing of doses 1–2 x MR tablets every 12–24 hours. Take tablets at the same time each day.
Dosage range *Adults* 400–800mg daily, depending on which product is used.
Onset of effect Within 90 minutes (MR tablets).
Duration of action Up to 12 hours for MR formulation.
Diet advice None.
Storage Keep in original container at room temperature out of the reach of children.
Missed dose Take as soon as you remember. If your next dose is due within 2 hours, take the next dose now (MR preparations). Return to your normal dose schedule thereafter.
Stopping the drug Do not stop without consulting your doctor; stopping the drug may lead to worsening of the underlying condition.

OVERDOSE ACTION

Seek immediate medical advice in all cases. Take emergency action if chest pains, confusion, or loss of consciousness occur.

POSSIBLE ADVERSE EFFECTS

Many adverse effects are related to blood levels of the drug. The most common effects are gastrointestinal symptoms such as nausea and vomiting, headache, and nervous symptoms such as agitation and insomnia. If you experience severe nausea, vomiting, diarrhoea, abdominal pain, or insomnia, discuss with your doctor. You should also consult your doctor if you have headaches or become unusually agitated. If palpitations occur, stop taking the drug and call your doctor immediately.

INTERACTIONS

General note Many drugs interact with theophylline. Some antibiotics, antidepressants, and anticonvulsants increase the drug's effect by increasing its blood level. Taken with theophylline, high doses of beta 2 agonists such as salbutamol increase the risk of low blood potassium levels. Discuss with your doctor.

SPECIAL PRECAUTIONS

Be sure to tell your doctor if:

- ◆ You have a liver problem.
- ◆ You have angina or irregular heart beat.
- ◆ You have high blood pressure.
- ◆ You have epilepsy.
- ◆ You have hyperthyroidism.
- ◆ You have porphyria.
- ◆ You have peptic ulcers.
- ◆ You have an exacerbation of lung disease, fever, or a viral infection.
- ◆ You have prostate enlargement.
- ◆ You smoke.
- ◆ You are taking other medicines.

Pregnancy Safety in pregnancy not established. Discuss with your doctor.

Breast-feeding Drug passes into breast milk and may affect the baby. Discuss with your doctor.

Infants and children Reduced dose necessary according to age and weight.

Over 60 Reduced dose may be necessary.

Driving and hazardous work No known problems.

Alcohol Avoid excess as this may alter levels of drug and increase gastrointestinal symptoms.

How to take your tablets Factors such as drug interactions, certain medical conditions (e.g. heart or liver failure), and smoking can affect theophylline levels. Levels also vary between brands, so you must always use the same brand.

PROLONGED USE

No problems expected.

Monitoring Checks on blood levels of drug and risk of heart rhythm disorders usually required.

TIMOLOL

Brand names Eysano, Timoptol, Timoptol LA, Tiopex, Travoprost

Used in the following combined preparations Azarga, Combigan, Cosopt, DuoTrav, Ganfort, Taptiqom, Xalacom

QUICK REFERENCE

Drug group Beta blocker (p.28) and drug for glaucoma (p.112)

Overdose danger rating High

Dependence rating Low

Prescription needed Yes

Available as generic Yes

GENERAL INFORMATION

Timolol is a non-cardioselective beta blocker used to treat angina. It may be given after a heart attack to prevent further damage to the heart. It is also used to treat hypertension (high blood pressure), but is not usually used to initiate treatment. The drug is commonly given as eye drops to people with certain types of glaucoma and is occasionally given to prevent migraine. Timolol can occasionally cause breathing difficulties, especially in people with respiratory diseases; this is more likely with the tablets but can also occur with the eye drops. Timolol may mask the body's response to low blood sugar; therefore, it is prescribed with caution to diabetic people on insulin.

INFORMATION FOR USERS

Your drug prescription is tailored for you. Do not alter dosage without checking with your doctor.

How taken/used Tablets, eye drops.

Frequency and timing of doses 1–3 x daily.

Adult dosage range *By mouth* 10–60mg daily (hypertension); 10–60mg daily (angina/hypertension); 10–20mg daily (after a heart attack); 10–20mg daily (migraine prevention).

Onset of effect Within 30 minutes (by mouth); 15–20 minutes (eye drops).

Duration of action Up to 24 hours.

Diet advice None.

Storage Keep in original container at room temperature out of the reach of children.

Missed dose Take as soon as you remember. If your next dose is due within 3 hours, take a single dose now and skip the next.

Stopping the drug Do not stop without consulting your doctor; stopping the drug may lead to worsening of the underlying condition.

OVERDOSE ACTION

Seek immediate medical advice in all cases of overdose by mouth. Take emergency action if breathing difficulties, palpitations, or loss of consciousness occur.

POSSIBLE ADVERSE EFFECTS

Eye drops commonly cause only irritation of the eyes; if this is severe, discuss with your doctor. Rarely, the drug may be absorbed from the eyes into the body and cause the systemic (whole-body) side effects that may occur with oral use. All systemic adverse effects should be reported to your doctor. The most common are lethargy, fatigue, and cold hands and feet. Nausea and vomiting are less common. Also uncommon are vivid dreams or nightmares, rash, dry eyes, and visual disturbances; stop taking the drug if any of these occur. Timolol by mouth can occasionally provoke or worsen heart problems and asthma. If you experience fainting (which may be a sign that the drug has slowed the heart beat or lowered blood pressure excessively) or palpitations, breathlessness, or wheezing, stop taking the drug and contact your doctor immediately.

INTERACTIONS

Calcium channel blockers may cause low blood pressure, a slow heartbeat, and heart failure if used with timolol.
Cardiac glycosides (e.g. digoxin) may increase the heart-slowing effect of timolol.
Antihypertensive drugs Timolol may enhance the blood-pressure-lowering effect.
Drugs for asthma (e.g. salbutamol, salmeterol, and other beta agonists) The effects of these drugs may be reduced by timolol.

SPECIAL PRECAUTIONS

Be sure to tell your doctor if:
- You have heart problems.
- You have kidney or liver problems.
- You have a lung disorder such as asthma, bronchitis, or emphysema.
- You have diabetes.
- You have psoriasis.
- You have an overactive thyroid gland.
- You are taking other medicines.

Pregnancy Safety in pregnancy not established. Discuss with your doctor.
Breast-feeding The drug passes into the breast milk, but normal doses are unlikely to affect the baby adversely. Discuss with your doctor.
Infants and children Not usually prescribed.
Over 60 Reduced dose may be necessary.
Driving and hazardous work Avoid until you have learned how timolol affects you because the tablets may cause dizziness or fatigue, and the eye drops may cause blurred vision.
Alcohol Avoid excessive intake. Alcohol may increase the blood-pressure-lowering effects of timolol.
Surgery and general anaesthetics Occasionally, timolol eye drops may need to be stopped before a general anaesthetic, but only do this after discussion with your doctor or dentist.

PROLONGED USE

No problems expected.

TIOTROPIUM

Brand names Braltus, Spiriva, Spiriva Respimat
Used in the following combined preparations Spiolto, Yanimo

QUICK REFERENCE

Drug group Bronchodilator (p.21)
Overdose danger rating Low
Dependence rating Low
Prescription needed Yes
Available as generic No

GENERAL INFORMATION

Tiotropium is a long-acting anticholinergic bronchodilator that relaxes the muscles surrounding the bronchioles (the airways in the lung). It is used in the maintenance treatment of chronic obstructive lung disorders, such as chronic bronchitis. The drug is not suitable for acute attacks of wheezing or in the emergency treatment of asthma, when salbutamol (p.396) should be used and urgent medical help sought. Tiotropium is taken by inhalation of a powder or solution, and it acts directly and locally on the inner surface of the lungs and not via the blood. The most common side effect is a dry mouth.

INFORMATION FOR USERS

Your drug prescription is tailored for you. Do not alter dosage without checking with your doctor.
How taken/used Powder in capsules for inhaler, solution for inhalation.
Frequency and timing of doses 1 capsule daily for inhaled powder; 2 puffs daily for inhalation solution. Use at the same time each day.
Adult dosage range Spiriva: 18mcg; Braltus: 10mcg (powder). Spiriva Respimat: 5mcg (solution).
Onset of effect 5–30 minutes.
Duration of action 24 hours.
Diet advice None.
Storage Keep in original container at room temperature out of the reach of children.
Missed dose Take as soon as you remember. If your next dose is due within 8 hours, take a single dose now and skip the next.
Stopping the drug Do not stop without consulting your doctor; symptoms may recur.
Exceeding the dose An occasional unintentional extra dose is unlikely to be a cause for concern. But if you notice any unusual symptoms,

or if a large overdose has been taken, notify your doctor.

POSSIBLE ADVERSE EFFECTS

Dry mouth is the most common adverse effect of tiotropium; sore throat and a cough are also common. If any of these are severe, discuss with your doctor. Rarely, the drug may cause nosebleeds, an altered sense of taste, changes in the voice, a fast heartbeat or palpitations, difficulty in passing urine, rash, and wheezing after inhalation. Consult your doctor if any of these symptoms occur. If you get the drug in your eye, it could trigger or worsen glaucoma, with symptoms such as eye pain, blurred vision, and visual haloes; if this happens, call your doctor immediately. If wheezing and breathlessness suddenly worsen after using the inhaler (paradoxical bronchospasm), stop taking the drug and call your doctor immediately.

INTERACTIONS

Anticholinergic drugs (e.g. atropine and ipratropium) The effects and toxicity of tiotropium are likely to be increased if it is used at the same time as these drugs.

SPECIAL PRECAUTIONS

Be sure to tell your doctor if:

- You are allergic to atropine or ipratropium.
- You have prostate problems.
- You have urinary retention.
- You have glaucoma.
- You have kidney problems.
- You have heart disease.
- You are taking other medicines.

Pregnancy Safety not established. Discuss with your doctor.

Breast-feeding Safety not established, but the amount present in breast milk is unlikely to harm your baby. Discuss with your doctor.

Infants and children Not recommended under 18 years.

Over 60 No known problems.

Driving and hazardous work Avoid until you have learned how the drug affects you as it can cause dizziness, blurred vision, or headache.

Alcohol No known problems.

Protecting your eyes Take care to avoid getting the drug into the eyes as it could trigger glaucoma or make existing glaucoma worse. If you develop eye or vision problems, contact your doctor immediately.

PROLONGED USE

No known problems.

TOLBUTAMIDE

Brand name None

Used in the following combined preparations None

QUICK REFERENCE

Drug group Drug for diabetes (p.80)

Overdose danger rating High

Dependence rating Low

Prescription needed Yes

Available as generic Yes

GENERAL INFORMATION

Tolbutamide is a sulfonylurea drug, but is shorter-acting than many others in this group. It is used to treat Type 2 diabetes, and acts by stimulating the beta cells in the pancreas to release insulin; it will only work, therefore, if functioning cells remain. For this reason, it is not effective in Type 1 diabetes, in which functioning cells are lacking.

Tolbutamide may also be given to people with impaired kidney function because it is less likely to build up in the body and excessively lower blood sugar. If additional control of blood glucose is needed, other oral drugs for diabetes, such as metformin or acarbose, can be added to tolbutamide.

As with other oral antidiabetic drugs, tolbutamide may need to be replaced with insulin during serious illnesses, injury, or surgery, when diabetic control is lost.

INFORMATION FOR USERS

Your drug prescription is tailored for you. Do not alter dosage without checking with your doctor.

How taken/used Tablets.

Frequency and timing of doses Taken with meals either once daily in the morning, or 2 x daily in the morning and evening.

Adult dosage range 500mg–2g daily.

Onset of effect Within 1 hour.

Duration of action 6–24 hours.

Diet advice An individualized diabetic diet must be maintained for the drug to be fully effective. Follow the advice of your doctor.

Storage Keep in original container at room temperature out of the reach of children. Protect from light.

Missed dose Take as soon as you remember. If your next dose is due within 2 hours, take a single dose now and skip the next.
Stopping the drug Do not stop taking the drug without consulting your doctor; stopping the drug may lead to worsening of the underlying condition.

OVERDOSE ACTION

Seek immediate medical advice in all cases. If you have warning signs of low blood sugar (e.g. faintness, dizziness, headache, confusion, sweating, or tremor), eat something sugary. Take emergency action if seizures or loss of consciousness occur.

POSSIBLE ADVERSE EFFECTS

Serious adverse effects are rare with tolbutamide. Symptoms such as dizziness, sweating, shaking, blurred vision, weakness, and confusion may indicate low blood sugar levels; if they occur, eat or drink something sugary and seek immediate medical help. Other common effects are nausea, indigestion, and diarrhoea; discuss with your doctor if severe. Rarely, headache, ringing in the ears, and weight gain may occur; if they are severe, discuss with your doctor. If you develop jaundice, fever, a rash, easy bruising, or sore throat, stop taking the drug and contact your doctor immediately.

INTERACTIONS

General note A range of drugs, including corticosteroids, oestrogens, diuretics, and rifampicin, may oppose the effect of tolbutamide and raise blood sugar levels. Others increase the risk of low blood sugar; these include sulfonamides, warfarin, chloramphenicol, aspirin and other non-steroidal anti-inflammatory drugs (NSAIDs), antidepressants, cimetidine, and some antibiotics and antifungals.
Beta blockers may mask the signs of low blood sugar, especially non-cardioselective beta blockers such as propranolol.

SPECIAL PRECAUTIONS

Be sure to tell your doctor if:
- You have long-term liver or kidney problems.
- You are allergic to sulfonamides.
- You have thyroid problems.
- You have porphyria or glucose-6-phosphate dehydrogenase (G6PD) deficiency.
- You are taking other medicines.

Pregnancy Not prescribed. Insulin is usually substituted. May cause birth defects if taken in the first 3 months of pregnancy. Discuss with your doctor.
Breast-feeding The drug passes into the breast milk and may affect the baby. Discuss with your doctor.
Infants and children Not prescribed.
Over 60 Risk of low blood sugar. Reduced dose may therefore be necessary.
Driving and hazardous work Usually no problem. However, avoid these activities if you have warning signs of low blood sugar (see Overdose action, above).
Alcohol Keep consumption low. Alcohol may upset diabetic control and cause flushing, nausea, nausea, vomiting, and signs of low blood sugar (see above).
Surgery and general anaesthetics Notify your doctor that you have diabetes before you undergo any surgery; insulin treatment may need to be substituted.

PROLONGED USE

No problems expected, but tolbutamide may lose its effect if the functioning of the pancreas becomes worse.
Monitoring Periodic monitoring of control of blood glucose levels is necessary.

TOLTERODINE

Brand names Blerone XL, Detrusitol, Detrusitol XL, Inconex XL, Mariosea XL, Neditol XL, Preblacon XL, Tolterma XL, Tolthen XL
Used in the following combined preparations None

QUICK REFERENCE

Drug group Drug for urinary disorders (p.110)
Overdose danger rating High
Dependence rating Low
Prescription needed Yes
Available as generic Yes

GENERAL INFORMATION

Tolterodine is an anticholinergic and antispasmodic drug similar to atropine (p.146). It is used to treat urinary frequency and incontinence in adults. It acts by reducing contraction of the bladder, allowing it to expand and hold more urine. It also stops spasms and delays the desire to empty the bladder. The usefulness of tolterodine is limited to some extent by its side effects, and dosage needs to be reduced in older adults. Children are more susceptible than adults to the drug's anticholinergic effects (p.7). Tolterodine can also trigger glaucoma.

INFORMATION FOR USERS

Your drug prescription is tailored for you. Do not alter dosage without checking with your doctor.

How taken/used Tablets, slow release (SR) capsules.

Frequency and timing of doses 1–2 x daily.

Dosage range 4mg daily, reduced to 2mg daily, if necessary, to minimize side effects.

Onset of effect 1 hour.

Duration of action 12 hours.

Diet advice None.

Storage Keep in original container at room temperature out of the reach of children.

Missed dose Take as soon as you remember. If your next dose is due within 2 hours, take a single dose now and skip the next.

Stopping the drug Do not stop without consulting your doctor; symptoms may recur.

OVERDOSE ACTION

Seek immediate medical advice in all cases. Take emergency action if symptoms such as breathing difficulty, seizures, or loss of consciousness occur.

POSSIBLE ADVERSE EFFECTS

Many of the drug's common adverse effects are the result of its anticholinergic action. Dry mouth, digestive upset, constipation, abdominal pain, headache, dry eyes, blurred vision, drowsiness, and nervousness are common effects. Discuss with your doctor if any of these are severe. Less commonly, the drug may cause chest pain, confusion, or urinary difficulties; consult your doctor if these occur. If you have an unexplained collapse, stop taking the drug and seek urgent medical help.

INTERACTIONS

General note All drugs that have an anticholinergic effect will have increased side effects when taken with tolterodine.

Domperidone and metoclopramide The effects of these drugs may be decreased by tolterodine.

Erythromycin, clarithromycin, itraconazole, ketoconazole, and miconazole These drugs may increase blood levels of tolterodine.

SPECIAL PRECAUTIONS

Be sure to tell your doctor if:

- You have liver or kidney problems.
- You have thyroid problems.
- You have heart problems, especially rhythm disturbances.
- You have hiatus hernia.
- You have prostate problems or urinary retention.
- You have ulcerative colitis.
- You have glaucoma.
- You have myasthenia gravis.
- You are taking other medicines.

Pregnancy Safety in pregnancy not established. May harm the developing fetus. Discuss with your doctor.

Breast-feeding Safety not established. Discuss with your doctor.

Infants and children Not recommended. Safety not established.

Over 60 Increased likelihood of side effects. Reduced dose may be required.

Driving and hazardous work Avoid. Tolterodine may cause drowsiness, disorientation, and blurred vision.

Alcohol Avoid. Alcohol increases the drug's sedative effects.

PROLONGED USE

No special problems. Effectiveness and continuing clinical need for the drug are usually reviewed after 3–6 months.

Monitoring Periodic eye tests for glaucoma may be performed.

TRAMADOL

Brand names Brimisol PR, Invodol SR, Mabron, Maneo, Marol, Maxitram SR, Tilodol SR, Tradorec XL, Tramquel SR, Tramulief, Zamadol, Zeridame SR, Zydol

Used in the following combined preparation Skudexa, Tramacet

QUICK REFERENCE

Drug group Analgesic (p.7)

Overdose danger rating High

Dependence rating Low

Prescription needed Yes

Available as generic Yes

GENERAL INFORMATION

Tramadol is a synthetic opioid analgesic that also acts on serotonin levels in the brain to relieve moderate to severe pain, either acute or chronic. The painkilling effect wears off after about 4 hours, but a modified-release (long-acting) form can provide relief for up to 24 hours.

Rarely, tramadol can be habit-forming, and dependence may occur. However, most people who take the drug for a short period do not become dependent and are able to stop taking it without difficulty.

Side effects of tramadol include a dry mouth, nausea, dizziness, and vomiting. Unlike morphine-like opioids, tramadol tends not to cause constipation.

INFORMATION FOR USERS

Your drug prescription is tailored for you. Do not alter dosage without checking with your doctor.

How taken/used Tablets, modified release/slow release (MR/SR) tablets, soluble tablets, capsules, MR/SR capsules, powder in sachets, injection.

Frequency and timing of doses Usually 1 x daily (MR/SR preparations) or up to 6 x daily (other preparations).

Adult dosage range Up to 400mg daily (by mouth); 600mg daily (injection).

Onset of effect 30–60 minutes (short-acting preparations by mouth), at least 2 hours (SR preparations by mouth); 15–30 minutes (injection).

Duration of action 4 hours (short-acting); 12 or 24 hours (long-acting).

Diet advice None.

Storage Keep in original container at room temperature out of the reach of children.

Missed dose Take as soon as you remember, and return to your normal dosing schedule as soon as possible.

Stopping the drug If the reason for taking tramadol no longer exists, you may stop taking the drug; first you will need to notify your doctor, who will advise you on how to stop taking it gradually. If you have been taking the drug for a long time, you may experience withdrawal effects.

OVERDOSE ACTION

Seek immediate medical advice in all cases. Take emergency action if breathing difficulties, severe drowsiness, seizures, or loss of consciousness occur.

POSSIBLE ADVERSE EFFECTS

Adverse effects such as tiredness and drowsiness seem to be more common with tramadol than with some other opioids. Other common adverse effects of tramadol include nausea, vomiting, dry mouth, dizziness, and headache; constipation is a less common effect. Discuss with your doctor if any of these symptoms are severe or if you experience confusion or hallucinations. If seizures, wheezing, or breathlessness occur, you must stop taking the drug and seek immediate medical attention.

INTERACTIONS

Antidepressants Tramadol may increase the risk of seizures if taken with antidepressants and antipsychotics.

Carbamazepine This drug may reduce blood levels and effects of tramadol.

Sedatives All drugs that have a sedative effect are likely to increase the sedative effects of tramadol. These drugs include antidepressants, antipsychotics, antihistamines, alcohol, benzodiazepines, and sleeping drugs.

SPECIAL PRECAUTIONS

Be sure to tell your doctor if:

- You have had a head injury.
- You have liver or kidney problems.
- You have heart or circulatory problems.
- You have a lung disorder such as asthma or bronchitis.
- You have thyroid disease.
- You have a history of epileptic seizures.
- You are taking other medicines.

Pregnancy Safety not established. Discuss with your doctor.

Breast-feeding The drug passes into the breast milk and may make the baby drowsy. Discuss with your doctor.

Infants and children Not recommended under 12 years.

Over 60 Reduced dose may be necessary.

Driving and hazardous work Avoid. Tramadol can cause drowsiness.

Alcohol Avoid. Alcohol increases the sedative effects of tramadol.

PROLONGED USE

Dependence may occur if tramadol is taken for long periods.

TRASTUZUMAB

Brand name Herceptin, Herzuma, Kanjinti, Ontruzant, Trazimera

Used in the following combined preparation Kadcyla

QUICK REFERENCE

Drug group Anticancer drug (p.94)

Overdose danger rating Low

Dependence rating Low

Prescription needed Yes

Available as generic No

GENERAL INFORMATION

Trastuzumab belongs to a group of drugs called monoclonal antibodies (p.95) and is used in the treatment of early and advanced breast cancer and some stomach cancers. Produced synthetically, it is similar to antibodies that the body makes naturally to fight infection and attacks cancer cells in a similar way.

Around one breast cancer in five involves cancer cells with excessive amounts of a protein called HER2 on their surface. HER2 stimulates the growth of these cancer cells, making the tumours aggressive and fast growing. Trastuzumab blocks the HER2 protein on the cancer cells, destroying them. Therefore, to see whether treatment would be appropriate, it is necessary for tests to be carried out to confirm the presence of HER2.

Trastuzumab may be given on its own or combined with other treatments. It is given by intravenous infusion, weekly or every 3 weeks.

INFORMATION FOR USERS

Trastuzumab is prescribed only under close medical supervision, taking account of your present condition and medical history.

How taken/used Intravenous infusion, subcutaneous injection.

Frequency and timing of doses Every 1–3 weeks. Infusions are usually given over a 90-minute period.

Adult dosage range As advised by doctors, according to your body weight.

Onset of effect Not known.

Duration of action Up to 24 weeks.

Diet advice None.

Storage Not applicable. The drug is not normally kept in the home.

Missed dose The drug is administered in hospital under close medical supervision. If for some reason you miss your dose, contact your doctor as soon as possible.

Stopping the drug Discuss with your doctor. Stopping the drug prematurely may lead to worsening of the underlying condition.

Exceeding the dose Overdosage is unlikely as treatment with trastuzumab is carefully monitored and supervised.

POSSIBLE ADVERSE EFFECTS

Infusion reactions such as fever and shivering are common, especially with the first infusion. Other common effects include nausea, vomiting, diarrhoea, weakness, abdominal pain, and muscle and joint pain. Discuss with your doctor if any of these are severe. If you experience wheezing, breathlessness, cough, palpitations, chest pain, dizziness, flulike symptoms, swelling of the lips or face, or an itchy rash, notify your doctor immediately. The drug treatment should be stopped if lip or facial swelling, itchy rash, or wheezing occur. Trastuzumab may also cause heart failure.

INTERACTIONS

Doxorubicin and other anticancer drugs There is an increased risk of heart failure when these are given with trastuzumab.

SPECIAL PRECAUTIONS

Be sure to tell your doctor if:

- You are allergic to trastuzumab.
- You have breathing difficulties.
- You have had heart failure, coronary artery disease, or high blood pressure.
- You have ever had chemotherapy before, especially with doxorubicin.
- You are pregnant or planning a pregnancy.
- You are taking other medicines.

Pregnancy Not recommended.

Breast-feeding Not advised during treatment and for 6 months after stopping.

Infants and children Not recommended under 18 years. Safety not established.

Over 60 No special problems.

Driving and hazardous work Trastuzumab can cause dizziness and drowsiness during treatment. If these symptoms occur, avoid hazardous activities until they have stopped.

Alcohol No known problems.

PROLONGED USE

Serious problems are rare.

Monitoring Treatment is carried out under specialist supervision. Patients are usually observed for at least 6 hours after the start of treatment and for 2 hours after subsequent treatments. Heart function should be assessed regularly with echocardiograms and ECGs during treatment.

TRIAMTERENE

Brand name Dytac
Used in the following combined preparations Dyazide (co-triamterzide), Frusene, Kalspare, Triam-Co

QUICK REFERENCE

Drug group Potassium-sparing diuretic (p.31)
Overdose danger rating Low
Dependence rating Low
Prescription needed Yes
Available as generic Yes (in combined products)

GENERAL INFORMATION

Triamterene belongs to a class of drugs called potassium-sparing diuretics. In combination with thiazide or loop diuretics, it is given to treat hypertension and oedema (fluid retention). Triamterene may be used either on its own or, more commonly, with a thiazide diuretic such as hydrochlorothiazide (p.269) as co-triamterzide, to treat oedema as a complication of heart failure, nephrotic syndrome, or cirrhosis of the liver. It has a mild effect on urine flow, which is apparent in 1–2 hours. For this reason, you should avoid taking it after about 4 pm. As with other potassium-sparing diuretics, unusually high levels of potassium may build up in the blood if the kidneys are functioning abnormally. Therefore, triamterene is prescribed with caution to people who have kidney failure.

INFORMATION FOR USERS

Your drug prescription is tailored for you. Do not alter dosage without checking with your doctor.

How taken/used Tablets, capsules.
Frequency and timing of doses 1–2 x daily after meals or on alternate days.
Adult dosage range 50–250mg daily.
Onset of effect 1–2 hours.
Duration of action 9–12 hours.
Diet advice Consume only small amounts of foods that are high in potassium, such as bananas, tomatoes, dried fruit, and "low salt" salt substitutes.
Storage Keep in original container at room temperature out of the reach of children.
Missed dose Take as soon as you remember. However, if it is late in the day, do not take the missed dose, or you may need to get up at night to pass urine. Take the next scheduled dose as usual.
Stopping the drug Do not stop without consulting your doctor; symptoms may recur.
Exceeding the dose An occasional unintentional extra dose is unlikely to be a cause for concern. But if you notice any unusual symptoms, or if a large overdose has been taken, tell your doctor.

POSSIBLE ADVERSE EFFECTS

Triamterene has few adverse effects. The main problem is the possibility of potassium being retained by the body, causing muscle weakness and heart rhythm problems; if these occur, stop taking the drug and consult your doctor. Triamterene may also colour your urine blue, but this is not a cause for concern. Digestive disturbances, headache, a rash, dry mouth, and thirst are other rare effects. Consult your doctor if digestive problems or headache are severe or if any of the other symptoms occur. You should also stop taking the drug if you develop a dry mouth, thirst, or a rash.

INTERACTIONS

Lithium Triamterene may increase the blood levels of lithium, leading to an increased risk of lithium toxicity.
Non-steroidal anti-inflammatory drugs (NSAIDs) These drugs may increase the risk of raised blood levels of potassium.
ACE inhibitors and angiotensin II blockers These drugs increase the risk of raised blood levels of potassium with triamterene.
Ciclosporin and tacrolimus may increase blood levels of potassium with triamterene.

SPECIAL PRECAUTIONS

Be sure to tell your doctor if:

- You have long-term liver or kidney problems.
- You have had kidney stones.
- You have gout.
- You are taking other medicines.

Pregnancy Not usually prescribed. May cause a reduction in the blood supply to the developing fetus. Discuss with your doctor.

Breast-feeding The drug passes into breast milk and may affect the baby. It could also reduce your milk supply. Discuss with your doctor.
Infants and children Not recommended.
Over 60 Increased likelihood of adverse effects. Reduced dose may therefore be necessary.
Driving and hazardous work No special problems with this drug.
Alcohol No known problems.

PROLONGED USE

Serious problems are unlikely with triamterene, but levels of salts such as sodium and potassium may occasionally become abnormal during prolonged use.
Monitoring Blood tests may be performed to check kidney function and levels of body salts.

TRIMETHOPRIM

Brand names None
Used in the following combined preparation [co-trimoxazole] Septrin

QUICK REFERENCE

Drug group Antibacterial drug (p.64)
Overdose danger rating Low
Dependence rating Low
Prescription needed Yes
Available as generic Yes

GENERAL INFORMATION

Trimethoprim is an antibacterial drug that became popular in the 1970s for preventing and treating infections of the urinary and respiratory tracts. The drug has been used for many years in combination with another antibacterial, sulfamethoxazole, in a preparation known as co-trimoxazole (p.202). Trimethoprim, however, has fewer adverse effects than co-trimoxazole and is equally effective in treating many conditions.

Although side effects of trimethoprim are not usually troublesome, tests to monitor blood composition are often advised when the drug is taken for prolonged periods.

INFORMATION FOR USERS

Your drug prescription is tailored for you. Do not alter dosage without checking with your doctor.
How taken/used Tablets, liquid.
Frequency and timing of doses 1–2 x daily.
Adult dosage range 400mg daily (treatment); 100mg daily (prevention).
Onset of effect 1–4 hours.
Duration of action Up to 24 hours.
Diet advice None.
Storage Keep in original container at room temperature out of the reach of children. Protect from light.
Missed dose Take as soon as you remember.
Stopping the drug Take the full course. Even if you feel better, the original infection may still be present and symptoms may recur if treatment is stopped too soon.
Exceeding the dose An occasional unintentional extra dose is unlikely to be a cause for concern. But if you notice any unusual symptoms, or if a large overdose has been taken, notify your doctor.

POSSIBLE ADVERSE EFFECTS

Trimethoprim on its own rarely causes side effects, but additional adverse effects may occur when it is taken as the combined preparation co-trimoxazole (comprising trimethoprim and sulfamethoxazole). The adverse effects covered here are for trimethoprim alone; for those of co-trimoxazole, see p.202. The adverse effects of trimethoprim include nausea, vomiting, rash, itching, sore throat, fever, spontaneous bleeding, and easy bruising. Discuss with your doctor if nausea and/or vomiting are severe. If any of the other side effects occur, stop taking the drug and contact your doctor promptly.

INTERACTIONS

Cytotoxic drugs Trimethoprim increases the risk of blood problems if taken with azathioprine or mercaptopurine. When taken with methotrexate, there is an increased risk of folate deficiency.
Ciclosporin Trimethoprim increases the risk of this drug causing kidney damage.
Phenytoin Taken with trimethoprim, this drug may increase the risk of folic acid deficiency, resulting in blood abnormalities. Trimethoprim may also increase the time taken for phenytoin to be eliminated from the body.
Warfarin Trimethoprim may increase the anticoagulant effect of warfarin.
Antimalarials containing pyrimethamine Drugs such as fansidar or maloprim may increase the risk of folic acid deficiency, resulting in

blood abnormalities, if they are taken with trimethoprim.
ACE inhibitors and angiotensin II blockers Trimethoprim increases the risk of high potassium levels in the blood when used with these drugs.
Digoxin Trimethoprim may increase the time taken for the body to eliminate digoxin.

SPECIAL PRECAUTIONS

Be sure to tell your doctor if:

- You have long-term liver or kidney problems.
- You have a blood disorder.
- You have porphyria.
- You are taking other medicines.

Pregnancy Not prescribed. May cause defects in the baby.
Breast-feeding The drug passes into the breast milk, but normal doses are unlikely to affect the baby adversely. Discuss with your doctor.
Infants and children Reduced dose necessary.
Over 60 Increased likelihood of adverse effects. Reduced dose may be required.
Driving and hazardous work No known problems.
Alcohol No known problems.

PROLONGED USE

Long-term use of trimethoprim may lead to folate deficiency, which, in turn, may lead to blood abnormalities. Folate supplements may be prescribed.
Monitoring Periodic blood tests to monitor blood composition are usually advised.

ULIPRISTAL

Brand names EllaOne
Used in the following combined preparations None

QUICK REFERENCE

Drug group Oral contraceptive (p.103)
Overdose danger rating Low
Dependence rating Low
Prescription needed Yes, but available for emergency use from a pharmacy without prescription
Available as generic No

GENERAL INFORMATION

Ulipristal is a synthetic progesterone used as an emergency contraceptive after unprotected sexual intercourse. It works by blocking the action of naturally produced progesterone, thereby inhibiting or delaying ovulation.

Ulipristal is only effective if taken within 120 hours (5 days) of intercourse and is solely for occasional use; the drug should not be used instead of regular contraception. You can use it while taking other oral contraceptives, but this may reduce their effectiveness. Ulipristal does not prevent pregnancy in every case: up to 2 per cent of women still become pregnant after using it. If after using ulipristal your next period is more than 7 days late or you have abnormal bleeding at the expected date of your period, the drug may have failed and you should have a pregnancy test. If the test is positive, you should see your doctor to check for the possibility of an ectopic pregnancy.

INFORMATION FOR USERS

Your drug prescription is tailored for you. Do not alter dosage without checking with your doctor.
How taken/used Tablets.
Frequency and timing of doses One tablet as soon as possible but within 120 hours (5 days) of unprotected sexual intercourse. If vomiting occurs within 3 hours, take another tablet immediately.
Adult dosage range 30mg per tablet.
Onset of effect 2 hours.
Duration of action Up to 120 hours.
Diet advice None.
Storage Keep at room temperature in original packaging to protect from light. Keep out of reach of children.
Missed dose Not applicable as treatment is one dose.
Stopping the drug Not applicable as treatment is one dose.
Exceeding the dose An occasional unintentional extra dose is unlikely to be a cause for concern. However, if you notice any unusual symptoms, notify your doctor.

POSSIBLE ADVERSE EFFECTS

Ulipristal generally causes few serious adverse effects. The most common are nausea, vomiting, and dizziness, although upper abdominal discomfort or pain, headache, tiredness, mood swings, muscle aches, and breast tenderness are also fairly common. Discuss with your doctor if these are severe. If you have lower abdominal or back pain or any other signs of pregnancy after taking the drug, you should consult your doctor immediately to check for the possibility of an ectopic pregnancy.

INTERACTIONS

General note Numerous drugs can interact with ulipristal to reduce its effectiveness, including phenytoin, phenobarbital, carbamazepine, rifampicin, ritonavir, antacids, H2 blockers (e.g. cimetidine), proton pump inhibitors (e.g. omeprazole), and St John's wort. If you have used any of these drugs with ulipristal, you should use a barrier contraceptive until your next menstrual period.
Oral contraceptives Ulipristal may reduce the effectiveness of oral contraceptives, so you should use a reliable barrier method of contraception until your next menstrual period.
Antifungals and antibiotics Certain antifungals (e.g. ketoconazole and itraconazole) and antibiotics (e.g. telithromycin and clarithromycin) may increase the activity of ulipristal, and concomitant use should be avoided.

SPECIAL PRECAUTIONS

Be sure to tell your doctor if:
◆ You are definitely already pregnant.
◆ You have severe asthma.
◆ You have liver disease.
◆ You have lactose intolerance.
◆ You are taking or have recently taken any other medicines, including over-the-counter medicines and herbal remedies.
Pregnancy Should not be taken if you are definitely already pregnant.
Breast-feeding Breast-feeding is not recommended in the 36 hours after use of ulipristal.
Infants and children Not recommended under age 16 years.
Over 60 Not needed for post-menopausal women.
Driving and hazardous work Avoid such activities until you know how the drug has affected you. Ulipristal may sometimes cause dizziness, drowsiness, blurred vision, and difficulty concentrating.
Alcohol No known problems.

PROLONGED USE

Ulipristal is intended for one-off use only for emergency postcoital contraception. Repeated use of the drug in the same menstrual cycle is not recommended as its safety and effectiveness are unknown.

Ulipristal is no longer licensed for long-term use in women with fibroids because of the risk of rare but severe liver injury.

VARENICLINE

Brand name Champix
Used in the following combined preparations None

QUICK REFERENCE

Drug group Smoking cessation aid
Overdose danger rating Medium
Dependence rating Low
Prescription needed Yes
Available as generic No

GENERAL INFORMATION

Varenicline is an effective aid to stopping smoking in adults. It works in a similar way to nicotine in the body and helps reduce tobacco cravings. It has been shown to be more effective than nicotine replacement therapy or bupropion, and, like these treatments, is also more likely to be successful in motivated individuals who are given additional expert advice and specialist support.

Treatment with varenicline is usually started 1–2 weeks before stopping smoking (the target stop date) and continued for a period of 12 weeks in total. The course may be repeated in people who have successfully given up but are at risk of relapsing. Adverse effects are common but not usually serious; however, the drug may rarely cause suicidal behaviour. You should discontinue treatment and seek immediate medical advice if you become agitated or depressed, or have suicidal thoughts, while taking varenicline.

INFORMATION FOR USERS

Your drug prescription is tailored for you. Do not alter dosage without checking with your doctor.
How taken/used Tablets.
Frequency and timing of doses Treatment started 1–2 weeks before target stop date. Initially 0.5mg once daily for 3 days, increased to 0.5mg 2 x daily for 4 days, then 1mg 2 x daily for 11 weeks (reduce to 0.5mg 2 x daily if higher dose not tolerated). Take doses at same time every day.
Adult dosage range 0.5–2mg daily.
Onset of effect 3–4 hours, but may take weeks for full effect to be noticeable.
Duration of action 24 hours.
Diet advice None.
Storage Keep in original container at room temperature and out of the reach of children.

Missed dose Take as soon as you remember unless your next dose is due within 12 hours, in which case omit the missed dose and take the next one as scheduled. Do not take a double dose to make up for a missed one.
Stopping the drug The drug can be stopped safely when no longer needed. However, stopping before the end of the course may increase the likelihood of a relapse.
Exceeding the dose An occasional unintentional extra dose is unlikely to cause problems, although an overdose may cause vomiting. Notify your doctor.

POSSIBLE ADVERSE EFFECTS

Headache, nausea, vomiting, tiredness, sleepiness or insomnia, and strange dreams are common adverse effects of varenicline. Discuss with your doctor if any of these effects are severe. Rarely, the drug may cause agitation, hallucinations, depression, or suicidal thoughts. If any of these occur, stop taking the drug and consult your doctor immediately.

INTERACTIONS

General note Stopping smoking, with or without varenicline, may alter the effects of a wide range of drugs, sometimes necessitating a dose adjustment; important examples include insulin, theophylline, and warfarin. Consult your doctor or pharmacist if you are on other medications or before you take a new medication.

SPECIAL PRECAUTIONS

Be sure to tell your doctor if:
- You have a history of psychiatric problems.
- You have had a head injury or have a history of seizures or epilepsy.
- You have severe kidney disease.
- You are pregnant or planning a pregnancy.
- You are taking other medicines.

Pregnancy Avoid. Safety in pregnancy not established. Discuss with your doctor.
Breast-feeding The drug passes into the breast milk. Safety not established. Discuss with your doctor.
Infants and children Not recommended.
Over 60 No special problems.
Driving and hazardous work Avoid until you have learned how varenicline affects you. The drug may cause dizziness and sleepiness.
Alcohol Avoid. Alcohol may increase the sedative effect of varenicline.

PROLONGED USE

A course of varenicline lasts 12 weeks. If necessary, the course may be repeated in those who have stopped smoking if they are likely to relapse.

VENLAFAXINE

Brand names Alventa XL, Depefex XL, Efexor XL, Politid XL, Suveniz XL, Venaxx XL, Venlalic XL, ViePax, and others
Used in the following combined preparations None

QUICK REFERENCE

Drug group Antidepressant drug (p.12)
Overdose danger rating High
Dependence rating Low
Prescription needed Yes
Available as generic Yes

GENERAL INFORMATION

Venlafaxine is an antidepressant with a chemical structure unlike that of any other available antidepressant. It combines the therapeutic properties of both tricyclic antidepressants and selective serotonin reuptake inhibitors (SSRIs), without anticholinergic adverse effects (p.7). Venlafaxine is used in the treatment of depression and generalized anxiety disorder. It acts to elevate mood, increase physical activity, and restore interest in everyday activities.

Nausea, dizziness, drowsiness or insomnia, and restlessness are common side effects. At high doses, the drug can raise blood pressure.

INFORMATION FOR USERS

Your drug prescription is tailored for you. Do not alter dosage without checking with your doctor.
How taken/used Tablets, XL preparations (modified release (MR) tablets and capsules).
Frequency and timing of doses 2 x daily (tablets); 1 x daily (XL preparations). The drug should be taken with food.
Dosage range 75–150mg daily for outpatients; up to 375mg daily in severely depressed people.
Onset of effect Can appear within days, although full antidepressant effect may not be felt for 2–6 weeks. Anxiety may take longer to respond.
Duration of action About 8–12 hours (tablets); 24 hours (XL preparations). Antidepressant effects may persist for up to 6 weeks following prolonged treatment.

Diet advice None.
Storage Keep in original container at room temperature out of the reach of children.
Missed dose Do not make up for a missed dose. Just take your next regularly scheduled dose.
Stopping the drug Do not stop the drug without consulting your doctor. Stopping abruptly can cause withdrawal symptoms.

OVERDOSE ACTION

Seek immediate medical advice in all cases. Take emergency action if seizures, slow or irregular pulse, or loss of consciousness occur.

POSSIBLE ADVERSE EFFECTS

The most common adverse effects are weakness, nausea, constipation, restlessness (which may take the form of anxiety, nervousness, tremor, abnormal dreams, agitation, or confusion), blurred vision, drowsiness, dizziness, and sexual dysfunction. Some of these effects may wear off in 1–2 weeks. Discuss with your doctor if they persist or are severe. Rarely, high blood pressure develops when high doses are taken; you should have your blood pressure monitored periodically. Palpitations may also rarely occur and should be reported to your doctor promptly. If there are suicidal thoughts or attempts, you should stop taking the drug and seek immediate medical help.

INTERACTIONS

Sedatives All drugs with a sedative effect may increase the sedative effect of venlafaxine.
Antihypertensive drugs Venlafaxine may reduce the effectiveness of these drugs.
Warfarin Venlafaxine may increase effect of warfarin; warfarin dose may need to be reduced.
Serotonergics including triptans, other SSRIs, tramadol, and St John's wort may interact dangerously with venlafaxine.
Monoamine oxidase inhibitors (MAOIs) Venlafaxine may interact with these drugs to produce a dangerous rise in blood pressure. At least 14 days should elapse between stopping MAOIs and starting venlafaxine.

SPECIAL PRECAUTIONS

Be sure to tell your doctor if:
◆ You have had an adverse reaction to any other antidepressants.
◆ You have long-term liver or kidney problems.
◆ You have diabetes.
◆ You have a heart problem, raised blood pressure, or a history of bleeding disorders.
◆ You have a history of epilepsy or mania.
◆ You have glaucoma.
◆ You have had problems with alcohol or drug misuse.
◆ You are taking other medicines.

Pregnancy Safety in pregnancy not established. Discuss with your doctor.
Breast-feeding Not recommended. Discuss with your doctor.
Infants and children Not recommended under 18 years.
Over 60 Increased likelihood of adverse effects. Reduced dose may therefore be necessary.
Driving and hazardous work Avoid until you know how venlafaxine affects you; it can cause dizziness, drowsiness, and blurred vision.
Alcohol Avoid. Alcohol may increase the sedative effects of this drug.

PROLONGED USE

Withdrawal symptoms (e.g. dizziness, headache, anxiety, nausea, and insomnia) may occur if the drug is not stopped gradually over at least 4 weeks. There is also a small risk of suicidal thoughts and self-harm in children and adolescents, although the drug is rarely used for this age group.
Monitoring Blood pressure should be measured periodically if high doses are prescribed. People with confusion, drowsiness, muscle cramps, or seizures should be monitored for low blood levels of sodium. Under-18s should be monitored for suicidal thoughts and self-harm.

VERAPAMIL

Brand names Cordilox, Securon, Univer, Verapress, Vera-Til, Vertab, Zolvera
Used in the following combined preparations Tarka

QUICK REFERENCE

Drug group Anti-angina drug (p.33), anti-arrhythmic drug (p.32), and antihypertensive drug (p.34)
Overdose danger rating Medium
Dependence rating Low
Prescription needed Yes
Available as generic Yes

GENERAL INFORMATION

Verapamil belongs to a group of drugs called calcium channel blockers, which interfere with the conduction of signals in the muscles of the heart and blood vessels. It is used in the treatment of hypertension, abnormal heart rhythms, and angina. The drug reduces the frequency of angina attacks, although it does not help relieve pain while an attack is in progress. Verapamil increases the ability to tolerate physical exertion and can be used safely by people with asthma. It is also prescribed for certain types of abnormal heart rhythm; the drug can be administered by injection as well as in tablet form for such disorders.

Verapamil is not generally prescribed for people with low blood pressure, slow heart beat, or heart failure because it may worsen these conditions.

INFORMATION FOR USERS

Your drug prescription is tailored for you. Do not alter dosage without checking with your doctor.

How taken/used Tablets, slow release (SR) tablets/capsules, liquid, injection.

Frequency and timing of doses 2–3 x daily (tablets, liquid); 1–2 x daily (SR tablets/capsules).

Adult dosage range 120–480mg daily.

Onset of effect 1–2 hours (tablets); 2–3 minutes (injection).

Duration of action 6–8 hours. During prolonged treatment some beneficial effects may last for up to 12 hours. SR tablets act for 12–24 hours.

Diet advice Avoid grapefruit juice, which may increase blood levels of verapamil.

Storage Keep in original container at room temperature out of the reach of children.

Missed dose Take as soon as you remember. If your next dose of the drug is due within 3 hours (tablets, liquid) or within 8 hours (SR tablets/capsules), take a single dose now and skip the next.

Stopping the drug Do not stop the drug without consulting your doctor; symptoms may recur.

Exceeding the dose An occasional unintentional extra dose is unlikely to be a cause for concern. Large overdoses may cause dizziness. Notify your doctor.

POSSIBLE ADVERSE EFFECTS

The main adverse effect of verapamil is constipation. It also commonly causes headache, nausea, vomiting, and ankle swelling. Discuss with your doctor if these are severe. Rare side effects include dizziness (which may be due to slowing of the heart rate), rash, and, after prolonged use, breast enlargement in males and an increase in gum tissue. Consult your doctor if you experience any of these adverse effects.

INTERACTIONS

Beta blockers When verapamil is taken with these drugs, there is a slight risk of abnormal heart beat and heart failure.

Carbamazepine, ciclosporin, dabigatran, digoxin, theophylline, sirolimus, and ivabradine The effects of these drugs may be increased by verapamil; their doses may need to be reduced or the combination may need to be avoided.

Rifampicin and barbiturates may reduce the effects of verapamil.

Clarithromycin and erythromycin may increase the effects of verapamil.

Simvastatin and atorvastatin There is an increased risk of muscle damage if these drugs are taken with verapamil.

Colchicine Verapamil may increase effects of colchicine; the combination should be avoided.

SPECIAL PRECAUTIONS

Be sure to tell your doctor if:

- You have a long-term liver problem.
- You have heart failure.
- You have myasthenia gravis.
- You have porphyria.
- You are taking other medicines.

Pregnancy Not usually prescribed. May inhibit labour if taken during later stages of pregnancy. Discuss with your doctor.

Breast-feeding The drug passes into the breast milk, but normal doses are unlikely to affect the baby adversely. Discuss with your doctor.

Infants and children Usually given on specialist advice only. Reduced dose necessary.

Over 60 No special problems.

Driving and hazardous work Avoid until you have learned how verapamil affects you because the drug can cause dizziness.

Alcohol Avoid; may further reduce blood pressure, causing dizziness or other symptoms.

Surgery and general anaesthetics Verapamil may need to be stopped before surgery. Consult your doctor or dentist.

PROLONGED USE

Rarely, gynaecomastia (breast enlargement in men) or enlargement of the gum tissues may occur with long-term use.

WARFARIN

Brand name None
Used in the following combined preparations None

QUICK REFERENCE

Drug group Anticoagulant drug (p.37)
Overdose danger rating High
Dependence rating Low
Prescription needed Yes
Available as generic Yes

GENERAL INFORMATION

Warfarin is an anticoagulant designed to prevent deep-vein thromboses: blood clots, particularly in the leg and pelvic veins, where blood flow is slowest. The clots could otherwise break off and travel to the lungs to cause pulmonary embolism. The drug is also used to reduce the risk of clots in the heart in people with atrial fibrillation (irregular heart rhythm) or artificial heart valves; these clots could travel to the brain and cause a stroke. Regular monitoring is needed to ensure proper maintenance, dosage, and safety with warfarin, using the International Normalized Ratio (INR) blood test. As the full benefits of warfarin are not felt for 2 to 3 days, a faster-acting drug such as heparin (p.268) is often used initially in people who have or who are at risk of developing a clot.

Due to its risk of excessive bleeding, and the advent of newer anticoagulants, the use of warfarin is in decline except in patients with artificial heart valves.

INFORMATION FOR USERS

Your drug prescription is tailored for you. Do not alter dosage without checking with your doctor.
How taken/used Tablets.
Frequency and timing of doses Once daily, taken at the same time each day.
Dosage range Large variation in starting and maintenance dose, according to patient factors, but usually 10mg for 2 days (starting dose); 3–9mg daily at same time, determined by blood tests (maintenance dose).
Onset of effect Within 24–48 hours; full effect after several days.
Duration of action 2–3 days.
Diet advice Avoid cranberry juice and avoid major diet changes (especially of salads and vegetables).
Storage Keep in original container at room temperature out of the reach of children. Protect from light.
Missed dose Take as soon as you remember. Take the following dose on your original dosing schedule.
Stopping the drug Do not stop taking the drug without consulting your doctor; stopping the drug may lead to worsening of the underlying condition.

OVERDOSE ACTION

Seek immediate medical advice in all cases. Take emergency action if severe bleeding or loss of consciousness occur.

POSSIBLE ADVERSE EFFECTS

Bleeding is the most common adverse effect of warfarin. If you notice serious bruising, very prolonged bleeding from a minor wound, or blood in your urine or faeces, contact your doctor immediately and stop taking the drug. Rarely, warfarin may cause nausea, vomiting, abdominal pain, diarrhoea, rash, and hair loss. Consult your doctor if any of these symptoms occur. If you develop fever or jaundice, you should stop taking the drug and contact your doctor urgently.

INTERACTIONS

General note A wide range of drugs interact with warfarin to affect the risk of bleeding; they include aspirin and other non-steroidal anti-inflammatory drugs (NSAIDs), diuretics, chemotherapy, oral contraceptives, lipid-lowering drugs, amiodarone, barbiturates, cimetidine, steroids, certain laxatives, antidepressants, antibiotics, and herbal medicines. Consult your pharmacist before using over-the-counter medicines. Inform your warfarin clinic of any changes to your medicines.

SPECIAL PRECAUTIONS

Be sure to tell your doctor if:

- You have long-term liver or kidney problems.
- You have high blood pressure.
- You have a history of peptic ulcers.
- You have a bleeding disorder.
- You are taking other medicines.

Pregnancy Not prescribed. Given in early pregnancy, the drug can cause malformations in the fetus. Taken near the time of delivery, it may cause the mother to bleed excessively. Discuss with your doctor, who will prescribe alternative treatment.

Breast-feeding The drug passes into the breast milk, but at normal doses adverse effects on the baby are unlikely. Discuss with your doctor.

Infants and children Reduced dose necessary.

Over 60 No special problems.

Driving and hazardous work Use caution. Even minor bumps can cause severe bruises and excessive bleeding.

Alcohol Avoid making major changes in alcohol consumption.

Surgery and general anaesthetics Warfarin may need to be stopped before surgery. Discuss with your doctor or dentist.

PROLONGED USE

No special problems.

Monitoring Regular INR blood tests are carried out. Dose is adjusted accordingly and recorded in a treatment book, which should be carried with you at all times. More frequent testing may be needed if there is a significant change in your health.

ZIDOVUDINE/LAMIVUDINE

Brand name [zidovudine] Retrovir; [lamivudine] Epivir, Zeffix

Used in the following combined preparations Combivir, Trizivir

QUICK REFERENCE

Drug group Drug for HIV and immune deficiency (p.98)

Overdose danger rating Medium

Dependence rating Low

Prescription needed Yes

Available as generic Yes (both drugs)

GENERAL INFORMATION

Zidovudine and lamivudine belong to the same class of drugs – nucleoside analogues – and are used in the treatment of HIV infection. The two drugs can be prescribed separately or combined in one tablet, which is usually prescribed with another class of drug (either a non-nucleoside reverse transcriptase inhibitor or a protease inhibitor) to treat HIV. This combination of three drugs is more effective at treating HIV than either a single or a double regime of drugs.

Although it is not a cure for HIV, combination antiretroviral therapy (ART) slows the production of the virus and, therefore, reduces the viral load and consequent damage done to the immune system. The drugs need to be taken regularly and on a long-term basis to remain effective.

INFORMATION FOR USERS

Your drug prescription is tailored for you. Do not alter dosage without checking with your doctor.

How taken/used Tablets, liquid, injection (zidovudine).

Frequency and timing of doses 1–2 x daily.

Adult dosage range One tablet; 15–30ml liquid; dosage for injection calculated according to body weight.

Onset of effect 1 hour.

Duration of action 12–24 hours.

Diet advice None.

Storage Keep in original container at room temperature out of the reach of children.

Missed dose Take as soon as you remember. If your next dose is due within 2 hours, take a single dose now and skip the next. It is very important not to miss doses on a regular basis as this can lead to the development of drug-resistant HIV.

Stopping the drug Do not stop taking the drug without consulting your doctor.

Exceeding the dose An occasional unintentional extra dose is unlikely to cause problems. But if you notice any unusual symptoms, or if a large overdose has been taken, notify your doctor.

POSSIBLE ADVERSE EFFECTS

The most common adverse effects of zidovudine and lamivudine are nausea, vomiting, and diarrhoea; fatigue is also common. Discuss with your doctor if these are severe. Less commonly, skin discoloration or anaemia (which can develop after prolonged use) may occur; discuss with your doctor if these are significant. If you develop severe abdominal pain, you should contact your doctor immediately. Prolonged use of the drugs may also cause other adverse effects (see below).

INTERACTIONS

General note A wide range of drugs may interact with zidovudine and lamivudine, causing either an increase in adverse effects or a reduction in the effect of the antiretrovirals. Check with your doctor or pharmacist before taking new drugs, including any from your dentist or a supermarket, and herbal medicines.

SPECIAL PRECAUTIONS

Be sure to tell your doctor if:

◆ You have liver or kidney problems.

◆ You have other infections, such as hepatitis B or C.

◆ You are taking other medicines.

Pregnancy Safety in pregnancy not established. If you are pregnant or planning pregnancy, discuss with your doctor.

Breast-feeding Safety not established. Breast-feeding is not recommended for HIV-positive mothers as the virus may pass to the baby.

Infants and children Reduced dose necessary under 12 years.

Over 60 Increased likelihood of adverse effects. Reduced dose may therefore be necessary.

Driving and hazardous work No special problems.

Alcohol No known problems.

PROLONGED USE

There is an increased risk of serious blood disorders, such as anaemia, with long-term use of zidovudine and lamivudine. There may also be a redistribution of fat from the limbs to the abdomen, back, and breasts. This may be accompanied by increases in blood levels of lipids and glucose.

Monitoring Regular blood checks will be carried out to monitor the viral load, blood count, and blood lipid and glucose levels.

ZOLEDRONIC ACID

Brand names Aclasta, Zerlinda, Zometa

Used in the following combined preparations None

QUICK REFERENCE

Drug group Drug for bone disorders (p.54) and anticancer drug (p.94)

Overdose danger rating Medium

Dependence rating Low

Prescription needed Yes

Available as generic No

GENERAL INFORMATION

Zoledronic acid is a bisphosphonate, one of a group of drugs used in the treatment of bone disorders. These drugs act directly on the bones, reducing the rate at which calcium is released from them and so making them less liable to fracture. The reduced calcium release can cause blood calcium levels to fall, which is useful if the level is high (e.g. due to cancer).

Zoledronic acid can only be given by infusion into a vein, and has a very long duration of action so that it can be used very infrequently. It is used to treat various bone disorders, including Paget's disease of the bone and osteoporosis in men and post-menopausal women – particularly those who have had a recent osteoporotic fracture or who are on long-term corticosteroids. Zoledronic acid is also used to prevent bone damage in patients with advanced cancer that has spread to bone.

INFORMATION FOR USERS

The drug is given only under medical supervision and is not for self-administration.

How taken/used Intravenous infusion.

Frequency and timing of doses *Advanced cancer involving bone* Every 3–4 weeks. *Paget's disease and high blood calcium associated with cancer* One-off dose, can be repeated if required. *Osteoporosis* Once yearly.

Adult dosage range 4–5mg.

Onset of effect Up to 3 months.

Duration of action Up to 1 year.

Diet advice None. Calcium and/or vitamin D supplements may be prescribed before or after treatment with zoledronic acid.

Storage Not applicable. The drug is not kept in the home.

Missed dose The drug is given in hospital under medical supervision. If you miss your dose, contact your doctor as soon as possible.

Stopping the drug Discuss with your doctor. Stopping the drug may lead to worsening of the underlying condition.

Exceeding the dose Overdosage is unlikely because the drug is given under close medical supervision. If you think you have received an overdose, tell your doctor as soon as possible.

POSSIBLE ADVERSE EFFECTS

The first dose of zoledronic acid may cause flulike symptoms, including bone pain, fever, and fatigue; some people also experience gastrointestinal problems, such as nausea and vomiting. These symptoms tend to be milder if further doses are given, but you should discuss with your doctor if they are severe. In addition, speak to your doctor if you have palpitations or severe headaches or dizziness. If you develop a rash, itching, facial swelling, tingling, muscle spasms, or pain in the jaw, you should notify your doctor immediately.

INTERACTIONS

None known.

SPECIAL PRECAUTIONS

Be sure to tell your doctor if:

- You have had a recent hip fracture.
- You have kidney problems.
- You are or may be pregnant or are planning a pregnancy.
- You have had a previous allergic reaction to any bisphosphonate drug.
- You are taking other medicines.

Pregnancy Not recommended. Safety not established. Discuss with your doctor.

Breast-feeding Not recommended. Safety not established. Discuss with your doctor.

Infants and children Not recommended.

Over 60 No special problems.

Driving and hazardous work No special problems.

Alcohol No special problems.

PROLONGED USE

There have been rare reports of atypical femoral fractures and ulceration of jaw bones in patients taking bisphosphonates including zoledronic acid. Patients undergoing bisphosphonate treatment are advised to report any thigh, hip, or groin pain to their doctor.

Monitoring Blood tests will be carried out to monitor your calcium levels. Your overall health will also be monitored.

ZOPICLONE

Brand names Zimovane, Zimovane LS

Used in the following combined preparations None

QUICK REFERENCE

Drug group Sleeping drug (p.9)

Overdose danger rating Medium

Dependence rating Medium

Prescription needed Yes

Available as generic Yes

GENERAL INFORMATION

Zopiclone is a hypnotic (sleeping drug) used for the short-term treatment of insomnia. Sleep problems can take the form of difficulty in falling asleep, frequent night-time awakenings, and/or early morning awakenings. Hypnotic drugs are given only when non-drug measures – for example, avoidance of caffeine – have proved ineffective. Unlike benzodiazepines, zopiclone has no anti-anxiety properties. Therefore, it may be suited for instances of insomnia that are not accompanied by anxiety, such as international travel or change in shift work routine.

Hypnotics are intended for occasional use only. Dependence can develop after as little as 1 week of continuous use.

INFORMATION FOR USERS

Your drug prescription is tailored for you. Do not alter dosage without checking with your doctor.

How taken/used Tablets.

Frequency and timing of doses Once daily at bedtime when required. Tablets should be swallowed whole, without sucking or chewing.

Dosage range 3.75–7.5mg.

Onset of effect Within 30 minutes.

Duration of action 4–6 hours.

Diet advice None.

Storage Keep in original container at room temperature out of the reach of children. Protect from light.

Missed dose If you fall asleep without having taken a dose and wake some hours later, do not take the missed dose.

Stopping the drug If you have been taking the drug continuously for less than 1 week, it can be safely stopped as soon as you feel you no longer need it. However, if you have been taking the drug for longer, consult your doctor.

Exceeding the dose An occasional, unintentional extra dose is unlikely to cause any problems. Large overdoses may cause prolonged sleep, drowsiness, lethargy, and poor muscle coordination and reflexes. Notify your doctor immediately.

POSSIBLE ADVERSE EFFECTS

The most common adverse effects are daytime drowsiness, which normally diminishes after the first few days of treatment, a bitter or metallic taste in the mouth, and headaches. Discuss drowsiness or headaches, or severe abnormal taste, with your doctor. Persistent daytime drowsiness or impaired coordination indicate an excessive dose; if they occur, you should notify your doctor immediately. Less commonly, zopiclone may cause dizziness, weakness, nausea, vomiting, and diarrhoea; if any of these symptoms are severe, discuss with your doctor. Rarely, the drug may cause amnesia, confusion, or a rash; if any of these occur, you should stop taking the drug and contact your doctor immediately. The drug may also cause depression and suicidal thoughts; if these symptoms occur, consult your doctor immediately.

INTERACTIONS

Sedatives All drugs, including alcohol, that have a sedative effect on the central nervous system are likely to increase the sedative effects of zopiclone. Such drugs include other sleeping and anti-anxiety drugs, antihistamines, antidepressants, opioid analgesics, and antipsychotics.

Erythromycin, clarithromycin, and ketoconazole may increase the levels and the effect of zopiclone, leading to adverse effects.

Carbamazepine, phenytoin, rifampicin, and St John's wort These treatments may reduce the effects of zopiclone.

SPECIAL PRECAUTIONS

Be sure to tell your doctor if:

- You have or have had any problems with alcohol or drug misuse.
- You have depression.
- You have myasthenia gravis.
- You have severe respiratory disease.
- You have liver or kidney problems.
- You are taking other medicines.

Pregnancy Safety in pregnancy not established. Use in late pregnancy may affect the baby and cause withdrawal symptoms. Discuss with your doctor.

Breast-feeding Safety in breast-feeding not established. The drug is present in breast milk. Discuss with your doctor.

Infants and children Not recommended.

Over 60 Increased likelihood of adverse effects. Reduced dose may therefore be necessary.

Driving and hazardous work Avoid such activities until you have learned how zopiclone affects you because the drug can cause drowsiness, reduced alertness, and slowed reactions.

Alcohol Avoid. Alcohol increases the sedative effects of this drug.

PROLONGED USE

Intended for occasional use only. Continuous use of zopiclone, or any other sleeping drug, for as little as 1 or 2 weeks may cause dependence. Withdrawal symptoms may occur when the drug is stopped. These may include insomnia, anxiety, tremor, confusion, and panic attacks. Withdrawal symptoms are less likely to occur when the drug is used for less than 4 weeks.

PART 3

DRUG FINDER AND INDEX

This part of the book consists of a combined drug finder and index, which helps you to find information on specific brand-name drugs and generic substances, as well as directing you to further information about them throughout the book.

DRUG FINDER AND INDEX

This section contains the names of more than 3,000 drug products and substances. It provides a quick reference for information on specific drugs and other medications.

WHAT IT CONTAINS

The alphabetical entries include all major generic drugs and many less widely used substances for treating and preventing disease. Each entry gives the name, the generic name for branded drugs, the drug class (if relevant), and the use. Inclusion of a drug or product does not imply the publisher's endorsement, nor does the exclusion of a particular drug or product indicate disapproval.

HOW THE REFERENCES WORK

References are to the pages in Part 2, containing the drug profiles of each principal generic drug, and to the section in Part 1 that describes the relevant drug group. Some entries for drugs that do not have a full profile contain a brief description here.

ABBREVIATIONS

For brevity and ease of reading, names of the following drug types have been abbreviated:
Disease-modifying anti-rheumatic drug – DMARD
Non-steroidal anti-inflammatory drug – NSAID

A

B

C

D

F

G

H

I

J

K

L

M

N

O

P

Q

R

S

W

X

Y

Z